W9-CGM-816

# Index of Applications

Enis Barış
Montréal
21.1.1988

# Fundamentals of Biostatistics

*second edition*

# Fundamentals of Biostatistics

## Bernard Rosner

*Harvard University*

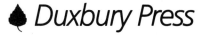 *Duxbury Press*

*Boston, Massachusetts*

# PWS PUBLISHERS

Prindle, Weber & Schmidt • ♣ • Duxbury Press • ♠ • PWS Engineering • ⚠ • Breton Publishers • ⚙
20 Park Plaza • Boston, Massachusetts 02116

Copyright ©1986 by PWS Publishers. Copyright ©1982 by PWS Publishers.

All rights reserved. No part of this book may be reproduced, stored in a retrieval system, or transcribed, in any form or by any means—electronic, mechanical, photocopying, recording, or otherwise—without prior written permission of PWS Publishers.

PWS Publishers is a division of Wadsworth, Inc.

**Library of Congress Cataloging-in-Publication Data**
Rosner, Bernard (Bernard A.)
   Fundamentals of biostatistics.

   Includes bibliographies and index.
1. Biometry.   2. Medical statistics.   I. Title.
QH323.5.R674   1986   574'.072   85-13088
ISBN 0-87150-981-4

ISBN 0-87150-981-4

Printed in the United States of America
86  87  88  89  90  —  10  9  8  7  6  5  4  3  2  1

**Editor:** Michael Payne
**Production Coordinator and designer:** S. London
**Manuscript Editor:** Ian List
**Typesetting:** Desmond Doyle Phototypesetters
**Printing and Binding Cover and Text:** R.R. Donnelley & Sons Company

*This book is dedicated to my wife Cynthia and
my children Sarah, David and Laura.*

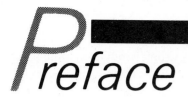

# Preface

I have written this introductory-level biostatistics text for upper-level undergraduate or graduate students interested in medicine or other health-related areas. This book requires no previous background in statistics, and its mathematical level assumes only a knowledge of algebra.

*Fundamentals of Biostatistics* evolved from a set of notes that I used in a course in biostatistics taught to Harvard University undergraduates and Harvard Medical School students over the past ten years. I wrote this book to help motivate students to master those statistical methods that are most often used in the medical literature. It is important from the student's viewpoint that the example material used to develop these methods be representative of what actually exists in the literature. Therefore most examples and exercises used in this book are either based on actual articles from the medical literature or on actual medical research problems that I have encountered during my consulting experience at the Harvard Medical School.

Most other introductory statistics texts either use a completely nonmathematical, cookbook approach or develop the material in a rigorous, sophisticated mathematical framework. In this book I have attempted to follow an intermediate course, minimizing the amount of mathematical formulation and yet giving complete explanations of all the important concepts. *Every* new concept is developed systematically through completely worked examples from current medical research problems. In addition, computer output is introduced where appropriate to illustrate these concepts.

The material in this book is suitable for either a one- or two-semester course in biostatistics. The material in Chapters 1 through 8 and Chapter 10 is suitable for a one-semester course. The instructor may select appropriate material from the other chapters as time permits.

The following changes have been made in the second edition:

•The number of exercises has more than doubled from the first edition, to over 1000 exercises overall. In particular, over 300 "drill" exercises have been added to facilitate immediate student comprehension of the material.

•The treatment of EDA has been augmented, including the presentation of box plots.

•Tables are supplied for the binomial and Poisson distributions to minimize computational complexity when working with these distributions.

•Extensive computer output is provided to reinforce the crucial concept of a sampling distribution. The treatment of the central limit theorem is handled in a similar fashion.

•A more thorough coverage is given to the important notions of estimation of power and sample size for one-sample problems in Chapter 7 and for two-sample problems in Chapters 8 and 10.

•The notion of an odds ratio for $2 \times 2$ tables is introduced, including appropriate methods of estimation and hypothesis testing.

•The Mantel-Haenszel test is introduced for the combination of data from more than one $2 \times 2$ table.

• The Kappa statistic is presented as a method for measuring reproducibility for discrete data.

•An introduction is given to multiple logistic regression as an analogue to multiple linear regression for binary outcome variables. Extensive computer output is used to motivate each of these methods.

•The Kruskal-Wallis test is presented as a nonparametric alternative to the one-way analysis of variance.

*Fundamentals of Biostatistics*, second edition, is organized as follows:

**Chapter 1** is an *introductory chapter* giving an outline of the development of an actual medical study that I was involved with. It provides a unique sense of the role of biostatistics in the medical research process.

**Chapter 2** concerns *descriptive statistics* and presents all the major numerical and graphical tools used for displaying medical data. This chapter is especially important for both consumers and producers of medical literature, since much of the actual communication of information is accomplished via descriptive material.

**Chapters 3 through 5** discuss *probability*. The basic principles of probability are developed, and the most common probability distributions, such as the binomial and normal distributions, are introduced. These distributions are used extensively in the later chapters of the book.

**Chapters 6 through 10** cover some of the basic methods of *statistical inference*.

**Chapter 6** introduces the concept of drawing random samples from populations. The difficult notion of a sampling distribution is also developed, including an introduction to the most common sampling distributions, such as the *t* and chi-square distributions. The basic methods of *estimation* are also presented, including an extensive discussion of confidence intervals.

**Chapters 7 and 8** contain the basic principles of *hypothesis testing*. The most elementary hypothesis tests for normally distributed data, such as the *t* test, are also fully discussed for the one- and two-sample problems.

**Chapter 9** covers the basic principles of *nonparametric statistics*. The assumptions of normality are relaxed, and distribution-free analogues are developed for the tests in Chapters 7 and 8.

**Chapter 10** contains the basic concepts of *hypothesis testing* as applied to categorical data, including some of the most widely used statistical procedures, such as the chi-square test and Fisher's exact test.

**Chapter 11** develops the principles of *regression analysis*. The case of simple linear regression is thoroughly covered, and extensions are provided for the multiple regression case. An important section on the limitations of the use of regression analysis is also included.

**Chapter 12** introduces the basic principles of the *analysis of variance* (ANOVA). The one-way and two-way analyses of variance are discussed.

The elements of study design are not formally covered in this book but are informally introduced in much of the example material. The concepts of matching, cohort studies, case-control studies, retrospective studies, prospective studies, and the sensitivity, specificity, and predictive value of screening tests are extensively discussed in the context of actual samples. In addition, specific sections on sample size estimation are provided for different statistical situations in Chapters 7, 8, and 10.

A flowchart of appropriate methods of statistical inference on page 575 provides an easy reference to the methods developed in this book. This flowchart is referred to at the end of each of Chapters 6 through 12 to give the student some perspective on how the methods in a particular chapter fit in with the overall collection of statistical methods introduced in this book.

In addition, an index summarizing all examples and problems used in this book is provided, grouped by *medical speciality*.

I am grateful to the Literary Executor of the late Sir Ronald A. Fisher, F.R.S., to Dr. Frank Yates, F.R.S., and to the Longman Group Ltd., London, for permission to reprint Table III from their book *Statistical Tables for Biological, Agricultural and Medical Research* (sixth edition, 1974).

I am indebted to Marie Sheehan and Harry Taplin, who have been invaluable in helping to type this manuscript. Michael Payne, Susan London, and Ian List were also instrumental in providing editorial advice in the preparation of the manuscript. I am grateful to Beow Yeap and Edward Freedman for their assistance in proofreading the manuscript. Finally, I am indebted to my many colleagues at the Channing Laboratory, most notably Edward Kass, Frank Speizer, Charles Hennekens, Frank Polk, Ira Tager, Jerome Klein, James Taylor, Stephen Zinner, Walter Willett, and Alvaro Munoz and to my other colleagues at the Harvard Medical School, most notably Frederick Mosteller, Eliot Berson, Robert Ackerman, Mark Abelson, Leo Chylack, Eugene Braunwald, and Arther Dempster, who provided the inspiration for writing this book.

Bernard Rosner
Boston, MA

# $\mathcal{C}$ontents

# 5 Continuous Probability Distributions                                          100

# 6 Estimation                                                                        137

# 7 Hypothesis Testing: One-Sample Inference                                          180

# 8 Hypothesis Testing: Two-Sample Inference

# 9 Nonparametric Methods

# $12$ Analysis of Variance    442

# $T$ables

# Fundamentals of Biostatistics

# 1 General Overview

**Statistics** is the science whereby inferences are made about specific random phenomena on the basis of relatively limited sample material. The field of statistics can be subdivided into two main areas: mathematical and applied statistics. **Mathematical statistics** concerns the development of new methods of statistical inference and requires a detailed knowledge of abstract mathematics for its implementation. **Applied statistics** concerns the application of the methods of mathematical statistics to specific subject areas, such as economics, psychology, and public health. **Biostatistics** is the branch of applied statistics that concerns the application of statistical methods to medical and biological problems.

A good way to learn about biostatistics and its role in the research process is to follow the flow of a research study from its inception at the planning stage to its completion, which usually occurs when a manuscript reporting the results of the study is published. I will now describe to you one such study in which I participated.

A friend called one morning and in the course of conversation mentioned to me that he had recently used a new, automated blood pressure device of the type seen in many banks, hotels, and department stores. The machine had read his average diastolic blood pressure on several occasions as 115 mm; the highest reading was 130 mm. I was horrified to hear of his experience, since if these readings were true, then my friend might be in imminent danger of having a stroke or developing some other serious cardiovascular disease. I referred him to a clinical colleague of mine, who used a standard blood pressure cuff and measured my friend's diastolic blood pressure as 90 mm. The contrast in the readings aroused my interest, and I began to routinely jot down the readings on the digital display every time I passed the machine at my local bank. I got the distinct impression that a large percentage of the reported readings were in the hypertensive range. Although one would expect that hypertensives would be more likely to use such a machine, I still believed that blood pressure readings obtained with the machine might not be comparable with standard methods of blood pressure measurement. I spoke to Dr. B. Frank Polk about my suspicion and succeeded in interesting him in a small-scale evaluation of such machines. We decided to send a human observer who was well trained in blood pressure measurement techniques to several of these machines. He would offer to pay the subjects 50¢ for the cost of using the machine if they would agree to fill out a short questionnaire and have their blood pressure measured by both the human observer and the machine.

At this stage we had to make several important decisions, each of which would prove to be vital to the success of the study. The decisions were based on the following questions:

1. How many machines should we test?
2. How many people should we test at each machine?
3. In what order should the measurements be taken—should the human observer or the machine be used first? Ideally, we would have preferred to avoid this problem by taking both the human and machine readings simultaneously, but this procedure was logistically impossible.
4. What other data should we collect on the questionnaire that might influence the comparison between methods?
5. How should the data be recorded to facilitate their computerization at a later date?
6. How should the accuracy of the computerized data be checked?

We resolved these problems as follows:

*1*. and *2*. We decided to test more than one machine (four to be exact), since we were not sure if the machines were comparable in quality. However, we wanted to sample enough subjects from each machine so that we would have an accurate comparison of the standard and automated methods for each machine. We tried to predict how large a discrepancy there might be between the two methods. Using the methods of sample size determination discussed in this book, we calculated that we would need 100 subjects at each site to have an accurate comparison.

*3*. We then had to decide in what order the measurements should be taken for each person. According to some reports, one problem that occurs with repeated blood pressure measurements is that persons tense up at the initial measurement, yielding higher blood pressures than at subsequent repeated measurements. Thus, we would not always want to use the automated or manual method first, since the effect of the method would get confused with the order-of-measurement effect. A conventional technique that we used here was to **randomize** the order in which the measurements were taken, so that for any person it was equally likely that the machine or the human observer would take the first measurement. This random pattern could be implemented by flipping a coin or, more likely, by using a table of **random numbers** as appears in Table 4 of the appendix.

*4*. We felt that the major extraneous factor that might influence the results would be body size, since we might have more difficulty getting accurate readings from persons with fatter arms than from those with leaner arms. We also wanted to get some idea of the type of people who use these machines; so we asked questions about age, sex, and previous hypertensive history.

*5*. To record the data, we developed a coding form that could be filled out on site and from which data could be easily entered on a computer terminal for subsequent analysis. Each person in the study was assigned an identification (ID) number by which the computer could uniquely identify that person. The data on the coding forms were then keyed and verified. That is, the same form was entered twice, and a comparison was made between the two records to make sure they were the same. If the records were not the same, then the form was reentered.

*6*. After data entry we ran some editing programs to ensure that the data were accurate. Checking each item on each form was impossible because of the large amount of data. Alternatively, we checked that the values for individual variables were within specified ranges and printed out aberrant values for manual checking. For example, we checked that all blood pressure readings were at least 50 and no more than 300 and printed out all readings that fell outside this range. This simple process enabled us to detect records that had been "offpunched"; that is, at some point in the data entry a column had been skipped, rendering all subsequent data on such records meaningless.

After completion of the data collection, data entry, and data editing phases, we were ready to look at the results of the study. The first step in this process is to get a general feel for the data by summarizing the information in the form of several descriptive statistics. This descriptive material can be numerical or graphical. If numerical, it can be in the form of a few summary statistics, which can be presented in tabular form or, alternatively, in the form of a **frequency distribution**, which lists each value in the data and how frequently it occurs. If graphical, the data are summarized pictorially and can be presented in one or more figures. The appropriate type of descriptive material will vary with the type of distribution considered. If the distribution is **continuous**, that is, if there are essentially an infinite number of possible values, as would be the case for blood pressure, then means and standard deviations might be the appropriate descriptive statistics. However, if the distribution is **discrete**, that is, if there are only a few possible values, as would be the case for sex, then percentages of people taking on each value would be the appropriate descriptive measure. In some cases both types of descriptive statistics are used for continuous distributions by condensing the range of possible values into a few groups and giving the percentage of people that fall into each group (e.g., the percentages of people that have blood pressures between 120 and 129 mm and between 130 and 139 mm).

In this study we decided first to look at mean blood pressure for each method at each of the four sites. Table 1.1 summarizes this information [1].

You might notice from this table that we did not obtain meaningful data from all of the 100 people interviewed at each site, since we could not obtain valid readings from the machine for many of the people. This type of missing data problem is very common in biostatistics and should be anticipated at the planning stage when deciding on sample sizes (which was not done in this study).

Our next step in the study was to determine whether the apparent differences in blood pressure between machine and human measurements at two of the locations (C, D) were "real" in some sense or were "due to chance." This type of question falls into the area of **inferential statistics**. We realized that although there was a 14-mm difference in mean systolic blood pressure between the two methods for the 98 people we interviewed at location C, this difference might not hold up if we interviewed 98 other people at a different time, and we wanted to have some idea

| Location | Number of people | Systolic blood pressures (mm Hg) | | | | | |
| --- | --- | --- | --- | --- | --- | --- | --- |
| | | Machine | | Human | | Difference | |
| | | Mean | Standard deviation | Mean | Standard deviation | Mean | Standard deviation |
| A | 98 | 142.5 | 21.0 | 142.0 | 18.1 | 0.5 | 11.2 |
| B | 84 | 134.1 | 22.5 | 133.6 | 23.2 | 0.5 | 12.1 |
| C | 98 | 147.9 | 20.3 | 133.9 | 18.3 | 14.0 | 11.7 |
| D | 62 | 135.4 | 16.7 | 128.5 | 19.0 | 6.9 | 13.6 |

(By permission of the American Heart Association, Inc.)

as to the **error in the estimate** of 14 mm. In technical jargon this group of 98 people represents a **sample** from the **population** of all people who use that machine. We are interested in the population and we wish to use the sample to help us learn something about the population. In particular, we wanted to know how different the **estimated** mean difference of 14 mm in our sample was likely to be from the **true** mean difference in the population of all people who might use this machine. More specifically, we wanted to know if it was still possible that there was no underlying difference between the two methods and that our results were due to chance. We refer to the 14-mm difference in our group of 98 people as an **estimator** of the true mean difference $(d)$ in the population. The problem of inferring characteristics of a population from a sample is the central concern of statistical inference and is a major topic in this text. To accomplish this aim, we needed to develop a **probability model**, which would tell us how likely it is that we would obtain a 14-mm difference between the two methods in a sample of 98 people if there were no real difference between the two methods over the entire population of users of the machine. If this probability were sufficiently small, then we would begin to believe that a real difference existed between the two methods. In this particular case, using a probability model based on the $t$ distribution, we were able to conclude that this probability was less than 1 in 1000 for each of machines C and D. This probability was sufficiently small for us to believe that there was a real difference between the automatic and manual methods of taking blood pressure for two of the four machines tested.

We used a statistical package to perform the preceding data analyses. A package is a collection of statistical programs that describe data and perform various statistical tests on the data. Currently the most widely used statistical packages include SAS, SPSS, BMDP, and MINITAB.

The final step in this study, after completing the data analysis, was to compile the results in the form of a publishable manuscript. Inevitably, because of space considerations, much of the material developed during the data analysis phase was weeded out and only the essential items were presented for publication.

I hope that the review of this study gives you some idea of what medical research is about and what the role of biostatistics is in this process. The material in this text will parallel the description of the data analysis phase of the study described. Chapter 2 summarizes different types of descriptive statistics. In Chapters 3 through 5, we learn some basic principles of probability and various probability models for use in later discussions of inferential statistics. In Chapters 6 through 12, we discuss the major topics of inferential statistics as used in biomedical practice. We will not formally be concerned with issues of study design or with data collection in this text.

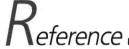

*R*eference

[*1*] Polk, B. F., Rosner, B., Feudo, R., and Vandenburgh, M. (1980) "An Evaluation of the Vita-Stat Automatic Blood Pressure Measuring Device," *Hypertension* **2(2)**: 221–227.

# 2 Descriptive Statistics

■ *2.1 INTRODUCTION*

The first step in looking at data is to describe the data at hand in some concise way. In smaller studies this step can be accomplished by listing each data point. In general, however, this procedure is tedious or impossible and, even if it were possible, would not give us an overall picture of what the data look like.

*Example 2.1*   *Cancer, Nutrition* Some investigators have proposed that consumption of vitamin A prevents cancer. To test this theory, we might use a dietary questionnaire to collect data on vitamin A consumption among 200 hospitalized cancer cases and among 200 controls. The controls would be matched on age and sex to the cancer cases and would be in the hospital at the same time for an unrelated disease. Now what do we do with these data?   ■

Before we formally attempt to answer the question, we would want to describe the vitamin A consumption among cases and controls. Consider Figure 2.1. The *bar graphs* give us a visual sense that the controls have a higher vitamin A consumption than the cases do, particularly in doses higher than the recommended daily allowance (RDA).

*Example 2.2*   *Pulmonary Disease* Medical researchers have often suspected that passive smokers, that is, persons who themselves do not smoke but who live or work in an environment where others smoke, might have impaired pulmonary function as a result. A research group in San Diego recently published results indicating that passive smokers did indeed have significantly lower pulmonary function than did comparable nonsmokers who did not work in smoky environments [1]. As supporting evidence, the authors measured the carbon monoxide (CO) concentrations in the working environments of passive smokers and of nonsmokers (where no smoking was permitted in the workplace) to see if the relative CO concentration changed over the course of the day. These results are displayed in the form of a **scatter plot** in Figure 2.2.   ■

Figure 2.2 clearly shows that the CO concentrations in the two working

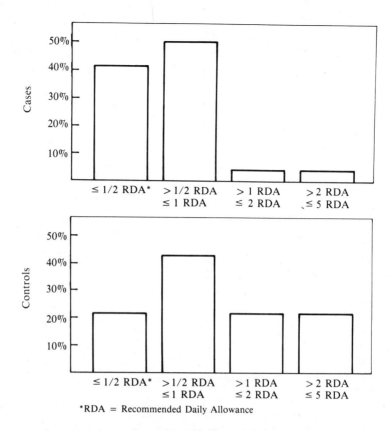

*Figure 2.1*

Daily vitamin A
consumption
among cancer cases
and controls

environments are about the same early in the day but diverge widely in the middle of the day and then converge again after the working day is over at 7 PM.

Graphical displays illustrate the important role of descriptive statistics, which is to quickly display data to give the researcher a clue as to the principal trends in the data and suggest hints as to where a more detailed look at the data, using the methods of inferential statistics, might be worthwhile. Descriptive statistics are also crucially important in conveying the final results of studies in written publications. Unless it is one of their primary interests, most readers will not have the time to critically evaluate the work of others, but will be influenced mainly by the descriptive statistics presented.

What makes a good graphical or numerical display? The principal guideline is that the material should be as self-contained as possible and should be understandable without reading the text. These attributes require clear labeling. The captions, units, and axes on graphs should be clearly labeled, and the statistical terms used in tables and figures should be well defined. The quantity of material presented is equally important. If bar graphs are constructed, then care must be taken that neither too many nor too few groups be displayed. The same is true of tabular material.

Many methods are available for summarizing data in both numerical and graphical form. In this chapter we will summarize the methods and give their strengths and weaknesses.

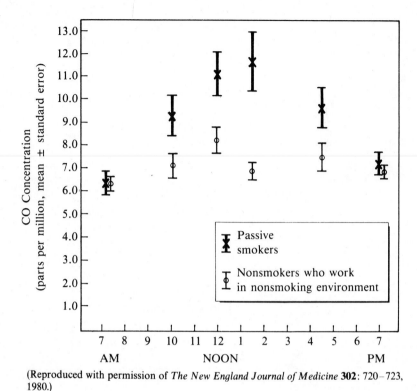

**_Figure 2.2_**
_Mean carbon monoxide concentration ( ± standard error) by time of day as measured in the working environment of passive smokers and nonsmokers who work in nonsmoking environments_

(Reproduced with permission of _The New England Journal of Medicine_ **302**: 720–723, 1980.)

# ■ 2.2 MEASURES OF CENTRAL LOCATION

The basic problem of statistics can be stated as follows: Suppose we have a sample of data $x_1, \ldots, x_n$, where $x_1$ corresponds to the first sample point and $x_n$ corresponds to the $n$th sample point. If we presume the sample is drawn from some population $P$, what inferences or conclusions can we make about $P$ from the sample?

Before we can answer such questions, we must summarize our data as succinctly as possible, since the number of sample points is frequently large and we can easily lose track of the overall picture by looking at all of the data at once. One type of measure useful for summarizing data is to define the center, or middle, of the sample. We will refer to this type of measure as a **measure of central location**.

## □ 2.2.1 The Arithmetic Mean

How to define the middle of a sample may seem obvious to you, but the more you think about it, the less obvious it becomes. Suppose we have a sample of birthweights of all live-born infants born at a private hospital in San Diego, California, during a 1-week period. This sample is shown in Table 2.1.

One measure of central location for this sample is the **arithmetic mean** (colloquially referred to as the average). The arithmetic mean (or mean or sample mean) is usually denoted by $\bar{x}$.

**Table 2.1**

_Sample of birthweights of live-born infants born at a private hospital in San Diego, California, during a 1-week period (g)_

| $i$ | $x_i$ | $i$ | $x_i$ | $i$ | $x_i$ | $i$ | $x_i$ |
|---|---|---|---|---|---|---|---|
| 1 | 3265 | 6 | 3323 | 11 | 2581 | 16 | 2759 |
| 2 | 3260 | 7 | 3649 | 12 | 2841 | 17 | 3248 |
| 3 | 3245 | 8 | 3200 | 13 | 3609 | 18 | 3314 |
| 4 | 3484 | 9 | 3031 | 14 | 2838 | 19 | 3101 |
| 5 | 4146 | 10 | 2069 | 15 | 3541 | 20 | 2834 |

**Definition 2.1**

The arithmetic mean is the sum of all the observations divided by the number of observations. It is written in statistical terms as

$$\bar{x} = \frac{1}{n} \sum_{i=1}^{n} x_i$$ ∎

The sign $\sum$ (sigma) in Definition 2.1 is referred to as a summation sign.

$$\sum_{i=1}^{n} x_i$$

is simply a short way of writing the quantity $(x_1 + x_2 + \cdots + x_n)$.

If $a$ and $b$ are integers, then

$$\sum_{i=a}^{b} x_i$$

means that

1. We substitute $a$ for $i$ and use $x_a$ as the first term in the summation.
2. We increase $i$ by 1 to $a + 1$ and add $x_{a+1}$ to $x_a$.
3. We repeat step 2 as many times as possible until $i = b$.

The term $x_b$ is the last term in the summation. Thus,

$$\sum_{i=a}^{b} x_i = x_a + x_{a+1} + \cdots + x_b$$

If $a = b$, then $\sum_{i=a}^{b} x_i = x_a$. One fundamental property of summation signs is that if each term in the summation is a multiple of the same constant $c$, then $c$ can be factored out from the summation, that is,

$$\sum_{i=1}^{n} cx_i = c\left(\sum_{i=1}^{n} x_i\right)$$

*Example 2.3*    If

$$x_1 = 2 \qquad x_2 = 5 \qquad x_3 = -4$$

find

$$\sum_{i=1}^{3} x_i \qquad \sum_{i=2}^{3} x_i \qquad \sum_{i=1}^{3} x_i^2 \qquad \sum_{i=1}^{3} 2x_i$$

*Solution*

$$\sum_{i=1}^{3} x_i = 2 + 5 - 4 = 3 \qquad \sum_{i=2}^{3} x_i = 5 - 4 = 1$$

$$\sum_{i=1}^{3} x_i^2 = 4 + 25 + 16 = 45 \qquad \sum_{i=1}^{3} 2x_i = 2 \sum_{i=1}^{3} x_i = 6 \qquad ■$$

It is important that you become familiar with summation signs, since they will be used extensively in the remainder of this text.

*Example 2.4*    What is the arithmetic mean for the sample of birthweights given in Table 2.1?

*Solution*
$$\bar{x} = (3265 + 3260 + \cdots + 2834)/20 = 3166.9 \text{ g} \qquad ■$$

The arithmetic mean is, in general, a very natural measure of central location. One of its principal limitations, however, is that it is overly sensitive to very extreme values. In this instance it may not be representative of the location of the great majority of the sample points. For example, if the first infant in Table 2.1 happened to be a premature infant weighing 500 g rather than 3265 g, then the arithmetic mean of the sample would be reduced to 3028.7 g. In this instance, 7 of the birthweights would be lower than the arithmetic mean, and 13 would be higher than the arithmetic mean. It is possible in very extreme cases for all but one of the sample points to be on one side of the arithmetic mean. The arithmetic mean is a poor measure of central location in these types of samples, since it does not reflect the center of the sample. Nevertheless, the arithmetic mean is by far the most widely used measure of central location.

## ☐ 2.2.2 The Median

An alternative measure of central location, which is perhaps second in popularity to the arithmetic mean, is the **median** or, more precisely, the **sample median**.

Suppose we have $n$ sample observations. If we place these observations in order from smallest to largest, then the median is defined as follows:

**Definition 2.2**

The **sample median** is

*1*. The $\left(\dfrac{n+1}{2}\right)$th largest observation if $n$ is odd

*2*. The average of the $\left(\dfrac{n}{2}\right)$th and $\left(\dfrac{n}{2}+1\right)$th largest observations if $n$ is even    ■

The rationale for these definitions is to ensure an equal number of sample points on both sides of the sample median. The median is defined differently when $n$ is even and odd because it is impossible to achieve this goal with one uniform definition. For samples with an odd sample size, there is a unique central point; for example, for samples of size 7, the fourth largest point is the central point in the sense that 3 points are both smaller and larger than it. For samples with an even sample size, there is no unique central point and we must average the middle 2 values. Thus, for samples of size 8, we would average the fourth and fifth largest points to obtain the median, since neither is the central point.

*Example 2.5*

*Solution*

Compute the sample median for the sample in Table 2.1.

We must first arrange the sample in ascending order as follows:

2069, 2581, 2759, 2834, 2838, 2841, 3031, 3101, 3200, 3245, 3248, 3260, 3265, 3314, 3323, 3484, 3541, 3609, 3649, 4146

Since $n$ is even, we want

Sample median = average of the 10th and 11th largest observations

$$= (3245 + 3248)/2$$

$$= 3246.5 \text{ g}$$

∎

*Example 2.6*

*Solution*

**Infectious Disease** Consider the data set in Table 2.2, which consists of white blood counts taken on admission of all patients entering a small hospital in Allentown, Pennsylvania, on a given day. Compute the median white blood count.

We first order the sample as follows: 3, 5, 7, 8, 8, 9, 10, 12, 35. Since $n$ is odd, the sample median is given by the fifth largest point, which equals 8. ∎

The principal strength of the sample median is that it is insensitive to very large or very small values. In particular, if the second patient in Table 2.2 had a white count of 65,000 rather than 35,000, the sample median would remain unchanged, since the fifth largest value is still 8000. Conversely, the arithmetic mean would increase dramatically from 10,778 in the original sample to 14,111 in the new sample. The principal weakness of the sample median is that it is determined mainly by the middle points in a sample and is less sensitive to the actual numerical values of the remaining data points.

*Table 2.2*

*Sample of admission white blood counts for all patients entering a hospital in Allentown, PA, on a given day ( × 1000)*

| $i$ | $x_i$ | $i$ | $x_i$ |
|-----|-------|-----|-------|
| 1 | 7 | 6 | 3 |
| 2 | 35 | 7 | 10 |
| 3 | 5 | 8 | 12 |
| 4 | 9 | 9 | 8 |
| 5 | 8 | | |

## ☐ *2.2.3 Comparison of the Arithmetic Mean and the Median*

If the arithmetic mean and the sample median are the same, then the sample is said to be **symmetric**; that is, the same number of points is on either side of the mean. Examples of distributions that we would expect to be roughly symmetric include the sample of birthweights in Table 2.1 and the distributions of systolic blood pressure measurements taken on all 30–39-year-old male factory workers in a given workplace.

If the arithmetic mean is greater than the sample median, then the sample is said to be **positively skewed**. Thus, most of the observations here would be to the left of the arithmetic mean, indicating that most of the observations would be

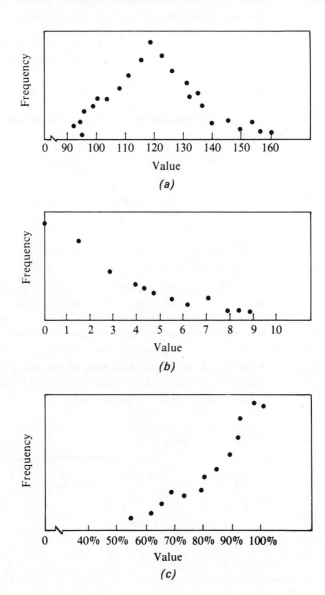

**Figure 2.3**
*Graphical displays of (a) symmetric (systolic blood pressure), (b) positively skewed (number of years used oral contraceptives), and (c) negatively skewed (relative humidity) distributions*

relatively small, with a few large observations to the right of $\bar{x}$. One such example would be the distribution of the number of years of oral contraceptive use by a group of women aged 20–29 participating in a prepaid health plan.

If the arithmetic mean is smaller than the sample median, then the distribution is said to be **negatively skewed**. Here most of the observations are larger than the arithmetic mean, with some very small observations to the left of $\bar{x}$. One example of a distribution that we would expect to be negatively skewed is a sample of relative humidities taken at a particular site in a humid climate at the same time of day over a number of days. In this sample most of the humidities will be at or close to 100%, with a few very low humidities on dry days. If we had very large samples of these three types of distributions and we plotted the frequency of occurrence of particular values versus the values themselves, then the plots of such distributions would appear as in Figure 2.3.

## ☐ 2.2.4 The Mode

Another widely used measure of central location is the **mode**.

_Definition 2.3_

The **mode** is the most frequently occurring value among all the observations in a sample.                                                                       ∎

_Example 2.7_   **_Family Planning_** Suppose we consider the sample of time intervals between successive menstrual periods for a group of 500 college women aged 18–21, as shown in Table 2.3. The frequency column gives the number of women who reported each of the respective durations. Twenty-eight days is the mode, since it is the most frequently occurring value.   ∎

_Example 2.8_   Compute the mode of the distribution in Table 2.2.

_Solution_      The mode is 8000 because it occurs more frequently than any other white count.   ∎

Some distributions have more than one mode. In fact, one useful method of classifying distributions is by the number of modes present. A distribution with one mode is referred to as **unimodal**; two modes, **bimodal**; three modes, **trimodal**; and so forth.

_Example 2.9_   Compute the mode of the distribution in Table 2.1.

_Solution_      There is no mode, since all the values occur exactly once.   ∎

**Table 2.3**
_Sample of time intervals between successive menstrual periods of college-aged women_

| Value | Frequency | Value | Frequency | Value | Frequency |
|-------|-----------|-------|-----------|-------|-----------|
| 24 | 5 | 29 | 96 | 34 | 7 |
| 25 | 10 | 30 | 63 | 35 | 3 |
| 26 | 28 | 31 | 24 | 36 | 2 |
| 27 | 64 | 32 | 9 | 37 | 1 |
| 28 | 185 | 33 | 2 | 38 | 1 |

Example 2.9 illustrates a common problem with the mode: It is not a useful measure of location if there are a large number of possible values, each of which occurs infrequently. In such cases the mode will either be far from the center of the sample or, in extreme cases, will not exist, as in Example 2.9. We will not use the mode very much in this text because its mathematical properties are, in general, rather intractable, and in most common situations it is inferior to the arithmetic mean.

## ☐ 2.2.5 The Geometric Mean

Much laboratory data, specifically data in the form of concentrations of one substance in another, as assessed by serial dilution techniques, are either multiples of 2 or are a constant multiplied by a power of 2; that is, they can have outcomes only of the form $2^k c$, $k = 0, 1, \ldots$, for some constant $c$. For example, the data in Table 2.4 represent the minimal inhibitory concentration (MIC) of penicillin G in the urine for *N. gonorrhoeae* in 74 patients [2]. The arithmetic mean would not be appropriate as a measure of central location in this situation because the distribution is very skewed. However, the data do have a certain symmetry, since the only possible values are of the form $2^k(0.03125)$ for $k = 0, 1, 2 \ldots$. One solution is to work with the distribution of the logs of the concentrations. The log concentrations have the property that successive possible concentrations differ by a constant; that is, $\log(2^{k+1}c) - \log(2^k c) = \log(2^{k+1}) + \log c - \log(2^k) - \log c = (k + 1)\log 2 - k \log 2 = \log 2$. Thus, the log concentrations are equally spaced from each other, and the resulting distribution is now not as skewed as the concentrations themselves. We could then compute the arithmetic mean in the log scale, that is,

$$\overline{\log x} = \frac{1}{n} \sum_{i=1}^{n} \log x_i$$

and use it as a measure of location. However, we usually prefer to work in the original scale by taking the antilogarithm of $\overline{\log x}$ to form the geometric mean, which leads to the following definition:

**Definition 2.4**

The **geometric mean** is the antilogarithm of $\overline{\log x}$, where

$$\overline{\log x} = \frac{1}{n} \sum_{i=1}^{n} \log x_i$$

∎

**Table 2.4**

Distribution of minimal inhibitory concentration (MIC) of penicillin G for *N. gonorrhoeae*

| (µg/ml) Concentration | Frequency | (µg/ml) Concentration | Frequency |
|---|---|---|---|
| $0.03125 = 2^0(0.03125)$ | 21 | $0.250 = 2^3(0.03125)$ | 19 |
| $0.0625 = 2^1(0.03125)$ | 6 | $0.50 = 2^4(0.03125)$ | 17 |
| $0.125 = 2^2(0.03125)$ | 8 | $1.0 = 2^5(0.03125)$ | 3 |

(Reproduced with permission from *JAMA* **220**: 205–208, 1972. Copyright 1972, American Medical Association.)

*Example 2.10*  
*Solution*

*Infectious Disease* Compute the geometric mean for the sample in Table 2.4.

*(1)* We compute
$$\overline{\log x} = [21 \log(0.03125) + 6 \log(0.0625) + 8 \log(0.125)$$
$$+ 19 \log(0.250) + 17 \log(0.50) + 3 \log(1.0)]/74 = -0.846$$

*(2)* The geometric mean = the antilogarithm of $-0.846 = 0.143$.  ∎

# ■ 2.3 SOME PROPERTIES OF THE ARITHMETIC MEAN

Suppose we have a sample $x_1, \ldots, x_n$, which we refer to as our original sample. Let us create a **translated sample** $x_1 + c, \ldots, x_n + c$ by adding a constant $c$ to each data point. Let $y_i = x_i + c$, $i = 1, \ldots, n$. Suppose we wish to compute the arithmetic mean of the translated sample. We can show that the following relationship holds:

**2.1** If

$$y_i = x_i + c, \quad i = 1, \ldots, n$$

then

$$\bar{y} = \bar{x} + c$$

Therefore, to find the arithmetic mean of the $y$'s, we need only to compute the arithmetic mean of the $x$'s and add the constant $c$.

This principle is useful because it is sometimes convenient to change the "origin" of our sample data, that is, compute the arithmetic mean after translation and transform back to the original origin.

*Example 2.11*

In Table 2.3 we can more conveniently work with numbers that are near 0 than with numbers near 28 to compute the arithmetic mean of the time interval between menstrual periods. Thus, we might first create a translated sample by subtracting 28 days from each of the outcomes in Table 2.3. We then would find the arithmetic mean of the translated sample and add 28 to get the actual arithmetic mean. The calculations are shown in Table 2.5.

**Table 2.5**

*Translated sample for duration between successive menstrual periods in college-aged women*

| Value | Frequency | Value | Frequency | Value | Frequency |
|-------|-----------|-------|-----------|-------|-----------|
| $-4$  | 5         | 1     | 96        | 6     | 7         |
| $-3$  | 10        | 2     | 63        | 7     | 3         |
| $-2$  | 28        | 3     | 24        | 8     | 2         |
| $-1$  | 64        | 4     | 9         | 9     | 1         |
| 0     | 185       | 5     | 2         | 10    | 1         |

$$\bar{y} = [(-4)(5) + (-3)(10) + \cdots + (10)(1)]/500 = 0.54$$
$$\bar{x} = \bar{y} + 28 = 0.54 + 28 = 28.54 \text{ days}$$  ∎

Similarly, systolic blood pressure scores are usually between 100 and 200. We can more easily subtract 100 from each blood pressure score, find the mean of the translated sample, and add 100 to obtain the mean of the original sample.

Of course, with the advent of the calculator, much of the tedium of routine calculation has been eliminated and the motivation for translation before performing calculations is not as great. Nevertheless, the chance of an error in data entry depends on the number of digits entered. If this number can be reduced by translation, then fewer errors are likely to appear in your final results.

What happens to the arithmetic mean if we change the units or scale we are working with? We can create a **rescaled sample**:

$$y_i = cx_i, \quad i = 1, \ldots, n$$

The following results hold:

**2.2** If

$$y_i = cx_i, \quad i = 1, \ldots, n$$

then

$$\bar{y} = c\bar{x}$$

Therefore, to find the arithmetic mean of the $y$'s, we need only to compute the arithmetic mean of the $x$'s and multiply it by the constant $c$.

*Example 2.12*　Express the mean birthweight for the data in Table 2.1 in ounces rather than grams.

*Solution*　We know that 1 oz = 28.35 g and that $\bar{x} = 3166.9$ g. Thus, if we were to express our data in terms of ounces, then we would have

$$c = \frac{1}{28.35} \quad \text{and} \quad \bar{y} = \frac{1}{28.35}(3166.9) = 111.71 \text{ oz} \qquad \blacksquare$$

Sometimes we wish to change both the origin and the scale of our data at the same time. We can apply **(2.1)** and **(2.2)** as follows:

**2.3** Let $x_1, \ldots, x_n$ be our original sample of data and let $y_i = c_1 x_i + c_2, i = 1, \ldots, n$, represent a transformed sample obtained by multiplying each original sample point by a factor $c_1$ and then shifting over by a constant $c_2$. If

$$y_i = c_1 x_i + c_2, \quad i = 1, \ldots, n$$

then

$$\bar{y} = c_1 \bar{x} + c_2$$

*Example 2.13*　If we have a sample of temperatures in °C with an arithmetic mean of 11.75°, convert this mean to °F:

*Solution*            Since the required transformation to convert the data to °F would be

$$y_i = \tfrac{9}{5}x_i + 32, \quad i = 1, \ldots, n$$

we have

$$\bar{y} = \tfrac{9}{5}(11.75) + 32 = 53.15°\mathrm{F} \qquad \blacksquare$$

# ■ 2.4 MEASURES OF SPREAD

Consider the two samples shown in Figure 2.4. They represent two samples of cholesterol measurements, each on the same person using different measurement techniques. They appear to have about the same center, and whatever measure of central location we use will probably be about the same in the two samples. In fact, the arithmetic means are both 200 mg%. However, the two samples visually appear to be radically different. Upon further inspection this difference lies in the greater **variability**, or **spread**, of the manual method relative to the automated method. We want to quantify the notion of variability. Many samples can be well described by the combination of a measure of central location and a measure of spread.

## ☐ 2.4.1 The Range

We can use several different measures to describe the variability of a sample. The simplest measure is perhaps the **range**.

Definition 2.5

The **range** is the difference between the largest and smallest observations in the sample. ■

*Example 2.14*    The range in the sample of birthweights in Table 2.1 is

$$4146 - 2069 = 2077\,\mathrm{g} \qquad \blacksquare$$

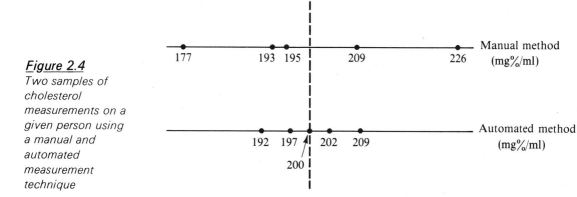

*Figure 2.4*
*Two samples of cholesterol measurements on a given person using a manual and automated measurement technique*

*Example 2.15*    Compute the ranges for the manual and automated method data in Figure 2.4 and compare the variability of the two methods.

*Solution*    The range for the manual method = 226 − 177 = 49 mg%. The range for the automated method = 209 − 192 = 17 mg%. The manual method clearly seems more variable.    ∎

One advantage of the range is that it is very easy to compute, once we have ordered the sample points. One striking disadvantage is that it is very sensitive to extreme observations. Hence, if the lightest infant in Table 2.1 were 500 g rather than 2069 g, then the range would increase dramatically to 4146 − 500 = 3646 g.

## ☐ 2.4.2 The Variance and Standard Deviation

The principal difference between the manual and automated method data in Figure 2.4 is that the automated method values are in some sense closer to the center of the sample than the manual method values are. If we define the center of the sample to be the arithmetic mean, then we need a measure that can summarize the difference (or deviations) between the individual sample points and the arithmetic mean, that is,

$$x_1 - \bar{x}, x_2 - \bar{x}, \ldots, x_n - \bar{x}$$

One simple measure that would seem to accomplish this goal is

$$d = \frac{\sum_{i=1}^{n} (x_i - \bar{x})}{n}$$

Unfortunately, this measure will not work because of the following principle:

 The sum of the deviations of the individual observations of a sample about the sample mean is always 0.

*Example 2.16*    Compute the sum of the deviations about the mean for the manual and automated data in Figure 2.4.

*Solution*    For the manual data,

$$d = (177 - 200) + (193 - 200) + (195 - 200) + (209 - 200) + (226 - 200)$$

$$= -23 - 7 - 5 + 9 + 26$$

$$= 0$$

For the automated data,

$$d = (192 - 200) + (197 - 200) + (200 - 200) + (202 - 200) + (209 - 200)$$

$$= -8 - 3 + 0 + 2 + 9$$

$$= 0$$    ∎

Thus, $d$ does not help us to distinguish the difference in spreads between the two methods.

A second idea is to use the squares of the deviations from the sample mean rather than the deviations themselves. We will refer to the resulting measure of spread as

$$s^2 = \frac{\sum_{i=1}^{n} (x_i - \bar{x})^2}{n}$$

The more usual form for this measure is with $(n-1)$ in the denominator rather than with $n$. The resulting measure is referred to as the **sample variance** (or **variance**).

## Definition 2.6

The **sample variance**, or **variance**, is defined as follows:

$$s^2 = \frac{\sum_{i=1}^{n} (x_i - \bar{x})^2}{(n-1)}$$ ∎

We shall present a rationale for using $(n-1)$ in the denominator rather than $n$ in our discussion of estimation in Chapter 6.

Another commonly used measure of spread is the **sample standard deviation**.

## Definition 2.7

The **sample standard deviation**, or **standard deviation**, is defined as follows:

$$s = \sqrt{\frac{\sum_{i=1}^{n} (x_i - \bar{x})^2}{(n-1)}} = \sqrt{\text{variance}}$$ ∎

*Example 2.17*

Compute the variance and standard deviation for the manual and automated method data in Figure 2.4.

*Solution*

*Manual method*

$$s^2 = [(177 - 200)^2 + (193 - 200)^2 + (195 - 200)^2 + (209 - 200)^2 + (226 - 200)^2]/4$$

$$= (529 + 49 + 25 + 81 + 676)/4 = 1360/4 = 340$$

$$s = \sqrt{340} = 18.4$$

*Automated method*

$$s^2 = [(192 - 200)^2 + (197 - 200)^2 + (200 - 200)^2 + (202 - 200)^2 + (209 - 200)^2]/4$$

$$= (64 + 9 + 0 + 4 + 81)/4 = 158/4 = 39.5$$

$$s = \sqrt{39.5} = 6.3$$

Thus, the manual method has a standard deviation roughly three times as large as that of the automated method. ∎

One problem in using the variance is that it is difficult to compute in its original form, since we must first compute the sample mean, then compute the deviation of each sample point about the sample mean, and then sum the squares of these deviations about the sample mean. This procedure introduces two extra steps, which make the computation both more cumbersome and more error prone, especially in light of the fact that many pocket calculators can accumulate both the sum and sum of squares of a sample in one pass. We thus have the following short forms for the variance:

**2 5**

The two **short forms** for the sample variance,

$$s^2 = \frac{\sum\limits_{i=1}^{n} (x_i - \bar{x})^2}{(n-1)}$$

are given by

$$\frac{\sum\limits_{i=1}^{n} x_i^2 - n\bar{x}^2}{(n-1)} \quad \text{and} \quad \frac{\sum\limits_{i=1}^{n} x_i^2 - \left(\sum\limits_{i=1}^{n} x_i\right)^2 \Big/ n}{(n-1)}$$

The first form is useful when we have already computed the sample mean, whereas the second form is useful if we have computed the sum and sum of squares of the observations without having computed the sample mean. Thus, we can compute the sample variance directly from the sum and the sum of squares of the individual observations.

Similarly, the two short forms for the standard deviation can be written as follows:

**2 6**

$$s = \sqrt{s^2} = \sqrt{\frac{\sum\limits_{i=1}^{n} x_i^2 - n\bar{x}^2}{(n-1)}}$$

$$= \sqrt{\frac{\sum\limits_{i=1}^{n} x_i^2 - \left(\sum\limits_{i=1}^{n} x_i\right)^2 \Big/ n}{(n-1)}}$$

*Example 2.18*

Compute the variance and standard deviation for the manual and automated data in Figure 2.4 using the short computational forms.

*Solution*

*Manual method* We first compute

$$\sum_{i=1}^{5} x_i = 177 + 193 + 195 + 209 + 226 = 1000$$

$$\sum_{i=1}^{5} x_i^2 = 177^2 + 193^2 + 195^2 + 209^2 + 226^2 = 201{,}360$$

$$s^2 = [201,360 - (1000)^2/5]/4 = (201,360 - 200,000)/4 = 1360/4 = 340$$

$$s = \sqrt{340} = 18.4$$

**Automated method**  We first compute

$$\sum_{i=1}^{5} x_i = 192 + 197 + 200 + 202 + 209 = 1000$$

$$\sum_{i=1}^{5} x_i^2 = 192^2 + 197^2 + 200^2 + 202^2 + 209^2 = 200,158$$

$$s^2 = [200,158 - (1000)^2/5]/4 = (200,158 - 200,000)/4 = 158/4 = 39.5$$

$$s = \sqrt{39.5} = 6.3$$

∎

# ■ 2.5 SOME PROPERTIES OF THE VARIANCE AND STANDARD DEVIATION

We can ask the same questions of the variance and standard deviation as we did for the arithmetic mean: namely, How are the variance and standard deviation affected by a change in origin or a change in the units we are working with? Suppose we have a sample $x_1, \ldots, x_n$ and all data points in the sample are shifted by a constant $c$; that is, we create a new sample $y_1, \ldots, y_n$ such that $y_i = x_i + c, i = 1, \ldots, n$.

If we refer to Figure 2.5, we would clearly expect that the variance and standard deviation would remain the same, since the relationship of the points in the sample relative to one another remains the same. This property is stated as follows:

**2.7**  Suppose we have two samples

$$x_1, \ldots, x_n \qquad \text{and} \qquad y_1, \ldots, y_n$$

where

$$y_i = x_i + c, \quad i = 1, \ldots, n$$

If we denote the respective sample variances of the two samples by

$$s_x^2 \qquad \text{and} \qquad s_y^2$$

then

$$s_y^2 = s_x^2$$

**Example 2.19**  Compare the variances and standard deviations for the menstrual period data in Tables 2.3 and 2.5.

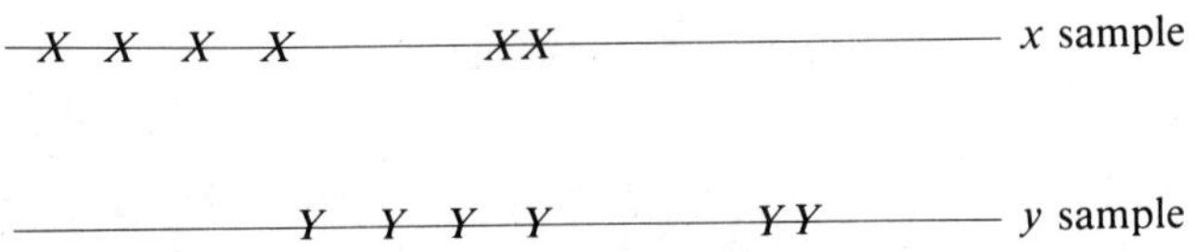

**Figure 2.5**
*Comparison of
the variances of
two samples,
where one sample
has an origin
shifted relative to
the other*

*Solution*    The variance and standard deviation of the two samples are the same, since the second sample was obtained from the first by subtracting 28 days from each data value; that is,

$$y_i = x_i - 28$$    ∎

Suppose we now change the units we use so that we create a new sample $y_1, \ldots, y_n$ such that $y_i = cx_i, i = 1, \ldots, n$. The following relationship holds between the variances of the two samples.

---

**2.8**    Suppose we have two samples

$$x_1, \ldots, x_n \quad \text{and} \quad y_1, \ldots, y_n$$

where

$$y_i = cx_i, \quad i = 1, \ldots, n, \quad c > 0$$

Then

$$s_y^2 = c^2 s_x^2 \qquad s_y = c s_x$$

---

*Example 2.20*    Compute the variance and standard deviation of the birthweight data in Table 2.1 in both grams and ounces.

*Solution*    The original data are given in grams; so we first compute the variance and standard deviation in these units. We have

$$\sum_{i=1}^{20} x_i = 63{,}338 \qquad \sum_{i=1}^{20} x_i^2 = 204{,}353{,}260$$

$$s^2 = [204{,}353{,}260 - (63{,}338)^2/20]/19 = 3{,}768{,}147.8/19 = 198{,}323.6 \text{ g}^2$$

$$s = 445.3 \text{ g}$$

To compute the variance and standard deviation in ounces, we note that

$$1 \text{ oz} = 28.35 \text{ g} \quad \text{or} \quad y_i = \frac{1}{28.35} x_i$$

Thus,

$$s^2 \text{ (oz)} = \frac{1}{(28.35)^2} s^2 \text{ (g)} = 246.8 \text{ oz}^2$$

$$s \text{ (oz)} = \frac{1}{28.35} s \text{ (g)} = 15.7 \text{ oz} \qquad \blacksquare$$

Thus, if the sample points change in scale by a factor of $c$, the variance changes by a factor of $c^2$ and the standard deviation changes by a factor of $c$. This relationship is the main reason why the standard deviation is more often used than the variance as a measure of scale, since the standard deviation and the arithmetic mean are in the same units, whereas the variance and the arithmetic mean are not. Thus, as illustrated in Examples 2.12 and 2.20, both the mean and the standard deviation change by a factor of 28.35 in the birthweight data of Table 2.1 when the units are expressed in terms of ounces rather than grams.

# ■ 2.6 THE COEFFICIENT OF VARIATION

It is useful to relate the arithmetic mean and the standard deviation together, since, for example, a standard deviation of 10 would mean something different conceptually if the arithmetic mean were 10 than if it were 1000. A special measure, called the **coefficient of variation**, is often used for this purpose.

**Definition 2.8**

The **coefficient of variation** ($CV$) is defined by

$$100\% \times (s/\bar{x}) \qquad \blacksquare$$

This measure remains the same regardless of what units are used because if the units are changed by a factor $c$, both the mean and standard deviation change by the factor $c$; the $CV$, which is the ratio between them, remains unchanged.

*Example 2.21*    Compute the coefficient of variation for the data in Table 2.1 when the birthweights are expressed in either grams or ounces.

*Solution*    We have

$$CV = 100\% \times (s/\bar{x}) = 100\% \times (445.3 \text{ g}/3166.9 \text{ g}) = 14.1\%$$

If the data were expressed in ounces, then

$$CV = 100\% \times (15.7 \text{ oz}/111.71 \text{ oz}) = 14.1\% \qquad \blacksquare$$

The coefficient of variation is most useful in comparing the variability of several different samples, each with different arithmetic means. This is because we usually expect a higher variability when the mean increases, and the $CV$ is a measure that accounts for this variability. Thus, if we are conducting a study where air pollution is measured at several sites and we wish to compare day-to-day variability at the different sites, we might expect a higher variability for the more highly polluted sites. A more accurate comparison could be made by comparing the *CV*'s at different sites than by comparing the standard deviations.

## 2.7 GROUPED DATA

Sometimes the sample size is prohibitively large to display all the raw data. Also, data are frequently collected in grouped form, since the required degree of accuracy to specify a measured quantity exactly is often lacking, because of either measurement error or imprecise patient recall. For example, systolic blood pressure measurements taken with a standard cuff are usually specified to the nearest 5 mm, since assessing them with any more precision is difficult using this instrument. Thus, a stated measurement of 120 mm may actually imply that the reading is some number $\geq 117.5$ mm and $< 122.5$ mm. Similarly, dietary recall is generally not very accurate and the most precise estimate of fish consumption might take the following form: 2–3 servings per day, 1 serving per day, 5–6 servings per week, 2–4 servings per week, 1 serving per week, $<1$ serving per week and $\geq 1$ serving per month, never.

Let us consider the data set in Table 2.6, which represents the birthweights from 100 consecutive deliveries at a Boston hospital.

Suppose we wish to display these data for publication purposes. How can we do this? If our data are on a computer, then the simplest way to display the data would be to generate a **frequency distribution** using one of the common statistical packages.

**Definition 2.9**

A **frequency distribution** is an ordered display of each value in a dataset together with its **frequency**, that is, the number of times that value occurs in the dataset. In addition, the percentage of sample points that take on a particular value is also typically given.  ∎

A frequency distribution of the sample of 100 birthweights in Table 2.6 was generated using the Statistical Analysis System (SAS) package and is displayed in Table 2.7.

The SAS frequency distribution program provides the frequency, cumulative frequency (CUM FREQ), percent, and cumulative percent (CUM PERCENT)

**Table 2.6**
*Sample of birthweights from 100 consecutive deliveries (oz)*

| | | | | | | | | | |
|---|---|---|---|---|---|---|---|---|---|
| 58 | 118 | 92 | 108 | 132 | 32 | 140 | 138 | 96 | 161 |
| 120 | 86 | 115 | 118 | 95 | 83 | 112 | 128 | 127 | 124 |
| 123 | 134 | 94 | 67 | 124 | 155 | 105 | 100 | 112 | 141 |
| 104 | 132 | 98 | 146 | 132 | 93 | 85 | 94 | 116 | 113 |
| 121 | 68 | 107 | 122 | 126 | 88 | 89 | 108 | 115 | 85 |
| 111 | 121 | 124 | 104 | 125 | 102 | 122 | 137 | 110 | 101 |
| 91 | 122 | 138 | 99 | 115 | 104 | 98 | 89 | 119 | 109 |
| 104 | 115 | 138 | 105 | 144 | 87 | 88 | 103 | 108 | 109 |
| 128 | 106 | 125 | 108 | 98 | 133 | 104 | 122 | 124 | 110 |
| 133 | 115 | 127 | 135 | 89 | 121 | 112 | 135 | 115 | 64 |

**Table 2.7**

*Frequency distribution of birthweight data in Table 2.6 using the Statistical Analysis System (SAS)*

SAMPLE OF BIRTHWEIGHTS FROM 100 CONSECUTIVE DELIVERIES (OZ.)

| BIRTHWT | FREQUENCY | CUM FREQ | PERCENT | CUM PERCENT |
|---------|-----------|----------|---------|-------------|
| 32 | 1 | 1 | 1.000 | 1.000 |
| 58 | 1 | 2 | 1.000 | 2.000 |
| 64 | 1 | 3 | 1.000 | 3.000 |
| 67 | 1 | 4 | 1.000 | 4.000 |
| 68 | 1 | 5 | 1.000 | 5.000 |
| 83 | 1 | 6 | 1.000 | 6.000 |
| 85 | 2 | 8 | 2.000 | 8.000 |
| 86 | 1 | 9 | 1.000 | 9.000 |
| 87 | 1 | 10 | 1.000 | 10.000 |
| 88 | 2 | 12 | 2.000 | 12.000 |
| 89 | 3 | 15 | 3.000 | 15.000 |
| 91 | 1 | 16 | 1.000 | 16.000 |
| 92 | 1 | 17 | 1.000 | 17.000 |
| 93 | 1 | 18 | 1.000 | 18.000 |
| 94 | 2 | 20 | 2.000 | 20.000 |
| 95 | 1 | 21 | 1.000 | 21.000 |
| 96 | 1 | 22 | 1.000 | 22.000 |
| 98 | 3 | 25 | 3.000 | 25.000 |
| 99 | 1 | 26 | 1.000 | 26.000 |
| 100 | 1 | 27 | 1.000 | 27.000 |
| 101 | 1 | 28 | 1.000 | 28.000 |
| 102 | 1 | 29 | 1.000 | 29.000 |
| 103 | 1 | 30 | 1.000 | 30.000 |
| 104 | 5 | 35 | 5.000 | 35.000 |
| 105 | 2 | 37 | 2.000 | 37.000 |
| 106 | 1 | 38 | 1.000 | 38.000 |
| 107 | 1 | 39 | 1.000 | 39.000 |
| 108 | 4 | 43 | 4.000 | 43.000 |
| 109 | 2 | 45 | 2.000 | 45.000 |
| 110 | 2 | 47 | 2.000 | 47.000 |
| 111 | 1 | 48 | 1.000 | 48.000 |
| 112 | 3 | 51 | 3.000 | 51.000 |
| 113 | 1 | 52 | 1.000 | 52.000 |
| 115 | 6 | 58 | 6.000 | 58.000 |
| 116 | 1 | 59 | 1.000 | 59.000 |
| 118 | 2 | 61 | 2.000 | 61.000 |
| 119 | 1 | 62 | 1.000 | 62.000 |
| 120 | 1 | 63 | 1.000 | 63.000 |
| 121 | 3 | 66 | 3.000 | 66.000 |
| 122 | 4 | 70 | 4.000 | 70.000 |
| 123 | 1 | 71 | 1.000 | 71.000 |
| 124 | 4 | 75 | 4.000 | 75.000 |
| 125 | 2 | 77 | 2.000 | 77.000 |
| 126 | 1 | 78 | 1.000 | 78.000 |
| 127 | 2 | 80 | 2.000 | 80.000 |
| 128 | 2 | 82 | 2.000 | 82.000 |
| 132 | 3 | 85 | 3.000 | 85.000 |
| 133 | 2 | 87 | 2.000 | 87.000 |
| 134 | 1 | 88 | 1.000 | 88.000 |
| 135 | 2 | 90 | 2.000 | 90.000 |
| 137 | 1 | 91 | 1.000 | 91.000 |
| 138 | 3 | 94 | 3.000 | 94.000 |
| 140 | 1 | 95 | 1.000 | 95.000 |
| 141 | 1 | 96 | 1.000 | 96.000 |
| 144 | 1 | 97 | 1.000 | 97.000 |
| 146 | 1 | 98 | 1.000 | 98.000 |
| 155 | 1 | 99 | 1.000 | 99.000 |
| 161 | 1 | 100 | 1.000 | 100.000 |

for each birthweight present in our sample. For any particular birthweight $b$, the cumulative frequency, or CUM FREQ, is the number of birthweights in the sample that are less than or equal to $b$. The cumulative percent (CUM PERCENT) = $100 \times$ CUM FREQ$/n$ = the percentage of birthweights less than or equal to $b$.

If the number of unique sample values is large, then a frequency distribution may still be too detailed a summary for publication purposes. Instead, we might consider lumping the data into broader categories. Some general instructions for categorizing the data are provided in the following guidelines:

*1.* We subdivide the data into $k$ intervals, starting at some lower bound $y_1$ and ending at some upper bound $y_{k+1}$.

*2.* The first interval is from $y_1$ inclusive to $y_2$ exclusive; the second interval is from $y_2$ inclusive to $y_3$ exclusive; ... ; the $k$th and last interval is from $y_k$ inclusive to $y_{k+1}$ exclusive. The rationale for this representation is to make certain that the group intervals include all possible values *and* do not overlap. These errors are common in the presentation of grouped data.

*3.* The group intervals are generally chosen to be equal, although the appropriateness of equal group sizes should be dictated more by subject matter considerations. Thus, equal intervals might be appropriate for the blood pressure or birthweight data but not for the dietary recall data, where the nature of the data dictates unequal group sizes corresponding to how most people remember what they eat.

*4.* A count is made of the number of units that fall in each interval, which is denoted by the **frequency** within that interval.

*5.* The midpoint of each group interval is computed for calculation of descriptive statistics. The midpoint of the first interval is denoted by

$$z_1 = \frac{y_1 + y_2}{2}$$

the midpoint of the second interval by

$$z_2 = \frac{y_2 + y_3}{2}, \ldots$$

and the midpoint of the last interval by

$$z_k = \frac{y_k + y_{k+1}}{2}$$

The intervals and their midpoints are depicted in Figure 2.6.

*6.* Finally, for the purpose of computing descriptive statistics, the group intervals and their midpoints and frequencies are then displayed concisely in a table such as Table 2.8.

**Figure 2.6**
*Subdivision of the real line for the purpose of forming group intervals*

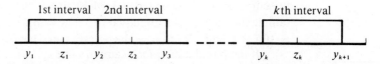

**Table 2.8**

General layout of
grouped data

|  | Midpoint of | |
| Group interval | group interval | Frequency |
| --- | --- | --- |
| $\geqslant y_1, < y_2$ | $z_1$ | $f_1$ |
| $\geqslant y_2, < y_3$ | $z_2$ | $f_2$ |
| $\vdots$ | $\vdots$ | $\vdots$ |
| $\geqslant y_i, < y_{i+1}$ | $z_i$ | $f_i$ |
| $\vdots$ | $\vdots$ | $\vdots$ |
| $\geqslant y_k, < y_{k+1}$ | $z_k$ | $f_k$ |

For example, we might display the raw data in Table 2.6 according to the format in Table 2.9.

If we are confronted with grouped data either in the form of published data from a secondary source or from our own data, then we want to be able to compute grouped means and variances that are analogous to the arithmetic mean and variance. Let us suppose that $f_i$ observations fall in the $i$th group interval, $i = 1, \ldots, k$, and that the midpoint of the $i$th interval is $z_i$, $i = 1, \ldots, k$, where $n = \sum_{i=1}^{k} f_i$ = total number of observations over all groups. The **grouped mean** is then defined as follows:

**Definition 2.10**

The **grouped mean** is defined by

$$\bar{x}_g \equiv \frac{\sum\limits_{i=1}^{k} f_i z_i}{\sum\limits_{i=1}^{k} f_i}$$

∎

**_Example 2.22_**  Compute the grouped mean for the data in Table 2.9.

**Table 2.9**

Grouped frequency
distribution of
birthweight (oz)
from 100
consecutive
deliveries

| Group interval | Midpoint | Frequency |
| --- | --- | --- |
| $\geqslant 29.5, \ \ < 69.5$ | 49.5 | 5 |
| $\geqslant 69.5, \ \ < 89.5$ | 79.5 | 10 |
| $\geqslant 89.5, \ \ < 99.5$ | 94.5 | 11 |
| $\geqslant 99.5, < 109.5$ | 104.5 | 19 |
| $\geqslant 109.5, < 119.5$ | 114.5 | 17 |
| $\geqslant 119.5, < 129.5$ | 124.5 | 20 |
| $\geqslant 129.5, < 139.5$ | 134.5 | 12 |
| $\geqslant 139.5, < 169.5$ | 154.5 | 6 |
|  |  | 100 |

**Solution**    We have

$$\bar{x}_g = \frac{\sum_{i=1}^{k} f_i z_i}{\sum_{i=1}^{k} f_i}$$

$$= [5(49.5) + 10(79.5) + 11(94.5) + \cdots + 6(154.5)]/100$$

$$= (11{,}045)/100$$

$$= 110.45 \text{ oz} \qquad \blacksquare$$

**Definition 2.11**

The **grouped variance** is defined by

$$s_g^2 \equiv \frac{\sum_{i=1}^{k} f_i(z_i - \bar{x}_g)^2}{\left[\left(\sum_{i=1}^{k} f_i\right) - 1\right]} \qquad \blacksquare$$

We can simplify the expression for the grouped variance as we did for the ungrouped variance, yielding the following two short forms for the grouped variance:

**2.9** **Short Forms for the Grouped Variance**

$$\textbf{Grouped variance} = \frac{\sum_{i=1}^{k} f_i z_i^2 - n\bar{x}_g^2}{(n-1)}$$

$$= \frac{\sum_{i=1}^{k} f_i z_i^2 - \left(\sum_{i=1}^{k} f_i z_i\right)^2 \Big/ n}{(n-1)}$$

**Example 2.23**    Compute the grouped variance for the data in Table 2.9.

**Solution**    We must compute

$$\sum_{i=1}^{k} f_i z_i^2 = 5(49.5)^2 + 10(79.5)^2 + \cdots + 6(154.5)^2 = 1{,}274{,}355$$

Thus,

$$s_g^2 = [1{,}274{,}355 - (11{,}045)^2/100]/99$$

$$= 54{,}434.75/99$$

$$= 549.85$$

and

$$s_g = \sqrt{549.85} = 23.45 \text{ oz} \qquad \blacksquare$$

# ■ *2.8 GRAPHICAL METHODS FOR GROUPED DATA*

In Section 2.7 we concentrated on methods for presenting grouped data in tabular form and on numerical measures for describing such data. In this section we will supplement these techniques by presenting certain commonly used graphical methods for displaying grouped data. The purpose of using graphical displays is to give a quick overall feel for the data, which is sometimes difficult to obtain with numerical measures.

## □ *2.8.1 The Bar Graph*

One of the most widely used methods for displaying grouped data is the bar graph.

■ A **bar graph** can be constructed as follows:

*1*. The data are divided into a number of groups using the guidelines that are provided in Section 2.7.

*2*. For each group a rectangle is constructed with base of a constant width and height proportional to the frequency within that group.

*3*. The rectangles are generally not contiguous and are equally spaced from each other.

A bar graph of daily vitamin A consumption among 200 cancer cases and 200 age- and sex-matched controls is presented in Figure 2.1.

## □ *2.8.2 The Histogram*

The bar graph tends to work well with grouped data when the groups are characterized by nonnumeric attributes, such as {current smoker/ex-smoker/never smoker} or {patient gets worse/patient gets better/patient stays the same}. If the groups are characterized by a numeric attribute, such as systolic blood pressure or birthweight, then a histogram is preferable. For a histogram, the position of the rectangle will correspond to the location of the group interval along the *x*-axis, and the size of the rectangle will correspond to the frequency within the group.

■ A **histogram** is constructed as follows:

*1*. The data are divided into groups as described in Section 2.7.

*2*. A rectangle is constructed for each group. The location of the base of the rectangle corresponds to the position of the ends of the group interval along the *x*-axis, and the **area** of the rectangle is proportional to the frequency within the group.

*3*. The scale used along either axis should allow all the rectangles to fit into the space allotted for the graph.

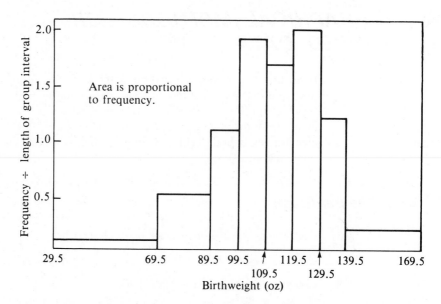

**Figure 2.7**

*Histogram for the birthweight data in Table 2.9*

Note that the area, rather than the height, is proportional to the frequency. If the length of each group interval is the same, then the area and the height are in the same proportions and the height will be proportional to the frequency as well. However, if one group interval is 5 times as large as another and the two group intervals have the same frequency, then the first group interval should have a height $\frac{1}{5}$ as large as the second group interval so that the areas will be the same. A common mistake in the literature is to construct histograms with group intervals of different lengths but with the height proportional to the frequency. This representation gives a misleading impression of the data. A histogram for the birthweight data in Table 2.9 is given in Figure 2.7.

## ☐ 2.8.3  The Stem and Leaf Plot

Two problems with histograms are that (1) they are somewhat difficult to construct and (2) we lose the sense of what the actual sample points are within the respective groups. One relatively recent type of graphical display that overcomes these problems is the stem and leaf plot.

■ A **stem and leaf** plot can be constructed as follows:

*1.* Separate each data point into a stem component and a leaf component, respectively, where the stem component consists of the number formed by all but the rightmost digit of the number, and the leaf component consists of the rightmost digit. Thus, the stem of the number 483 is 48, and the leaf is 3.

*2.* Write the smallest stem in the dataset in the upper-left-hand corner of the plot.

*3.* Write the second stem, which equals the first stem + 1, below the first stem.

*4.* Continue with step 3 until you reach the highest stem in the dataset.

*5.* Draw a vertical bar to the right of the column of stems.

*6.* For each number in the dataset, find the appropriate stem and write the leaf to the right of the vertical bar.

The collection of leaves thus formed will take on the general shape of the distribution of the sample points. Furthermore, we can preserve the actual sample values and yet have a grouped display for data, which is a distinct advantage over a histogram. Finally, we can usually construct a stem and leaf plot more quickly than a histogram from raw data, since we do not have to count the number of data points in each group interval. We can also easily compute the median and the range from a stem and leaf plot. A stem and leaf plot is given in Figure 2.8 for the birthweight data in Table 2.6. Thus, the point 5|8 represents 58, 11|8 represents 118, and so forth. Notice how we get an overall feel for the distribution without losing the individual values.

There are variations of stem and leaf plots where the leaf can consist of more than one digit. This variation might be appropriate for the birthweight data in Table 2.1, since the number of three-digit stems required would be very large relative to the number of data points. In this case we will let the leaf consist of the rightmost two digits and the stem the leftmost two digits, and we will underline the pairs of digits to the right of the vertical bar so that we can distinguish between two different leaves. The stem and leaf display for the data in Table 2.1 is presented in Figure 2.9.

Another common variation on the ordinary stem and leaf plot if the number of leaves is large is to allow more than one line for each stem. Similarly, one can position the largest stem at the top of the plot and the smallest stem at the bottom of the plot. In Figure 2.10 some graphical displays using the SAS UNIVARIATE procedure are given to illustrate this technique.

Note that each stem is allowed two lines, with the leaves from 5 to 9 on the upper line and the leaves from 0 to 4 on the lower line. Furthermore, the leaves are ordered on each line, and a count of the number of leaves on each line is provided under the # column to allow easy computation of the median and other descriptive statistics. Thus, the number 7 in the # column on the upper line for stem 12 indicates that there are 7 birthweights from 125 to 129 oz in the sample, whereas the number 13 indicates that there are 13 birthweights from 120 to 124 oz. Finally, a multiplication factor is given in the bottom of the display to allow for the repre-

| | |
|---|---|
| 3 | 2 |
| 4 | |
| 5 | 8 |
| 6 | 7 8 4 |
| 7 | |
| 8 | 6 3 5 8 9 5 9 7 8 9 |
| 9 | 2 6 5 4 8 3 4 1 9 8 8 |
| 10 | 8 5 0 4 7 8 4 2 1 4 9 4 5 3 8 9 6 8 4 |
| 11 | 8 5 8 2 2 6 3 5 1 0 5 9 5 0 5 2 5 |
| 12 | 0 8 7 4 3 4 1 2 6 1 4 5 2 2 8 5 2 4 7 1 |
| 13 | 2 8 4 2 2 7 8 8 3 3 5 5 |
| 14 | 0 1 6 4 |
| 15 | 5 |
| 16 | 1 |

**Figure 2.8**
*Stem and leaf plot for the birthweight data (oz) in Table 2.6*

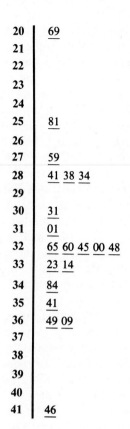

```
20 │ 69
21 │
22 │
23 │
24 │
25 │ 81
26 │
27 │ 59
28 │ 41 38 34
29 │
30 │ 31
31 │ 01
32 │ 65 60 45 00 48
33 │ 23 14
34 │ 84
35 │ 41
36 │ 49 09
37 │
38 │
39 │
40 │
41 │ 46
```

**Figure 2.9**
*Stem and leaf plot for the birthweight data (g) in Table 2.1*

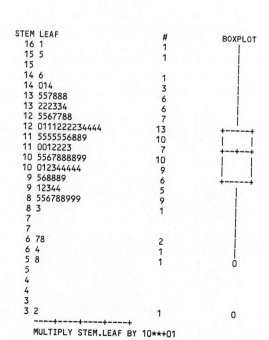

```
STEM  LEAF                      #      BOXPLOT
16   1                          1
15   5                          1
15
14   6                          1
14   014                        3
13   557888                     6
13   222334                     6
12   5567788                    7
12   0111222234444             13
11   5555556889                10
11   0012223                    7
10   5567888899                10
10   012344444                  9
 9   568889                     6
 9   12344                      5
 8   556788999                  9
 8   3                          1
 7
 7
 6   78                         2
 6   4                          1
 5   8                          1
 5
 4
 4
 3
 3   2                          1
   ----+----+----+----+
   MULTIPLY STEM.LEAF BY 10**+01
```

**Figure 2.10**
*Stem and leaf and box plots for the birthweight data (oz) in Table 2.6 as generated by the SAS UNIVARIATE procedure*

sentation of decimal numbers in stem and leaf form. In particular, if no multi-plication factor (*m*) is present, then we assume that all numbers have actual value stem leaf; whereas if *m* is present, then the actual value of the number is assumed to be stem.leaf $\times 10^m$. Thus, for example, since the multiplication factor is $10^1$, the value 6 4 on the stem and leaf plot represents the number $6.4 \times 10^1 = 64$ oz.

## ☐ 2.8.4 Box Plots

In Section 2.2.3 we discussed the comparison of the arithmetic mean and the median as a method for looking at the skewness of a distribution. We can also accomplish this goal by a graphical technique known as the **box plot**. To describe a box plot, we need to introduce the concept of the **hinges** of a sample. To accomplish this, it is first necessary to understand the notion of the depth of the medium.

**Definition 2.12**

The **depth** (*m*) of the median for a sample of size *n* is

1. $\dfrac{n}{2}$ if *n* is even

2. $\dfrac{n+1}{2}$ if *n* is odd

The upper and lower hinges can be thought of conceptually as the approximate 75th and 25th percentiles of the sample, that is, the points $\frac{3}{4}$ and $\frac{1}{4}$ along the way in the ordered sample. ∎

**Definition 2.13**

The **upper hinge** of a sample is

1. The $\dfrac{(m+1)}{2}$th largest point if *m* is odd

2. The average of the $\dfrac{m}{2}$th and $\left(\dfrac{m}{2}+1\right)$th largest points if *m* is even

where *m* = depth of the median. The **lower hinge** is defined similarly, starting from the smallest points in the sample. ∎

*Example 2.24*
*Solution*

Compute the upper and lower hinges for the birthweight data in Table 2.6.

Since $n = 100$, it follows that the depth of the median (*m*) = 50. Since *m* is even, the upper hinge is given by the average of the $\frac{50}{2}$th and $(\frac{50}{2} + 1)$th largest sample values or the average of the 25th and 26th largest points in the sample. Referring to the stem and leaf plot in Figure 2.10, if we count down from the top we note that $1 + 1 + 1 + 3 + 6 + 6 + 7 = 25$ points are in the upper 12 row or above. Thus, the 25th largest point is the smallest number in the upper 12 row, which equals 125 oz. Also, the 26th largest point = largest number in the lower 12 row = 124 oz. Thus, the upper hinge = $(125 + 124)/2 = 124.5$ oz.

Similarly, the lower hinge = average of the 25th and 26th smallest points in the sample. Counting up from the bottom, we note that $1 + 1 + 1 + 2 + 1 + 9 + 5 = 20$ points are in the lower 9 row or below, and 26 points are in the upper 9 row or below. Thus, the 25th smallest point = 2nd largest value in the upper 9 row = 98; the 26th smallest point = the largest value in the upper 9 row = 99. Therefore, the lower hinge = $(98 + 99)/2 = 98.5$ oz. ∎

How can we use the hinges to judge the symmetry of a distribution?

1. If the distribution is symmetric, then the upper and lower hinges should be approximately equally spaced from the median.
2. If the upper hinge is further away from the median than the lower hinge is, then the distribution is positively skewed.
3. If the lower hinge is further away from the median than the upper hinge is, then the distribution is negatively skewed.

These relationships are illustrated graphically in a box plot. If we refer to Figure 2.10, we see that the top of the box corresponds to the upper hinge, whereas the bottom of the box corresponds to the lower hinge. A horizontal line is also drawn at the median value. Furthermore, in the SAS implementation of the box plot, the sample mean is indicated by a + sign.

**Example 2.25**

What can we learn about the symmetry properties of the distribution of birthweights from the box plot in Figure 2.10?

**Solution**

Referring to Figure 2.10, since the lower hinge is further away from the median than the upper hinge is, we see that the distribution is slightly negatively skewed. This pattern is true of many birthweight distributions. ∎

In addition to giving us an appreciation of the symmetry properties of a sample, a box plot can also be used to give us a feel for the spread of a sample and can help us to identify possible outlying values, that is, values that seem inconsistent with the rest of the points in the sample. In the context of box plots, outlying values are defined as follows:

**Definition 2.14**

An **outlying value** is a value $x$ such that either

1. $x >$ upper hinge $+ 1.5 \times$ (upper hinge $-$ lower hinge) or
2. $x <$ lower hinge $- 1.5 \times$ (upper hinge $-$ lower hinge)

**Definition 2.15**

An **extreme outlying value** is a value $x$ such that either

1. $x >$ upper hinge $+ 3.0 \times$ (upper hinge $-$ lower hinge) or
2. $x <$ lower hinge $- 3.0 \times$ (upper hinge $-$ lower hinge)

The box plot is then completed by:

1. Drawing a vertical bar from the upper hinge to the largest nonoutlying value in the sample
2. Drawing a vertical bar from the lower hinge to the smallest nonoutlying value in the sample
3. Individually identifying the outlying and extreme outlying values in the sample by 0's and *'s, respectively

**Example 2.26**

Using the box plot in Figure 2.10, comment on the spread of the sample in Table 2.6 and the presence of outlying values.

**Solution**

Since the upper and lower hinges are 124.5 and 98.5 oz, respectively, we note that an outlying value $x$ must satisfy the following relations:

$$x > 124.5 + 1.5 \times (124.5 - 98.5) = 124.5 + 39.0 = 163.5$$

or

$$x < 98.5 - 1.5 \times (124.5 - 98.5) = 98.5 - 39.0 = 59.5$$

Similarly, an extreme outlying value $x$ must satisfy the following relations:

$$x > 124.5 + 3.0 \times (124.5 - 98.5) = 124.5 + 78.0 = 202.5$$

or

$$x < 98.5 - 3.0 \times (124.5 - 98.5) = 98.5 - 78.0 = 20.5$$

Thus, the values 32 and 58 oz are outlying values, but not extreme outlying values. These values are identified by 0's on the box plot. A vertical bar extends from 64 oz (the smallest nonoutlying value) to the lower hinge and from 161 oz (the largest nonoutlying value = largest value in the sample) to the upper hinge. We probably would check for the accuracy of the two identified outlying values.  ∎

Note that the methods used to identify outlying values are controversial, and the method given in Definitions 2.14 and 2.15 is not widely accepted by all statisticians. Nevertheless, it is given here to facilitate the understanding of box plots.

Many more details on stem and leaf plots, box plots, and other exploratory data methods are given in Tukey [3].

# ■ 2.9 SUMMARY

In this chapter we have learned several **numerical and graphical methods for describing data** for the purpose of:

*1.* Quickly summarizing a dataset for ourselves

*2.* Presenting results to others

In general, we can describe a dataset numerically in terms of a **measure of location** and a **measure of spread**. Several alternatives were introduced for each of these measures, including the **arithmetic mean, median, mode,** and **geometric mean** as possible choices for measures of location, and the **standard deviation** and **range** as possible choices for measures of spread. Criteria were discussed for choosing the appropriate measures in particular circumstances. We have also introduced several graphical techniques for summarizing data, including traditional methods, such as the **bar graph** and **histogram**, and some more modern methods characteristic of *exploratory data analysis*, or EDA, such as the **stem and leaf plot** and **box plot**.

How do the descriptive methods in this chapter fit in with the methods of statistical inference discussed later in this book? Specifically, if we find some interesting trends using descriptive methods, then we need some method for telling us how "significant" these trends are. For this purpose we will introduce several commonly used **probability models** in Chapters 3 through 5 and then explore approaches for testing the validity of these models using the methods of **statistical inference** in Chapters 6 through 12.

# Problems

## Pathology

The data in Table 2.10 are measurements from a group of 10 normal males and 11 males with left heart disease taken at autopsy at a particular hospital. Measurements were made on several variables at that time, and the table presents the measurements on total heart weight (THW) and total body weight (BW). Assume that the diagnosis of left heart disease is made independently of these variables.

**2.1** Compute the mean and median for each variable in each disease group.

**2.2** Compute the variance, standard deviation, range, and coefficient of variation for each variable in each disease group.

**2.3** Group the data in some appropriate way and compute the grouped mean, grouped variance, and grouped standard deviation for each variable in each disease group.

**2.4** Plot a histogram of each variable in each disease group with the groupings created in Problem 2.3.

**2.5** Construct a stem and leaf plot for each variable in each disease group.

**2.6** Can you qualitatively compare THW in the normal and abnormal groups from your answers to Problems 2.1 through 2.5? What about BW? (We will be covering this topic formally in our later work on *t* tests.)

**2.7** Is there any qualitative evidence of a relation between THW and BW *within* each of the disease groups? (*Hint*: A plot of THW versus BW may help here. We will be covering this topic formally in our work on regression analysis.)

**2.8** What are the principal differences (if any) between the groups as surmised from your answers to Problems 2.1 through 2.7?

## Infectious Disease

The data in Table 2.11 are a sample from a larger dataset collected on persons discharged from a selected Pennsylvania hospital as part of a retrospective chart review of antibiotic usage in hospitals [4].

**Table 2.10** *Autopsy data*

| | Left heart disease males | | | Normal males | | |
|---|---|---|---|---|---|---|
| Observation number | THW (g) | BW (kg) | | Observation number | THW (g) | BW (kg) |
| 1 | 450 | 54.6 | | 1 | 245 | 40.8 |
| 2 | 760 | 73.5 | | 2 | 350 | 67.4 |
| 3 | 325 | 50.3 | | 3 | 340 | 53.3 |
| 4 | 495 | 44.6 | | 4 | 300 | 62.2 |
| 5 | 285 | 58.1 | | 5 | 310 | 65.5 |
| 6 | 450 | 61.3 | | 6 | 270 | 47.5 |
| 7 | 460 | 75.3 | | 7 | 300 | 51.2 |
| 8 | 375 | 41.1 | | 8 | 360 | 74.9 |
| 9 | 310 | 51.5 | | 9 | 405 | 59.0 |
| 10 | 615 | 41.7 | | 10 | 290 | 40.5 |
| 11 | 425 | 59.7 | | | | |

**2.9** Compute the mean and median for duration of hospitalization for the 25 patients.

**2.10** Compute the standard deviation and range for the duration of hospitalization for the 25 patients.

**2.11** It is of clinical interest to know if the duration of hospitalization is affected by whether or not a patient has received antibiotics. Can you answer this question using either numerical or graphical methods?

Suppose we change the origin for a dataset by adding a constant to each observation.

**2.12** What is the effect on the median?

**2.13** What is the effect on the mode?

**2.14** What is the effect on the geometric mean?

**2.15** What is the effect on the range?

Suppose we change the scale for a dataset by multiplying each observation by a positive constant.

**2.16** What is the effect on the median?

**2.17** What is the effect on the mode?

**2.18** What is the effect on the geometric mean?

**2.19** What is the effect on the range?

### Renal Disease

For a study on kidney disease, the following measurements were made on a sample of women working in several factories in Switzerland. They represent concentrations of bacteria in a standard-size urine specimen. High concentrations of these bacteria may indicate possible kidney failure. The data are presented in Table 2.12.

***Table 2.11*** *Hospital stay data*

| ID no. | Duration of hospital stay | Age | Sex (1 = M, 2 = F) | First temp. following admission | First WBC ($\times 10^3$) following admission | Received antibiotic (1 = yes, 2 = no) | Received bacterial culture (1 = yes, 2 = no) | Service (1 = med., 2 = surg.) |
|---|---|---|---|---|---|---|---|---|
| 1 | 5 | 30 | 2 | 99.0 | 8 | 2 | 2 | 1 |
| 2 | 10 | 73 | 2 | 98.0 | 5 | 2 | 1 | 1 |
| 3 | 6 | 40 | 2 | 99.0 | 12 | 2 | 2 | 2 |
| 4 | 11 | 47 | 2 | 98.2 | 4 | 2 | 2 | 2 |
| 5 | 5 | 25 | 2 | 98.5 | 11 | 2 | 2 | 2 |
| 6 | 14 | 82 | 1 | 96.8 | 6 | 1 | 2 | 2 |
| 7 | 30 | 60 | 1 | 99.5 | 8 | 1 | 1 | 1 |
| 8 | 11 | 56 | 2 | 98.6 | 7 | 2 | 2 | 1 |
| 9 | 17 | 43 | 2 | 98.0 | 7 | 2 | 2 | 1 |
| 10 | 3 | 50 | 1 | 98.0 | 12 | 2 | 1 | 2 |
| 11 | 9 | 59 | 2 | 97.6 | 7 | 2 | 1 | 1 |
| 12 | 3 | 4 | 1 | 97.8 | 3 | 2 | 2 | 2 |
| 13 | 8 | 22 | 2 | 99.5 | 11 | 1 | 2 | 2 |
| 14 | 8 | 33 | 2 | 98.4 | 14 | 1 | 1 | 2 |
| 15 | 5 | 20 | 2 | 98.4 | 11 | 2 | 1 | 2 |
| 16 | 5 | 32 | 1 | 99.0 | 9 | 2 | 2 | 2 |
| 17 | 7 | 36 | 1 | 99.2 | 6 | 1 | 2 | 2 |
| 18 | 4 | 69 | 1 | 98.0 | 6 | 2 | 2 | 2 |
| 19 | 3 | 47 | 1 | 97.0 | 5 | 1 | 2 | 1 |
| 20 | 7 | 22 | 1 | 98.2 | 6 | 2 | 2 | 2 |
| 21 | 9 | 11 | 1 | 98.2 | 10 | 2 | 2 | 2 |
| 22 | 11 | 19 | 1 | 98.6 | 14 | 1 | 2 | 2 |
| 23 | 11 | 67 | 2 | 97.6 | 4 | 2 | 2 | 1 |
| 24 | 9 | 43 | 2 | 98.6 | 5 | 2 | 2 | 2 |
| 25 | 4 | 41 | 2 | 98.0 | 5 | 2 | 2 | 1 |

**Table 2.12** *Concentration of bacteria in the urine in a sample of female factory workers in Switzerland*

| Concentration | Frequency |
|---|---|
| $10^0$ | 521 |
| $10^1$ | 230 |
| $10^2$ | 115 |
| $10^3$ | 74 |
| $10^4$ | 69 |
| $10^5$ | 62 |
| $10^6$ | 43 |
| $10^7$ | 30 |
| $10^8$ | 21 |
| $10^9$ | 10 |
| $10^{10}$ | 2 |

**2.20** Compute the arithmetic mean for this sample.

**2.21** Compute the geometric mean for this sample.

**2.22** Which do you think is a more appropriate measure of location?

## Ophthalmology

Table 2.13 comes from a paper giving the distribution of astigmatism in 1033 young men, aged 18–22, who were accepted for military service in Great Britain [5]. Let us assume that the astigmatism is rounded to the nearest 10th of a diopter.

**Table 2.13** *Distribution of astigmatism in 1033 young men aged 18–22*

| Degree of astigmatism (diopters) | Frequency |
|---|---|
| 0.0 or less than 0.2 | 458 |
| 0.2–0.3 | 268 |
| 0.4–0.5 | 151 |
| 0.6–1.0 | 79 |
| 1.1–2.0 | 44 |
| 2.1–3.0 | 19 |
| 3.1–4.0 | 9 |
| 4.1–5.0 | 3 |
| 5.1–6.0 | 2 |
| | 1033 |

(Reprinted with permission of the Editor, the authors and the Journal from the *British Medical Journal*, May 7, 1394–1398, 1960.)

**2.23** Compute the grouped mean.

**2.24** Compute the grouped standard deviation.

**2.25** Plot a histogram to properly illustrate these data.

## Cardiovascular Disease

The mortality rates from heart disease (per 100,000 population) for each of the 50 states and the District of Columbia in 1973 are given in descending order in Table 2.14 [6].

Suppose we consider this data set as a sample of size 51 $(x_1, x_2, \ldots, x_{51})$. If

$$\sum_{i=1}^{51} x_i = 17{,}409 \qquad \left(\sum_{i=1}^{51} x_i\right)^2 = 303{,}073{,}281$$

$$\sum_{i=1}^{51} x_i^2 = 6{,}191{,}677$$

then:

**2.26** Compute the arithmetic mean of this sample.

**2.27** Compute the median of this sample.

**2.28** Compute the standard deviation of this sample.

**2.29** The national mortality rate for heart disease in 1973 was 360.8 per 100,000. Why does this figure *not* correspond to your answer of Problem 2.26?

**2.30** Does the differential in raw rates between Florida (417.4) and Georgia (311.8) actually imply that the risk of dying from heart disease is greater in Florida than in Georgia? Why or why not?

## Cardiovascular Disease

The data in Table 2.15 are a sample of cholesterol levels taken from 24 hospital employees who were on a standard American diet and who agreed to adopt a vegetarian diet for a 1-month period. Serum cholesterol measurements were made before adopting the diet and 1 month after.

**2.31** Compute the mean change in cholesterol.

**2.32** Compute the standard deviation of the change in cholesterol levels.

**2.33** Construct a stem and leaf plot of the cholesterol changes.

**2.34** Compute the median change in cholesterol.

**2.35** Construct a box plot of the cholesterol changes to the right of the stem and leaf plot.

**2.36** Comment on the symmetry of the distribution of change scores based on your answers to Problems 2.31 through 2.35.

Some authors contend that cholesterol measurements are better expressed in the log scale, since they are skewed in the original scale.

**2.37** Compute the arithmetic mean and geometric mean of the "before" cholesterol measurements.

**2.38** Draw stem and leaf and box plots of the "before" cholesterol measurements in the raw and log scales.

**2.39** Based on your answers to Problems 2.37 and 2.38, do you feel this distribution is more symmetric in the raw or log scale?

### Hypertension

An experiment was performed to look at the effect of position on level of blood pressure [7]. In the experiment 32 subjects had their blood pressures measured while lying down with their arms at their sides and again standing with their arms supported at heart level. The data are given in Table 2.16.

**2.40** Compute the arithmetic mean and median for the difference in systolic and diastolic blood pressure, respectively, between the positions (recumbent and standing).

**2.41** Construct stem and leaf and box plots for each type of blood pressure in each position.

**2.42** Based on your answers to Problems 2.40 and 2.41, comment on the effect of position on the levels of systolic and diastolic blood pressure.

### Nutrition

Table 2.17 shows the distribution of dietary vitamin A intake as reported by 14 students who filled out a dietary questionnaire in class. The total intake is a combination of intake from individual food items and from vitamin pills. The units are in IU/100 (International Units/100).

**2.43** Compute the mean and median from these data.

**2.44** Compute the standard deviation and coefficient of variation from these data.

**Table 2.14** *Mortality rates from heart disease (per 100,000 population) for the 50 states and the District of Columbia in 1973*

| | | | | | |
|---|---|---|---|---|---|
| 1 | West Virginia | 445.4 | 27 | Louisiana | 349.4 |
| 2 | Pennsylvania | 442.7 | 28 | Connecticut | 340.3 |
| 3 | Maine | 427.3 | 29 | Oregon | 338.7 |
| 4 | Missouri | 422.9 | 30 | Washington | 334.2 |
| 5 | Illinois | 420.8 | 31 | Minnesota | 332.7 |
| 6 | Florida | 417.4 | 32 | Michigan | 330.2 |
| 7 | Rhode Island | 414.4 | 33 | Alabama | 329.1 |
| 8 | Kentucky | 407.6 | 34 | North Carolina | 328.4 |
| 9 | New York | 406.7 | 35 | DC | 327.1 |
| 10 | Iowa | 396.9 | 36 | South Carolina | 322.4 |
| 11 | Arkansas | 396.8 | 37 | Montana | 319.1 |
| 12 | New Jersey | 395.2 | 38 | Maryland | 315.9 |
| 13 | Massachusetts | 394.0 | 39 | Georgia | 311.8 |
| 14 | Kansas | 391.7 | 40 | Virginia | 311.2 |
| 15 | Oklahoma | 391.0 | 41 | California | 310.6 |
| 16 | Ohio | 377.7 | 42 | Wyoming | 306.8 |
| 17 | South Dakota | 376.2 | 43 | Texas | 300.6 |
| 18 | Wisconsin | 369.8 | 44 | Idaho | 297.4 |
| 19 | Vermont | 369.2 | 45 | Colorado | 274.6 |
| 20 | Nebraska | 368.9 | 46 | Arizona | 265.4 |
| 21 | Tennessee | 361.4 | 47 | Nevada | 236.9 |
| 22 | New Hampshire | 358.2 | 48 | Utah | 214.2 |
| 23 | Indiana | 356.4 | 49 | New Mexico | 194.0 |
| 24 | North Dakota | 353.3 | 50 | Hawaii | 169.0 |
| 25 | Delaware | 351.6 | 51 | Alaska | 83.9 |
| 26 | Mississippi | 351.6 | | | |

**Table 2.15** *Serum cholesterol levels before and after adopting a vegetarian diet*

| Subject | Before | After | Before–after |
|---------|--------|-------|--------------|
| 1 | 195 | 146 | 49 |
| 2 | 145 | 155 | −10 |
| 3 | 205 | 178 | 27 |
| 4 | 159 | 146 | 13 |
| 5 | 244 | 208 | 36 |
| 6 | 166 | 147 | 19 |
| 7 | 250 | 202 | 48 |
| 8 | 236 | 215 | 21 |
| 9 | 192 | 184 | 8 |
| 10 | 224 | 208 | 16 |
| 11 | 238 | 206 | 32 |
| 12 | 197 | 169 | 28 |
| 13 | 169 | 182 | −13 |
| 14 | 158 | 127 | 31 |
| 15 | 151 | 149 | 2 |
| 16 | 197 | 178 | 19 |
| 17 | 180 | 161 | 19 |
| 18 | 222 | 187 | 35 |
| 19 | 168 | 176 | −8 |
| 20 | 168 | 145 | 23 |
| 21 | 167 | 154 | 13 |
| 22 | 161 | 153 | 8 |
| 23 | 178 | 137 | 41 |
| 24 | 137 | 125 | 12 |

**2.45** Suppose we express the data in IU rather than IU/100. What are the mean, standard deviation, and coefficient of variation in the new units?

**Table 2.17** *Distribution of dietary vitamin A intake as reported by 14 students*

| Student number | Intake (IU/100) | Student number | Intake (IU/100) |
|----------------|-----------------|----------------|-----------------|
| 1 | 31.1 | 8 | 48.1 |
| 2 | 21.5 | 9 | 24.4 |
| 3 | 74.7 | 10 | 13.4 |
| 4 | 95.5 | 11 | 37.1 |
| 5 | 19.4 | 12 | 21.3 |
| 6 | 64.8 | 13 | 78.5 |
| 7 | 108.7 | 14 | 17.7 |

**Table 2.16** *Effect of position on blood pressure*

| | Blood pressure (mm Hg) | | | |
|---------|-----------------------------|------|------------------------------------|------|
| Subject | Recumbent, arm at side | | Standing, arm at heart level | |
| B. R. A. | 99* | 71† | 105* | 79† |
| J. A. B. | 126 | 74 | 124 | 76 |
| F.L.B. | 108 | 72 | 102 | 68 |
| V. P. B. | 122 | 68 | 114 | 72 |
| M. F. B. | 104 | 64 | 96 | 62 |
| E. H. B. | 108 | 60 | 96 | 56 |
| G. C. | 116 | 70 | 106 | 70 |
| M. M. C. | 106 | 74 | 106 | 76 |
| T. J. F. | 118 | 82 | 120 | 90 |
| R. R. F. | 92 | 58 | 88 | 60 |
| C. R. F. | 110 | 78 | 102 | 80 |
| E. W. G. | 138 | 80 | 124 | 76 |
| T. F. H. | 120 | 70 | 118 | 84 |
| E. J. H. | 142 | 88 | 136 | 90 |
| H. B. H. | 118 | 58 | 92 | 58 |
| R. T. K. | 134 | 76 | 126 | 68 |
| W. E. L. | 118 | 72 | 108 | 68 |
| R. L. L. | 126 | 78 | 114 | 76 |
| H. S. M. | 108 | 78 | 94 | 70 |
| V. J. M. | 136 | 86 | 144 | 88 |
| R. H. P. | 110 | 78 | 100 | 64 |
| R. C. R. | 120 | 74 | 106 | 70 |
| J. A. R. | 108 | 74 | 94 | 74 |
| A. K. R. | 132 | 92 | 128 | 88 |
| T. H. S. | 102 | 68 | 96 | 64 |
| O. E. S. | 118 | 70 | 102 | 68 |
| R. E. S. | 116 | 76 | 88 | 60 |
| E. C. T. | 118 | 80 | 100 | 84 |
| J. H. T. | 110 | 74 | 96 | 70 |
| F. P. V. | 122 | 72 | 118 | 78 |
| P. F. W. | 106 | 62 | 94 | 56 |
| W. J. W. | 146 | 90 | 138 | 94 |

*Systolic blood pressure
†Diastolic blood pressure
(Reprinted with permission of the *American Journal of Medicine*.)

**2.46** Construct a stem and leaf plot of the data on some convenient scale.

**2.47** Do you think the mean or median is a more appropriate measure of location for this dataset?

# *References*

[*1*]  White, J. R. and Froeb, H. E. (1980) "Small-Airways Dysfunction in Nonsmokers Chronic-
       ally Exposed to Tobacco Smoke," *New England Journal of Medicine* **302(33)**: 720–723.

[*2*]  Pedersen, A., Wiesner, P., Holmes, K., Johnson, C., and Turck, M. (1972) "Spectinomycin
       and Penicillin G in the Treatment of Gonorrhea," *JAMA* **220(2)**: 205–208.

[*3*]  Tukey, J. (1977) *Exploratory Data Analysis* (Reading, Mass: Addison-Wesley).

[*4*]  Townsend, T., Shapiro, M., Rosner, B., and Kass, E. H. (1979) "Use of Antimicrobial
       Drugs in General Hospitals I. Description of Population and Definition of Methods,"
       *Journal of Infectious Diseases* **139(6)**, 688–697.

[*5*]  Sorsby, A., Sheridan, M., Leary, G. A., and Benjamin, B. (1960) "Vision, Visual Acuity and
       Ocular Refraction of Young Men in a Sample of 1033 Subjects," *British Medical Journal*,
       1394–1398.

[*6*]  *Monthly Vital Statistics Report, Summary Report, Final Mortality Statistics* (1973)
       National Center of Health Statistics, **23(11)** Supplement (2), February 10, 1975.

[*7*]  Kossmann, C. E. (1946) "Relative Importance of Certain Variables in the Clinical Deter-
       mination of Blood Pressure," *American Journal of Medicine* **1**: 464–467.

# 3 Probability

## ■ 3.1 INTRODUCTION

In Chapter 2 we outlined various techniques for concisely describing data. We will usually want to do more with our data than describe it. In particular, we might want to test certain specific inferences about the behavior of the data.

*Example 3.1*

*Cancer* One theory concerning the etiology of breast cancer states that women in a given age group who give birth to their first child relatively late in life (after 30) are at greater risk for eventually developing breast cancer over some time period *t* than are women who give birth to their first child early in life (before 20). Because women in the upper social classes tend to have children later in life, this theory has been used to explain why these women have a higher risk of developing breast cancer than women in the lower social classes. If we wanted to test this hypothesis, we might identify 2000 women from a particular census tract who are currently ages 45–54 and have never had breast cancer, of whom 1000 had their first child before the age of 20 (call this group A) and 1000 after the age of 30 (call this group B). We might then follow these 2000 women for 5 years and ask if they had a new case of breast cancer during this period. Suppose that we have 4 new cases of breast cancer out of 1000 in group A and 5 new cases out of 1000 in group B. ■

Is this sufficient evidence to confirm a difference in risk between the two groups? Most people would feel uneasy about coming to this conclusion on the basis of such a limited amount of data.

Suppose we had a more ambitious plan and sampled 10,000 women from groups A and B, respectively, and found 40 new cases in group A and 50 new cases in group B and asked the same question. We might be more comfortable with the conclusion because of the larger sample size, but we would still admit that there was some possibility that this apparent difference in the rates could be due to chance.

The problem is that we need a conceptual framework to make these decisions but have not explicitly stated what that framework is. We will see that this framework is provided by the underlying concept of **probability**. In this chapter we will define probability and will introduce some rules for working with probabilities.

# ■ 3.2  DEFINITION OF PROBABILITY

*Example 3.2*

*Obstetrics* Suppose we are interested in the probability of a male live childbirth (or live-birth) among all livebirths in the United States. Conventional wisdom tells us that this probability should be close to 0.5. We can explore this subject by looking at some vital statistics data, as presented in Table 3.1 [1]. We find that the probability of a male livebirth based on 1965 data is 0.51247, based on 1965–1969 data 0.51248, and based on 1965–1974 data 0.51268. In principle, we could expand the sample size indefinitely and obtain an increasingly more precise estimate of this probability.  ■

This principle leads us to the following definition of probability.

**Definition 3.1**

We define the **sample space** as the set of all possible outcomes. We will refer to probabilities of events, where an **event** is any set of outcomes that are of interest to us. The **probability** of an event is the relative frequency of this set of outcomes over an indefinitely large (or infinite) number of trials.  ■

*Example 3.3*

*Pulmonary Disease* The tuberculin skin test is a routine screening test for the detection of tuberculosis. Let us categorize the results of this test as either positive, negative, or uncertain. If we state that the probability of a positive test is 0.1, we mean that if a large number of such tests were performed, about 10% of them would be positive. The actual percentage of positive tests will be increasingly close to 0.1, the larger the number of tests we perform.  ■

*Example 3.4*

*Cancer* The probability of developing a new case of breast cancer in 1 year in 40-year-old women who have never had breast cancer is 0.001. This probability means that over a large sample of 40-year-old women who have never had breast cancer, approximately 1 in 1000 will develop the disease over 1 year, with this percentage becoming increasingly close to 0.001 as the number of women sampled increases.  ■

In real life, of course, we cannot perform experiments an infinite number of times and must content ourselves with, at best, estimating probabilities from large samples, as was done in Examples 3.2, 3.3, and 3.4. In many situations we will not even be able to use a large sample, but instead will make a reasonable guess at the probability based on previous experience or on other work in the field. We will then look at our data to see how closely it conforms to our guess.

*Table 3.1*

*Probability of a male livebirth during the period 1965–1974*

| Time period | Number of male livebirths (a) | Total number of livebirths (b) | Probability of a male livebirth (a/b) |
|---|---|---|---|
| 1965 | 1,927,054 | 3,760,358 | 0.51247 |
| 1965–1969 | 9,219,202 | 17,989,361 | 0.51248 |
| 1965–1974 | 17,857,857 | 34,832,051 | 0.51268 |

**Example 3.5**    *Cancer* The probability of developing a new case of stomach cancer over a 1-year period for 45–49-year-old women based on Connecticut Tumor Registry data from 1963–1965 is 14 per 100,000 [2]. Suppose we have studied cancer rates in a small group of Connecticut nurses over this period and wish to compare how close the rates from this limited sample are to the tumor registry figures. The figure 14 per 100,000 would be our best estimate of the probability prior to collecting our data, and we would then see how closely our new sample data conformed with this probability.    ∎

We can deduce from Definition 3.1 and from the preceding examples that probabilities have the following basic properties:

**3.1**
> *1*. The probability of any event $E$, denoted by $Pr(E)$, always satisfies $0 \leqslant Pr(E) \leqslant 1$. $\leqslant 1$.
>
> *2*. If outcomes $A$ and $B$ are two events that cannot both happen at the same time, then $Pr(A \text{ or } B \text{ occurs}) = Pr(A) + Pr(B)$.

**Example 3.6**    *Hypertension* Let $A$ be the event that a person has normotensive diastolic blood pressure (bp) readings (i.e., diastolic bp $<90$), and let $B$ be the event that a person has borderline diastolic bp readings (i.e., bp $\geqslant 90$ and $<95$). Suppose that $Pr(A) = 0.7$, $Pr(B) = 0.1$. Let $C$ be the event that a person has diastolic bp $<95$. Then,

$$Pr(C) = Pr(A) + Pr(B) = 0.8$$

because the events $A$ and $B$ cannot occur at the same time.    ∎

**Definition 3.2**

We define two events $A$ and $B$ as being **mutually exclusive** if they cannot both happen at the same time.    ∎

Thus, the events $A$ and $B$ in Example 3.6 are mutually exclusive.

**Example 3.7**    *Hypertension* Let $x$ be diastolic bp, $C$ be the event that $x \geqslant 90$, and $D$ be the event that $75 \leqslant x \leqslant 100$. The events $C$ and $D$ are *not* mutually exclusive, since they both occur when $90 \leqslant x \leqslant 100$.    ∎

# ■ *3.3 SOME USEFUL PROBABILISTIC NOTATION*

**Definition 3.3**

We will use the symbol { } as shorthand for the phrase "the event."    ∎

**Definition 3.4**

We define $A \cup B$ as the event that either $A$ or $B$ occurs or they both occur.    ∎

Figure 3.1 diagrammatically depicts $A \cup B$ both for the case where $A$ and $B$ are and are not mutually exclusive.

**Example 3.8**    *Hypertension* Let the events $A$ and $B$ be defined as in Example 3.6; that is, $A = \{x < 90\}$, $B = \{90 \leqslant x < 95\}$, where $x =$ diastolic bp. Then, $A \cup B = \{x < 95\}$.    ∎

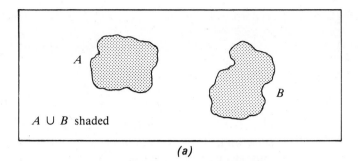

**(a)**

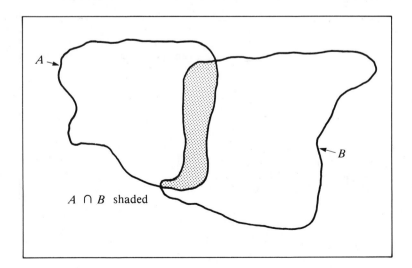

**(b)**

**Figure 3.1**
*Diagrammatic representation of A ∪ B: (a) A, B mutually exclusive; (b) A, B not mutually exclusive*

**Example 3.9**

**Hypertension** Let the events $C$ and $D$ be defined as in Example 3.7; that is,

$$C = \{x \geqslant 90\} \qquad D = \{75 \leqslant x \leqslant 100\}$$

Then,

$$\{C \cup D\} = \{x \geqslant 75\} \qquad\qquad ■$$

**Definition 3.5**

We define $\{A \cap B\}$ as the event that both $A$ and $B$ occur simultaneously. $\{A \cap B\}$ is depicted diagrammatically in Figure 3.2. ■

**Figure 3.2**
*Diagrammatic representation of A ∩ B*

*Example 3.10*    **Hypertension** Let the events $C$ and $D$ be defined as in Example 3.7; that is,

$$C = \{x \geqslant 90\} \qquad D = \{75 \leqslant x \leqslant 100\}$$

Then,

$$\{C \cap D\} = \{90 \leqslant x \leqslant 100\} \qquad\blacksquare$$

Notice that $\{A \cap B\}$ is not well defined for the events $A$ and $B$ in Example 3.6, since both $A$ and $B$ cannot occur simultaneously. This situation is true for any mutually exclusive events.

**Definition 3.6**

We define $\bar{A}$ as the event that $A$ does not occur. It is sometimes referred to as the **complement** of $A$. Notice that $Pr(\bar{A}) = 1 - Pr(A)$, since $\bar{A}$ occurs only when $A$ does not occur. The event $\bar{A}$ is depicted diagrammatically in Figure 3.3. $\qquad\blacksquare$

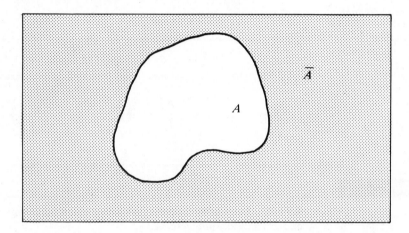

**Figure 3.3**
*Diagrammatic representation of $\bar{A}$*

*Example 3.11*    **Hypertension** Let the events $A$ and $C$ be defined as in Examples 3.6 and 3.7; that is,

$$A = \{x < 90\} \qquad C = \{x \geqslant 90\}$$

Then, $C = \bar{A}$, since $C$ can only occur when $A$ does not occur. Notice that

$$Pr(C) = Pr(\bar{A}) = 1 - 0.7 = 0.3$$

Thus, if 70% of people have diastolic bp $< 90$, then 30% of people must have diastolic bp $\geqslant 90$.

$\blacksquare$

# 3.4 INDEPENDENT AND DEPENDENT EVENTS

In the preceding section we spoke of events in general. We now will refer to certain specific types of events.

*Example 3.12*   **Hypertension, Genetics**  Suppose we are conducting a hypertension screening program in the home. Let us then consider all possible pairs of diastolic bp measurements of the mother and father within a given family, where we assume that the mother and father are not genetically related. This sample space consists of all pairs of numbers of the form $(X, Y)$, where $X > 0, Y > 0$. We might be interested in certain specific events in this context. In particular, we might be interested in whether the mother or father is hypertensive, which we describe respectively by the events $A = \{$mother's bp $\geqslant 95\}$, $B = \{$father's bp $\geqslant 95\}$. These events are depicted graphically in Figure 3.4.

Suppose we know that $Pr(A) = 0.1$, $Pr(B) = 0.2$. What can we say about $Pr(A \cap B) = Pr($mother's bp $\geqslant 95$ and father's bp $\geqslant 95) = Pr($both mother and father are hypertensive)? We can say nothing unless we are willing to make certain assumptions.  ■

**Definition 3.7**

Two events $A$ and $B$ are referred to as **independent events** if

$$Pr(A \cap B) = Pr(A) \cdot Pr(B)$$  ■

*Example 3.13*   **Hypertension, Genetics**  Compute the probability that both the mother and father are hypertensive if the events in Example 3.12 are independent.

*Solution*   If $A$ and $B$ are independent events, then

$$Pr(A \cap B) = Pr(A) \cdot Pr(B) = (0.1)(0.2) = 0.02$$  ■

One way to interpret this example is to assume that the hypertensive status of the mother does not depend at all on the hypertensive status of the father. Thus,

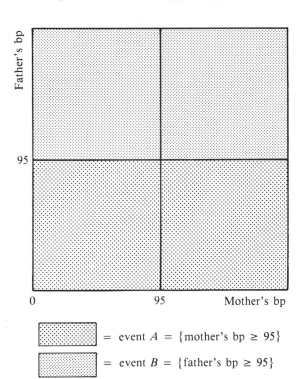

*Figure 3.4*
*Possible blood pressure measurements of the mother and father within a given family*

□ = event $A = \{$mother's bp $\geq 95\}$

□ = event $B = \{$father's bp $\geq 95\}$

if these events are independent, then in 10% of all households where the father is hypertensive the mother is also hypertensive, and in 10% of all households where the father is *not* hypertensive the mother is hypertensive. We would expect these two events to be independent if the primary determinants of elevated blood pressure were genetic. However, if the primary determinants of elevated blood pressure were, to some extent, environmental, then we would expect that the mother would be more likely to have elevated blood pressure ($A$ true) if the father had elevated blood pressure ($B$ true) than if the father did not have elevated blood pressure ($B$ not true). In this latter case the events would not be independent. We will discuss the implications of this situation further on in this chapter.

If two events are not independent, then they are said to be dependent.

**Definition 3.8**

Two events $A$, $B$ are **dependent** if

$$Pr(A \cap B) \neq Pr(A) \cdot Pr(B)$$    ∎

Example 3.14 is a classic example of dependent events.

**Example 3.14**    ***Hypertension, Genetics***  Let us consider all possible diastolic blood pressure measurements from a mother and her first-born child. Let

$$A = \{\text{mother's bp} \geqslant 95\} \qquad B = \{\text{first-born child's bp} \geqslant 80\}$$

Suppose

$$Pr(A \cap B) = 0.05 \qquad Pr(A) = 0.1 \qquad Pr(B) = 0.2$$

Then

$$Pr(A \cap B) = 0.05 > Pr(A) \cdot Pr(B) = 0.02$$

and the events $A$, $B$ would be dependent.    ∎

We would expect this outcome, since the mother and first-born child both share the same environment and are genetically related. In other words, the first-born child is more likely to have elevated blood pressure in households where the mother is hypertensive than in households where the mother is not hypertensive.

**Example 3.15**    ***Venereal Disease***  Suppose two doctors $A$ and $B$ diagnose all patients coming into a VD clinic for syphilis. Let the events $A^+ = \{\text{doctor } A \text{ makes a positive diagnosis}\}$, $B^+ = \{\text{doctor } B \text{ makes a positive diagnosis}\}$. Suppose that doctor $A$ diagnoses 10% of all patients as positive, doctor $B$ diagnoses 17% of all patients as positive, and both doctors diagnose 8% of all patients as positive. Are the events $A^+$, $B^+$ independent?

**Solution**    We are given that

$$Pr(A^+) = 0.1 \qquad Pr(B^+) = 0.17 \qquad Pr(A^+ \cap B^+) = 0.08$$

Thus,

$$Pr(A^+ \cap B^+) = 0.08 > Pr(A^+) \cdot Pr(B^+) = 0.1(0.17) = 0.017$$

and the events are **dependent**. We would expect this result, since there should be a similarity between how two doctors diagnose patients for syphilis.  ∎

# ■ 3.5 THE ADDITION LAW OF PROBABILITY

We have seen from the definition of probability that if $A$ and $B$ are mutually exclusive events, then $Pr(A \cup B) = Pr(A) + Pr(B)$. We shall now develop a more general formula for $Pr(A \cup B)$ when the events $A$ and $B$ are not necessarily mutually exclusive.

**3.2**    **Addition Law of Probability**

If $A$ and $B$ are any events, then

$$Pr(A \cup B) = Pr(A) + Pr(B) - Pr(A \cap B)$$

This situation is depicted diagrammatically in Figure 3.5. Thus, to compute $Pr(A \cup B)$, we add the probabilities of $A$ and $B$ separately and then subtract the overlap, which is $Pr(A \cap B)$.

*Example 3.16*

*Venereal Disease* Let us consider the data given in Example 3.15. Suppose we refer a patient for further lab tests if either doctor $A$ or $B$ makes a positive diagnosis. What is the probability that a patient will be referred for further lab tests?

*Solution*

We can represent the event that either doctor makes a positive diagnosis by $\{A^+ \cup B^+\}$. We know that

$$Pr(A^+) = 0.1 \qquad Pr(B^+) = 0.17 \qquad Pr(A^+ \cap B^+) = 0.08$$

Thus, from the addition law of probability, we have

$$Pr(A^+ \cup B^+) = Pr(A^+) + Pr(B^+) - Pr(A^+ \cap B^+) = 0.1 + 0.17 - 0.08 = 0.19$$

Thus, 19% of all patients will be referred for further lab tests.  ∎

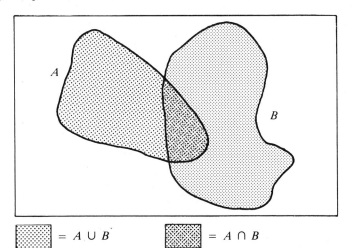

*Figure 3.5*
*Diagrammatic representation of the addition law of probability*

It is of interest to note special cases of the addition law. First, if the events $A$ and $B$ are *mutually exclusive*, then $Pr(A \cap B) = 0$ and the addition law reduces to $Pr(A \cup B) = Pr(A) + Pr(B)$. This property is one of those given in **(3.1)** for probabilities over any two mutually exclusive events. Second, if the events $A$ and $B$ are *independent*, then by definition $Pr(A \cap B) = Pr(A) \cdot Pr(B)$ and $Pr(A \cup B)$ can be rewritten as $Pr(A) + Pr(B) - Pr(A) \cdot Pr(B)$. If we collect terms, then this leads us to the following important special case of the addition law.

**3.3**    ### Addition Law of Probability for Independent Events

If two events $A$ and $B$ are independent, then

$$Pr(A \cup B) = Pr(A) + Pr(B) \cdot [1 - Pr(A)]$$

We can interpret this special case of the addition law as follows: The event $A \cup B$ can be separated into two mutually exclusive events: $\{A \text{ occurs}\}$ and $\{B \text{ occurs and } A \text{ does not occur}\}$. Furthermore, because of the independence of $A$ and $B$, we can write the probability of the latter event as $Pr(B) \cdot [1 - Pr(A)]$. This probability is depicted diagrammatically in Figure 3.6.

*Example 3.17*    *Hypertension*  Let us refer to Example 3.12, where

$$A = \{\text{mother's bp} \geqslant 95\} \quad \text{and} \quad B = \{\text{father's bp} \geqslant 95\}$$

$Pr(A) = 0.1$, $Pr(B) = 0.2$, and we assume that $A$ and $B$ are independent events. Suppose we define a "hypertensive household" as one where either the mother or the father is hypertensive, and we define hypertension for the mother and father respectively in terms of the events $A$ and $B$. What is the probability of a hypertensive household?

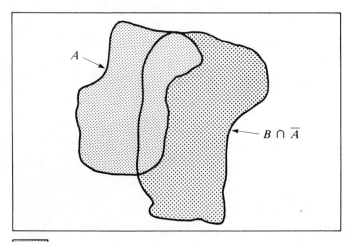

*Figure 3.6*

*Diagrammatic representation of the addition law of probability for independent events*

☐ = $A$

☐ = $\{B \text{ occurs and } A \text{ does not occur}\} = B \cap \overline{A}$

**Solution**               $Pr$(hypertensive household) is

$$Pr(A \cup B) = Pr(A) + Pr(B) \cdot [1 - Pr(A)] = 0.1 + 0.2(0.9) = 0.28$$

Thus, 28% of all households will be hypertensive.                                      ■

# ■ *3.6 CONDITIONAL PROBABILITY*

We introduced the concepts of independent and dependent events in Section 3.4. We now wish to express the concept of dependence in more quantitative terms. In particular, if two events $A$ and $B$ are not independent, then we want some idea as to how dependent the two events are relative to each other. Consider the following example.

*Example 3.18*    **Pulmonary Disease** In many places of employment, prospective employees are customarily given a screening test for tuberculosis (TB) before starting employment. The definitive test for the detection of TB is the chest X-ray. Unfortunately, the chest X-ray is somewhat expensive to administer and exposure to the radiation from the X-ray is an undesirable side effect of the test. A common procedure to avoid giving everyone a chest X-ray is to perform a less expensive test, the skin test, with the hope that only persons who are positive on the skin test can possibly have TB. The ideal situation would be if the probability of having TB among all persons with positive skin tests (SKT) were 1 and the probability of having TB among all persons with negative skin tests were 0. The two events {SKT$^+$}, {TB} would then be completely dependent; that is, the result of the screening test would automatically determine the disease state. The opposite extreme is achieved when the events {SKT$^+$}, {TB} are completely independent. In this case the probability of TB is the same whether or not the skin test is positive, and the skin test would not be useful in screening for TB and should not be given.    ■

We can quantify these concepts in the following way. Let $A = \{\text{SKT}^+\}$, $B = \{\text{TB}\}$ and suppose that we are interested in the probability of TB ($B$) given that the skin test is positive ($A$). We can write this probability as $Pr(A \cap B)/Pr(A)$.

**Definition 3.9**

We define the quantity $Pr(A \cap B)/Pr(A)$ as the **conditional probability of B given A**, which we write as $Pr(B|A)$.    ■

However, from Section 3.4 we know that, by definition, if two events are independent, then $Pr(A \cap B) = Pr(A) \cdot Pr(B)$. If we divide both sides by $Pr(A)$, we have $Pr(B) = Pr(A \cap B)/Pr(A) = Pr(B|A)$. Similarly, we can show that if $A$ and $B$ are independent events, then $Pr(B|\bar{A}) = Pr(B|A) = Pr(B)$. This relationship leads us to the following alternative interpretation of independence in terms of conditional probabilities:

**3.4**    *1.* If $A$ and $B$ are independent events, then $Pr(B|A) = Pr(B)$.
*2.* If two events $A$, $B$ are dependent, then $Pr(B|A) \neq Pr(B) \neq Pr(B|\bar{A})$ and $Pr(A \cap B) \neq Pr(A) \cdot Pr(B)$.

---

**Definition 3.10**

We define the **relative risk (RR)** of $B$ given $A$ as

$$Pr(B|A)/Pr(B|\bar{A}) \qquad \blacksquare$$

Notice that if two events $A$, $B$ are independent, then the relative risk will be 1. If two events $A$, $B$ are dependent, then the relative risk will be different from 1. Heuristically, we can think of the dependence between events as increasing the further the relative risk is from 1.

**Example 3.19**

*Pulmonary Disease* Suppose that 1 person in 10,000 from those with negative skin tests have TB, or $Pr(B|\bar{A}) = 0.0001$, whereas 1 person in 100 from those with positive skin tests have TB, or $Pr(B|A) = 0.01$. The two events would be highly dependent here, since

$$RR = Pr(B|A)/Pr(B|\bar{A}) = 0.01/0.0001 = 100$$

In words, persons with positive skin tests are 100 times as likely to have TB than persons with negative skin tests. This is the rationale for using the skin test as a screening test for TB. If the events $A$ and $B$ were independent, then the relative risk would be 1; that is, persons with positive or negative skin tests would be equally likely to have TB and the test would not be useful as a screening test. $\qquad \blacksquare$

**Example 3.20**

*Venereal Disease* Using the data in Example 3.15, find the conditional probability that doctor $B$ makes a positive diagnosis of syphilis given that doctor $A$ makes a positive diagnosis. What is the conditional probability that doctor $B$ makes a positive diagnosis of syphilis given that doctor $A$ makes a negative diagnosis? What is the relative risk of $\{B^+\}$ given $\{A^+\}$?

**Solution**

We have that

$$Pr(B^+|A^+) = Pr(B^+ \cap A^+)/Pr(A^+) = 0.08/0.1 = 0.80$$

Thus, doctor $B$ will confirm doctor $A$'s positive diagnosis 80% of the time. Similarly,

$$Pr(B^+|A^-) = Pr(B^+ \cap A^-)/Pr(A^-) = Pr(B^+ \cap A^-)/0.9$$

We must compute $Pr(B^+ \cap A^-)$. We know that if doctor $B$ diagnoses a patient as positive, then doctor $A$ either does or does not diagnose the patient as positive. Thus,

$$Pr(B^+) = Pr(B^+ \cap A^+) + Pr(B^+ \cap A^-)$$

since the events $\{B^+ \cap A^+\}$ and $\{B^+ \cap A^-\}$ are mutually exclusive. If we subtract $Pr(B^+ \cap A^+)$ from both sides of the equation, then

$$Pr(B^+ \cap A^-) = Pr(B^+) - Pr(B^+ \cap A^+) = 0.17 - 0.08 = 0.09$$

Therefore,

$$Pr(B^+|A^-) = 0.09/0.9 = 0.1$$

Thus, when doctor $A$ diagnoses a patient as negative, doctor $B$ will contradict the diagnosis 10% of the time. The relative risk of the event $\{B^+\}$ given $\{A^+\}$ is

$$Pr(B^+|A^+)/Pr(B^+|A^-) = 0.8/0.1 = 8$$

This indicates that doctor $B$ is 8 times as likely to diagnose a patient as positive when doctor $A$ diagnoses the patient as positive than when doctor $A$ diagnoses the patient as negative. These results quantify the dependence between the two doctors' diagnoses. ∎

We can relate the conditional ($Pr(B|A)$, $Pr(B|\bar{A})$) and unconditional ($Pr(B)$) probabilities mentioned previously in the following way:

**3.5**   For any events $A$ and $B$,

$$Pr(B) = Pr(B|A) \cdot Pr(A) + Pr(B|\bar{A}) \cdot Pr(\bar{A})$$

This formula tells us that the unconditional probability of $B$ is the sum of the conditional probability of $B$ given $A$ *times* the unconditional probability of $A$ *plus* the conditional probability of $B$ given $A$ *not* occurring *times* the unconditional probability of $A$ *not* occurring.

*Example 3.21*   **Pulmonary Disease**  Let $A$ and $B$ be defined as in Example 3.19 and suppose that 1% of the general population will have a positive skin test. What is the probability of tuberculosis in the general population?

*Solution*

$$Pr(B) = Pr(TB) = Pr(TB|SKT^+) \cdot Pr(SKT^+) + Pr(TB|SKT^-) \cdot Pr(SKT^-)$$

$$= (0.01)(0.01) + (10^{-4})(0.99)$$

$$= 0.000199 \simeq 0.0002$$

$$= 2 \times 10^{-4}$$

Thus, the unconditional probability of TB in the general population ($2 \times 10^{-4}$) is a weighted average of the conditional probability of TB given a positive skin test ($0.01 = 100 \times 10^{-4}$) and the conditional probability of TB given a negative skin test ($10^{-4}$). ∎

In **(3.5)** we expressed the probability of the event $B$ in terms of the two events $A$ and $\bar{A}$. In many instances the probability of an event $B$ will need to be expressed in terms of more than two events, which we denote by $A_1, A_2, \ldots, A_k$. We will assume that these events are mutually exclusive and that at least one of the events must occur; that is, their union encompasses the entire sample space. In this case we can generalize **(3.5)** in the total probability rule:

**3.6**   **Total Probability Rule**

Let $A_1, \ldots, A_k$ be mutually exclusive events such that at least one of the events must occur. The unconditional probability of $B$ ($Pr(B)$) can then be written as a weighted average of the conditional probabilities of $B$ given $A_i$ ($Pr(B|A_i)$) as follows:

$$Pr(B) = \sum_{i=1}^{k} Pr(B|A_i) \times Pr(A_i)$$

An application of the total probability rule is given in the following example:

*Example 3.22*   **Ophthalmology**  We are planning a 5-year study of cataract in a population of 5000 people 60 years of age and older. We know from census data that 45% of this population are ages 60–64,

28% are ages 65–69, 20% are ages 70–74, and 7% are age 75 or older. We also know from the Framingham Eye Study that 2.4%, 4.6%, 8.8%, and 15.3% of the people in those respective age groups will develop cataract over the next 5 years [3]. What percent of our population will develop cataract over the next 5 years and how many cataracts does this percent represent?

**Solution**    Let $A_1 = \{$ages 60–64$\}$, $A_2 = \{$ages 65–69$\}$, $A_3 = \{$ages 70–74$\}$, $A_4 = \{$age 75+$\}$. These events are mutually exclusive, and one of these events must occur for each person in our population. Furthermore, from the conditions of the problem, we know that $Pr(A_1) = 0.45$, $Pr(A_2) = 0.28$, $Pr(A_3) = 0.20$, $Pr(A_4) = 0.07$, $Pr(B|A_1) = 0.024$, $Pr(B|A_2) = 0.046$, $Pr(B|A_3) = 0.088$, and $Pr(B|A_4) = 0.153$. Finally, using the total probability rule, we have

$$Pr(B) = Pr(B|A_1) \times Pr(A_1) + Pr(B|A_2) \times Pr(A_2) + Pr(B|A_3) \times Pr(A_3) + Pr(B|A_4) \times Pr(A_4)$$

$$= (0.024)(0.45) + (0.046)(0.28) + (0.088)(0.20) + (0.153)(0.07)$$

$$= 0.052$$

Thus, 5.2% of our population will develop cataract over the next 5 years, which represents a total of $5000 \times 0.052 = 260$ persons with cataract.    ∎

# ■ *3.7 BAYES' RULE*

The tuberculosis skin test example given in Example 3.18 illustrates the general concept of the predictive value of a screening test, which can be defined as follows:

**Definition 3.11**
___

The **predictive value positive** (PV$^+$) of a screening test is the probability that a person has disease given that the test is positive

$$Pr(\text{disease}|\text{test}^+)$$

The **predictive value negative** (PV$^-$) of a screening test is the probability that a person does *not* have disease given that the test is negative

$$Pr(\text{no disease}|\text{test}^-)$$    ∎

**Example 3.23**    **Pulmonary Disease** Find the predictive values positive and negative for the tuberculosis skin test given the data in Example 3.18.

**Solution**    We see that

$$PV^+ = Pr(B|A) = 0.01$$

whereas

$$PV^- = Pr(\bar{B}|\bar{A}) = 1 - Pr(B|\bar{A}) = 0.9999$$

Thus, if the skin test is negative, the person is virtually certain not to have disease (PV$^- \approx 1$); whereas if the skin test is positive, the person still has only a small chance of having disease (PV$^+ = 0.01$).    ∎

We can also regard a symptom, or set of symptoms, as a screening test for disease. The higher the predictive value of the screening test or symptoms, the more valuable the test. Ideally, we would like to find a set of symptoms such that both PV$^+$ and PV$^-$ are 1. Then, we would be able to accurately diagnose disease for each patient.

Clinicians often cannot directly measure the predictive value of a set of symptoms. However, they can measure how often specific symptoms occur in diseased and normal persons. These measures are defined as follows:

**Definition 3.12**

The **sensitivity** of a symptom (or set of symptoms or screening test) is the probability that the symptom is present given that the person has disease.                                    ∎

**Definition 3.13**

The **specificity** of a symptom (or set of symptoms or screening test) is the probability that the symptom is not present given that the person does not have disease.                    ∎

**Definition 3.14**

A **false negative** is defined as a person who tests out as negative but who is actually positive. A **false positive** is defined as a person who tests out as positive but who is actually negative.    ∎

It is important that both the sensitivity and specificity be high for a symptom to be effective in predicting disease.

**Example 3.24**    *Cancer* Suppose that the disease is lung cancer and the symptom is cigarette smoking. If we assume that 90% of persons with lung cancer and 50% of persons without lung cancer (essentially the entire general population) are smokers, then the sensitivity and specificity are 0.9 and 0.5, respectively. We obviously cannot use cigarette smoking by itself as a diagnostic tool for predicting lung cancer, because there will be too many false positives (normal persons who are smokers).                                    ∎

**Example 3.25**    *Cancer* Suppose that the disease is breast cancer in women and the symptom is having a family history of breast cancer (i.e., either a mother or a sister with breast cancer). If we assume that 5% of persons with breast cancer have a family history of breast cancer whereas only 2% of persons without breast cancer have such a history, then the sensitivity is 0.05 and the specificity is 0.98 (1 − 0.02). We cannot use a family history of breast cancer by itself to diagnose breast cancer because there will be too many false negatives (i.e., people without a family history who have the disease).                                    ∎

How can we use the sensitivity and specificity of a symptom (or set of symptoms), which are quantities a physician can estimate, to compute predictive values, which are quantities a physician needs to make appropriate diagnoses? This procedure is given by Bayes' rule, as follows:

**3.7**    *Bayes' Rule*

Let $A$ = symptom and $B$ = disease. From definitions 3.11, 3.12, and 3.13, we have

$$\text{Predictive value positive} = \text{PV}^+ = Pr(B|A)$$

$$\text{Sensitivity} = Pr(A|B)$$

$$\text{Specificity} = Pr(\bar{A}|\bar{B})$$

Let $Pr(B)$ = probability of disease in the general population $\equiv x$. These quantities are related by the following formula:

$$PV^+ = x \cdot \text{sensitivity}/[x \cdot \text{sensitivity} + (1 - x) \cdot (1 - \text{specificity})]$$

which can be expressed in symbols as follows:

$$Pr(B|A) = [Pr(A|B) \cdot Pr(B)]/[Pr(A|B) \cdot Pr(B) + Pr(A|\bar{B}) \cdot Pr(\bar{B})]$$

Similarly, we can write

$$PV^- = (1 - x) \cdot \text{specificity}/[(1 - x) \cdot \text{specificity} + x \cdot (1 - \text{sensitivity})]$$

**Example 3.26**    *Hypertension*  Suppose that 84% of hypertensives and 23% of normotensives are classified as hypertensive by an automated blood pressure machine. What is the predictive value positive and predictive value negative of the machine, assuming that 20% of the adult population is hypertensive?

**Solution**    We have that sensitivity = 0.84, specificity = $1 - 0.23 = 0.77$. Thus, from Bayes' rule it follows that

$$PV^+ = (0.2)(0.84)/[(0.2)(0.84) + (0.8)(0.23)]$$

$$= 0.168/0.352$$

$$= 0.48$$

Similarly,

$$PV^- = (0.8)(0.77)/[(0.8)(0.77) + (0.2)(0.16)]$$

$$= 0.616/0.648$$

$$= 0.95$$

Thus, a negative result from the machine is very predictive, since we are 95% sure that such a person is normotensive. However, a positive result is not very predictive, since we are only 48% sure that such a person is hypertensive. ∎

In Example 3.26 there were only two possible disease states: hypertensive and normotensive. In clinical medicine there are often more than two possible disease states. We would like to be able to predict the most likely disease state given a specific symptom (or set of symptoms). We will assume that the probability of having these symptoms for each disease state is known from clinical experience as is the probability of each of the disease states in the general population. This objective leads us to the generalized Bayes' rule:

## 3.8    Generalized Bayes' Rule

Let $B_1, B_2, \ldots, B_k$ be a set of disease states such that at least one disease state must occur and no two disease states can occur at the same time. Let $A$ represent the presence of a symptom or set of symptoms. Then

$$Pr(B_i|A) = Pr(A|B_i)Pr(B_i) \bigg/ \left[ \sum_{j=1}^{k} Pr(A|B_j)Pr(B_j) \right]$$

*Example 3.27*    **Pulmonary Disease** Suppose that a 60-year-old male who has never smoked cigarettes presents himself to a physician with symptoms consisting of a chronic cough and occasional breathlessness. The physician becomes concerned and orders the patient admitted to the hospital for a lung biopsy. Suppose that the results of the lung biopsy are consistent with either lung cancer or sarcoidosis, a fairly common, nonfatal lung disease. In this case

$$\text{Symptoms } A = \{\text{chronic cough, results of lung biopsy}\}$$

$$\text{Disease state } B_1 = \text{normal}$$

$$B_2 = \text{lung cancer}$$

$$B_3 = \text{sarcoidosis}$$

Suppose that

$$Pr(A|B_1) = 0.001 \qquad Pr(A|B_2) = 0.9 \qquad Pr(A|B_3) = 0.9$$

and that in 60-year-old, never-smoking males

$$Pr(B_1) = 0.99 \qquad Pr(B_2) = 0.001 \qquad Pr(B_3) = 0.009$$

The first set of probabilities $Pr(A|B_i)$ could be obtained from clinical experience with the previous diseases, whereas the latter set of probabilities $Pr(B_i)$ would have to be obtained from age-sex-smoking specific prevalence rates for the diseases in question. The interesting question now is what are the probabilities $Pr(B_i|A)$ of the three disease states given the previous symptoms?

*Solution*    We have from Bayes' rule that

$$Pr(B_1|A) = Pr(A|B_1)Pr(B_1) \bigg/ \left[ \sum_{j=1}^{3} Pr(A|B_j)Pr(B_j) \right]$$

$$= (0.001)(0.99)/[(0.001)(0.99) + 0.9(0.001) + 0.9(0.009)]$$

$$= 0.00099/0.00999 = 0.099$$

$$Pr(B_2|A) = 0.9(0.001)/[(0.001)(0.99) + 0.9(0.001) + 0.9(0.009)]$$

$$= 0.00090/0.00999 = 0.090$$

$$Pr(B_3|A) = 0.9(0.009)/[(0.001)(0.99) + 0.9(0.001) + 0.9(0.009)]$$

$$= 0.00810/0.00999 = 0.811$$

Thus, although the unconditional probability of sarcoidosis is very low (0.009), the conditional probability of the disease given these symptoms and this age-sex-smoking group is 0.811. Also, although the symptoms are consistent with both lung cancer and sarcoidosis, the latter is much more likely among patients in this age-sex-smoking group.                                    ∎

*Example 3.28*   **Pulmonary Disease** Now, suppose that the patient discussed in Example 3.27 was a smoker of two packs of cigarettes per day for 40 years. Then, let us assume that $Pr(B_1) = 0.98$, $Pr(B_2) = 0.015$, $Pr(B_3) = 0.005$ in this type of person. What are the probabilities of the three disease states given these symptoms for this type of patient?

*Solution*

$$Pr(B_1|A) = (0.001)(0.98)/[(0.001)(0.98) + 0.9(0.015) + 0.9(0.005)]$$

$$= 0.00098/0.01898 = 0.052$$

$$Pr(B_2|A) = 0.9(0.015)/0.01898 = 0.01350/0.01898 = 0.711$$

$$Pr(B_3|A) = 0.9(0.005)/0.01898 = 0.237$$

Thus, in this type of patient, lung cancer is the most likely diagnosis.   ∎

## ■ 3.8 PREVALENCE AND INCIDENCE

In clinical medicine the terms *prevalence* and *incidence* are used to denote probabilities in a special context, which we will use frequently in this text.

*Definition 3.15*

The **prevalence** of a disease is the probability of currently having that disease regardless of the duration of time one has had the disease. It is obtained by dividing the number of people who currently have the disease by the number of people in the study population.

*Example 3.29*   **Hypertension** The prevalence of hypertension in 1974 among all persons 17 years of age and older was reported to be 15.7% as assessed by a government study [4]. It was computed by dividing the number of persons who had elevated blood pressure and were 17 years of age and older (22,626) by the total number of people 17 years of age and older in the study population (144,380).   ∎

*Definition 3.16*

The **incidence** of a disease is the probability an individual with no prior disease will develop a new case of the disease over some specified time period.   ∎

*Example 3.30*   **Cancer** The annual incidence rate of breast cancer in 40–44-year-old Connecticut women over the time period January 1, 1970, through December 31, 1970, was approximately 1 per 1000 [2]. This rate means that about 1 woman in 1000 of the 40–44-year-old women who have never had breast cancer on January 1, 1970, will develop a new case of breast cancer by December 31, 1970.   ∎

## ■ 3.9 SUMMARY

In this chapter we learned what probabilities are and how to work with them using the **addition** and **multiplication** laws. We made an important distinction between **independent** events, which are unrelated to each other, and **dependent** events, which tend to occur simultaneously. We introduced the general concepts of **conditional probability** and **relative risk** to quantify the dependence between two events. These ideas were then applied to the special area of screening populations for disease.

In particular, the notions of **sensitivity, specificity,** and **predictive value,** which are used to define the accuracy of screening tests, were developed as applications of conditional probability. On some occasions only sensitivities and specificities are available and we wish to compute the predictive value of screening tests. This task can be accomplished using **Bayes' theorem.** Indeed, Bayes' theorem can be used generally to change the direction of conditional probabilities. Finally, we defined the terms **prevalence** and **incidence,** which are probabilistic parameters that are often used to describe the magnitude of disease in a population.

In the next two chapters, we will apply these general principles of probability to derive some of the important probabilistic models often used in biomedical research, including the **binomial, Poisson,** and **normal** models. Using these models, we will eventually be able to test hypotheses concerning our data.

# $P$roblems

Let $A = \{$serum cholesterol $= 250–299\}$, $B = \{$serum cholesterol $\geq 300\}$, $C = \{$serum cholesterol $\leq 280\}$.

**3.1** Are the events $A$ and $B$ mutually exclusive?

**3.2** Are the events $A$ and $C$ mutually exclusive?

**3.3** Suppose $Pr(A) = 0.2$, $Pr(B) = 0.1$. What is $Pr($serum cholesterol $\geq 250)$?

**3.4** What does $A \cup C$ mean?

**3.5** What does $A \cap C$ mean?

**3.6** What does $B \cup C$ mean?

**3.7** What does $B \cap C$ mean?

**3.8** Are the events $B$ and $C$ mutually exclusive?

**3.9** What does the event $\bar{B}$ mean? What is its probability?

Let us consider a family with a mother, father, and two children. Let $A_1 = \{$mother has influenza$\}$, $A_2 = \{$father has influenza$\}$, $A_3 = \{$first child has influenza$\}$, $A_4 = \{$second child has influenza$\}$, $B = \{$at least one child has influenza$\}$, $C = \{$at least one parent has influenza$\}$, $D = \{$at least one person in the family has influenza$\}$.

**3.10** What does $A_1 \cup A_2$ mean?

**3.11** What does $A_1 \cap A_2$ mean?

**3.12** Are $A_3$ and $A_4$ mutually exclusive?

**3.13** What does $A_3 \cup B$ mean?

**3.14** What does $A_3 \cap B$ mean?

**3.15** Express $C$ in terms of $A_1, A_2, A_3, A_4$.

**3.16** Express $D$ in terms of $B$ and $C$.

**3.17** What does $\bar{A}_1$ mean?

**3.18** What does $\bar{A}_2$ mean?

**3.19** Represent $\bar{C}$ in terms of $A_1, A_2, A_3, A_4$.

**3.20** Represent $\bar{D}$ in terms of $B$ and $C$.

Refer to Problem 3.10. Suppose that an influenza epidemic strikes a city. In 10% of families the mother has influenza; in 10% of families the father has influenza; and in 2% of families both the mother and father have influenza.

**3.21** Are the events $A_1, A_2$ independent?

Suppose that the gender of successive offspring in the same family are independent events and that the probability of a male or female offspring is 0.5.

**3.22** What is the probability of two successive female offspring?

**3.23** What is the probability that exactly one of two successive children will be female?

**3.24** Suppose that three successive offspring are male. What is the probability that a fourth child will be male?

Refer to Problem 3.21.

**3.25** What is the probability that at least one parent will get influenza?

Suppose that there is a 20% chance that each child will get influenza, whereas in 10% of two-child families, both children get the disease.

**3.26** What is the probability that at least one child will get influenza?

## Hypertension

Multiple drugs are often used in treating hypertension.

Suppose that 10% of patients taking antihypertensive agent *A* experience gastrointestinal (GI) side effects, whereas 20% of patients taking antihypertensive agent *B* experience such side effects.

*3.27* If the side effects of the two agents are assumed to be independent events, then what is the probability that a patient taking the two agents simultaneously will experience GI side effects?

Refer to Problem 3.21.

*3.28* What is the conditional probability that the father has influenza given that the mother has influenza?

*3.29* What is the conditional probability that the father has influenza given that the mother does not have influenza?

## Occupational Health

A study is conducted in male workers 50–69 years old working in a chemical plant. We are interested in comparing the mortality experience of the workers in the plant with national mortality rates. Suppose that of the 500 workers in this age group in the plant, 35% are 50–54, 30% are 55–59, 20% are 60–64, and 15% are 65–69.

*3.30* If the annual national mortality rates are 0.9% in 50–54-year-old men, 1.4% in 55–59-year-old men, 2.2% in 60–64-year-old men, and 3.3% in 65–69-year-old men, then what is the projected annual mortality rate in the plant as a whole?

The SMR (standardized mortality ratio) is often used in occupational studies as a measure of risk. It is defined as 100% *times* the observed number of events in the exposed group *divided by* the expected number of events in the exposed group (based on some reference population).

*3.31* If 15 deaths are observed over 1 year among the 500 workers, then what is the SMR?

## Pulmonary Disease

Pulmonary embolism is a relatively common condition that necessitates hospitalization and also often occurs in patients hospitalized for other reasons. An oxygen tension (arterial $P_{O_2}$) $< 90$ mm Hg is one of the important criteria used in diagnosing this condition. Suppose that the sensitivity of this test is 95%, the specificity is 75%, and the estimated prevalence is 20% (i.e., a doctor estimates that a patient has a 20% chance of pulmonary embolism before performing the test).

*3.32* What is the predictive value positive of this test? What does it mean in words?

*3.33* What is the predictive value negative of this test? What does it mean in words?

*3.34* Answer Question 3.32 if the estimated prevalence is 80%.

*3.35* Answer Question 3.33 if the estimated prevalence is 80%.

## Genetics

Suppose that a disease is inherited via a **dominant** mode of inheritance and that one of two parents is affected with the disease whereas one is not. The implications of this situation are that the probability is $\frac{1}{2}$ that any particular offspring will get the disease.

*3.36* What is the probability that in a family with two children, both siblings are affected?

*3.37* What is the probability that exactly one sibling is affected?

*3.38* What is the probability that neither sibling will be affected?

*3.39* Suppose that the older child is affected. What is the probability that the younger child will be affected?

*3.40* If *A*, *B* are two events such that *A* = {older child is affected}, *B* = {younger child is affected}, then are the events *A*, *B* independent?

Suppose that a disease is inherited via an **autosomal recessive** mode of inheritance. The implications of this type of inheritance are that the children in a family each have a probability of $\frac{1}{4}$ of inheriting the disease.

*3.41* What is the probability that in a family with two children, both siblings are affected?

*3.42* What is the probability that exactly one sibling is affected?

*3.43* What is the probability that neither sibling is affected?

Suppose that a disease is inherited via a **sex-linked** mode of inheritance. The implications of this mode are that each male offspring has a 50% chance of inheriting the disease, whereas the female offspring have no chance at all of getting the disease.

*3.44* In a family with one male and one female offspring, what is the probability that both siblings are affected?

*3.45* What is the probability that exactly one sibling is affected?

*3.46* What is the probability that neither sibling is affected?

*3.47* Answer Problem 3.44 for families with two male siblings.

*3.48* Answer Problem 3.45 for families with two male siblings.

*3.49* Answer Problem 3.46 for families with two male siblings.

Suppose that in a family with two male siblings, both siblings are affected with a genetically inherited disease. Suppose also that, although the genetic history of the family is unknown, only a dominant, recessive, or sex-linked mode of inheritance is possible.

*3.50* Let us assume that the dominant, recessive, and sex-linked modes of inheritance follow the probability laws given in Problems 3.36, 3.41, and 3.44 and that, without prior knowledge about the family in question, each is equally likely to occur. What is the probability of each mode of inheritance in this family?

*3.51* Answer Problem 3.50 for a family with two male siblings where only one sibling is affected.

*3.52* Answer Problem 3.50 for a family with one male and female sibling where both siblings are affected.

*3.53* Answer Problem 3.52 where only the male sibling is affected.

### Environmental Health, Pediatrics

*3.54* Suppose that a company plans to build a lead smelter in a community and that the city council wishes to assess the health effects of the smelter. In particular, there is concern from previous literature that children living very close to the smelter will experience unusually high rates of lead poisoning in the first 3 years of life. Suppose that the projected rates of lead poisoning over this time period are 50 per 100,000 for those children living within 2 km of the smelter, 20 per 100,000 for children living >2 km but ⩽5 km from the smelter, and 5 per 100,000 for children living >5 km from the smelter. If 80% of the children live more than 5 km from the smelter, 15% live >2 km but ⩽5 km from the smelter, and the remainder live ⩽2 km from the smelter, then what is the overall probability that a child from this community will get lead poisoning?

### Obstetrics

The following data are derived from the 1973 Final Natality Statistics Report issued by the National Center for Health Statistics [5]. These data are pertinent to live births only.

Suppose that infants are classified as low if they have a birthweight ⩽2500 g and as normal if they have a birthweight ⩾2501 g. Suppose that infants are also classified by period of gestation in the following four categories: <20 weeks, 20–27 weeks, 28–36 weeks, >36 weeks. We assume that the probabilities of the different periods of gestation are given in Table 3.2.

*Table 3.2* Relationship between birthweight and gestational age

| Period of gestation | Probability |
|---|---|
| <20 weeks | 0.0004 |
| 20–27 weeks | 0.0059 |
| 28–36 weeks | 0.0855 |
| >36 weeks | 0.9082 |

We also assume that the probability of being low given that the period of gestation is <20 weeks is 0.540, the probability of being low given that the period of gestation is 20–27 weeks is 0.813, the probability of being low given that the period of gestation is 28–36 weeks is 0.379, and the probability of being low given that the period of gestation is >36 weeks is 0.035.

*3.55* What is the probability of having a low infant?

*3.56* Show that the events (period of gestation ⩽27 weeks) and (low) are not independent.

*3.57* What is the probability of having a period of gestation ⩽36 weeks given that a child is low?

### Cerebrovascular Disease

One problem with using the angiogram to diagnose stroke is the slight risk of mortality associated with this test (<1%). Some investigators have attempted to use the PET scanner (which measures blood flow in the brain) to detect stroke disease noninvasively as an alternative to the angiogram. A comparison was made on the same patients between these two methodologies for detecting stroke, with the results given in Table 3.3.

*Table 3.3* Comparison of a noninvasive test for detecting stroke with an angiogram

| Angiogram | Noninvasive test | Frequency |
|---|---|---|
| − | − | 21 |
| − | + | 8 |
| + | − | 3 |
| + | + | 32 |

Let us regard the angiogram as the definitive test.

*3.58* What is the sensitivity of the noninvasive test?

*3.59* What is the specificity of the noninvasive test?

*3.60* What is the predictive value positive of the noninvasive test if we assume that the patients in this series are typical of patients for whom the confirmation of a stroke diagnosis is necessary?

**3.61** What is the predictive value negative of the non-invasive test under the same assumptions as in Problem 3.60?

### Pulmonary Disease

A recent paper by Colley et al. looked at the relationship between parental smoking and the incidence of pneumonia and/or bronchitis in children in the first year of life [6]. One important finding of the paper was that 7.8% of children with nonsmoking parents had episodes of pneumonia and/or bronchitis in the first year of life, whereas, respectively, 11.4% of children with one smoking parent and 17.6% of children with two smoking parents had such an episode. Suppose that in the general population both parents are smokers in 40% of households, one parent smokes in 25% of households, and neither parent smokes in 35% of households.

**3.62** What percent of children in the general population will have pneumonia and/or bronchitis in the first year of life?

A group of families in which both parents smoke at the time of the first prenatal visit decide, after counseling by the nurse practitioner, to give up smoking. Suppose that in 10% of these families both parents resume smoking and in 30% of these families one parent resumes smoking. In the remainder of the families both parents have not resumed smoking at the time of birth of the child. Let us assume also that the smoking status of the parents at the time of the birth is maintained during the first year of life of the child.

**3.63** What is the probability of pneumonia and/or bronchitis in children from families in this group?

**3.64** What percent of cases of pneumonia and/or bronchitis have been prevented by this type of counseling in families where both parents smoke?

### Diabetes

The prevalence of diabetes in adults at least 20 years old has been studied in Tecumseh, Michigan [7]. The age-sex specific prevalence (per 1000) is given in Table 3.4.

**3.65** Suppose we plan a new study in a town that consists of 48% males and 52% females. Of the males, 40% are ages 20–39, 32% are 40–54, and 28% are 55+. Of the females, 44% are ages 20–39, 37% are 40–54, and 19% are 55+. If we assume that the Tecumseh prevalence holds, what is the expected prevalence of diabetes in the new study?

**Table 3.4** *Age-sex specific prevalence of diabetes in Tecumseh, Michigan (per 1000)*

| Age group (years) | Sex | |
|---|---|---|
| | Male | Female |
| 20–39 | 5 | 7 |
| 40–54 | 23 | 31 |
| 55+ | 57 | 89 |

(Reprinted with permission from the *American Journal of Epidemiology* **116(6)**: 971–980.)

**3.66** What proportion of diabetics in the new study would be expected in each of the six age-sex groups?

### Pulmonary Disease

The familial aggregation of respiratory disease is a well-established clinical phenomenon. However, whether this aggregation is due to genetic or environmental factors or both is somewhat controversial. An investigator wishes to study a particular environmental factor, namely, the relationship of cigarette smoking habits in the parents to the presence or absence of asthma in their oldest child living in the household in the 5–9-year-old age range (referred to below as their offspring). Suppose that the investigator finds that: (i) if both the mother and father are current smokers, then the probability of their offspring having asthma is 0.15; (ii) if the mother is a current smoker and the father is not, then the probability of their offspring having asthma is 0.13; (iii) if the father is a current smoker and the mother is not, then the probability of their offspring having asthma is 0.05; (iv) if neither parent is a current smoker, then the probability of their offspring having asthma is 0.04.

**3.67** Suppose that the smoking habits of the parents are independent and that the probability that the mother is a current smoker is 0.4 whereas the probability that the father is a current smoker is 0.5. What is the probability that both the father and the mother are current smokers?

**3.68** What is the probability that the father is a current smoker if the mother is not a current smoker?

Suppose, alternatively, that if the father is a current smoker, then the probability that the mother is a current smoker is 0.6; whereas if the father is not a current smoker, then the probability that the mother is a current smoker is 0.2. Also assume that items (i), (ii), (iii), and (iv) above hold.

**3.69** If the probability that the father is a current smoker is 0.5, what is the probability that the father is a current smoker *and* that the mother is not a current smoker?

**3.70** Are the current smoking habits of the father and the mother independent? Why or why not?

**3.71** Find the unconditional probability that the off-spring will have asthma under the assumptions in *3.69* and *3.70*.

**3.72** Suppose that a child has asthma. What is the probability that the father is a current smoker?

**3.73** What is the probability that the mother is a current smoker if the child has asthma?

**3.74** Answer question 3.72 if the child does not have asthma.

**3.75** Answer question 3.73 if the child does not have asthma.

**3.76** Are the child's asthma status and the father's smoking status independent? Why or why not?

**3.77** Are the child's asthma status and the mother's smoking status independent? Why or why not?

## Cancer

Table 3.5 shows the annual incidence rates for colon cancer, lung cancer, and stomach cancer in males ages 50 years and older from the Connecticut Tumor Registry, 1963–1965 [2].

***Table 3.5*** *Average annual incidence per 100,000 males for colon, lung, and stomach cancer from the Connecticut Tumor Registry, 1963–1965* [2]

| | Ages | | |
|---|---|---|---|
| *Type of cancer* | *50–54* | *55–59* | *60–64* |
| Colon | 35.7 | 60.3 | 98.9 |
| Lung | 76.1 | 137.5 | 231.7 |
| Stomach | 20.8 | 39.1 | 46.0 |

(Reprinted from *Cancer Incidence in Five Continents* **II**, 1970, with permission of Springer-Verlag, Berlin.)

**3.78** What is the probability that a 57-year-old, disease-free male will develop lung cancer over the next year?

**3.79** What is the probability that a 55-year-old, disease-free male will develop colon cancer over the next 5 years?

**3.80** Suppose we have a cohort of 1000 50-year-old men who have never had cancer. How many colon cancers would we expect to develop in this cohort over a 15-year period?

**3.81** Answer Problem 3.80 for lung cancer.

**3.82** Answer Problem 3.80 for stomach cancer.

## Pulmonary Disease

Smoking cessation is an important dimension in public health programs aimed at prevention of cancer and heart and lung diseases. For this purpose data were accumulated starting in 1962 on a group of current smoking men as part of the Normative Aging Study, a longitudinal study of the Veterans Administration in Boston. No interventions were attempted on this group of men, but the following data were obtained as to annual quitting rates among initially healthy men who remained healthy during the entire period [8]:

| *Time period* | *Light smokers ($\leqslant$ one pack per day) average annual quitting rate per 100 persons* | *Heavy smokers ( > one pack per day) average annual quitting rate per 100 persons* |
|---|---|---|
| 1962–1966 | 3.1 | 2.0 |
| 1967–1970 | 7.1 | 5.0 |
| 1971–1975 | 4.7 | 4.1 |

Note that the quitting rates increased during the period of 1967 to 1970, which was around the time of the first Surgeon General's report on cigarette smoking.

**3.83** Suppose a man was a light smoker on January 1, 1962. What is the probability that he quit smoking by the end of 1975 (a 14-year period)?

**3.84** Answer Question 3.83 for a heavy smoker on January 1, 1962 (assuming that he remained a heavy smoker until just prior to quitting).

## Cardiovascular Disease

An experiment was set up by a group from the University of Utah to use Bayes' rule to help make clinical diagnoses [9]. In particular, a detailed medical history questionnaire and electrocardiogram were administered to each patient referred to a cardiovascular laboratory and suspected of having congenital heart disease. From the experience of this laboratory and from estimates based on other published data, two sets of probabilities were generated:

*1.* The unconditional probability of each of several disease states (refer to prevalence column in Table 3.6)

*2.* The conditional probability of specific symptoms given specific disease states (refer to the rest of Table 3.6)

Thus, the probability that a person has chest pain given that he or she is normal is 0.05. Similarly, the proportion of persons with isolated pulmonary hypertension is 0.020. A subset of the data is given in Table 3.6.

We will assume that these diagnoses are the only ones possible and that a patient can have one and only one diagnosis.

*3.85* What is the probability of having a symptom of chest pain given that you have isolated pulmonary hypertension?

*3.86* What is the probability of being more than 20 years old in this clinic?

*3.87* Suppose we assume that the probability of any two symptoms are independent given a specific diagnosis (e.g., the probability of being >20 years old and having mild cynanosis given that one is normal is $0.50 \times 0.01 = 0.005$). What is the probability of being diagnosed as normal given that you have the following symptoms: (i) age 1–20 years, (ii) repeated respiratory infections, and (iii) easy fatigue?

*3.88* What is the *most likely* diagnosis given that you have all the following symptoms: (i) mild cyanosis, (ii) age >20 years, (iii) EKG axis more than 110°? What is the second most likely diagnosis?

Suppose we use the symptom of an EKG axis of more than 110° as a screening criterion for diagnosing atrial

**Table 3.6** *Prevalence of symptoms and diagnoses for patients suspected of having congenital heart disease*

| Diagnosis | Prevalence | Symptoms | | | | | | |
|---|---|---|---|---|---|---|---|---|
| | | $X_1$ | $X_2$ | $X_3$ | $X_4$ | $X_5$ | $X_6$ | $X_7$ |
| $Y_1$ | 0.155 | 0.49 | 0.50 | 0.01 | 0.10 | 0.05 | 0.05 | 0.01 |
| $Y_2$ | 0.126 | 0.50 | 0.50 | 0.02 | 0.50 | 0.02 | 0.40 | 0.70 |
| $Y_3$ | 0.084 | 0.55 | 0.05 | 0.25 | 0.90 | 0.05 | 0.10 | 0.95 |
| $Y_4$ | 0.020 | 0.45 | 0.45 | 0.01 | 0.95 | 0.10 | 0.10 | 0.95 |
| $Y_5$ | 0.098 | 0.10 | 0.00 | 0.20 | 0.70 | 0.01 | 0.05 | 0.40 |
| $Y_6$ | 0.391 | 0.70 | 0.15 | 0.01 | 0.30 | 0.01 | 0.15 | 0.30 |
| $Y_7$ | 0.126 | 0.60 | 0.10 | 0.30 | 0.70 | 0.10 | 0.20 | 0.70 |

$Y_1$ = normal
$Y_2$ = atrial septal defect without pulmonary stenosis or pulmonary hypertension*
$Y_3$ = ventricular septal defect with valvular pulmonary stenosis
$Y_4$ = isolated pulmonary hypertension*
$Y_5$ = transposed great vessels
$Y_6$ = ventricular septal defect without pulmonary hypertension*
$Y_7$ = ventricular septal defect with pulmonary hypertension*
$X_1$ = age 1–20 years old
$X_2$ = age >20 years old
$X_3$ = mild cyanosis
$X_4$ = easy fatigue
$X_5$ = chest pain
$X_6$ = repeated respiratory infections
$X_7$ = EKG axis more than 110°

*Pulmonary hypertension is defined as pulmonary artery pressure $\geqslant$ systemic arterial pressure.
(Reprinted with permission of *The American Medical Association* from *The Journal of the American Medical Association* **177(3)**: 177–183, 1961. Copyright 1961, American Medical Association.)

septal defect without pulmonary stenosis or pulmonary hypertension.

**3.89** What is the sensitivity of this test?

**3.90** What is the specificity of this test?

### Pulmonary Disease

Research into cigarette smoking habits, smoking prevention, and cessation programs necessitates accurate measurement of smoking behavior. However, decreasing social acceptability of smoking appears to engender significant underreporting. Chemical markers for cigarette use can provide objective indicators of smoking behavior. One widely used noninvasive marker is the level of saliva thiocyanate (SCN). In a Minneapolis school district 1332 students in the eighth grade (ages 12–14) participated in a study [10] whereby they

> *1*. Viewed a film illustrating how recent cigarette use could be readily detected from small samples of saliva
>
> *2*. Provided a personal sample of saliva thiocyanate
>
> *3*. Provided a self-report on the number of cigarettes smoked per week

The results are given in Table 3.7.

Suppose we regard the self-reports as completely accurate and as representative of the amount that eighth-grade students smoke in the general community. We are considering using an SCN level of $\geq 100 \, \mu g/ml$ as a test criterion for identifying cigarette smokers. Let us regard a student as positive if he or she smokes 1 or more cigarettes per week.

**3.91** What is the sensitivity of the test for light-smoking students (i.e., students who smoke $\leq 14$ cigarettes per week)?

**3.92** What is the sensitivity of the test for moderate-smoking students (i.e., students who smoke 15–44 cigarettes per week)?

**3.93** What is the sensitivity of the test for heavy-smoking

**Table 3.7** *Relationship between saliva thiocyanate levels (SCN) and self-reported cigarettes smoked per week*

| Self-reported cigarettes smoked in last week | Number of students | Percent with SCN $\geq 100 \, \mu g/ml$ |
|---|---|---|
| None | 1163 | 3.3 |
| 1–4 | 70 | 4.3 |
| 5–14 | 30 | 6.7 |
| 15–24 | 27 | 29.6 |
| 25–44 | 19 | 36.8 |
| 45+ | 23 | 65.2 |

(Reprinted with permission from the *American Journal of Public Health* **71(12)**: 1320, 1981.)

students (i.e., students who smoke $\geq 45$ cigarettes per week)?

**3.94** What is the specificity of the test?

**3.95** What is the predictive value positive of the test?

**3.96** What is the predictive value negative of the test?

Suppose we regard the self-reports of all students who report some cigarette consumption as valid but estimate that 10% of students who report no cigarette consumption actually smoke 1–4 cigarettes per week and an additional 2% smoke 5–14 cigarettes per week.

**3.97** If we assume that the percentage of students with SCN $\geq 100 \, \mu g/ml$ in these two subgroups is the same as in those who truly report 1–4 and 5–14 cigarettes per week, then what effect would this underreporting have on the predictive value positive of the test (i.e., would the true predictive value positive be the same, higher, or lower than that computed in *3.95*)?

**3.98** Compute the predictive value positive under these altered assumptions.

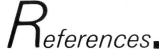

*R*eferences

[*1*] *Monthly Vital Statistics Report, Advance Report Final Natality Statistics* (1974) National Center for Health Statistics, **24(11)** Supplement 2, February 13, 1976.

[*2*] Doll, R., Muir, C., and Waterhouse, J., eds. (1970) *Cancer Incidence in Five Continents* **II** (Berlin: Springer-Verlag).

[3] Podgor, M. J., Leske, M. C., and Ederer, F. (1983) "Incidence Estimates for Lens Changes, Macular Changes, Open-Angle Glaucoma, and Diabetic Retinopathy," *American Journal of Epidemiology* **118(2)**: 206–212.

[4] *Advance Data from Vital and Health Statistics*, National Center for Health Statistics, **2**, November 8, 1976.

[5] *Monthly Vital Statistics Report, Final Natality Statistics* (1973) National Center for Health Statistics, **23 (11)** Supplement, January 30, 1975.

[6] Colley, J. R. T., Holland, W. W., and Corkhill, R. T. (1974) "Influence of Passive Smoking and Parental Phlegm on Pneumonia and Bronchitis in Early Childhood," *Lancet* **II**: 1031.

[7] Butler, W. J., Ostrander, L. D. Jr., Carman, W. J., and Lamphiear, D. E. (1982) "Diabetes Mellitus in Tecumseh, Michigan: Prevalence, Incidence and Associated Conditions," *American Journal of Epidemiology* **116(6)**: 971–980.

[8] Garvey, A. J., Bossé, R., Glynn, R. J., and Rosner, B. (1983) "Smoking Cessation in a Prospective Study of Healthy Adult Males: Effects of Age, Time Period, and Amount Smoked," *American Journal of Public Health* **73(4)**: 446–450.

[9] Warner, H., Toronto, A., Veasey, L. G., and Stephenson, R. (1961) "A Mathematical Approach to Medical Diagnosis," *JAMA* **177(3)**: 177–183.

[10] Luepker, R. V., Pechacek, T. F., Murray, D. M., Johnson, C. A., Hund, F., and Jacobs, D. R. (1981) "Saliva Thiocyanate: A Chemical Indicator of Cigarette Smoking in Adolescents," *American Journal of Public Health* **71(12)**: 1320.

# 4 *Discrete Probability Distributions*

■ *4.1  INTRODUCTION*

In Chapter 3 the definition of probability and some of the basic tools used in working with probabilities were introduced. We now wish to look at problems that can be put in a probabilistic framework. That is, by assessing the probabilities of certain events from actual past data, we can use specific probability models that fit our problems.

*Example 4.1*    *Ophthalmology*  Retinitis pigmentosa is a progressive ocular disease that in some cases eventually results in blindness. The three main genetic forms of the disease are the dominant mode, the recessive mode, and the sex-linked mode. Each mode has a different rate of progression, with the dominant mode being the slowest to progress and the sex-linked mode the fastest. Suppose a man does not have a clear idea of the prior history of disease in his family but he does know that 1 of his 2 male children is affected, whereas his 1 female child is not affected. Can this information help us to identify the genetic type?    ■

We can apply the **binomial distribution** to calculate the probability of this event occurring (1 out of 2 males affected, 0 out of 1 females affected) under each of the genetic modes mentioned and then use these results to infer what is the most likely genetic mode. In fact, we can use this distribution to make an inference for any family where we know that $k_1$ out of $n_1$ male children are affected and $k_2$ out of $n_2$ female children are affected.

*Example 4.2*    *Cancer*  A second example of a commonly used probability model concerns a recent cancer scare in young children in Woburn, Massachusetts. A recent news story reported an "excessive" number of cancer deaths in young children in this town and speculated whether or not this high rate was due to the dumping of industrial wastes in the northeastern portion of town [1]. Suppose that 5 cases of leukemia were reported in a town where we would normally expect 1. Is this difference sufficient evidence for concluding that there is an association between the industrial wastes and the cancer cases?    ■

We can use the **Poisson distribution** to calculate the probability of five or more cases if typical national rates for cancer were present in this town. If this probability were sufficiently small, then we would conclude that there was an association; otherwise, we would conclude that a longer surveillance of the town was necessary before arriving at a conclusion.

In this chapter we first introduce the general concept of a discrete random variable and then give an in-depth description of the binomial and Poisson distributions.

# ■ 4.2 RANDOM VARIABLES

In the previous chapter we dealt with very specific events, such as: (1) the outcome of a tuberculin skin test or (2) blood pressure measurements taken on different members of a family. We now want to introduce ideas that will enable us to refer, in general terms, to different types of events having the *same probabilistic structure*. For this purpose we introduce the concept of a random variable.

**Definition 4.1**

A **random variable** is a numerical quantity that takes different values depending on chance.    ■

We will be dealing with two types of random variables in this text: discrete and continuous random variables.

**Definition 4.2**

A **discrete random variable** is a variable for which there exists a discrete set of values with nonzero probability.    ■

**Example 4.3**    *Otolaryngology*    Otitis media is a disease of the middle ear and is one of the most frequent reasons for visiting a doctor in the first 2 years of life other than a routine well-baby visit. Let $X$ be the random variable that represents the number of episodes of otitis media in the first 2 years of life. Then $X$ is a discrete random variable, which takes on the values 0, 1, 2, . . . .    ■

**Example 4.4**    *Hypertension*    Many new drugs have been introduced in the last decade to bring hypertension under control, that is, to reduce high blood pressure to normotensive levels. Suppose a physician agrees to use a new antihypertensive drug on a trial basis on the first 4 untreated hypertensives whom she encounters in her practice before deciding whether to adopt the drug for routine use. Let $X$ = the number of patients out of 4 who are brought under control. Then $X$ is a discrete random variable, which takes on the values 0, 1, 2, 3, 4.    ■

**Definition 4.3**

A **continuous random variable** is any random variable that is not discrete, that is, whose values naturally form a continuum.    ■

**Example 4.5**    *Environmental Health*    The possible health effects on workers exposed to low levels of radiation over long periods of time are an issue of recent public health interest. One problem in assessing this situation is how to measure the cumulative exposure of a worker. A recent study was performed at the Portsmouth Naval Shipyard, whereby each exposed worker wore a badge, or dosimeter, which measured their annual radiation exposure in rem [2]. The cumulative exposure over a worker's lifetime could then be obtained by summing the yearly exposures. The cumulative lifetime exposure is a good example of a continuous random variable, since it varied in this study from 0.000 rem to 91.414 rem, which we would regard as taking on an essentially infinite number of values.                                                                                         ∎

# ■ 4.3 THE PROBABILITY MASS FUNCTION

The values taken by a random variable and its associated probabilities can be expressed by a rule, or relationship, which is called a probability mass function.

**Definition 4.4**

A **probability mass function** is a mathematical relationship, or rule, that assigns to any value $r$ of a discrete random variable $X$ the probability $Pr(X = r)$. This assignment is made for all values $r$ that have positive probability. The probability mass function is sometimes also referred to as a **probability distribution**.                                                                     ∎

The probability mass function can be displayed in the form of a table giving the values and their associated probabilities and/or it can be expressed as a mathematical formula giving the probability of all possible values.

*Example 4.6*

**Hypertension** Let us consider the situation in Example 4.4. Suppose that from previous experience with the drug, the drug company expects that for any clinical practice the probability that 0 patients out of 4 will be brought under control is 0.008, 1 patient out of 4 is 0.076, 2 patients out of 4 is 0.265, 3 patients out of 4 is 0.411, and all 4 patients is 0.240. This probability mass function, or probability distribution, is displayed in Table 4.1.

**Table 4.1**
*Probability mass function for the hypertension control example*

| $Pr(X = r)$ | 0.008 | 0.076 | 0.265 | 0.411 | 0.240 |
|---|---|---|---|---|---|
| $r$ | 0 | 1 | 2 | 3 | 4 |

Notice that for any probability mass function, the probability of any particular value must be between 0 and 1 and the sum of the probabilities of all values must exactly equal 1. Thus, $0 \leqslant Pr(X = r) \leqslant 1$, $\Sigma Pr(X = r) = 1$, where the summation is taken over all possible values that have positive probability.

*Example 4.7*

**Hypertension** In Table 4.1, for any clinical practice, the probability that between 0 and 4 hypertensives are brought under control = 1, that is,

$$0.008 + 0.076 + 0.265 + 0.411 + 0.240 = 1$$                                                                 ∎

## □ 4.3.1 Relationship of Probability Distributions to Sample Distributions

In Chapters 1 and 2, we discussed the concept of a **frequency distribution** in the context of a sample: a list of each value in the dataset and a corresponding count of how frequently the values occur. If we divide each count by the total number of points in the sample, then the frequency distribution can be considered as a sample analogue to a probability distribution. In particular, we can think of a probability distribution as a model based on an infinitely large sample, giving the fraction of data points in a sample that *should* be allocated to each specific value. Since the frequency distribution gives the actual proportion of points in a sample that correspond to specific values, we can validate the appropriateness of the model by comparing the observed sample frequency distribution to the probability distribution. The formal statistical procedure for making this comparison is called a **goodness-of-fit test,** which we discuss in Chapter 10.

*Example 4.8*

*Hypertension* How can we use the probability mass function in Table 4.1 to see if the drug behaves with the same efficacy in actual practice as predicted by the drug company? The drug company might distribute the drug to 100 physicians and ask each of them to treat their first 4 untreated hypertensives with the drug. Each physician would then report his or her results to the drug company, and the combined results could be compared with the expected results in Table 4.1. For example, suppose that out of 100 physicians who agree to participate, 19 are able to bring all of their first 4 untreated hypertensives under control, 48 are able to bring 3 of the 4 hypertensives under control, 24 are able to bring 2 out of 4 under control, 9 are able to bring only 1 of 4 under control, and none of the physicians bring 0 out of 4 hypertensives under control. We can compare the observed frequency distribution with the probability distribution given in Table 4.1. This comparison is shown in Table 4.2.

The distributions look reasonably similar. The role of statistical inference is to compare the two distributions to judge if the differences between the two can be attributed to chance or whether real differences exist between the drug's performance in actual clinical practice and expectations from previous drug company experience.    ■

*Table 4.2*

*Comparison of the observed frequency distribution and expected probability distribution for the hypertension control example*

| r | Probability distribution $Pr(X = r)$ | Frequency distribution |
|---|---|---|
| 0 | 0.008 | 0.000 = 0/100 |
| 1 | 0.076 | 0.090 = 9/100 |
| 2 | 0.265 | 0.240 = 24/100 |
| 3 | 0.411 | 0.480 = 48/100 |
| 4 | 0.240 | 0.190 = 19/100 |

A question often asked is where does a probability mass function come from. In some instances we can obtain previous data on the same type of random variable we are studying and can compute our probability mass function from these data. In other instances previous data may not be available, but we may try to use the probability mass function from some well-known distribution and see how well it fits with some sample data. In fact, we used this approach in Table 4.2, where we derived our probability mass function from the binomial distribution and then compared it with the observed frequency distribution.

# ■ 4.4 THE EXPECTED VALUE OF A RANDOM VARIABLE

If a random variable has a large number of values with positive probability, then the probability mass function is not a useful summary measure. Indeed, we are faced with the same problem as in trying to summarize a sample by enumerating each of the data values.

We can develop measures of location and spread for a random variable in much the same way as we developed them for samples. The analogue to the arithmetic mean $\bar{x}$ is referred to as the **expected value** or **population mean** and is denoted by $E(X)$ or $\mu$. The expected value represents the "average" value of the random variable. It is obtained by multiplying each of the possible values by its respective probability and summing over all the values that have positive probability.

**Definition 4.5**

The **expected value of a discrete random variable** is defined as

$$`E(X) \equiv \mu = \sum_{i=1}^{k} x_i Pr(x_i)$$

where the $x_i$'s are the values for which the random variable takes on positive probability. ■

*Example 4.9* **Hypertension** Find the expected value for the random variable depicted in Table 4.1.

*Solution* We have

$$E(X) = 0(0.008) + 1(0.076) + 2(0.265) + 3(0.411) + 4(0.240) = 2.80$$

Thus, on the average we would expect about 2.8 hypertensives to be brought under control for every 4 that are treated. ■

*Example 4.10* **Otolaryngology** Consider the random variable mentioned in Example 4.3 representing the number of episodes of otitis media in the first 2 years of life. Suppose this random variable has a probability mass function as given in Table 4.3.

**Table 4.3**
*Probability mass function for the number of episodes of otitis media in the first 2 years of life*

| *r* | 0 | 1 | 2 | 3 | 4 | 5 | 6 |
|---|---|---|---|---|---|---|---|
| *Pr(X = r)* | 0.129 | 0.264 | 0.271 | 0.185 | 0.095 | 0.039 | 0.017 |

What is the expected number of episodes of otitis media in the first 2 years of life?

*Solution* We have

$$E(X) = 0(0.129) + 1(0.264) + 2(0.271) + 3(0.185) + 4(0.095) + 5(0.039) + 6(0.017)$$

$$= 2.04$$

Thus, on the average we would expect a child to have 2 episodes of otitis media in the first 2 years of life. ■

In Example 4.8 we compared the probability mass function for the random variable representing the number of previously untreated hypertensives brought under control with the actual number of hypertensives brought under control in 100 clinical practices. In much the same way, we can compare the expected value of a random variable with the actual sample mean in a data set ($\bar{x}$).

*Example 4.11*    **Hypertension** Compare the number of hypertensives brought under control in the 100 clinical practices ($\bar{x}$) with the expected number of hypertensives brought under control ($\mu$).

*Solution*    From Table 4.2 we have

$$\bar{x} = [0(0) + 1(9) + 2(24) + 3(48) + 4(19)]/100 = 2.77$$

hypertensives controlled per clinical practice while $\mu = 2.80$. This agreement is rather good. The specific methods for comparing the observed and expected average values of a random variable ($\bar{x}$ and $\mu$) will be covered in our work on statistical inference in Chapter 7. Notice that $\bar{x}$ could be written in the form

$$\bar{x} = 0(0/100) + 1(9/100) + 2(24/100) + 3(48/100) + 4(19/100)$$

that is, as a weighted average of observed probabilities. The expected value, in comparison, can be written as a weighted average of theoretical probabilities:

$$\mu = 0(0.008) + 1(0.076) + 2(0.265) + 3(0.411) + 4(0.240)$$

Thus, the two quantities are actually obtained in the same way, one as a weighted average of "observed" probabilities and the other as a weighted average of "theoretical" probabilities.  ∎

## ■ 4.5 THE VARIANCE OF A RANDOM VARIABLE

The analogue to the sample variance ($s^2$) for a random variable is referred to as the **variance of the random variable** or **population variance** and is denoted by $Var(X)$. The variance represents the spread of all values that have positive probability relative to the expected value. In particular, the variance is obtained by multiplying the squared distance of each possible value from the expected value by its respective probability and summing over all the values that have positive probability.

**Definition 4.6**

The **variance of a discrete random variable** denoted by $X$ is defined by

$$Var(X) \equiv \sigma^2 = \sum_{i=1}^{k} (x_i - \mu)^2 Pr(X = x_i)$$

where the $x_i$ are the values for which the random variable takes on positive probability. The **standard deviation of a random variable** $X$, denoted by $sd(X)$ or $\sigma$, is defined by the square root of its variance.  ∎

There is also a short form for the population variance, which is similar to the equation presented for the sample variance.

**4.1**  A **short form for the population variance** is given by

$$\sigma^2 = E(X - \mu)^2 = \sum_{i=1}^{k} x_i^2 Pr(x_i) - \mu^2$$

*Example 4.12*  **Otolaryngology**  Compute the variance and standard deviation for the random variable depicted in Table 4.3.

*Solution*  We know from Example 4.10 that $\mu = 2.04$. Furthermore, we have

$$\sum_{i=1}^{k} x_i^2 Pr(x_i) = 0^2(0.129) + 1^2(0.264) + 2^2(0.271) + 3^2(0.185)$$

$$+ 4^2(0.095) + 5^2(0.039) + 6^2(0.017)$$

$$= 0(0.129) + 1(0.264) + 4(0.271) + 9(0.185)$$

$$+ 16(0.095) + 25(0.039) + 36(0.017)$$

$$= 6.12$$

Thus, $Var(X) = \sigma^2 = 6.12 - (2.04)^2 = 1.96$. The standard deviation of $X = \sigma = \sqrt{1.96} = 1.40$. ∎

How can we get a feel for what the standard deviation of a random variable means? The following often-used principle is true for many, but not all, random variables:

**4.2**  Approximately 95% of the probability mass falls within two standard deviations of the mean of a random variable.

This statement holds exactly for normally distributed random variables, which we will discuss in the next chapter, and approximately for certain other random variables.

*Example 4.13*  **Otolaryngology**  Find $a, b$ such that approximately 95% of infants will have between $a$ and $b$ episodes of otitis media in the first 2 years of life.

*Solution*  The random variable depicted in Table 4.3 has mean ($\mu$) = 2.04 and standard deviation ($\sigma$) = 1.40. The interval $\mu \pm 2\sigma$ is given by

$$2.04 \pm 2(1.4) = 2.04 \pm 2.80$$

or from $-0.76$ to $4.84$. Since only positive integer values are possible for this random variable, we have a valid range from $a = 0$ to $b = 4$ episodes. From Table 4.3 we see that the probability of having ⩽4 episodes is

$$0.129 + 0.264 + 0.271 + 0.185 + 0.095 = 0.944$$  ∎

The rule allows us to quickly summarize the range of values that have most of the probability mass for a random variable without specifying each individual value. In Chapter 6 we will specify more precisely the type of random variable for which **(4.2)** is applicable.

# ■ *4.6 THE CUMULATIVE DISTRIBUTION FUNCTION OF A RANDOM VARIABLE*

Many random variables are displayed in tables or figures in terms of a cumulative distribution function rather than a distribution of probabilities of individual values as in Table 4.1. The basic concept is to assign to each individual value the sum of probabilities of all values that are no larger than the value being considered. This function is defined as follows:

**Definition 4.7**

The **cumulative distribution function** of a random variable $X$ is denoted by $F(x)$ and is defined by $Pr(X \leqslant x)$.

**Example 4.14**   *Otolaryngology*   Compute the cumulative distribution function for the otitis media random variable in Table 4.3 and display it graphically.

**Solution**   The cumulative distribution function is given by

$$F(x) = 0 \qquad \text{if} \qquad x < 0$$

$$F(x) = 0.129 \qquad \text{if} \qquad 0 \leqslant x < 1$$

$$F(x) = 0.393 \qquad \text{if} \qquad 1 \leqslant x < 2$$

$$F(x) = 0.664 \qquad \text{if} \qquad 2 \leqslant x < 3$$

$$F(x) = 0.849 \qquad \text{if} \qquad 3 \leqslant x < 4$$

$$F(x) = 0.944 \qquad \text{if} \qquad 4 \leqslant x < 5$$

$$F(x) = 0.983 \qquad \text{if} \qquad 5 \leqslant x < 6$$

$$F(x) = 1.0 \qquad \text{if} \qquad x \geqslant 6$$

The function can be displayed as shown in Figure 4.1.   ■

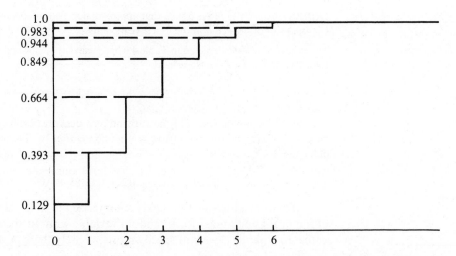

**Figure 4.1**
*Cumulative distribution function for the number of episodes of otitis media in the first 2 years of life*

The cumulative distribution for a discrete random variable looks like a series of steps. The steps become smaller as the number of values increases, and the graph approaches that of a smooth curve.

# ◼ 4.7 THE BINOMIAL DISTRIBUTION

In Sections 4.2 through 4.6 we introduced the concept of a discrete random variable in very general terms. In the remainder of this chapter, we will focus on some specific discrete random variables that occur frequently in medical and biological work. In this section we will concentrate on the binomial distribution. Some examples of this distribution follow.

**Example 4.15**    *Infectious Disease*   One of the most common laboratory tests performed on any routine medical examination is the blood test. The two main aspects to a blood test are (a) counting the number of white blood cells (referred to as the "white count") and (b) differentiating the white blood cells that do exist into five categories, namely, neutrophils, lymphocytes, monocytes, eosinophils, and basophils (referred to as the "differential"). Both the white count and the differential are extensively used for clinical diagnoses. We will concentrate here on the differential, particularly on the distribution of the number of neutrophils $k$ out of 100 white blood cells (which is the typical number counted). We will see that the number of neutrophils follows a binomial distribution.      ◼

**Example 4.16**    *Infectious Disease*   Suppose that a group of 100 males aged 60–64 received a new flu vaccine in 1959 and that 5 of them died within the next year. Is this event unusual or can this kind of death rate be expected from persons of this age-sex group? The distribution of the number of males who will die in the next year follows a binomial distribution.      ◼

**Example 4.17**    *Pulmonary Disease*   An investigator notices that children develop chronic bronchitis in the first year of life in 3 of 20 households where both parents are chronic bronchitics, as compared with the national incidence rate of chronic bronchitis, which is 5% in the first year of life. Is this difference "real" or can it be attributed to chance? The number of households where the infants develop chronic bronchitis follows a binomial distribution.      ◼

All of these examples have a common structure: we have a sample of $n$ independent trials, each of which can have only two possible outcomes, which we denote as a "success" and a "failure." Furthermore, the probability of a success at each trial is assumed to be some constant $p$, and hence the probability of a failure at each trial is $1 - p = q$. We will use the term "success" in a general way without any specific contextual meaning.

For Example 4.15, $n = 100$ and a "success" occurs when a cell is a neutrophil. For Example 4.16, $n = 100$ and a "success" occurs when a person dies within the next year. For Example 4.17, $n = 20$ and a "success" occurs when a child has disease within the first year of life. We are concerned with the probability of $k$ successes in $n$ trials for any $k = 0, 1, \ldots, n$.

**Example 4.18**    *Infectious Disease*   Let us reconsider Example 4.15 with 5 cells rather than 100 and ask the more limited question: What is the probability that the second and fifth cells considered will be neutrophils and the remaining cells nonneutrophils given that the probability that any one cell is a neutrophil is 0.6?

*Solution*    If we denote a neutrophil by an $x$ and a nonneutrophil by a $o$, then we are asking the question, what is the probability of the outcome $oxoox = Pr(oxoox)$? Since the probabilities of success and failure are given respectively by 0.6 and 0.4, and the outcomes for different cells are presumed to be independent, then this probability is

$$q \cdot p \cdot q \cdot q \cdot p = p^2 q^3 = (0.6)^2 \cdot (0.4)^3$$    ∎

*Example 4.19*    **Infectious Disease**  Now consider the more general question: What is the probability that any 2 cells out of 5 will be neutrophils?

*Solution*    We note that the arrangement $oxoox$ is only one of many possible orderings that result in 2 neutrophils. The 10 possible orderings are given in Table 4.4.

**Table 4.4**
*Possible orderings*
*for 2 neutrophils*
*out of 5 cells*

| | | |
|---|---|---|
| xxooo | oxxoo | ooxox |
| xoxoo | oxoxo | oooxx |
| xooxo | oxoox | |
| xooox | ooxxo | |

The probability of any of the orderings in Table 4.4 is the same as that for the ordering $oxoox$, namely, $(0.6)^2(0.4)^3$. Thus, the probability of obtaining 2 neutrophils in 5 cells is $10(0.6)^2(0.4)^3$.    ∎

Suppose that we number the cells as 1, 2, 3, 4, 5 and note that the first cell can be any of 1, 2, 3, 4, 5 and can thus be chosen in 5 ways. Once we have chosen the first cell, it can no longer be a candidate for the second cell; thus the second cell can be chosen in 4 ways. There are thus $5 \times 4 = 20$ ways of selecting 2 cells out of 5 where the order of selection is important. These selections are given in Table 4.5.

**Table 4.5**
*Twenty possible*
*selections of 2 cells*
*out of 5 where the*
*order of selection is*
*important*

| | | | | |
|---|---|---|---|---|
| 1 2 | 2 1 | 3 1 | 4 1 | 5 1 |
| 1 3 | 2 3 | 3 2 | 4 2 | 5 2 |
| 1 4 | 2 4 | 3 4 | 4 3 | 5 3 |
| 1 5 | 2 5 | 3 5 | 4 5 | 5 4 |

We can now ask the question, how many ways can we select $k$ objects out of $n$ where the order matters? We note that the first object has been selected in any one of $n = (n + 1) - 1$ ways. Given that the first object has been selected, we can select the second object in any one of $n - 1 = (n + 1) - 2$ ways; ... ; the $k$th object can be selected in any one of $n - k + 1 = (n + 1) - k$ ways.

If we consider the number of ways of selecting $n$ objects out of $n$ where order matters, then by the preceding principle we have

$$n(n - 1) \times \cdots \times [(n + 1) - n] = n(n - 1) \times \cdots \times 2 \times 1$$

The special symbol generally used for this quantity is $n!$, which is called $n$ factorial and is defined as follows:

| Definition 4.8 |

$n! = n$ **factorial** is defined as

$$n(n-1) \times \cdots \times 2 \times 1 \qquad \blacksquare$$

*Example 4.20*     Evaluate 5 factorial.

*Solution*     We have

$$5! = (5)(4)(3)(2)(1) = 120 \qquad \blacksquare$$

The quantity $0!$ has no inherent meaning, but for the consistency of our later discussions we will define it to be 1.

Now let us ask the question, how many ways can we select 2 cells out of 5 where order is not important, which is obviously the case in real life. We note that for each selection of 2 cells (say, cells 2 and 5), there are $2 \times 1$ ways of ordering these cells among themselves, namely, 25 and 52. Thus, the number of ways of selecting 2 cells out of 5 without respect to order = the number of ways of selecting 2 cells out of 5 where order is important/$(2 \times 1) = 10$.

The number of ways of selecting 2 cells out of 5 without respect to order is referred to as the number of **combinations** of 5 things taken 2 at a time and is denoted by ${}_5C_2$ or $\binom{5}{2} = 10$. The 10 combinations of 5 things taken 2 at a time are shown in Table 4.6.

*Table 4.6*
*Ten possible*
*selections of 2 cells*
*out of 5 where the*
*order of selection*
*is not important*

| 1 2 | 2 3 | 3 4 | 4 5 |
|-----|-----|-----|-----|
| 1 3 | 2 4 | 3 5 |     |
| 1 4 | 2 5 |     |     |
| 1 5 |     |     |     |

We can generalize this discussion to evaluate the number of combinations of $n$ things taken $k$ at a time. We note that for every selection of $k$ distinct items out of $n$, there are $k(k-1) \times \cdots \times (2) \times (1) = k!$ ways of ordering the items among themselves. Thus, we have the following definition:

| Definition 4.9 |

The number of **combinations** of $n$ things taken $k$ at a time is

$$_nC_k = \binom{n}{k} = [n(n-1) \times \cdots \times (n-k+1)]/k!$$

By algebraic manipulation, this equation becomes

$$_nC_k = n!/[k!(n-k)!] \qquad \blacksquare$$

*Example 4.21*      Evaluate $_7C_3$.

*Solution*

$$_7C_3 = \frac{7 \times 6 \times 5}{3 \times 2 \times 1} = 7 \times 5 = 35$$ ∎

Note that the number of terms in the numerator is always equal to $k$. A special situation arises upon evaluating $\binom{n}{0}$. By definition, $\binom{n}{0} = n!/(0!n!)$ and we defined $0!$ to be 1. Hence, $\binom{n}{0} = 1$ for any $n$.

We will frequently need to compute $\binom{n}{k}$ for $k = 0, 1, \ldots, n$. The combinatorials have the following symmetry property, which makes this calculation easier than it appears at first glance.

---

**4.3**   For any nonnegative integers $n, k$ where $n \geqslant k$,

$$\binom{n}{k} = \binom{n}{n-k}$$

---

Hence we only need to evaluate combinatorials $\binom{n}{k}$ for $k \leqslant n/2$. If $k > n/2$, then we can use the relationship $\binom{n}{n-k} = \binom{n}{k}$.

*Example 4.22*      Evaluate

$$\binom{7}{0}, \binom{7}{1}, \ldots, \binom{7}{7}$$

*Solution*      We have

$$\binom{7}{0} = 1 \quad \binom{7}{1} = 7 \quad \binom{7}{2} = \frac{7 \cdot 6}{2 \cdot 1} = 21 \quad \binom{7}{3} = \frac{7 \cdot 6 \cdot 5}{3 \cdot 2 \cdot 1} = 35$$

$$\binom{7}{4} = \binom{7}{3} = 35 \quad \binom{7}{5} = \binom{7}{2} = 21 \quad \binom{7}{6} = \binom{7}{1} = 7 \quad \binom{7}{7} = \binom{7}{0} = 1 \quad ∎$$

Suppose that we now consider the neutrophils problem more generally, with $n$ trials rather than 5 trials, and we ask the question, what is the probability of $k$ successes (rather than 2 successes) in these $n$ trials? The probability that the $k$ successes will occur at $k$ **specified** trials within the $n$ trials and that the remaining trials will be failures is given by $p^k(1-p)^{n-k}$. To compute the probability of $k$ successes in any of the $n$ trials, we must multiply this probability by the number of ways in which we can select $k$ trials for the successes and $n-k$ trials for the failures (as was done in Table 4.4). Thus, the probability of $k$ successes in $n$ trials, or $k$ neutrophils in $n$ cells, is

$$\binom{n}{k} p^k (1-p)^{n-k} = \binom{n}{k} p^k q^{n-k}$$

**4.4** The distribution of the number of successes in $n$ trials, where the probability of success on each trial is $p$, is known as the **binomial distribution** and has a probability mass function given by

$$Pr(X = k) = \binom{n}{k} p^k q^{n-k}, \qquad k = 0, 1, \ldots, n$$

We will refer to $Pr(X = k)$ as the general binomial probability.

# ■ 4.8 COMPUTATION OF BINOMIAL PROBABILITIES

## ☐ 4.8.1 Use of Binomial Tables

We will frequently need to evaluate a number of binomial probabilities for the same $n$ and $p$, which would be tedious if we had to calculate each probability from **(4.4)**. Instead, for small $n$ ($n \leqslant 20$) and selected values of $p$, we can refer to Table 1 in the appendix, where the individual binomial probabilities are calculated. In this table the number of trials ($n$) is provided in the first column, the number of successes ($k$) out of the $n$ trials is given in the second column, and the probability of success for an individual trial ($p$) is given in the first row. Binomial probabilities are provided for $n = 2, 3, \ldots, 20$, $p = 0.05, 0.10, \ldots, 0.50$.

*Example 4.23*   **Infectious Disease**  Evaluate the probability of 2 lymphocytes out of 10 white blood cells if the probability that any one cell is a lymphocyte is 0.2.

*Solution*   We refer to Table 1 with $n = 10$, $k = 2$, $p = 0.20$. The appropriate probability, given in the $k = 2$ row and $p = 0.20$ column under $n = 10$, is 0.3020.   ■

*Example 4.24*   **Pulmonary Disease**  Let us analyze the bronchitis data given in Example 4.17. Specifically, how likely are infants in at least 3 out of 20 households to develop chronic bronchitis if the probability of developing disease in any one household is 0.05?

*Solution*   Suppose the underlying rate of disease in the offspring is 0.05. The probability of observing $k$ cases out of 20 with disease is given by

$$\binom{20}{k} (0.05)^k (0.95)^{20-k}, \qquad k = 0, 1, \ldots, 20$$

We ask the question, what is the probability of observing at least 3 cases? The answer is given by

$$Pr(X \geqslant 3) = \sum_{k=3}^{20} \binom{20}{k} (0.05)^k (0.95)^{20-k}$$

$$= 1 - \sum_{k=0}^{2} \binom{20}{k} (0.05)^k (0.95)^{20-k}$$

We can evaluate these 3 probabilities in the sum using the binomial table (Table 1). We refer to $n = 20$, $p = 0.05$ and note that $Pr(X = 0) = 0.3585$, $Pr(X = 1) = 0.3774$, $Pr(X = 2) = 0.1887$.

Thus,

$$Pr(X \geqslant 3) = 1 - (0.3585 + 0.3774 + 0.1887) = 0.0754$$

Thus, $X \geqslant 3$ is an unusual event, but not very unusual. If 3 infants out of 20 were to develop the disease, we would probably decline to judge whether the familial aggregation was real until a larger sample was available. ∎

One question that arises is how to use the binomial tables if the probability of success on an individual trial ($p$) is greater than 0.5. If we recall that $\binom{n}{k} = \binom{n}{n-k}$ and we let $X$ be a binomial random variable with parameters $n$ and $p$, $Y$ be a binomial random variable with parameters $n$ and $q = 1 - p$, then **(4.4)** can be rewritten as

**4.5**
$$Pr(X = k) = \binom{n}{k}p^k q^{n-k} = \binom{n}{n-k}q^{n-k}p^k = Pr(Y = n - k)$$

In words, the probability of obtaining $k$ successes for a binomial random variable $X$ with parameters $n$ and $p$ is the same as the probability of obtaining $n - k$ successes for a binomial random variable $Y$ with parameters $n$ and $q$. Clearly, if $p > 0.5$, then $q = 1 - p < 0.5$, and we can use Table 1 with sample size $n$, referring to the $n - k$ row and the $q$ column to obtain the appropriate probability.

*Example 4.25*　**Infectious Disease** Evaluate the probabilities of obtaining $k$ neutrophils out of 5 cells for $k = 0, 1, 2, 3, 4, 5$, where the probability that any one cell is a neutrophil is 0.6.

*Solution*　Since $p > 0.5$, we refer to the random variable $Y$ with parameters $n = 5$, $p = 1 - 0.6 = 0.4$. We have

$$Pr(X = 0) = \binom{5}{0}(0.6)^0(0.4)^5 = \binom{5}{5}(0.4)^5(0.6)^0 = Pr(Y = 5)$$

$= 0.0102$ upon referring to the $k = 5$ row and $p = 0.40$ column under $n = 5$. Similarly,

$Pr(X = 1) = Pr(Y = 4) = 0.0768$ upon referring to the 4 row and 0.40 column under $n = 5$

$Pr(X = 2) = Pr(Y = 3) = 0.2304$ upon referring to the 3 row and 0.40 column under $n = 5$

$Pr(X = 3) = Pr(Y = 2) = 0.3456$ upon referring to the 2 row and 0.40 column under $n = 5$

$Pr(X = 4) = Pr(Y = 1) = 0.2592$ upon referring to the 1 row and 0.40 column under $n = 5$

$Pr(X = 5) = Pr(Y = 0) = 0.0778$ upon referring to the 0 row and 0.40 column under $n = 5$

∎

## ☐ 4.8.2 Recursion Rule for Binomial Probabilities

In many instances we will want to evaluate binomial probabilities for $n > 20$ and/or for values of $p$ not given in Table 1. For sufficiently large $n$ we can use the normal distribution to approximate the binomial distribution and use tables of the normal distribution to evaluate binomial probabilities. This procedure is usually less tedious than evaluating binomial probabilities directly using **(4.4)**. We will study this procedure in detail in Chapter 5. Alternatively, if our sample size is not large enough to allow us to use the normal approximation and/or if the value of $p$ is not in Table 1, then we can use a *recursion rule* to evaluate binomial probabilities. This rule is particularly useful if we wish to evaluate many binomial probabilities for the same $n$ and $p$. The recursion rule will allow us to easily evaluate $Pr(X = k + 1)$ once we know $Pr(X = k)$. Thus, once we have computed the probability of 0 successes, we can easily compute the probability of 1 success, 2 successes, and so forth without computing any combinatorials. The recursion rule is given as follows:

| 4.6 |
|---|

### Recursion Rule for Binomial Probabilities

$$Pr(X = k + 1) = [(n - k)/(k + 1)] \times (p/q) \times Pr(X = k),$$

$$k = 0, 1, \ldots, n - 1$$

*Example 4.26*

*Infectious Disease* Let us now analyze the flu vaccine data given in Example 4.16. Specifically, how likely are at least 5 out of 100 60–64-year-old males who receive a flu vaccine to die in the next year?

*Solution*

We must first find the expected annual death rate in 60–64-year-old males. From a 1959 U.S. life table, we find that 60–64-year-old men have an approximate probability of death in the next year of 0.028 [3]. Thus, from the binomial distribution the probability that $k$ out of 100 men will die during the next year is given by $\binom{100}{k}(0.028)^k(0.972)^{100-k}$. We want to know if 5 deaths in a sample of 100 men is an "unusual" event. One criterion for this evaluation might be to find the probability of getting at least 5 deaths in this group $= Pr(X \geqslant 5)$ given that the probability of death for an individual man is 0.028. We can express this probability as

$$\sum_{k=5}^{100} \binom{100}{k}(0.028)^k(0.972)^{100-k}$$

This sum of 96 probabilities is tedious to compute and thus we instead compute

$$Pr(X < 5) = \sum_{k=0}^{4} \binom{100}{k}(0.028)^k(0.972)^{100-k}$$

and then evaluate $Pr(X \geqslant 5) = 1 - Pr(X < 5)$. We cannot use the binomial tables, since $n > 20$. Therefore, we evaluate this sum of 5 binomial probabilities by the recursion rule. We have

$$Pr(X = 0) = \binom{100}{0}(0.028)^0(0.972)^{100} = (0.972)^{100} = 0.05843$$

$$Pr(X = 1) = \left(\frac{100 - 0}{0 + 1}\right)\left(\frac{0.028}{0.972}\right)(0.05843) = 0.16832$$

$$Pr(X = 2) = \left(\frac{99}{2}\right)\left(\frac{0.028}{0.972}\right)(0.16832) = 0.24001$$

$$Pr(X = 3) = \left(\frac{98}{3}\right)\left(\frac{0.028}{0.972}\right)(0.24001) = 0.22585$$

$$Pr\,(X = 4) = \left(\frac{97}{4}\right)\left(\frac{0.028}{0.972}\right)(0.22585) = 0.15777$$

Hence,

$$Pr(X < 5) = 0.05843 + 0.16832 + 0.24001 + 0.22585 + 0.15777 = 0.85038$$

and $$Pr(X \geqslant 5) = 1 - Pr(X < 5) = 0.14962 \approx 0.15$$

Thus, 5 deaths in 100 is a slightly unusual, but not a very unusual, event. If there were 10 deaths rather than 5, then using the same approach we have

$$Pr(X \geqslant 10) = 1 - Pr(X < 10) = 0.0005$$

which is very unlikely and would probably be grounds for halting the use of the vaccine in the absence of any other evidence.    ∎

# ■ 4.9 EXPECTED VALUE AND VARIANCE OF THE BINOMIAL DISTRIBUTION

The expected value and the variance of the binomial distribution is important both in terms of our general knowledge about the binomial distribution and for our later work on estimation and hypothesis testing. From Definition 4.5 we know that the general formula for the expected value of a discrete random variable is

$$\sum_{i=1}^{k} x_i Pr(x_i)$$

In the special case of a binomial distribution, the only values that take on positive probability are 0, 1, 2, . . . , $n$, and these values take on the probabilities

$$\binom{n}{0} p^0 q^n, \binom{n}{1} p^1 q^{n-1}, \ldots$$

Thus, $$E(X) = \sum_{k=0}^{n} k \binom{n}{k} p^k q^{n-k}$$

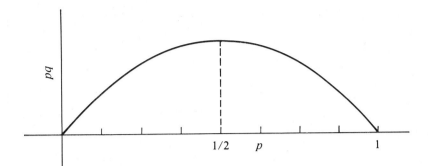

**Figure 4.2**
*Plot of pq vs. p*

We can show that this summation can be reduced to the simple expression $np$. Similarly, using Definition 4.6, we can show that

$$Var(X) = \sum_{k=0}^{n} (k - np)^2 \binom{n}{k} p^k q^{n-k} = npq$$

which leads directly to the following result:

**4.7**  The **expected value and variance of a binomial distribution** are $np$ and $npq$, respectively.

These results make good sense, since the expected number of successes in $n$ trials is simply the probability of success on one trial multiplied by $n$, which equals $np$. Furthermore, we note that for a given number of trials $n$, the binomial distribution has the highest variance when $p = \frac{1}{2}$, as shown in Figure 4.2. The variance of the distribution decreases as $p$ moves away from $\frac{1}{2}$ in either direction, becoming 0 when $p = 0$ or 1. This result makes sense, since when $p = 0$ there must be 0 successes in $n$ trials and when $p = 1$ there must be $n$ successes in $n$ trials, and there is no variability in either instance. Furthermore, when $p$ is near 0 or near 1, the distribution of the number of successes is clustered near 0 and $n$, respectively, and there is comparatively little variability as compared with the situation when $p = \frac{1}{2}$. This point is depicted in Figure 4.3.

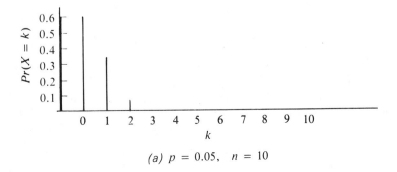

**Figure 4.3**
*The binomial distribution for various values of p when n = 10*

*(a) $p = 0.05$,  $n = 10$*

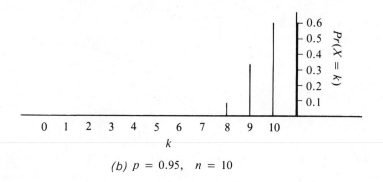

(b) $p = 0.95$,   $n = 10$

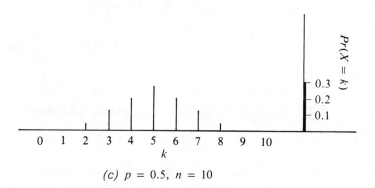

**Figure 4.3**
*(Continued)*                     (c) $p = 0.5$, $n = 10$

# ■ 4.10 THE POISSON DISTRIBUTION

The Poisson distribution is perhaps the second most frequently used discrete distribution after the binomial distribution. This distribution is usually associated with rare events.

*Example 4.27*  **Infectious Disease** Consider the distribution of the number of deaths attributed to typhoid fever over a long period of time, for example, 1 year. If we assume that the probability of a new death from typhoid fever in any one day is very small and that the number of cases reported in any two distinct periods of time are independent random variables, then the number of deaths over a 1-year period will follow a Poisson distribution.  ■

*Example 4.28*  **Bacteriology** The preceding example concerns a rare event occurring over time. We can also consider rare events not over time but on a surface area, such as the distribution of the number of bacterial colonies growing on an agar plate. Suppose we have a 100-cm$^2$ agar plate and that the probability of finding any bacterial colonies at any 1 point $a$ (or more precisely in a small area around $a$) is very small and that the events of finding bacterial colonies at any 2 points $p_1$, $p_2$ are independent. The number of bacterial colonies over the entire agar plate will follow a Poisson distribution.  ■

Suppose we consider Example 4.27. Let us ask the question, what is the distribution of the number of deaths due to typhoid fever from time 0 to time *T* (where *T* is some long period of time, such as 1 year or 20 years)?

We must make three assumptions about the incidence of the disease. Suppose we consider any general *small* subinterval of the time period *T*, denoted by $\Delta t$.

*Assumption 1*    We will assume that

   *(a)* The probability of observing 1 death is directly proportional to the length of the time interval $\Delta t$. That is, $Pr(1 \text{ death}) \approx \lambda \Delta t$ for some constant $\lambda$.

   *(b)* The probability of observing 0 deaths over $\Delta t$ is approximately $1 - \lambda \Delta t$.

   *(c)* The probability of observing more than 1 death over this time interval is essentially 0.  ■

*Assumption 2*    We assume that the number of deaths per unit time is the same throughout the entire time interval *T*. Thus, an increase in the incidence of the disease as time goes on within the time period *T* would violate this assumption. Note that *T* should not be overly long, since this assumption is less likely to hold as *T* increases.  ■

*Assumption 3*    *Independence*   If a death occurs within one time subinterval, it has no bearing on the probability of death in the next time subinterval. This assumption would be violated in an epidemic situation, because if a new case of disease occurs, then subsequent deaths are likely to build up over a short period of time until after the epidemic subsides.  ■

Based on these assumptions, we can derive the Poisson probability distribution, which is given as follows:

**4.8**    The probability of *k* events occurring in a time period *T* for a Poisson random variable with parameter $\lambda$ is

$$Pr(X = k) = e^{-\mu}\mu^k/k!, \qquad k = 0, 1, 2, \ldots$$

where $\mu = \lambda T$ and e is approximately 2.71828.

Thus, the Poisson distribution depends on two parameters, the length of the time interval *T* and the underlying parameter $\lambda$. Note that the parameter $\lambda$ represents the *expected number of events per unit time*, whereas the parameter $\mu$ represents the *expected number of events over the time period T*. One important difference between the Poisson distribution and the binomial distribution concerns the numbers of trials and events. For a binomial distribution there are a finite number of trials *n* and the number of events can be no larger than *n*. For a Poisson distribution the number of trials is essentially infinite and the number of events (or number of deaths) can be indefinitely large, although for very large *k* the probability of *k* events will get very small.

*Example 4.29*    *Infectious Disease*   Let us consider the typhoid fever example. Suppose the number of deaths attributable to typhoid fever over a 1-year period is Poisson with parameter $\mu = 4.6$. What is the probability distribution of the number of deaths over a 6-month period? a 3-month period?

*Solution*
Since $\mu = 4.6$, $T = 1$, it follows that $\lambda = 4.6$. For a 6-month period we have that $\lambda = 4.6$, $T = 0.5$. Thus, $\mu = \lambda T = 2.3$. Therefore,

$$Pr(0 \text{ deaths}) = e^{-2.3} = 0.100$$

$$Pr(1 \text{ death}) = \frac{(2.3)}{1!} e^{-2.3} = 0.231$$

$$Pr(2 \text{ deaths}) = \frac{(2.3)^2}{2!} e^{-2.3} = 0.265$$

$$Pr(3 \text{ deaths}) = \frac{(2.3)^3}{3!} e^{-2.3} = 0.203$$

$$Pr(4 \text{ deaths}) = \frac{(2.3)^4}{4!} e^{-2.3} = 0.117$$

$$Pr(5 \text{ deaths}) = \frac{(2.3)^5}{5!} e^{-2.3} = 0.054$$

$$Pr(\geqslant 6 \text{ deaths}) = 1 - (0.100 + 0.231 + 0.265 + 0.203 + 0.117 + 0.054) = 0.030$$

For a 3-month period we have that $\lambda = 4.6$, $T = 0.25$, $\mu = \lambda T = 1.15$. Therefore,

$$Pr(0 \text{ deaths}) = e^{-1.15} = 0.317$$

$$Pr(1 \text{ death}) = \frac{1.15}{1!} e^{-1.15} = 0.364$$

$$Pr(2 \text{ deaths}) = \frac{(1.15)^2}{2!} e^{-1.15} = 0.209$$

$$Pr(3 \text{ deaths}) = \frac{(1.15)^3}{3!} e^{-1.15} = 0.080$$

$$Pr(\geqslant 4 \text{ deaths}) = 1 - (0.317 + 0.364 + 0.209 + 0.080) = 0.030$$

These distributions are plotted in Figure 4.4. Note that the distribution tends to become more symmetric as the time interval increases or, more specifically, as $\mu$ increases. ∎

We can also apply the Poisson distribution to Example 4.28, where we discuss the distribution of the number of bacterial colonies in an agar plate of area $A$. If we are willing to assume that the probability of finding 1 colony in an area of size $\Delta A$ at any point on the plate is $\lambda \Delta A$ for some $\lambda$ and that the number of bacterial colonies found at 2 different points of the plate are independent random variables, then the probability of finding $k$ bacterial colonies in an area of size $A$ is given by $e^{-\mu} \mu^k / k!$, where $\mu = \lambda A$.

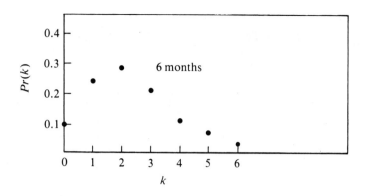

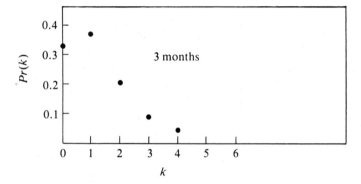

**Figure 4.4**
*Distribution of the number of deaths attributable to typhoid fever over various time intervals*

**Example 4.30**     **Bacteriology** If $A = 100 \text{ cm}^2$, $\lambda = 0.02$, calculate the probability distribution of the number of bacterial colonies.

**Solution**     We have that $\mu = \lambda A = 100\,(0.02) = 2$. Thus,

$$Pr(0 \text{ colonies}) = e^{-2} = 0.135$$

$$Pr(1 \text{ colony}) = e^{-2}(2)^1/1! = 2e^{-2} = 0.271$$

$$Pr(2 \text{ colonies}) = e^{-2}(2)^2/2! = 2e^{-2} = 0.271$$

$$Pr(3 \text{ colonies}) = e^{-2}(2)^3/3! = \frac{4}{3}e^{-2} = 0.180$$

$$Pr(4 \text{ colonies}) = e^{-2}(2)^4/4! = \frac{2}{3}e^{-2} = 0.090$$

$$Pr(\geqslant 5 \text{ colonies}) = 1 - (0.135 + 0.271 + 0.271 + 0.180 + 0.090) = 0.053$$

Clearly, the larger $\lambda$ is, the more bacterial colonies or deaths due to typhoid fever or whatever we would expect to find.     ∎

# ■ 4.11 COMPUTATION OF POISSON PROBABILITIES

## ☐ 4.11.1 Use of Poisson Tables

We often need to evaluate a number of Poisson probabilities for the same parameter $\mu$. This task would be tedious if we had to repeatedly apply formula 4.8. Instead, for $\mu \leqslant 20$ we can refer to Table 2 in the appendix, in which individual Poisson probabilities are specifically calculated. In this table the Poisson parameter $\mu$ is given in the first row, the number of events ($k$) is given in the first column, and the corresponding Poisson probability is given in the $k$ row and $\mu$ column.

**Example 4.31**    Compute the probability of obtaining at least 5 events for a Poisson distribution with parameter $\mu = 3$.

**Solution**    We refer to Table 2 under the 3.0 column. We find that

$$Pr(0) = 0.0498$$

$$Pr(1) = 0.1494$$

$$Pr(2) = 0.2240$$

$$Pr(3) = 0.2240$$

$$Pr(4) = 0.1680$$

Thus,

$$Pr(X \geqslant 5) = 1 - Pr(X \leqslant 4)$$

$$= 1 - (0.0498 + 0.1494 + 0.2240 + 0.2240 + 0.1680)$$

$$= 1 - 0.8152 = 0.1848 \qquad ■$$

## ☐ 4.11.2 Recursion Rule for Poisson Probabilities

In many instances we will want to evaluate a collection of Poisson probabilities for the same $\mu$, but $\mu$ will not be given in Table 2. For large $\mu$ ($\mu \geqslant 5$) we can use a normal approximation, as given in Chapter 5. Otherwise, we can use the following recursion rule, which is similar to that given for binomial probabilities.

**4.9**    **Recursion Rule for Poisson Probabilities**

If $Pr(k)$ is the Poisson probability of observing $k$ events with underlying parameter $\mu$, then

$$Pr(k + 1) = [\mu/(k + 1)]Pr(k)$$

**Example 4.32**    **Infectious Disease**  Let us apply the recursion rule to the distribution of deaths due to typhoid fever over a 3-month period given in Example 4.29.

*Solution*     First, we compute the probability of 0 deaths $= Pr(0) = e^{-1.15} = 0.3166$. Then,

$$Pr(1) = (1.15/1)Pr(0) = 1.15(0.3166) = 0.3641$$

$$Pr(2) = (1.15/2)Pr(1) = (0.575)(0.3641) = 0.2094$$

$$Pr(3) = (1.15/3)Pr(2) = (1.15/3)(0.2094) = 0.0803$$

$$\vdots$$

# ■ 4.12 EXPECTED VALUE AND VARIANCE OF THE POISSON DISTRIBUTION

In many instances we cannot predict whether the assumptions for the Poisson distribution given in Section 4.10 are satisfied. Fortunately, the relationship between the expected value and variance of the Poisson distribution provides an important guideline that will help us in identifying random variables that follow this distribution. This relationship can be stated as follows:

| 4.10 | The **expected value and variance of a Poisson distribution** with parameter $\mu$ is $\mu$. |

This fact is useful to know, since if we have a dataset from a discrete distribution where the *mean and variance are about the same*, then we can preliminarily identify it as a Poisson distribution and use various tests to confirm this hypothesis.

*Example 4.33*     **Infectious Disease**  The number of deaths attributable to polio during the years 1968–1976 are given in Table 4.7 [4, 5]. Comment on the applicability of the Poisson distribution to this dataset.

**Table 4.7**

*Number of deaths attributable to polio during the years 1968–1976*

| Year | 1968 | 1969 | 1970 | 1971 | 1972 | 1973 | 1974 | 1975 | 1976 |
|---|---|---|---|---|---|---|---|---|---|
| Number of deaths | 24 | 13 | 7 | 18 | 2 | 10 | 3 | 9 | 16 |

*Solution*     The mean and variance of the annual number of deaths due to polio during the period 1968–1976 are 11.3 and 51.5, respectively. The Poisson distribution clearly will not fit well here, since the variance is 4.6 times as large as the mean. The larger variance is probably due to the clustering of polio deaths at certain times and geographical locations, which leads to a violation of both the independence assumption and the assumption of constant incidence over time. ■

Suppose we are studying a rare event phenomenon and wish to apply the Poisson distribution. A question that often arises is how to estimate the parameter $\mu$ of the Poisson distribution in this context. Since the expected value of the Poisson distribution is $\mu$, we can estimate $\mu$ by the observed mean number of events, if such data are available. If the data are not available, we can use other data sources to estimate $\mu$.

*Example 4.34*    **Occupational Health**    A public health issue arose recently concerning the possible carcinogenic potential of food ingredients containing ethylene dibromide (EDB). In some instances foods were removed from public consumption if they were shown to have excessive quantities of EDB. A study was previously performed looking at the mortality experience of 161 white male employees of two plants in Texas and Michigan who were exposed to EDB over the time period 1940–1975 [6]. Seven deaths due to cancer were observed among these employees. For this time period 5.8 cancer deaths were expected as calculated from overall mortality rates for U.S. white males. Assess if the observed number of cancer deaths was excessive in this group.

*Solution*    We estimate the parameter $\mu$ from the expected number of cancer deaths from U.S. white male mortality rates; that is, $\mu = 5.8$. We then calculate $Pr(X \geqslant 7)$, where $X$ is a Poisson random variable with parameter 5.8. We use the relationship

$$Pr(X \geqslant 7) = 1 - Pr(X \leqslant 6)$$

Since 5.8 is not in Table 2, we use the recursion rule. We have

$$Pr(X = 0) = \frac{e^{-5.8}(5.8)^0}{0!} = e^{-5.8} = 0.0030$$

$$Pr(X = 1) = \frac{5.8}{1} \times 0.0030 = 0.0174$$

$$Pr(X = 2) = \frac{5.8}{2} \times 0.0174 = 0.0505$$

$$Pr(X = 3) = \frac{5.8}{3} \times 0.0505 = 0.0976$$

$$Pr(X = 4) = \frac{5.8}{4} \times 0.0976 = 0.1415$$

$$Pr(X = 5) = \frac{5.8}{5} \times 0.1415 = 0.1641$$

$$Pr(X = 6) = \frac{5.8}{6} \times 0.1641 = 0.1586$$

Thus,

$$Pr(X \geqslant 7) = 1 - Pr(X \leqslant 6)$$

$$= 1 - (0.0030 + \cdots + 0.1586)$$

$$= 1 - 0.6327 = 0.3673$$

Clearly, the observed number of cancer deaths is not excessive in this group.    ∎

# ■ 4.13 POISSON APPROXIMATION TO THE BINOMIAL DISTRIBUTION

We have seen in the preceding section that the Poisson distribution appears to fit well in some applications. Another important use for the Poisson distribution is as an approximation to the binomial distribution. Consider the binomial distribution for large $n$ and small $p$. The mean of this distribution is given by $np$ and the variance by $npq$. We note that $q \approx$ (is approximately equal to) 1 for small $p$, and thus $npq \approx np$. Therefore, the mean and variance of the binomial distribution are almost equal in this case, which suggests the following rule:

| 4.11 | **Poisson Approximation to the Binomial Distribution** |

The binomial distribution with large $n$ and small $p$ can be accurately approximated by a Poisson distribution with parameter $\mu = np$.

The rationale for using this approximation is that the Poisson distribution is easier to work with than the binomial distribution. The binomial distribution involves expressions such as $\binom{n}{k}$ and $(1 - p)^{n-k}$, which are cumbersome for large $n$.

_Example 4.35_    **_Cancer, Genetics_** Suppose we are interested in the genetic susceptibility to breast cancer. We find that 4 out of 1000 women aged 40–49 whose mothers have had breast cancer develop breast cancer over the next year of life. We would expect from large population studies that 1 in 1000 women of this age group will develop a new case of the disease over this period of time. How unusual is this event?

_Solution_    We could compute the exact binomial probability

$$Pr(X \geqslant 4) = 1 - Pr(X \leqslant 3)$$

$$= 1 - \left[\binom{1000}{0}(0.001)^0(0.999)^{1000} + \binom{1000}{1}(0.001)^1(0.999)^{999}\right.$$

$$\left. + \binom{1000}{2}(0.001)^2(0.999)^{998} + \binom{1000}{3}(0.001)^3(0.999)^{997}\right]$$

Instead, we use the Poisson approximation with $\lambda = 1000(0.001) = 1$, which is obtained as follows:

$$Pr(X \geqslant 4) = 1 - [Pr(0) + Pr(1) + Pr(2) + Pr(3)]$$

Using Table 2 under the $\mu = 1.0$ column, we find that

$$Pr(0) = 0.3679$$

$$Pr(1) = 0.3679$$

$$Pr(2) = 0.1839$$

$$Pr(3) = 0.0613$$

Thus,

$$Pr(X \geqslant 4) = 1 - (0.3679 + 0.3679 + 0.1839 + 0.0613)$$

$$= 1 - 0.9810 = 0.0190$$

This event is indeed unusual and suggests a genetic susceptibility to breast cancer among female offspring of women who have had breast cancer.    ∎

How large should $n$ be or how small should $p$ be before the approximation is "adequate"? A conservative rule is to use the approximation when $n \geqslant 100$ and $p \leqslant 0.01$. As an example we give the exact binomial probability and the Poisson approximation for $n = 100$, $p = 0.01$, $k = 0, 1, 2, 3, 4, 5$ in Table 4.8. The two probability distributions agree to within 0.002 in all instances.

**Table 4.8**

_An example of the Poisson approximation to the binomial distribution for_ $n = 100$, $p = 0.01$, $k = 0, 1, \ldots, 5$

| $k$ | Exact binomial probability | Poisson approximation | $k$ | Exact binomial probability | Poisson approximation |
|---|---|---|---|---|---|
| 0 | 0.366 | 0.368 | 3 | 0.061 | 0.061 |
| 1 | 0.370 | 0.368 | 4 | 0.015 | 0.015 |
| 2 | 0.185 | 0.184 | 5 | 0.003 | 0.003 |

## ■ 4.14   SUMMARY

In this chapter we learned about **random variables** and distinguished between **discrete** and **continuous** random variables. We focused in detail on specific attributes of random variables, including the notions of **probability mass function** (or **probability distribution**), **cumulative distribution function, expected value,** and **variance**. These notions were shown to be related to similar concepts for finite samples, which we discussed in Chapter 2. In particular, we noted that the sample frequency distribution is a sample realization of a probability distribution, whereas the sample mean ($\bar{x}$) and variance ($s^2$) are sample analogues of the expected value and variance, respectively, of a random variable. We will explore the relationship between attributes of probability models and finite samples in more detail in Chapter 6.

Finally, we introduced some specific probability models focusing in depth on the **binomial** and **Poisson** distributions. The binomial distribution was shown to be applicable if we have a binary outcome, that is, only two possible outcomes. We label these two outcomes as success and failure, where the probability of success is the same for each trial. The Poisson distribution is a classic model used to describe the distribution of rare events.

We will continue our study of probability models in Chapter 5, focusing on continuous random variables.

# Problems

Using the data in Problem 3.21, let $X$ be the random variable representing the number of adults with influenza.

**4.1** What is the probability mass function for this random variable?

**4.2** What is its expected value?

**4.3** What is its variance?

**4.4** What is the cumulative distribution function?

Let $X$ be the random variable representing the number of hypertensive adults in Example 3.13.

**4.5** Derive the probability mass function for $X$.

**4.6** What is its expected value?

**4.7** What is its variance?

**4.8** What is the cumulative distribution function?

Refer to Example 3.15. Let $Y$ be a random variable representing the number of doctors who diagnose a patient as positive for syphilis.

**4.9** What is the probability mass function for $Y$?

**4.10** What is its expected value?

**4.11** What is its variance?

**4.12** What is the cumulative distribution function?

Suppose we wish to check the accuracy of self-reported diagnoses of angina by getting further medical records on a subset of the cases.

**4.13** If we have 50 reported cases of angina and we wish to select 5 for further review, then how many ways can we select these cases if the order of selection matters?

**4.14** Answer Problem 4.13 if the order of selection does not matter.

**4.15** Evaluate the number of ways of selecting 4 objects out of 10 if the order of selection matters.

**4.16** Evaluate the number of ways of selecting 4 objects out of 10 if the order of selection does *not* matter. What term is used to denote this quantity?

**4.17** Evaluate $_{10}C_0, _{10}C_1, \ldots, _{10}C_{10}$.

**4.18** Evaluate 9!

Suppose that the probability that a person will develop hypertension over a lifetime is 20%.

**4.19** What is the probability distribution of the number of hypertensives over a lifetime among 20 students graduating from the same high school class?

**4.20** Suppose that 6 out of 15 students in a grade school class develop influenza, whereas nationwide 20% of grade school students develop influenza. Is there evidence of an excessive number of cases in the class? That is, what is the probability of obtaining at least 6 cases in this class if the nationwide rate holds true.

**4.21** What is the expected number of students in the class who will develop influenza?

Refer to Example 4.16.

**4.22** What is the probability that exactly 4 persons out of 50 aged 60–64 will die after receiving flu vaccine if the probability that 1 person will die is 0.028?

**4.23** What is the probability that at least 4 persons will die after receiving the vaccine?

**4.24** What is the expected number of deaths following the flu vaccine?

**4.25** What is the standard deviation of the number of deaths following the flu vaccine?

**4.26** What is the probability of obtaining exactly 6 events for a Poisson distribution with parameter $\mu = 4.0$?

**4.27** What is the probability of obtaining at least 6 events for a Poisson distribution with parameter $\mu = 4.0$?

**4.28** What is the expected value and variance for a Poisson distribution with parameter $\mu = 4.0$?

## Occupational Health

Many investigators have suspected that workers in the tire industry have an unusual incidence of cancer.

**4.29** Suppose the expected number of deaths due to bladder cancer for all workers in a tire plant on January 1, 1964, over the next 20 years (1/1/64–12/31/83) based on U.S. mortality rates is 1.8. If the Poisson distribution is assumed to hold and there are 6 reported deaths due to bladder cancer among the tire workers, then how unusual is this event?

**4.30** Suppose a similar analysis is done for stomach cancer. In this plant 4 deaths due to stomach cancer are observed for the workers, whereas 2.5 are expected based on U.S. mortality rates. How unusual is this event?

## Cardiovascular Disease

The rate of myocardial infarction (MI) in 50–59-year-old, disease-free women is approximately 2 per 1000 per year or 10 per 1000 over 5 years. Suppose that 3 MI's are reported over 5 years among 1000 women initially disease-free who have been taking postmenopausal hormones.

**4.31** Use the binomial distribution to see if this experience represents an unusually small number of events based on the overall rate.

**4.32** Answer Problem 4.31 using the Poisson approximation to the binomial distribution.

**4.33** Compare your answers in Problems 4.31 and 4.32.

### Infectious Disease

One hypothesis is that gonorrhea tends to cluster in central cities.

**4.34** Suppose that 10 gonorrhea cases are reported over a 3-month period among 10,000 persons living in an urban county. The statewide incidence of gonorrhea is 50 per 100,000 over this period. Is the number of gonorrhea cases in this county unusual for this time period?

### Cardiovascular Disease

**4.35** A new hypothesis in the etiology of heart disease is that aspirin intake of 325 mg per day reduces subsequent cardiovascular mortality in men with a prior heart attack. Suppose that in a pilot study of 50 men who received 1 tablet per day (325 mg), only 2 die over a 3-year period from cardiovascular disease. How likely is it that not more than 2 men will die if the underlying 3-year mortality rate is 10% in such men?

### Otolaryngology

Suppose we assume that the number of episodes per year of otitis media, a common disease of the middle ear in early childhood, follows a Poisson distribution with parameter $\lambda = 1.6$.

**4.36** Find the probability of getting 3 or more episodes of otitis media in the first 2 years of life.

**4.37** Find the probability of not getting any episodes of otitis media in the first year of life.

An interesting question in pediatrics is whether the tendency for children to have many episodes of otitis media is inherited in a family.

**4.38** What is the probability that 2 siblings will both have 3 or more episodes of otitis media in the first 2 years of life?

**4.39** What is the probability that exactly 1 of the siblings will have 3 or more episodes in the first 2 years of life?

**4.40** What is the probability that neither sibling will have 3 or more episodes in the first 2 years of life?

**4.41** What is the expected number of siblings in a 2-sibling family that will have 3 or more episodes in the first 2 years of life?

### Pediatrics

A hospital administrator wants to construct a special-care nursery for low-birthweight infants ($\leqslant 2500$ g) and wants to have some idea as to the number of beds she should allocate to the nursery. She is willing to assume that the recovery period of each baby is exactly 4 days and thus is interested in the expected number of premature births over the period.

**4.42** If the number of premature births in any 4-day period is binomially distributed with parameters $n = 25$ and $p = 0.1$, then find the probability of 0, 1, 2, . . . , 7 premature births over this period.

**4.43** The administrator wishes to allocate $x$ beds where the probability of having more than $x$ premature births over a 4-day period is less than 5%. What should $x$ be?

**4.44** Answer Problem 4.43 for 1%.

### Hypertension

Hypertension has often been claimed to have a "familial aggregation." That is, if 1 person in a family is hypertensive, then his or her siblings are more likely to be hypertensive. Suppose that the prevalence of hypertension among 50–59 year olds in the general population is 18%. Suppose we identify sibships of size 3 in a community where all members of the sibship are 50–59 years old.

**4.45** What is the probability that 0, 1, 2, or 3 hypertensives will be identified in such sibships if the hypertensive status of 2 siblings in the same family are independent events?

**4.46** Suppose that among 25 sibships of this type, 5 have at least 2 affected siblings. How does this situation agree with the independence assumption in Problem 4.45?

### Cancer

The incidence rate of malignant melanoma is suspected to be increasing over time. To document this rate change, a mail questionnaire was sent to 100,000 American nurses in 1976 and 1978, asking about any current or previous tumors. Thirty new cases of malignant melanoma were found to have developed over the 2-year period among women with no previous cancers in 1976.

**4.47** If the annual incidence rate from cancer registry

data is 10 per 100,000, then what is the expected number of new cases over 2 years?

**4.48** Do the preceding results agree or disagree with the cancer registry data? Specifically, what is the probability of observing at least 30 new cases over a 2-year period if the cancer registry incidence rate is correct?

### Environmental Health, Obstetrics
Suppose that the rate of major congenital malformations in the general population is 2.5 per 100 deliveries. A study is set up to investigate if the offspring of Vietnam veteran fathers are at special risk of having congenital malformations.

**4.49** If 100 infants are identified in a birth registry as being offspring of a Vietnam veteran father and 4 have a major congenital malformation, then is there an excess risk of malformations in this group?

Using these same birth registry data, let us look at the effect of maternal use of marijuana on the rate of major congenital malformations.

**4.50** Of 75 offspring of mothers who used marijuana, 8 are found to have a major congenital malformation. Is there an excess risk of malformations in this group?

### Accident Epidemiology
Suppose the annual number of traffic fatalities at a given intersection follows a Poisson distribution with parameter $\mu = 10$.

**4.51** What is the probability of observing exactly 10 traffic fatalities in 1984?

**4.52** What is the probability of observing exactly 25 traffic fatalities over the 2-year period from January 1, 1984, to December 31, 1985?

**4.53** Suppose that the traffic intersection is redesigned with better lighting, and 12 traffic fatalities are observed over the next 2 years. Is this rate a meaningful improvement over the previous rate of traffic fatalities?

### Hypertension
A recent national study found that treating people appropriately for high blood pressure reduced their overall mortality by 20%. Treating people adequately for hypertension has been difficult, since it is estimated that 50% of the hypertensives do not know they have high blood pressure; 50% of those that do know are inadequately treated by their physicians; and 50% that are appropriately treated fail to comply with this treatment by taking the appropriate number of pills.

**4.54** What is the probability that among 10 true hyper-

tensives at least 50% are being treated appropriately and are complying with this treatment?

**4.55** What is the probability that at least 7 of the 10 hypertensives know they have high blood pressure?

**4.56** If the preceding 50% rates were decreased to 40% by a massive education program, then what effect would this rate change have on the overall mortality rate among true hypertensives?

### Pulmonary Disease, Environmental Health
Suppose the number of people seen for violent asthma attacks in the emergency ward of a hospital over a 1-day period is usually Poisson distributed with parameter $\lambda = 1.5$.

**4.57** What is the probability of observing 5 or more cases over a 2-day period?

On a particular 2-day period, the air pollution levels increase dramatically and the distribution of attacks over a 1-day period is now estimated to be Poisson distributed with parameter $\lambda = 3$.

**4.58** Answer Problem 4.57 under these assumptions.

**4.59** If 10 days out of every year are high-pollution days, what is the expected number of asthma cases seen in the emergency ward over a 1-year period?

### Renal Disease
The presence of bacteria in a urine sample (bacteriuria) is sometimes associated with symptoms of kidney disease in women. Suppose we assume that a determination of bacteriuria has been made over a large population of women at one point in time and that 5% of those sampled are positive for bacteriuria.

**4.60** If we selected a sample of size 5 from this population, what would be the probability that 1 or more women would be positive for bacteriuria?

**4.61** Suppose we sample 100 women from this population. What is the probability that 3 or more women would be positive for bacteriuria?

One interesting phenomenon of bacteriuria is that there is a "turnover"; that is, if we measure bacteriuria on the same woman at 2 different points in time, then we do not necessarily get the same result. Let us assume that $\frac{1}{5}$ of all women who are bacteriuric at time 0 are again bacteriuric at time 1 (1 year later), whereas only 4.2% of women who were not bacteriuric at time 0 *are* bacteriuric at time 1. Let $X$ be the random variable representing the number of bacteriuric events over the 2 time periods for 1 woman and let us still assume that the probability that a woman will be positive for bacteriuria at any one exam is 5%.

**4.62** What is the probability distribution of $X$?

**4.63** What is the mean of $X$?

**4.64** What is the variance of $X$?

## Demography

The dataset enumerated in Table 4.9 is an example of current life table data for males living in the United States in 1960 [3]. $P_x$ represents the probability of living for the next year given that one is currently $x$ years old. The $\ell_x$ column is obtained from the formula

$$\ell_0 = 100{,}000 \qquad \ell_x = \ell_0 \times P_0 \times P_1 \times \cdots \times P_{x-1},$$

$$x = 1, 2, \ldots, 100$$

Let us assume that the *current* death rates hold not only for the year 1960 but for all the subsequent years as well.

**4.65** What is the probability of living to age 65 given that one is 21 in 1960?

**4.66** What is the probability of dying exactly between the ages of 56 and 57 given that one is 21 in 1960?

**4.67** Suppose 100 persons of age 21 in 1960 live in a particular town and that 5 of them die before reaching the age of 30. Is this event unusual? Specifically, how likely are 5 or more persons to die before reaching the age of 30?

**4.68** What is the probability distribution and expected value of the lifetime of a person who is age 80 in 1960?

**4.69** Suppose we are not willing to assume that the $P_x$'s remain constant in years subsequent to 1960. Can we still answer Problems 4.65 through 4.68? If not, what additional information do we need?

## Pediatrics, Otolaryngology

Otitis media is a disease that occurs frequently in the first few years of life and is one of the most common reasons for physician visits after the routine check-up.

**Table 4.9** *Current life table for U.S. males in 1960*

| $x$ | $\ell_x$ | $x$ | $\ell_x$ | $x$ | $\ell_x$ | $x$ | $\ell_x$ |
|---|---|---|---|---|---|---|---|
| 0 | 100,000 | 25 | 94,631 | 50 | 86,199 | 75 | 38,950 |
| 1 | 97,087 | 26 | 94,466 | 51 | 85,325 | 76 | 36,210 |
| 2 | 96,911 | 27 | 94,306 | 52 | 84,369 | 77 | 33,468 |
| 3 | 96,800 | 28 | 94,148 | 53 | 83,333 | 78 | 30,732 |
| 4 | 96,714 | 29 | 93,990 | 54 | 82,222 | 79 | 28,006 |
| 5 | 96,643 | 30 | 93,826 | 55 | 81,039 | 80 | 25,300 |
| 6 | 96,580 | 31 | 93,656 | 56 | 79,783 | 81 | 22,619 |
| 7 | 96,522 | 32 | 93,479 | 57 | 78,451 | 82 | 19,983 |
| 8 | 96,469 | 33 | 93,293 | 58 | 77,032 | 83 | 17,439 |
| 9 | 96,420 | 34 | 93,097 | 59 | 75,513 | 84 | 15,045 |
| 10 | 96,375 | 35 | 92,889 | 60 | 73,887 | 85 | 12,845 |
| 11 | 96,333 | 36 | 92,666 | 61 | 72,151 | 86 | 10,819 |
| 12 | 96,290 | 37 | 92,426 | 62 | 70,308 | 87 | 8980 |
| 13 | 96,242 | 38 | 92,166 | 63 | 68,361 | 88 | 7333 |
| 14 | 96,182 | 39 | 91,883 | 64 | 66,316 | 89 | 5876 |
| 15 | 96,107 | 40 | 91,572 | 65 | 64,177 | 90 | 4609 |
| 16 | 96,014 | 41 | 91,230 | 66 | 61,947 | 91 | 3534 |
| 17 | 95,905 | 42 | 90,854 | 67 | 59,631 | 92 | 2648 |
| 18 | 95,779 | 43 | 90,441 | 68 | 57,235 | 93 | 1939 |
| 19 | 95,641 | 44 | 89,988 | 69 | 54,770 | 94 | 1387 |
| 20 | 95,491 | 45 | 89,492 | 70 | 52,244 | 95 | 970 |
| 21 | 95,330 | 46 | 88,950 | 71 | 49,665 | 96 | 665 |
| 22 | 95,158 | 47 | 88,359 | 72 | 47,040 | 97 | 446 |
| 23 | 94,981 | 48 | 87,709 | 73 | 44,375 | 98 | 293 |
| 24 | 94,803 | 49 | 86,992 | 74 | 41,676 | 99 | 187 |
|  |  |  |  |  |  | 100 | 0 |

**Table 4.10** *Number of infants (out of 2500) who remain disease-free at the end of each month during the first year of life*

| i | Disease-free infants at the end of month i |
|---|---|
| 00 | 2500 |
| 1 | 2425 |
| 2 | 2375 |
| 3 | 2300 |
| 4 | 2180 |
| 5 | 2000 |
| 6 | 1875 |
| 7 | 1700 |
| 8 | 1500 |
| 9 | 1300 |
| 10 | 1250 |
| 11 | 1225 |
| 12 | 1200 |

A study was conducted to assess the frequency of otitis media in the general population in the first year of life. Table 4.10 gives the number of infants out of 2500 infants who were first seen at birth and who remained disease-free by the end of the $i$th month of life, $i = 0, 1, \ldots, 12$. (*Assume that no infants have been lost to follow-up.*)

**4.70** What is the probability that an infant will have 1 or more episodes of otitis media by the end of the 6th month of life? the first year of life?

**4.71** What is the probability that an infant will have 1 or more episodes of otitis media by the end of the 9th month of life given that no episodes have been observed by the end of the 3rd month of life?

**4.72** Suppose we define an "otitis prone family" as one where at least 3 siblings out of 5 develop otitis media in the first 6 months of life. What proportion of 5-sibling families are otitis prone if we assume that the disease occurs independently for different siblings in a family?

**4.73** What is the expected number of otitis prone families out of 100 5-sibling families?

## Pulmonary Disease

Each year approximately 4% of current smokers attempt to quit smoking, and 50% of those who try to quit are successful in the sense that they abstain from smoking for at least 1 year from the date they quit.

**4.74** What is the probability that a current smoker will quit for at least 1 year?

**4.75** What is the probability that among 100 current smokers, at least 5 will quit smoking for at least 1 year?

An educational program was conducted among smokers who attempt to quit to maximize the likelihood that such individuals would continue to abstain for the long term.

**4.76** Suppose that of 20 people who enter the program when they first stop smoking, 15 will abstain from smoking 1 year later. Can the program be considered successful?

## Cancer, Epidemiology

A frequent design for biomedical investigations is the case-control study. A group of **cases** is isolated on the basis of having a particular disease (such as lung cancer patients on a medical register), and a group of **controls** is chosen (e.g., patients on the same register with cancer of the esophagus) such that every case is *matched* with 1 or more controls. That is, the case and control(s) are matched in every sense except that the controls do not have the disease trait. We can then look at whether or not some other factor (such as smoking) is associated with the disease trait. Obtaining "exact" matches is usually impossible, and we select several characteristics to use for matching, such as age and sex. Suppose the group of cases and controls is as given in Table 4.11.

Suppose that the match is performed so that each control has the same age group and sex as its corresponding case. An example of a 1-to-1 match would be

| Case number | 1 | 2 | 3 | 4 | 5 |
|---|---|---|---|---|---|
| Control number | 24 | 51 | 18 | 14 | 22 |

An example of a 2-to-1 match would be

| Case number | 1 | 2 | 3 | 4 | 5 |
|---|---|---|---|---|---|
| Control number | 24, 26 | 51, 49 | 18, 21 | 14, 06 | 22, 27 |

Assume that the order within each group of matched controls in a many-to-one matching does not matter.

**4.77** How many ways can 1-to-1 matches be assigned for age and sex?

**4.78** Suppose the designers of the study get lazy and

match only for age. How many ways can this matching be done?

**4.79** If the groups were matched only on age, then what is the probability that the groups will be matched for sex as well if each match is equally likely?

**4.80** Answer Problem 4.77 for 2-to-1 matches.

**4.81** Answer Problem 4.78 for 2-to-1 matches.

**4.82** Answer Problem 4.79 for 2-to-1 matches.

**4.83** Answer Problem 4.77 for 3-to-1 matches.

**4.84** Answer Problem 4.78 for 3-to-1 matches.

**4.85** Answer Problem 4.79 for 3-to-1 matches.

An experiment is designed to test the potency of a drug on 20 rats. Previous animal studies have shown that a 10-mg dose of the drug is lethal 5% of the time within the first 4 hours; of the animals alive at 4 hours, 10% will die in the next 4 hours.

**4.86** What is the probability that 3 or more rats will die in the first 4 hours?

**4.87** Suppose 2 rats die in the first 4 hours. What is the probability that 2 or fewer rats will die in the next 4 hours?

**4.88** What is the probability that 0 rats will die in the 8-hour period?

**4.89** What is the probability that 1 rat will die in the 8-hour period?

**4.90** What is the probability that 2 rats will die in the 8-hour period?

**4.91** Can you write a general formula for the probability that $x$ rats will die in the 8-hour period? Evaluate this formula for $x = 0, 1, \ldots, 10$. (Do not do this computation by hand. Use either a calculator or a computer.)

*Infectious Disease*

An outbreak of acute gastroenteritis occurred at a nursing home in Baltimore, Maryland, in December 1980 [7]. A total of 46 out of 98 residents of the nursing home became ill. Persons living in the nursing home shared rooms: 13 rooms contained 2 occupants, 4 rooms contained 3 occupants, and 15 rooms contained 4 occupants. One question that arises is whether or not a geographical clustering of disease occurred for persons living in the same room.

**4.92** If the binomial distribution holds, what is the probability distribution of the number of affected persons in rooms with 2 occupants? That is, what is the probability of finding 0 affected persons? 1 affected person? 2 affected persons?

**4.93** Answer Problem 4.92 for the probability distribution of the number of affected persons in rooms with 3 occupants.

**4.94** Answer Problem 4.92 for the probability distribution of the number of affected persons in rooms with 4 occupants.

**4.95** One useful summary measure of geographical clustering is the number of rooms with 2 or more affected occupants. If the binomial distribution holds, what is the expected number of rooms with 2 or more affected occupants over the entire nursing home?

**Table 4.11**    *Selection of controls for a case-control study*

| Cases | | | Controls | | | |
|---|---|---|---|---|---|---|
| Case number | Age | Sex | Control number | Age group | Sex | Frequency |
| 1 | 36 | M | 01–15 | 21–30 | M | 15 |
| 2 | 50 | F | 16–21 | 21–30 | F | 6 |
| 3 | 24 | F | 22–27 | 31–40 | M | 6 |
| 4 | 22 | M | 28–45 | 31–40 | F | 18 |
| 5 | 35 | M | 46–48 | 41–50 | M | 3 |
| | | | 49–54 | 41–50 | F | 6 |
| | | | 55–66 | 51–60 | M | 12 |
| | | | 67–69 | 51–60 | F | 3 |
| | | | 70–78 | 61–70 | M | 9 |
| | | | 79–84 | 61–70 | F | 6 |

_Table 4.12_ Number of affected persons and total number of persons in a room for
an outbreak of acute gastroenteritis in a nursing home in Baltimore, Maryland

| Persons in room | Total number of rooms | Number of rooms with | | | | |
|---|---|---|---|---|---|---|
| | | 0 affected persons | 1 affected person | 2 affected persons | 3 affected persons | 4 affected persons |
| 2 | 13 | 5 | 4 | 4 | 0 | 0 |
| 3 | 4 | 1 | 2 | 0 | 1 | 0 |
| 4 | 15 | 2 | 4 | 3 | 5 | 1 |

(Reprinted with permission of the _American Journal of Epidemiology_ **116(6)**: 940–948, 1982.)

A summary of the number of affected persons and the total number of persons in a room is given in Table 4.12.

_4.96_ Compare the observed number of rooms with 2 or more affected occupants with the expected number of rooms with 4 persons in a room. Does this comparison give any evidence that clustering of disease occurs within rooms?

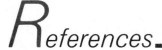

# References

[1] _Boston Globe_, October 7, 1980.

[2] Rinsky, R. A., Zumwalde, R. O., Waxweiler, R. J., Murray, W. E., Bierbaum, P. J., Landrigan, P. J., Terpilak, M., and Cox, C. (1981) "Cancer Mortality at a Naval Nuclear Shipyard." _The Lancet_, January 31: 231–235.

[3] _United States Life Tables_: 1959–1961, _Life Tables_: 1956–1961 **1 (1)**. U.S. Department of Health, Education, and Welfare, 1964.

[4] _Monthly Vital Statistics Report, Annual Summary for the United States_ (1973) National Center for Health Statistics, **22 (13)** June 27, 1974.

[5] _Monthly Vital Statistics Report, Annual Summary for the United States_ (1977) National Center for Health Statistics, **26 (13)** December 7, 1978.

[6] Ott, M. G. Scharnweber, H. C., and Langner, R. (1980) "Mortality Experience of 161 Employees Exposed to Ethylene Dibromide in Two Production Units," _British Journal of Industrial Medicine_ **37**: 163–168.

[7] Kaplan, J. E., Schonberger, L. B., Varano, G., Jackman, N., Bied, J., and Gary, G. W. (1982) "An Outbreak of Acute Nonbacterial Gastroenteritis in a Nursing Home: Demonstration of Person-to-Person Transmission by Temporal Clustering of Cases," _American Journal of Epidemiology_ **116(6)**: 940–948.

# 5 Continuous Probability Distributions

## ■ 5.1 INTRODUCTION

In this chapter we discuss continuous probability distributions. In particular, we will be discussing the normal distribution, which is the most widely used distribution in statistical work.

The normal, or Gaussian or "bell-shaped," distribution is the cornerstone of most of the methods of estimation and hypothesis testing that are developed in the rest of this text. Many random variables, such as the distribution of birthweights or blood pressures in the general population, tend to approximately follow a normal distribution. In addition, many random variables that are not themselves normal are closely approximated by a normal distribution when summed many times. In such cases use of the normal distribution is desirable, since tables for the normal distribution are more widely available than those for many other distributions.

*Example 5.1*　　*Infectious Disease* The number of neutrophils in a sample of 2 white blood cells is not normally distributed, but the number in a sample of 100 white blood cells is very close to being normally distributed. ■

## ■ 5.2 GENERAL CONCEPTS

We want to develop an analogue for a continuous random variable to the concept of a probability mass function, which we developed for a discrete random variable (Section 4.3). Thus, we would like to know which values are more probable than others and how probable they are.

*Example 5.2*　　*Hypertension* Suppose we consider the distribution of diastolic blood pressure measurements in 35–44-year-old men. In actual practice this distribution is discrete because only a finite number of blood pressure values are possible, since the measurement is only accurate to within 2 mm or in some cases 5 mm. However, we will assume that there is no measurement error and hence the random variable can take on a continuum of possible values. One consequence of this assumption is that the probabilities of specific blood pressure measurement values such as 117.3 are 0 and, thus, we cannot use the concept of a probability mass function. Instead, we speak in terms of the probability that blood pressure falls within a range of values. Thus, the probabilities of blood pressures (denoted by $X$) falling in the ranges of $90 \leq X < 95$, $95 \leq X < 100$, and $X \geq 100$ might be 15%, 5%, and 2%, respectively. We might denote persons whose blood pressures fell in these ranges as borderline, mild hypertensive, and severe hypertensive, respectively. ∎

Although the probability of exactly obtaining any value is 0, we still have the intuitive notion that certain ranges of values occur more frequently than others. This notion can be quantified using the concept of a probability density function.

**Definition 5.1** _____

The **probability density function** of the random variable $X$ is a curve such that the area under the curve between any two points $a$ and $b$ is equal to the probability that the random variable $X$ falls between $a$ and $b$. Thus, the total area under the curve over the possible range of values for the random variable is 1. ∎

The probability density function will take on high values in regions of high probability and low values in regions of low probability.

**Example 5.3**   *Hypertension*   The probability density function for diastolic blood pressure in 35–44-year-old men is given in Figure 5.1. Areas *A*, *B*, and *C* correspond to the probabilities of being borderline, mild hypertensive, and severe hypertensive, respectively. Furthermore, the most likely range of values for diastolic blood pressure occurs around 80 mm, with the values becoming increasingly unlikely as we move further away from 80. ∎

The cumulative distribution function is defined similarly to that for a discrete random variable (Section 4.6).

**Definition 5.2** _____

The **cumulative distribution function** for the random variable $X$ evaluated at the point $a$ is defined as the probability that $X$ will take on values $\leq a$. It is represented by the area under the probability density function to the left of $a$. ∎

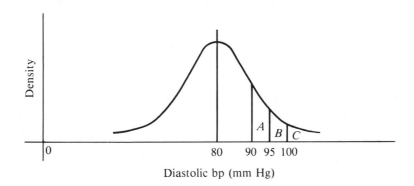

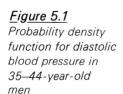

**Figure 5.1**
*Probability density function for diastolic blood pressure in 35–44-year-old men*

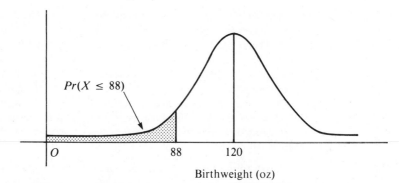

**Figure 5.2**
Cumulative
distribution function
evaluated at 88 oz
for the distribution
of birthweights in
the general
population

$Pr(X \leq 88)$

Birthweight (oz)

**Example 5.4**   **Obstetrics** The probability density function for the random variable representing the distribution of birthweights (oz) in the general population is given in Figure 5.2. The cumulative distribution function evaluated at 88 oz $= Pr(X \leq 88)$ is represented by the area under this curve to the left of 88 oz. The region $X \leq 88$ oz has a special meaning in obstetrics, since 88 oz is the cutoff point usually used by obstetricians for identifying low-birthweight infants. Such infants are generally at higher risk for various unfavorable outcomes, such as mortality in the first year of life. ∙   ∎

The expected value and variance for continuous random variables have the same meaning as for discrete random variables (Sections 4.4 and 4.5). However, the mathematical definition of these terms is beyond the scope of this book.

**Definition 5.3**

The **expected value** $\equiv E(X) \equiv \mu$ of a continuous random variable $X$ is the average value acquired by the random variable.   ∎

**Definition 5.4**

The **variance** $\equiv Var(X) \equiv \sigma^2$ of a continuous random variable $X$ is the average squared distance of each value of the random variable from its expected value. The standard deviation $\equiv sd(X) \equiv \sigma$ is the $\sqrt{\text{variance}}$.   ∎

**Example 5.5**   **Hypertension** The expected value and standard deviation of the distribution of diastolic blood pressures in 35–44-year-old men are 80 mm and 12 mm, respectively.   ∎

# ∎ 5.3 THE NORMAL DISTRIBUTION

We will now discuss the most widely used continuous distribution—the normal distribution. This distribution is also frequently referred to as the Gaussian distribution after the well-known mathematician Gauss.

**Example 5.6**   **Hypertension** The distribution of body weights or of diastolic blood pressures for a group of 35–44-year-old males will follow a normal distribution. So will the distribution of tree diameters of a certain species of tree from some defined forest area.   ∎

Many other distributions that are not themselves normal can be made normal upon transforming the data onto a different scale.

*Example 5.7*    ***Cardiovascular Disease*** The distribution of serum triglyceride concentrations from this same group of 35–44-year-old males is likely to be positively skewed. However, the log transformation of these measurements will usually follow a normal distribution.  ■

Generally speaking, any random variable that can be expressed as a sum of many other random variables can be well approximated by a normal distribution.

*Example 5.8*    ***Infectious Disease*** The distribution of the number of lymphocytes in a differential of 100 white blood cells (refer to Example 4.15 for the definition of a differential) will tend to be normally distributed, since this random variable is a sum of 100 random variables, each representing whether or not an individual cell is a lymphocyte.  ■

Thus, because of its omnipresence, the normal distribution is vital to statistical work, and most of the estimation procedures and hypothesis tests that we will propose are based on the assumption that the random variable we are considering has an underlying normal distribution.

Another important area of application of the normal distribution is as an approximating distribution to other distributions. The normal distribution is generally more convenient to work with than any other distribution is, particularly regarding hypothesis testing. Thus, if we can find an accurate normal approximation to some other distribution, we will be eager to use it.

**Definition 5.5**

We will define the **normal distribution** by its **probability density function**, which is given as follows:

$$f(x) = [1/(\sqrt{2\pi}\sigma)] \exp\left[-\frac{1}{2\sigma^2}(x - \mu)^2\right], \qquad -\infty < x < \infty$$

for some parameters $\mu$, $\sigma$, where $\sigma > 0$.  ■

The exp function merely implies that the quantity to the right in brackets is raised to the "*e*" power. A plot of this probability density function is given in Figure 5.3.

The density function follows a bell-shaped curve, with the most frequently occurring value at $\mu$. The curve is symmetric about $\mu$, with points of inflection on

*Figure 5.3*
*Probability density function for a normal distribution with mean $\mu$ and variance $\sigma^2$*

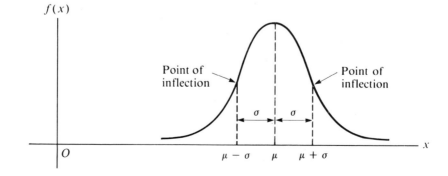

each side of $\mu$ at $\mu - \sigma$ and $\mu + \sigma$, respectively. A point of inflection is a point where the slope of the curve changes direction. In Figure 5.3 the slope of the curve increases to the left of $\mu - \sigma$ and then starts to decrease to the right of $\mu - \sigma$ and continues to decrease until reaching $\mu + \sigma$, after which it starts increasing again. Thus, the distances from $\mu$ to the points of inflection provide a good visual sense of the magnitude of the parameter $\sigma$.

You may wonder why we have used the parameters $\mu$ and $\sigma^2$ in defining the normal distribution when we have formerly defined the expected value and variance of an arbitrary distribution as $\mu$ and $\sigma^2$. Indeed, we can show from the definition of the normal distribution that $\mu$ and $\sigma^2$ are, respectively, the expected value and variance of this distribution.

*Example 5.9*    For diastolic blood pressure we might expect $\mu = 80$ mm, $\sigma = 12$ mm; for birthweight we might expect $\mu = 120$ oz, $\sigma = 15$ oz; for tree diameters we might expect $\mu = 8$ in., $\sigma = 2$ in. ∎

Interestingly, the entire shape of the normal distribution is determined by the two parameters $\mu$ and $\sigma^2$. If we compare two normal distributions with the same variance $\sigma^2$ and different means $\mu_1, \mu_2$, where $\mu_2 > \mu_1$, then their density functions will appear as in Figure 5.4.

Similarly, we can compare two normal distributions with the same mean but different variances ($\sigma_2^2 > \sigma_1^2$), which are shown in Figure 5.5. Note that the area under any normal density function must be 1. Thus, the two normal distributions shown in Figure 5.5 must cross, since otherwise one curve would remain completely above the other and the areas under both curves could not simultaneously be 1.

**Definition 5.6**

We will generally refer to a **normal distribution with mean $\mu$ and variance $\sigma^2$** as a $N(\mu, \sigma^2)$ distribution. ∎

Note that the second parameter is always the variance $\sigma^2$ and not the standard deviation $\sigma$.

**Definition 5.7**

We will refer to a normal distribution with mean 0 and variance 1 as a **standard**, or **unit**, normal distribution. This distribution is denoted by $N(0, 1)$. ∎

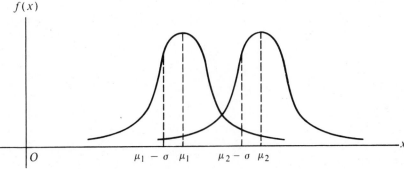

*Figure 5.4*
*Comparison of two normal distributions with the same variance and different means*

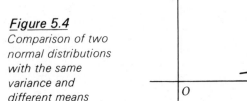

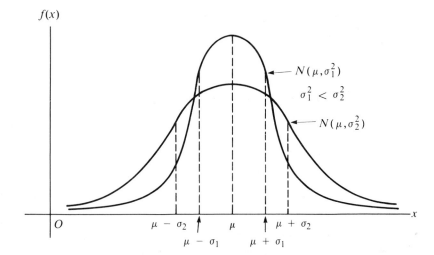

**Figure 5.5**
*Comparison of two normal distributions with the same mean and different variances*

We will see that any information we desire concerning a $N(\mu, \sigma^2)$ can be obtained from appropriate manipulations of a $N(0, 1)$ distribution.

# ■ 5.4 EMPIRICAL AND SYMMETRY PROPERTIES OF THE STANDARD NORMAL DISTRIBUTION

To familiarize ourselves with the $N(0, 1)$ distribution, we will review some of its empirical and symmetry properties. First, the probability density function in this case reduces to

**5.1**
$$f(x) = \frac{1}{\sqrt{2\pi}} e^{(1/2)x^2}, \quad -\infty < x < +\infty$$

This distribution is symmetrical about 0, since $f(x) = f(-x)$, and is depicted in Figure 5.6.

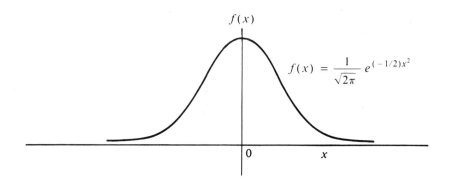

$$f(x) = \frac{1}{\sqrt{2\pi}} e^{(-1/2)x^2}$$

**Figure 5.6**
*Probability density function for a standard normal distribution*

We can show that about 67% of the area under the normal density lies between $+1$ and $-1$, about 95% of the area lies between $+2$ and $-2$, and about 99% lies between $+2.5$ and $-2.5$.

We can express these relationships more precisely by saying that

$$Pr(-1 < X < +1) = 0.6827 \qquad Pr(-1.96 < X < +1.96) = 0.95$$
$$Pr(-2.576 < X < +2.576) = 0.99$$

Thus, the standard normal distribution slopes off very rapidly, and absolute values greater than 3 are unlikely. These relationships are depicted in Figure 5.7.

Tables of the area under the normal density function, or so-called normal tables, take advantage of the symmetry properties of the normal distribution and generally are concerned with areas for positive values of $x$.

### Definition 5.8

We denote the cumulative distribution function for a standard normal distribution by

$$\Phi(x) = Pr(X \leqslant x)$$

where $X$ follows a $N(0, 1)$ distribution. This function is depicted in Figure 5.8.    ■

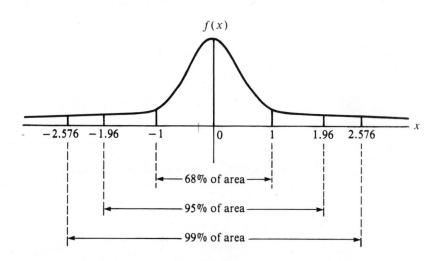

**Figure 5.7**
*Empirical properties of the standard normal distribution*

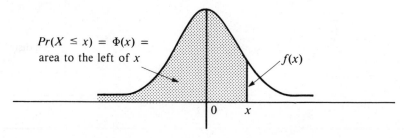

**Figure 5.8**
*Cumulative distribution function ($\Phi(x)$) for a standard normal random variable*

Generally, we will not make a distinction between the probabilities $Pr(X \leqslant x)$ and $Pr(X < x)$ when $X$ follows a normal distribution. The reason is that they represent the same quantity, because the probability of individual values is 0, that is, $Pr(X = x) = 0$.

**Definition 5.9**

We will use the symbol $\sim$ as shorthand for the phrase "**is distributed as**". Thus, $X \sim N(0, 1)$ means that the random variable $X$ is distributed as a $N(0, 1)$ distribution. ∎

## 5.4.1 Use of Normal Tables

Under column A in Table 3 of the appendix, we present $\Phi(x)$ for various positive values of $x$ for a standard normal distribution. We depict this cumulative distribution function in Figure 5.9. Notice that the area to the left of 0 is 0.5. Furthermore, the area to the left of $x$ approaches 0 as $x$ becomes small and approaches 1 as $x$ becomes large.

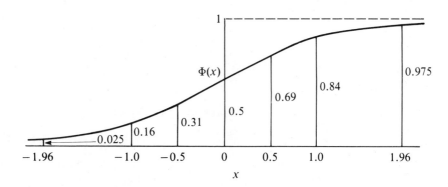

**Figure 5.9**
*Cumulative distribution function for a standard normal distribution ($\Phi(x)$)*

**Example 5.10**    If

$$X \sim N(0, 1)$$

then find

$$Pr(X \leqslant 1.96) \quad \text{and} \quad Pr(X \leqslant 1)$$

**Solution**    From Table 3, column A, we have

$$\Phi(1.96) = 0.975 \quad \text{and} \quad \Phi(1) = 0.8413$$    ∎

**5.2**    **Symmetry Properties of the Standard Normal Distribution**
From the symmetry properties of the standard normal distribution, we have

$$\Phi(-x) = Pr(X \leqslant -x) = Pr(X \geqslant x) = 1 - Pr(X \leqslant x) = 1 - \Phi(x)$$

This symmetry is depicted in Figure 5.10.

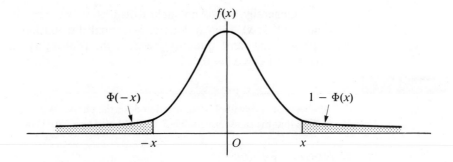

**Figure 5.10**
*Illustration of the
symmetry properties
of the normal
distribution*

The right-hand tail of the standard normal distribution $= Pr(X \geqslant x)$ is provided in column B of Table 3.

**Example 5.11**    Calculate

$$Pr(X \leqslant -1.96)$$

if

$$X \sim N(0, 1)$$

**Solution**

$$Pr(X \leqslant -1.96) = Pr(X \geqslant 1.96)$$

$$= 0.0250 \text{ from column B of Table 3} \qquad \blacksquare$$

Furthermore, for any numbers $a, b$, we have $Pr(a \leqslant X \leqslant b) = Pr(X \leqslant b) - Pr(X \leqslant a)$ and we thus can evaluate $Pr(a \leqslant X \leqslant b)$ for any $a, b$ from Table 3.

**Example 5.12**    Compute

$$Pr(-1 \leqslant X \leqslant 1.5)$$

if

$$X \sim N(0, 1)$$

**Solution**    $$Pr(-1 \leqslant X \leqslant 1.5) = Pr(X \leqslant 1.5) - Pr(X \leqslant -1)$$

$$= Pr(X \leqslant 1.5) - Pr(X \geqslant 1)$$

$$= 0.9332 - 0.1587$$

$$= 0.7745 \qquad \blacksquare$$

**Example 5.13**    **Pulmonary Disease**  Forced Vital Capacity (FVC) is a standard measure of pulmonary function and represents the volume of air a person can expel in 6 seconds. A topic of current research interest is to look at potential risk factors that may affect FVC in grade school children, such as cigarette smoking, air pollution, or the type of stove used in the home. One problem is that pulmonary function is affected by age, sex, and height, and these variables must be corrected for before looking at other risk factors. One way to accomplish these adjustments for a particular child is to find the mean $\mu$ and standard deviation $\sigma$ for the same age (in 1-year age groups), sex, and height (in 2-inch height groups) from large national surveys and compute a so-called **standardized FVC**, which is defined as $(x - \mu)/\sigma$, where $x$ is the original FVC. The standardized FVC would then approximately follow a $N(0, 1)$ distribution. Suppose that a child is considered in poor pulmonary health if his or her standardized FVC $< -1.5$. What percentage of children are in poor pulmonary health?

**Solution**     We want

$$Pr(X < -1.5) = Pr(X > 1.5)$$

$$= 0.0668$$

Thus, about 7% of children are in poor pulmonary health.     ∎

In many instances we will be concerned with tail areas on either side of 0 for a standard normal distribution. For example, the *normal range* for a biological quantity is often defined by a range within $x$ standard deviations of the mean for some specified value of $x$. The probability of a value falling in this range is given by $Pr(-x \leqslant X \leqslant x)$ for a standard normal distribution. This quantity is tabulated in column D of Table 3 for various values of $x$.

**Example 5.14**     **Pulmonary Disease** Suppose a child is considered to have normal lung growth if his or her standardized FVC is within 1.5 standard deviations of the mean. What proportion of children are within the normal range?

**Solution**     We wish to compute $Pr(-1.5 \leqslant X \leqslant 1.5)$. Under 1.50 in Table 3, column D, this quantity is given as 0.8664. Thus, about 87% of children are considered to have normal lung growth using this definition.     ∎

Finally, in column C of Table 3, we provide the area under the standard normal density from 0 to $X = 0.5 \times$ the corresponding entry in column D, since these areas will occasionally prove useful in our work on statistical inference.

**Example 5.15**     Find the area under the standard normal density from 0 to 1.45.

**Solution**     We refer to column C of Table 3 under 1.45. The appropriate area is given by 0.4265.     ∎

Of course, the areas given under columns A, B, C, and D are somewhat redundant in that *all* computations concerning the standard normal distribution could be performed using any one of these columns. In particular, we have seen that $B(x) = 1 - A(x)$. Also, from the symmetry of the normal distribution, we can easily show that $C(x) = A(x) - 0.5$, $D(x) = 2 \cdot C(x) = 2 \cdot A(x) - 1.0$. However, this redundancy is deliberate, since for some applications one or the other of these columns will be more convenient to use.

We will frequently want to refer to the percentiles of a standard normal distribution in our work on statistical inference. For this purpose we introduce the following definition:

**Definition 5.10**

The **100% × pth percentile** of a standard normal distribution is denoted by $z_p$. It is defined by the relationship.

$$Pr(X < z_p) = p, \quad \text{where } X \sim N(0, 1)$$

$z_p$ is depicted graphically in Figure 5.11.

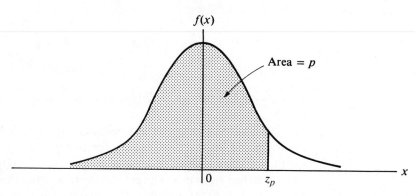

**Figure 5.11**
*Graphical display of the p th percentile of a standard normal distribution ($z_p$)*

**Example 5.16**　Compute

$$z_{.975}, \quad z_{.95}, \quad z_{.5}, \quad \text{and } z_{.025}$$

**Solution**　We have from Table 3 that

$$\Phi(1.96) = 0.975$$

$$\Phi(1.645) = 0.95$$

$$\Phi(0) = 0.5$$

$$\Phi(-1.96) = 1 - \Phi(1.96) = 1 - 0.975 = 0.025$$

Thus,

$$z_{.975} = 1.96$$

$$z_{.95} = 1.645$$

$$z_{.5} = 0$$

$$z_{.025} = -1.96$$

■

# ■ 5.5 *CONVERSION FROM A N($\mu$, $\sigma^2$) DISTRIBUTION TO A N(0, 1) DISTRIBUTION*

**Example 5.17**　*Hypertension* Suppose we define a borderline hypertensive as a person whose diastolic blood pressure is between 90 and 100 mm inclusive, and we assume that we are dealing with 35–44-year-old males whose blood pressures are normally distributed with mean 80 and variance 144. What is the probability that a randomly selected person from this population will be a borderline hypertensive? We can restate this question more precisely as follows: If

$$X \sim N(80, 144)$$

then what is

$$Pr(90 < X < 100)$$

(The solution is given on page 112.) ∎

More generally, we can ask the question: If $X \sim N(\mu, \sigma^2)$, then what is $Pr(a < X < b)$ for any $a, b$? The basic idea is to convert this probability statement about an $N(\mu, \sigma^2)$ distribution to an equivalent probability statement about an $N(0, 1)$ distribution. Let us consider the random variable $Z = (X - \mu)/\sigma$. We can show that the following relationship holds:

**5.3**  If

$$X \sim N(\mu, \sigma^2) \quad \text{and} \quad Z = (X - \mu)/\sigma$$

then $Z \sim N(0, 1)$.

We now wish to convert $Pr(a < X < b)$ into a probability statement about $Z$, since $Z$ is a standard normal random variable and we have tables available only for the standard normal distribution.

We can easily show that $a < X < b$ if and only if $(a - \mu)/\sigma < Z < (b - \mu)/\sigma$. This procedure is known as **standardization of a normal variable**. This fact together with (**5.3**) leads us to the following key relationship:

**5.4**  *Evaluation of Probabilities for Any Normal Distribution via Standardization*

If

$$X \sim N(\mu, \sigma^2) \quad \text{and} \quad Z \sim N(0, 1)$$

then

$$Pr(a < X < b) = Pr\left(\frac{a - \mu}{\sigma} < Z < \frac{b - \mu}{\sigma}\right)$$

$$= \Phi[(b - \mu)/\sigma] - \Phi[(a - \mu)/\sigma]$$

Since the $\Phi$ function, which is the cumulative distribution function for a standard normal distribution, is given in column A of Table 3, we can now evaluate probabilities for *any* normal distribution. This procedure is depicted in Figure 5.12.

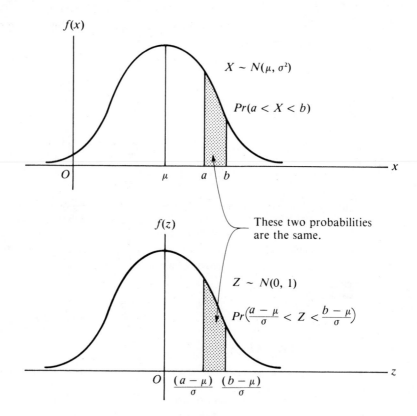

**Figure 5.12**
*Evaluation of
probabilities for any
normal distribution
via standardization*

## Solution to Example 5.17

We now calculate the probability of being a borderline hypertensive among the group of 35–44-year-old males. We have

$$Pr(90 < X < 100) = Pr\left(\frac{90 - 80}{12} < Z < \frac{100 - 80}{12}\right)$$

$$= Pr(0.83 < Z < 1.67)$$

$$= \Phi(1.67) - \Phi(0.83)$$

$$= 0.9525 - 0.7967$$

$$= 0.156$$

Thus, 15.6% of this population will be borderline hypertensive.    ∎

**Example 5.18**  **Botany**  Suppose we assume that tree diameters of a certain species of tree from some defined forest area are normally distributed with mean 8 inches and standard deviation 2 inches. Find the probability of a tree having an unusually large diameter, which we define as $>12$ inches.

**Solution**  We have $X \sim N(8, 4)$ and we require

$$Pr(X > 12) = 1 - Pr(X < 12)$$

$$= 1 - Pr\left(Z < \frac{12 - 8}{2}\right)$$

$$= 1 - Pr(Z < 2.0) = 1 - 0.977$$

$$= 0.023$$

Thus, 2.3% of trees from this area have an unusually large diameter. ∎

The general principle is that for any probability statement concerning normal random variables of the form $Pr(a < X < b)$, we subtract the population mean $\mu$ from each boundary point and divide by the standard deviation $\sigma$ to obtain an equivalent probability statement for the standard normal random variable $Z$,

$$Pr[(a - \mu)/\sigma < Z < (b - \mu)/\sigma]$$

We then use the standard normal tables to evaluate this latter probability.

---

*Example 5.19*

**Cerebrovascular Disease** Making the diagnosis of stroke strictly on the basis of clinical symptoms is difficult. A standard diagnostic test used in clinical medicine for the detection of stroke in patients is the angiogram. This test has some risks for the patient, and several non-invasive techniques have been developed that are hoped to be as effective as the angiogram. One such method utilizes the measurement of cerebral blood flow (CBF) in the brain, since stroke patients tend to have lower levels of CBF than normals. Suppose we assume that in the general population CBF is normally distributed with mean 75 and standard deviation 17. We classify a patient as being at risk for having stroke if his or her CBF is less than 40. What proportion of normal patients will be mistakenly classified as being at risk for stroke?

*Solution*

Let $X$ be the random variable representing CBF. Then $X \sim N(75, 17^2) = N(75, 289)$. We want to find $Pr(X < 40)$. We standardize the limit of 40 so as to use the standard normal distribution. The standardized limit is $(40 - 75)/17 = -2.06$. Thus, if $Z$ represents the standardized normal random variable $= (X - \mu)/\sigma$, then

$$Pr(X < 40) = Pr(Z < -2.06)$$

$$= \Phi(-2.06)$$

$$= 1 - \Phi(2.06) = 1 - 0.9803$$

$$\approx 0.020$$

Thus, about 2.0% of normal patients will be incorrectly classified as being at risk for stroke. ∎

*Example 5.20*

**Ophthalmology** Glaucoma is a disease of the eye that is manifested by high intraocular pressure. The distribution of intraocular pressure in the general population is approximately normal with mean 16 mm and standard deviation 3 mm. If a normal intraocular pressure is considered to be between 12 mm and 20 mm, then what percentage of the general population would fall within this range?

**Solution**

We wish to calculate $Pr(12 \leqslant X \leqslant 20)$, where $X \sim N(16, 9)$. We must first standardize the limits 12 and 20 so as to use the standard normal tables to evaluate this probability. The standardized limits are $(12 - 16)/3 = -1.33$ and $(20 - 16)/3 = +1.33$. Thus, we evaluate $Pr(-1.33 \leqslant Z \leqslant 1.33)$, where $Z$ follows a standard normal distribution. We have

$$Pr(-1.33 \leqslant Z \leqslant 1.33) = Pr(Z \leqslant 1.33) - Pr(Z < -1.33)$$

$$= Pr(Z \leqslant 1.33) - [1 - Pr(Z \leqslant 1.33)]$$

$$= 2Pr(Z \leqslant 1.33) - 1$$

$$= 2(0.9082) - 1$$

$$= 0.816$$

Alternatively, we could evaluate $Pr(-1.33 \leqslant Z \leqslant 1.33)$ directly from the 1.33 row under column D of Table 3, yielding a probability of 0.8165. Thus, 81.6% of the population have intra-ocular pressures in the normal range. These calculations are depicted in Figure 5.13.  ■

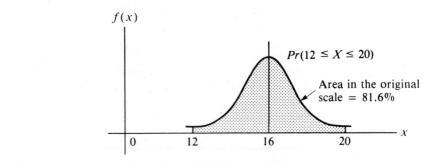

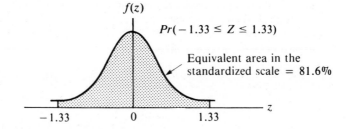

**Figure 5.13**
*Calculation of the proportion of persons with intraocular pressures in the normal range*

# ■ 5.6 NORMAL APPROXIMATION TO THE BINOMIAL DISTRIBUTION

Suppose we have a binomial distribution with parameters $n$ and $p$. If $n$ is large and $p$ is either near 0 or near 1, then the binomial distribution will be very positively or negatively skewed, respectively. See Figure 5.14(a) and (b). Similarly, when $n$ is small, for any $p$, the distribution will tend to be skewed. See Figure 5.14(c).

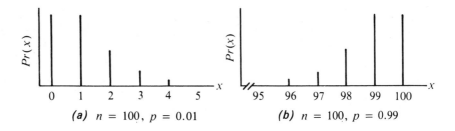

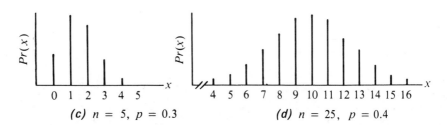

**Figure 5.14**
Symmetry properties
of the binomial
distribution

However, if $n$ is moderately large and $p$ is not too extreme, then the binomial distribution will tend to be symmetric and will be well approximated by a normal distribution. See Figure 5.14(d).

We know from Chapter 4 that the mean and variance of a binomial distribution are $np$ and $npq$, respectively. A natural approximation to use is a normal distribution with the *same* mean and variance, that is, $N(np, npq)$. Suppose we wish to compute $Pr(a \le X \le b)$ for some integers $a$, $b$, where $X$ is binomially distributed with parameters $n$ and $p$. We might approximate this probability by the area under the normal curve from $a$ to $b$. However, we can empirically show that a better approximation to this probability is given by the area under the normal curve from $a - \frac{1}{2}$ to $b + \frac{1}{2}$. This will generally be the case when we approximate any discrete distribution by the normal distribution. We thus have the following rule:

---

**5.5** **Normal Approximation to the Binomial Distribution**

If $X$ is a binomial random variable with parameters $n$ and $p$, then we approximate $Pr(a \le X \le b)$ by the area under a $N(np, npq)$ curve from $(a - \frac{1}{2})$ to $(b + \frac{1}{2})$. This rule implies that for the special case $a = b$, we approximate the binomial probability $Pr(X = a)$ by the area under the normal curve from $(a - \frac{1}{2})$ to $(a + \frac{1}{2})$. The only exception to this rule is that we approximate $Pr(X = 0)$ and $Pr(X = n)$ by the area under the normal curve to the left of $\frac{1}{2}$ and to the right of $n - \frac{1}{2}$, respectively.

---

*Example 5.21*    Suppose we have a binomial distribution with parameters $n = 25$, $p = 0.4$. How can we approximate $Pr(7 \le X \le 12)$?

*Solution*    We have $np = 25(0.4) = 10$, $npq = 25(0.4)(0.6) = 6.0$. Thus, we approximate this distribution by a normal random variable $Y$ with mean 10 and variance 6. We specifically want to compute the area under this normal curve from 6.5 to 12.5. We have

$$Pr(6.5 \leqslant X \leqslant 12.5) = \Phi\left(\frac{12.5 - 10}{\sqrt{6}}\right) - \Phi\left(\frac{6.5 - 10}{\sqrt{6}}\right)$$

$$= \Phi(1.02) - \Phi(-1.43)$$

$$= \Phi(1.02) - [1 - \Phi(1.43)]$$

$$= \Phi(1.02) + \Phi(1.43) - 1$$

$$= 0.8461 + 0.9236 - 1$$

$$= 0.770$$

This approximation is depicted in Figure 5.15.    ∎

**Figure 5.15**
*The approximation of the binomial random variable X with parameters n = 25, p = 0.4 by the normal random variable Y with mean 10 and variance 6*

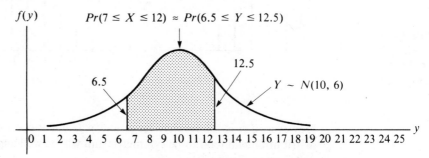

**Example 5.22**

**Infectious Disease** Suppose we wish to compute the probability that between 50 and 75 of 100 white blood cells will be neutrophils, where the probability that any one cell is a neutrophil is 0.6. We choose these values as proposed limits to the range of neutrophils in normal persons and we wish to predict what proportion of persons will be normal according to this definition.

**Solution**

The exact probability is given by

$$\sum_{k=50}^{75} \binom{100}{k} (0.6)^k (0.4)^{100-k}$$

We will use the normal approximation to approximate the exact probability. The mean of the binomial distribution in this case is $100(0.6) = 60$, and the variance is $100(0.6)(0.4) = 24$. Thus, we find the area between 49.5 and 75.5 for an $N(60, 24)$ distribution. This area is

$$\Phi\left(\frac{75.5 - 60}{\sqrt{24}}\right) - \Phi\left(\frac{49.5 - 60}{\sqrt{24}}\right)$$

$$= \Phi(3.16) - \Phi(-2.14)$$

$$= \Phi(3.16) - \Phi(-2.14)$$

$$= \Phi(3.16) + \Phi(2.14) - 1$$

$$= 0.9992 + 0.9838 - 1$$

$$= 0.983$$

Thus, 98.3% of the people will be normal.    ∎

*Example 5.23*    **Infectious Disease** Suppose we define a person as abnormally high if the number of neutrophils is $\geq 76$ and abnormally low if the number of neutrophils is $\leq 49$. Calculate the proportion of people that are abnormally high and low.

*Solution*    The probability of being abnormally high is given by $Pr(X \geq 76) \approx Pr(Y \geq 75.5)$, where $X$ is a binomial random variable with parameters $n = 100$, $p = 0.6$ and $Y \sim N(60, 24)$. This latter probability is

$$1 - \Phi\left(\frac{75.5 - 60}{\sqrt{24}}\right)$$

$$= 1 - \Phi(3.16)$$

$$= 0.001$$

Similarly, the probability of being abnormally low is

$$Pr(X \leq 49) \approx Pr(Y \leq 49.5)$$

$$= \Phi\left(\frac{49.5 - 60}{\sqrt{24}}\right)$$

$$= 1 - \Phi(2.14)$$

$$= 1 - \Phi(2.14)$$

$$= 1 - 0.9838$$

$$= 0.016$$

Thus, 0.1% of persons will be abnormally high and 1.6% of persons will be abnormally low. These probabilities are depicted in Figure 5.16.    ∎

### Under what conditions should we use this approximation?

We will use the normal distribution with mean $np$ and variance $npq$ to approximate a binomial distribution with parameters $n$ and $p$ when $npq \geq 5$.

This condition will be satisfied if $n$ is moderately large and $p$ is not too small. To illustrate this condition, we have plotted the binomial probability distribution for $p = 0.1$, $n = 10, 20, 50$, and 100 in Figure 5.17(a) through (d) and $p = 0.2$,

*Figure 5.16*
*Normal approximation to the distribution of neutrophils*

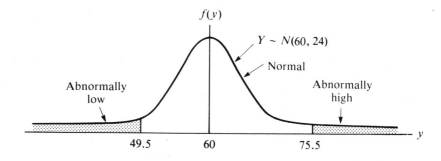

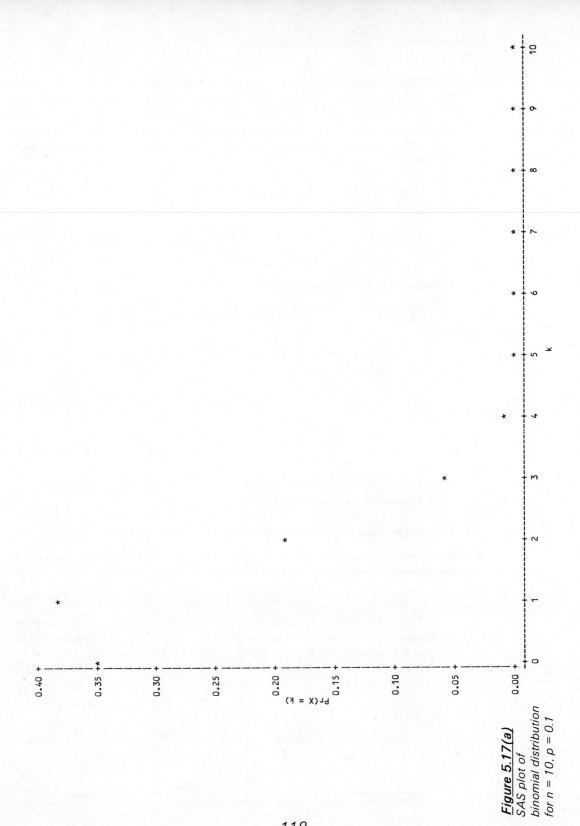

*Figure 5.17(a)*
SAS plot of
binomial distribution
for n = 10, p = 0.1

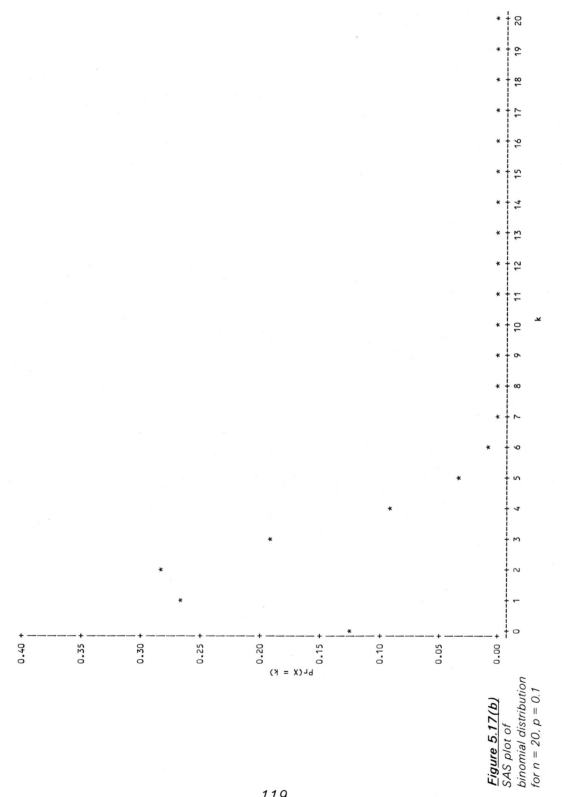

*Figure 5.17(b)*
*SAS plot of*
*binomial distribution*
*for n = 20. p = 0.1*

119

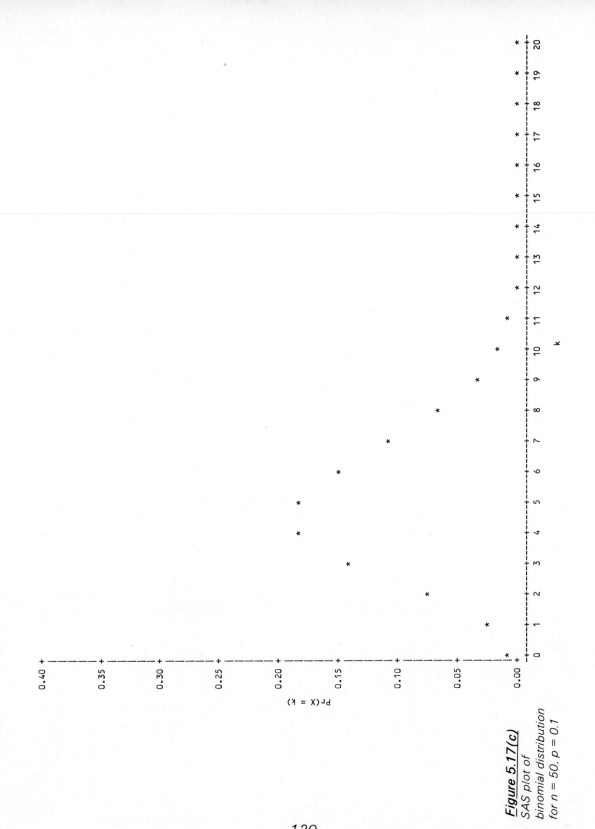

*Figure 5.17(c)*
*SAS plot of*
*binomial distribution*
*for n = 50, p = 0.1*

120

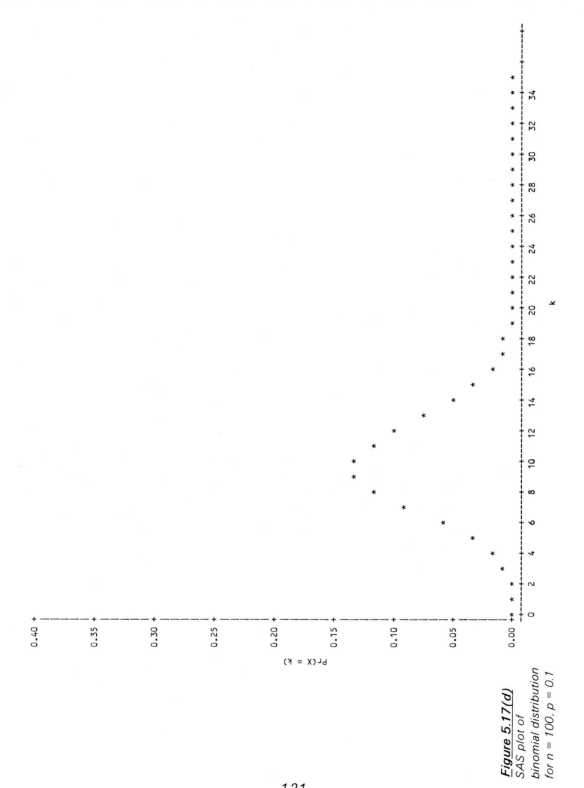

*Figure 5.17(d)*
SAS plot of
binomial distribution
for n = 100, p = 0.1

121

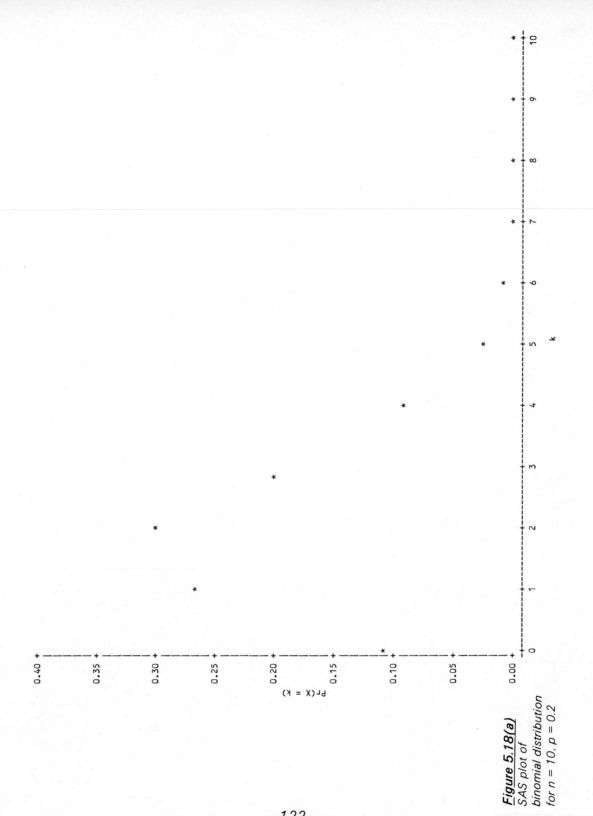

*Figure 5.18(a)*
SAS plot of
binomial distribution
for n = 10, p = 0.2

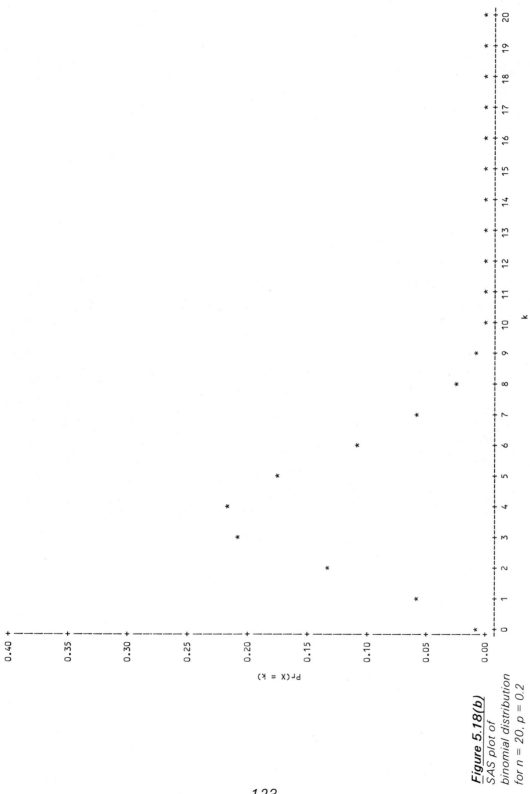

**_Figure 5.18(b)_**
_SAS plot of_
_binomial distribution_
_for n = 20, p = 0.2_

123

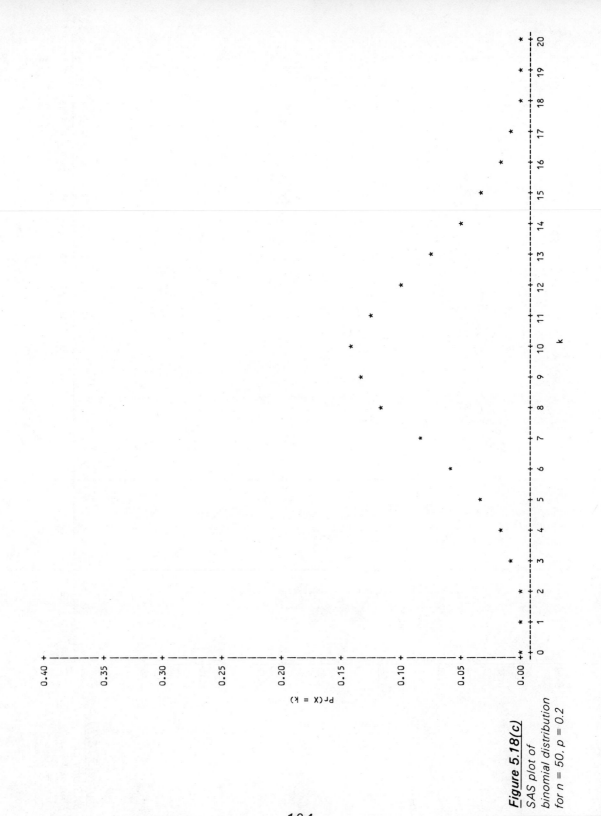

*Figure 5.18(c)*

SAS plot of
binomial distribution
for $n = 50$, $p = 0.2$

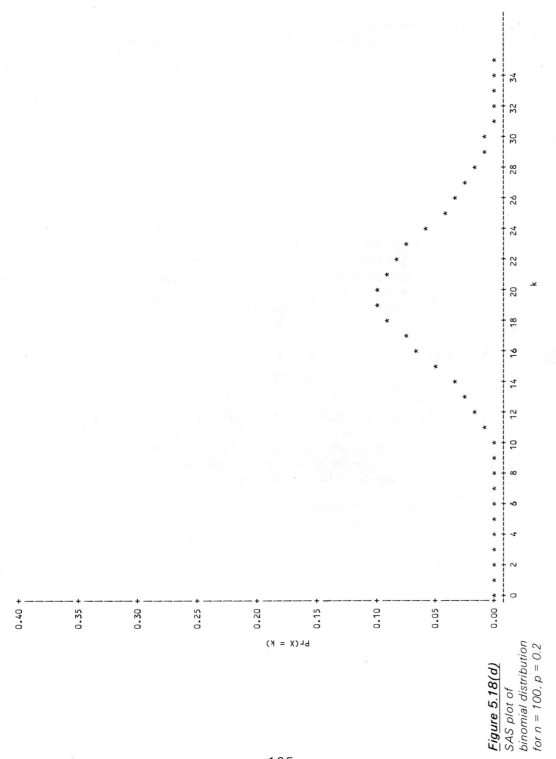

*Figure 5.18(d)*
*SAS plot of*
*binomial distribution*
*for n = 100, p = 0.2*

125

$n = 10, 20, 50,$ and $100$ in Figure 5.18(a) through (d) using a Statistical Analysis System plotting routine (PROC PLOT). Notice that the normal approximation to the binomial distribution does not fit well in Figure 5.17(a), $n = 10$, $p = 0.1$ ($npq = 0.9$), or Figure 5.17(b), $n = 20$, $p = 0.1$ ($npq = 1.8$). The approximation is marginally adequate in Figure 5.17(c), $n = 50$, $p = 0.1$ ($npq = 4.5$), where the right-hand tail is only slightly longer than the left-hand tail. The approximation is quite good in Figure 5.17(d), $n = 100$, $p = 0.1$ ($npq = 9.0$), where the distribution appears to be quite symmetric. Similarly, for $p = 0.2$, although the normal approximation is not good for $n = 10$ [Figure 5.18(a), $npq = 1.6$], it becomes marginally adequate for $n = 20$ [Figure 5.18(b), $npq = 3.2$] and quite good for $n = 50$ [Figure 5.18(c), $npq = 8.0$] and $n = 100$ [Figure 5.18(d), $npq = 16.0$].

Note that the conditions under which the normal approximation to the binomial distribution works well (namely, $npq \geqslant 5$), which correspond to $n$ moderate and $p$ not too large or too small, are generally *not* the same as the conditions for which the Poisson approximation to the binomial distribution works well [$n$ large ($\geqslant 100$) and $p$ very small ($p \leqslant 0.01$)]. However, occasionally both of these criteria will be met. In such cases, for example, when $n = 1000$, $p = 0.01$, the two approximations will yield about the same results. The normal approximation is preferable because it is easier to apply.

# ◼ 5.7 NORMAL APPROXIMATION TO THE POISSON DISTRIBUTION

The normal distribution can be used to approximate discrete distributions other than the binomial distribution and, in particular, can be used to approximate the Poisson distribution. We will use the same technique as for the binomial distribution; that is, we will equate the means and variances of the Poisson distribution and the approximating normal distribution.

| 5.6 | **Normal Approximation to the Poisson Distribution** |
|---|---|

We will approximate a Poisson distribution with parameter $\mu$ by a normal distribution with mean and variance both equal to $\mu$. We will use this approximation for $\mu \geqslant 5$ and will approximate $Pr(X = x)$ by the area under a $N(\mu, \mu)$ density from $x - \frac{1}{2}$ to $x + \frac{1}{2}$ for $x > 0$ or by the area to the left of $\frac{1}{2}$ for $x = 0$.

We plot the Poisson distribution for $\mu = 2, 5, 10,$ and $20$ using the SAS plotting program (PROC PLOT) in Figure 5.19(a) through (d), respectively. The normal approximation is clearly inadequate for $\mu = 2$ [Figure 5.19(a)], marginally adequate for $\mu = 5$ [Figure 5.19(b)], and adequate for $\mu = 10$ [Figure 5.19(c)] and $\mu = 20$ [Figure 5.19(d)].

*Example 5.24*    **Bacteriology**    Let us consider again the distribution of the number of bacteria in a petri plate of area $A$. Let us assume that the probability of observing $x$ bacteria is given exactly by a Poisson distribution with parameter $\mu = \lambda A$, where $\lambda = 0.1$ and $A = 100 \text{ cm}^2$. Suppose we observe 20 bacteria in this area. How unusual is this event?

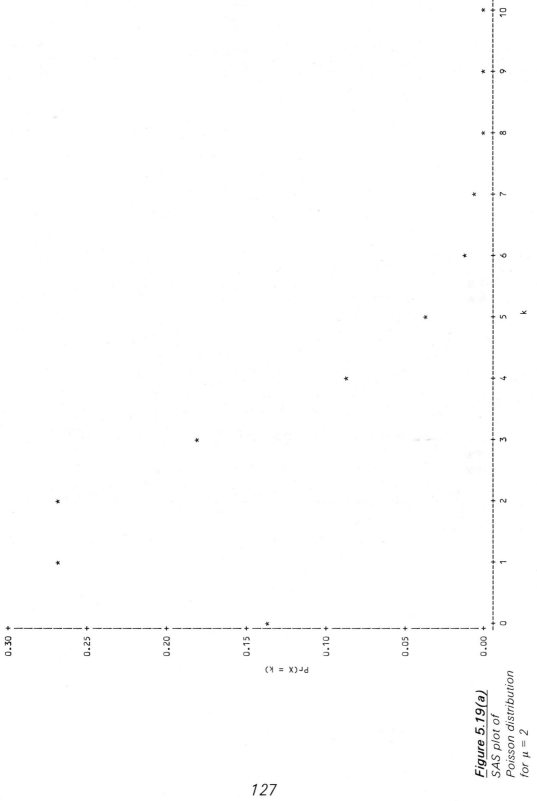

*Figure 5.19(a)*
SAS plot of
Poisson distribution
for μ = 2

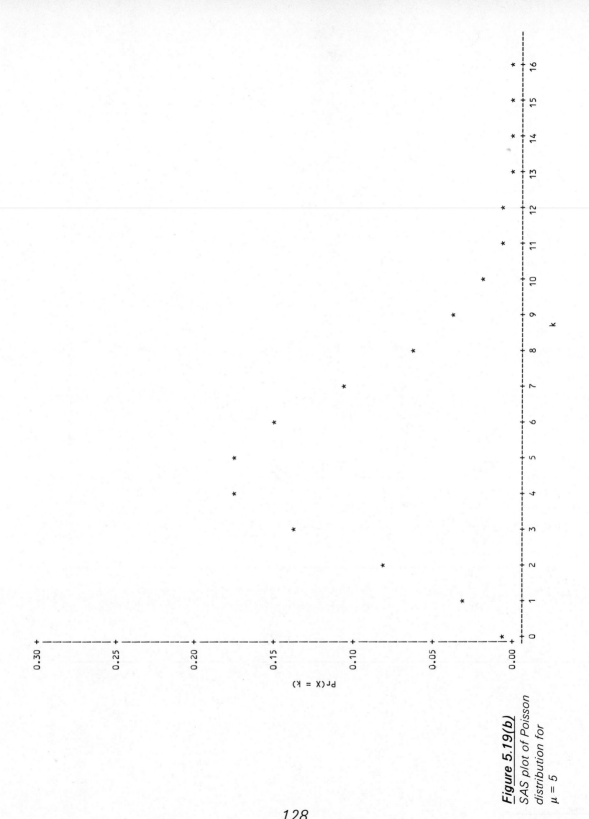

Pr(X = k)

k

*Figure 5.19(b)*
SAS plot of Poisson
distribution for
μ = 5

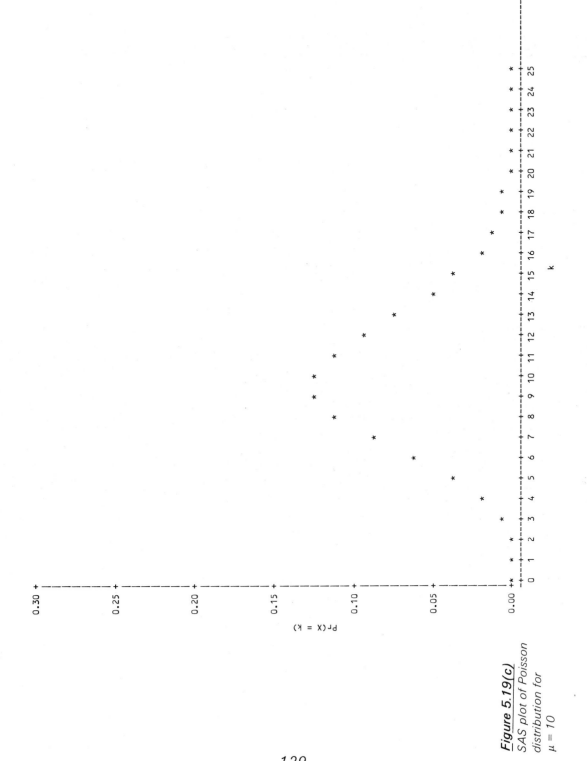

*Figure 5.19(c)*
*SAS plot of Poisson distribution for*
*μ = 10*

129

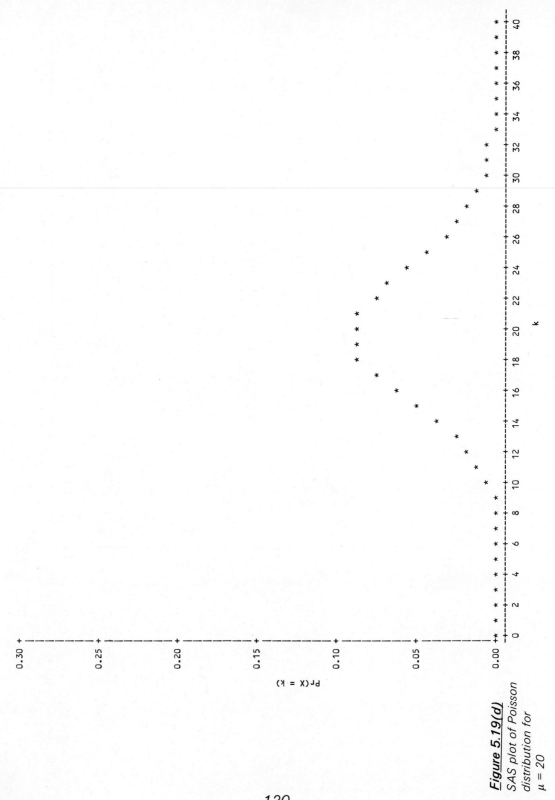

**Figure 5.19(d)**

SAS plot of Poisson distribution for $\mu = 20$

*Solution*   We must compute

$$Pr(X \geqslant 20) \approx Pr(Y \geqslant 19.5)$$

where

$$Y \sim N(\lambda A, \lambda A) = N(10, 10)$$

We have

$$Pr(Y \geqslant 19.5) = 1 - Pr(Y \leqslant 19.5)$$

$$= 1 - \Phi\left(\frac{19.5 - 10}{\sqrt{10}}\right)$$

$$= 1 - \Phi\left(\frac{9.5}{\sqrt{10}}\right)$$

$$= 1 - \Phi(3.00)$$

$$= 1 - 0.9987$$

$$= 0.0013$$

Thus, we would expect to find 20 or more colonies in 100 cm$^2$ only 1.3 times in 1000 plates, a rare event indeed. ∎

# ■ *5.8 SUMMARY*

In this chapter we learned about continuous random variables. The concept of a **probability density function** was introduced, which is the analogue to a probability mass function for discrete random variables. In addition, generalizations of the concepts of expected value, variance, and cumulative distribution were presented for continuous random variables.

We then looked in detail at the **normal distribution**, the most important continuous distribution. The normal distribution is used often in statistical work, since many random phenomena follow this probability law, particularly those that can be expressed as a sum of many random variables. We saw that the normal distribution was indexed by two parameters, the mean $\mu$ and the variance $\sigma^2$. Fortunately, all computations concerning any normal random variable can be accomplished using the **standard**, or **unit**, normal probability law, which has mean 0 and variance 1. **Normal tables** were introduced to enable us to work with the standard normal distribution. Finally, since the normal distribution is easy to use, it is often employed to approximate other distributions. We focused in particular on the normal approximations to the binomial and Poisson distributions.

In the next three chapters, we will use the normal distribution extensively as a foundation for our work on statistical inference.

# Problems

## Cardiovascular Disease

Since serum cholesterol is related to age and sex, some investigators prefer to express it in terms of z-scores. If $X$ = raw serum cholesterol, then $Z = \dfrac{X - \mu}{\sigma}$, where $\mu$ is the mean and $\sigma$ is the standard deviation of serum cholesterol for a given age-sex group. Suppose we regard $Z$ as a standard normal distribution.

**5.1** What is $Pr(z < 0.5)$?

**5.2** What is $Pr(z > 0.5)$?

**5.3** What is $Pr(-1.0 < z < 1.5)$?

Suppose we regard a person as having high cholesterol if $z > 2.0$ and borderline cholesterol if $1.5 < z < 2.0$.

**5.4** What proportion of persons have high cholesterol?

**5.5** What proportion of persons have borderline cholesterol?

**5.6** What are the deciles of the standard normal distribution, that is, the $10, 20, 30, \ldots, 90$ percentiles?

**5.7** What are the quartiles of the standard normal distribution?

## Hypertension

Blood pressure in childhood tends to increase with age, but differently for boys and girls. Suppose that for both boys and girls mean systolic blood pressure is 95 mm Hg at 3 years of age and increases 1.5 mm per year up to the age of 13. Furthermore, starting at age 13, the mean increases by 2 mm per year for boys and 1 mm per year for girls up to the age of 18. Finally, assume that blood pressure is normally distributed and that the standard deviation is 12 mm Hg for all age-sex groups.

**5.8** What is the probability that an 11-year-old boy will have a blood pressure greater than 130 mm Hg?

**5.9** What is the probability that a 15-year-old girl will have a blood pressure between 100 and 120 mm Hg?

**5.10** What proportion of 17-year-old boys have systolic blood pressure between 120 and 140 mm Hg?

**5.11** What is the probability that of 200 15-year-old boys, at least 10 will have systolic blood pressure of 130 mm Hg or greater?

**5.12** What level of systolic blood pressure is at the 80th percentile for 7-year-old boys?

**5.13** What level of systolic blood pressure is at the 70th percentile for 12-year-old girls?

**5.14** Suppose that a task force of pediatricians decides that children over the 95th percentile, but not over the 99th percentile, for their age-sex group should be encouraged to take preventive nonpharmacologic measures to reduce their blood pressure, whereas those children over the 99th percentile should receive antihypertensive drug therapy. Construct a table giving the appropriate levels of blood pressure to identify these groups for boys and girls for each year of age from 3 to 18.

## Nutrition

Suppose that total carbohydrate intake in 12–14-year-old males is normally distributed with mean 124 g/1000 cal and standard deviation 20 g/1000 cal.

**5.15** What percentage of boys in this age range have carbohydrate intake above 140 g/1000 cal?

**5.16** What percentage of boys in this age range have carbohydrate intake below 90 g/1000 cal?

Suppose boys in this age range that live below the poverty level have a mean carbohydrate level of 121 g/1000 cal with a standard deviation of 19 g/1000 cal.

**5.17** Answer Problem 5.15 for boys in this age range and economic environment.

**5.18** Answer Problem 5.16 for boys in this age range and economic environment.

## Cancer

The incidence of breast cancer in 40–59-year-old women is approximately 1 new case per 1000 per year.

**5.19** What is the incidence of breast cancer over 10 years in women initially 40 years old?

**5.20** Suppose we are planning a study based on an enrollment of 10,000 women. What is the probability of obtaining at least 120 new breast cancer cases over a 10-year follow-up period?

## Gynecology

There has been much speculation regarding the role of intrauterine devices (IUDs) in the development of pelvic inflammatory disease (PID). Of particular interest is the type of IUD called the Dalkon Shield.

**5.21** Suppose that 2% of 800 PID case women of childbearing age are curent users of the Dalkon Shield at the time of diagnosis compared with 1% in the general population of women of childbearing age. Is this frequency of use among **PID** cases excessive?

## Pulmonary Disease
Many investigators have studied the relationship between asbestos exposure and death due to chronic obstructive pulmonary disease (COPD).

*5.22* Suppose that among workers exposed to asbestos in a shipyard in 1960, 33 have died over a 10-year period from COPD, whereas only 24 such deaths could be expected based on statewide mortality rates. Is the number of deaths due to COPD in this group excessive?

*5.23* Twelve cases of leukemia are reported in persons living in a particular census tract over a 5-year period. Is this number of cases abnormal if only 6.7 cases would be expected based on national cancer incidence rates?

## Obstetrics
Suppose we assume that birthweights are normally distributed with a mean of 3400 g and a standard deviation of 700 g.

*5.24* Find the probability of a low-birthweight child, where low birthweight is defined as $\leq 2500$ g.

*5.25* Find the probability of a very low birthweight child, where very low birthweight is defined as $\leq 2000$ g.

*5.26* If we assume that successive deliveries by the same woman have the same probability of being low birthweight, then what is the probability that a woman with exactly 3 deliveries will have 2 or more low-birthweight deliveries?

## Cardiovascular Disease, Pulmonary Disease
The duration of cigarette smoking has been linked to many diseases, including lung cancer and various forms of heart disease. Suppose we know that among men aged 30–34 who have ever smoked, the mean number of years they smoked is 12.8 with a standard deviation of 5.1 years. For women in this age group, the mean number of years they smoked is 9.3 with a standard deviation of 3.2.

*5.27* If we assume that the duration of smoking is normally distributed, then what proportion of men in this age group have smoked for more than 20 years?

*5.28* Answer Problem 5.27 for women.

## Renal Disease
The presence of bacteria in a urine sample (bacteriuria) is sometimes associated with symptoms of kidney disease. Suppose we assume that a determination of bacteriuria has been made over a large population at one point in time and that 5% of the persons sampled are positive for bacteriuria.

*5.29* Suppose that we sample 1000 persons from this population. What is the probability that 50 or more persons would be positive for bacteriuria?

## Cancer
Previous census data have indicated that approximately 0.2% of women aged 45–54 will have had cervical cancer at some point in their lives. However, the general feeling is that the rate of cervical cancer has increased.

*5.30* If we perform a new study by mail questionnaire and find that 300 out of 100,000 women have had cervical cancer, then is this proportion consistent with the census rate?

## Ophthalmology
A study was conducted of patients with retinitis pigmentosa, an ocular condition where pigment appears over the retina, resulting in substantial loss of vision in many cases. The study was based on 94 patients who were seen annually at a baseline visit and at three annual follow-up visits. In this study, 90 patients provided visual field measurements at each of the four examinations and are the subjects of the following data analyses. Visual field was transformed to the $\log_e$ scale to better approximate normality and yielded the data given in Table 5.1.

**Table 5.1** *Visual field measurements in retinitis pigmentosa patients*

| Year of examination | Mean* | Standard deviation | n |
|---|---|---|---|
| Year 0 (baseline) | 8.15 | 1.23 | 90 |
| Year 3 | 8.01 | 1.33 | 90 |
| Year 0–year 3 | 0.14 | 0.66 | 90 |

*$\log_e$ (area of visual field) in degrees squared
(Reprinted with permission of the *American Journal of Ophthalmology* **99**: 240–251, 1985.)

*5.31* If we assume the change in visual field over 3 years is normally distributed when using the $\log_e$ scale, then what is the proportion of patients who showed a decline in visual field over 3 years?

*5.32* What percentage of patients would be expected to show a decline of at least 20% in visual field over 3 years? (*Note*: In the $\log_e$ scale this is equivalent to a decline of at least $\log_e(1/0.8) = 0.223$).

**5.33** Answer Problem 5.32 for a 50% decline over 3 years.

### Cardiovascular Disease

Serum cholesterol is an important risk factor for coronary disease. We can show that $\log_e$ (serum cholesterol) is approximately normally distributed with mean 5.39 and standard deviation 0.23.

**5.34** If the clinically normal range for cholesterol is 150–250 mg%/ml, then what proportion of people have abnormally low levels of cholesterol?

**5.35** What proportion of people have abnormally high levels of cholesterol?

**5.36** Some investigators feel that only cholesterol levels of over 300 mg%/ml indicate a high risk for heart disease. What proportion of the subpopulation with abnormally high levels does this group represent?

**5.37** What proportion of the general population does the group with cholesterol levels over 300 mg%/ml represent?

### Cancer

A recent study of the Massachusetts Department of Health found 46 deaths due to cancer among women in the city of Bedford over the period 1974–1978, where 30 deaths had been expected from statewide rates [1].

**5.38** Write an expression for the probability of observing exactly $k$ deaths over this period if the statewide rates are correct.

**5.39** Can the occurrence of 46 deaths be attributed to chance? Specifically, what is the probability of observing at least 46 deaths if the statewide rates are correct?

### Nutrition, Cancer

Beta carotene is a substance that is hypothesized to prevent cancer. A dietary survey was undertaken for the purpose of measuring the level of beta carotene intake in the typical American diet. Let us assume that the distribution of $\log_e$ carotene is normal with mean 8.34 and standard deviation 1.00. (Units are in $\log_e$ IU.)

**5.40** What percentage of persons have dietary carotene levels below 2000 IU? (*Note:* $\log_e 2000 = 7.60$.)

**5.41** What percentage of persons have dietary carotene levels below 1000 IU? (*Note:* $\log_e 1000 = 6.91$.)

**5.42** Some studies suggest that carotene levels over 10,000 IU may protect against cancer. What percentage of persons have a dietary intake of at least 10,000 IU?

Suppose that each person took a carotene supplement pill of dosage 5000 IU in addition to his or her normal diet. Let us assume that the resulting distribution of $\log_e$ carotene is normally distributed with mean 9.12 and standard deviation 1.00.

**5.43** What percentage of persons would have an intake from diet and supplements of at least 10,000 IU?

### Hypertension

Suppose we desire to recruit persons for a hypertensive treatment study and we feel that 10% of the population to be sampled is hypertensive.

**5.44** If we require 100 persons for our study and we assume perfect cooperation, then how many persons do we need to sample to be 80% sure of ascertaining 100 hypertensives?

**5.45** How many people do we need to sample to be 90% sure of ascertaining 100 hypertensives?

### Hypertension

People are classified as hypertensive if their systolic blood pressure is higher than a specified level for their age group, according to the scheme in Table 5.2.

**Table 5.2** *Mean and standard deviation of systolic blood pressure (mm Hg) in specific age groups*

| Age group | Mean | Standard deviation | Specified hypertension level |
|-----------|------|--------------------|------------------------------|
| 1–14 | 105.0 | 5.0 | 115.0 |
| 15–44 | 125.0 | 10.0 | 140.0 |

Assume that systolic blood pressure is normally distributed with mean and standard deviation given in Table 5.2 for the age groups 1–14 and 15–44, respectively. Define a *family* as a group of 2 people in the age group 1–14 and 2 people in the age group 15–44. A family is classified as hypertensive if *any one* family member is hypertensive.

**5.46** What proportion of 1–14-year-olds are hypertensive?

**5.47** What proportion of 15–44-year-olds are hypertensive?

**5.48** What proportion of families are hypertensive? (Assume that the hypertensive status of different members of the family are independent random variables.)

**5.49** Suppose an apartment building has 200 families living in it. What is the probability that between 10 and 25 families are hypertensive?

## Nutrition

The distribution of serum levels of alpha tocopherol (serum vitamin E) is approximately normal with mean 860 $\mu$g/dl and standard deviation 340 $\mu$g/dl.

**5.50** What percentage of persons have serum alpha tocopherol levels between 400 and 1000 $\mu$g/dl?

**5.51** Suppose a person is identified as having toxic levels of alpha tocopherol if his or her serum level is > 2000 $\mu$g/dl. What percentage of persons will be so identified?

**5.52** A study is undertaken for evidence of toxicity of 2000 persons who regularly take vitamin E supplements. The investigators found that 4 persons have serum alpha tocopherol levels > 2000 $\mu$g/dl. Is this an unusual number of persons with toxic levels of serum alpha tocopherol?

## Pulmonary Disease

Forced expiratory volume (FEV) is an index of pulmonary function that measures the volume of air expelled after 1 second of constant effort. FEV is known to be influenced by age, sex, and cigarette smoking. Let us assume that in 45–54-year-old nonsmoking males FEV is normally distributed with mean 4.0 liters and standard deviation 0.5 liter. In comparably aged currently smoking males FEV is normally distributed with mean 3.5 liters and standard deviation 0.6 liter.

**5.53** If we regard an FEV of less than 2.5 liters as showing some functional impairment (occasional breathlessness, inability to climb stairs, etc.), then what is the probability that a currently smoking male has functional impairment?

**5.54** Answer Problem 5.53 for a nonsmoking male.

Many persons are not functionally impaired now but their pulmonary function usually declines with age and they eventually will be functionally impaired. Let us assume that the *decline* in FEV over $n$ years is normally distributed with mean $0.03n$ and standard deviation $0.02n$.

**5.55** What is the probability that a 45-year-old man with FEV of 4.0 liters will be functionally impaired by the age of 75?

**5.56** Answer Problem 5.55 for a 25-year-old man with FEV of 4.0 liters.

## Epidemiology

A major problem in performing longitudinal studies in medicine is that persons initially entered into a study are lost to follow-up for various reasons.

**5.57** Suppose we wish to evaluate our data after 2 years and anticipate that the probability a patient will be available for study after 2 years is 90%. How many patients should we enter into the study to be 80% sure of having at least 100 patients left at the end of this period?

**5.58** How many patients should we enter if we want to be 90% sure of having at least 150 patients after 4 years if the probability of remaining in the study after 4 years is 80%?

## Infectious Disease

The differential is a standard measurement made during a blood test. It consists of classifying white blood cells into the following 5 categories: (a) basophils, (b) eosinophils, (c) monocytes, (d) lymphocytes, and (e) neutrophils. The usual practice is to look at 100 randomly selected cells under a microscope and count the number of cells within each of the 5 categories. Let us assume that a normal adult will have the following proportions of the categories: basophils, 0.5%; eosinophils, 1.5% monocytes, 4%; lymphocytes, 34%; and neutrophils, 60%.

**5.59** An excess of eosinophils is sometimes consistent with a violent allergic reaction. What is the exact probability that a normal adult will have 5 or more eosinophils?

**5.60** An excess of lymphocytes is consistent with various forms of viral infection, such as hepatitis. What is the probability that a normal adult will have 40 or more lymphocytes?

**5.61** What is the probability that a normal adult will have 50 or more lymphocytes?

**5.62** How many lymphocytes would have to appear in the differential before you would feel that the "normal" pattern was violated?

**5.63** An excess of neutrophils is consistent with several types of bacterial infection. Suppose an adult has $x$ neutrophils. How large would $x$ have to be in order that the probability of a normal adult having $x$ or more neutrophils was $\leqslant 5\%$?

**5.64** How large would $x$ have to be in order that the probability of a normal adult having $x$ or more neutrophils was $\leqslant 1\%$?

## Pulmonary Disease

**5.65** The usual annual death rate from asthma in England over the period 1862–1962 for persons aged 5–34 has been approximately 1 per 100,000. Suppose that in 1963 twenty deaths are observed in a group of

1,000,000 people in this age group living in Britain. Is this number of deaths inconsistent with the preceding 100-year rate? In particular, what is the probability of observing 20 or more deaths in 1 year in a group of 1,000,000 people? (*Note*: This finding is both statistically and medically interesting, since it was found that the excess risk could be attributed to certain aerosols used by asthmatics in Britain during the period 1963–1967. The rate returned to normal during the period 1968–1972, when these types of aerosols were no longer used. For further information see Speizer et al. [3].)

### Blood Chemistry

In pharmacologic research a variety of clinical chemistry measurements are routinely monitored closely for evidence of side effects of the medication under study. Suppose typical blood glucose levels are normally distributed with mean 90 mg/dl and standard deviation 38 mg/dl.

**5.66** If the normal range is from 65–120 mg/dl, then what percentage of values will fall in the normal range?

**5.67** In some studies only values that are at least 1.5 times as high as the upper limit of normal are identified as abnormal. What percentage of values would fall in this range?

**5.68** Answer Problem 5.67 for 2.0 times the upper limit of normal.

**5.69** Frequently, tests that yield abnormal results are repeated for confirmation. What is the probability that for a normal person a test will be at least 1.5 times as high as the upper limit of normal on two separate occasions?

**5.70** Suppose that in a pharmacologic study involving 6000 patients, 75 patients have blood glucose levels at least 1.5 times the upper limit of normal on one occasion. What is the probability that this result could be due to chance?

### Hypertension

Blood pressure measurements are known to be variable, and repeated measurements are essential to accurately characterize a person's blood pressure status. Suppose we measure a person on $n$ visits with $k$ measurements per visit and use the average of all $nk$ measurements ($\bar{x}$) to classify a person as to blood pressure status. Specifically, if $\bar{x} \geqslant 95$ mm, then we denote the person as hypertensive; if $\bar{x} < 90$ mm, then we denote the person as normotensive; and if $\bar{x} \geqslant 90$ mm and $<95$ mm, then we denote the person as borderline. We also assume that a person's "true" blood pressure is $\mu$, representing an average over a large number of visits with a large number of measurements per visit, and that $\bar{x}$ is normally distributed with mean $\mu$ and variance $= 27.7/n + 7.9/(nk)$.

**5.71** If a person's true blood pressure is 100, then what is the probability that we will accurately classify the person (as hypertensive) if a single measurement is taken at 1 visit?

**5.72** Is the probability in Problem 5.71 a measure of sensitivity, specificity, or predictive value?

**5.73** If a person's true blood pressure is 85 mm, then what is the probability that we will accurately classify the person (as normotensive) if 3 measurements are taken at each of 2 visits?

**5.74** Is the probability in Problem 5.73 a measure of sensitivity, specificity, or predictive value?

**5.75** Suppose we decide to take 2 measurements per visit. How many visits do we need so that the reliability measures in Problems 5.71 and 5.73 would each be at least 95%?

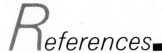

eferences

[*1*] *Boston Globe*, April 25, 1980.

[*2*] Berson, L. L., Sandberg, M. A., Rosner, B., Birch, D. G., and Hanson, A. H. (1985) "Natural Cause of Retinitis Pigmentosa Over a Three-Year Interval," *American Journal of Ophthalmology* **94**: 240–251.

[*3*] Speizer, F. E., Doll, R., Heaf, P., and Strang, L. B. (1968) "Investigation into Use of Drugs Preceding Death from Asthma," *British Medical Journal* **1**, February 8: 339–343.

# 6 Estimation

## ■ 6.1 INTRODUCTION

In Chapters 3 through 5 we were concerned with exploring the properties of different probability models. In so doing, we always assumed that the specific probability distributions were known.

*Example 6.1*     **Infectious Disease** We assumed that the number of neutrophils in a sample of 100 white blood cells was binomially distributed with parameter $p = 0.6$. ■

*Example 6.2*     **Bacteriology** We assumed that the number of bacterial colonies on a 100-cm$^2$ agar plate was Poisson distributed with parameter $\mu = 0.02$. ■

*Example 6.3*     **Hypertension** We assumed that the distribution of diastolic blood pressure measurements in 35–44-year-old men was normal with mean $\mu = 80$ mm and $\sigma = 12$ mm. ■

In general, we have been assuming that the properties of the underlying distributions from which our data are drawn are known and the only question that remains is what can be predicted about the behavior of the data given a knowledge of these properties.

*Example 6.4*     **Hypertension** Using the data in Example 6.3, we could predict that about 95% of all diastolic blood pressures from 35–44-year-old men should fall between 56 mm and 104 mm. ■

The problem to be addressed in the remainder of this text, and the more basic statistical problem, is that we have a data set and we want to **infer** the properties of the underlying distribution from this data set. This inference usually involves **inductive** rather than **deductive** reasoning; that is, in principle we must at least try a variety of different probability models and see which model "fits" our data best.

Statistical inference can be further subdivided into the two main areas of estimation and hypothesis testing. **Estimation** is concerned with predicting the values of specific population parameters; **hypothesis testing** is concerned with testing whether the value of a population parameter is equal to some specific value. We will be concerned with problems of estimation in this chapter and with problems of hypothesis testing in Chapters 7 through 10.

Some typical problems that fall into the realm of estimation follow.

*Example 6.5*    **Hypertension** Suppose we measure the systolic blood pressures of a group of Polynesian villagers and we believe the underlying distribution is normal. How can we estimate the parameters of this distribution ($\mu$, $\sigma^2$) if no previous data are available on these people?    ∎

*Example 6.6*    **Pulmonary Disease** Suppose we look at persons living within a low-income census tract in some urban area and we wish to estimate the prevalence of tuberculosis (TB) in the community. We assume that the number of cases among $n$ persons sampled will be binomially distributed with some parameter $p$. How do we estimate the parameter $p$?

In the previous two examples, we were interested in obtaining specific numbers as estimates of our parameters, which are often referred to as **point estimates**. Sometimes we want to specify a range within which the parameter values are likely to fall. If this range is narrow, then we may feel that our point estimate is a good one. This type of problem falls into the realm of **interval estimation**.

*Example 6.7*    **Ophthalmology** A study is proposed to screen a group of 1000 persons ages 65 or older to identify persons with "low vision," that is, persons with a visual acuity of 20–50 or worse in both eyes, even with the aid of glasses. Suppose we assume that the number of such people ascertained in this manner is binomially distributed with parameters $n = 1000$ and unknown $p$. We would like to obtain a point estimate of $p$ and to provide an interval about this point estimate to see how accurate our point estimate is. For example, we would feel better about a point estimate of 5% if this interval were 0.04–0.06 than if it were 0.01–0.10.    ∎

# ■ 6.2 THE RELATIONSHIP BETWEEN POPULATION AND SAMPLE

*Example 6.8*    **Obstetrics** Suppose we wish to characterize the distribution of birthweights of all liveborn infants that were born in the United States in 1980. Let us assume that the underlying distribution of these measurements has an expected value (or mean) $\mu$ and variance $\sigma^2$. We wish to estimate $\mu$ and $\sigma^2$ exactly. This task is impossible with such a large group. Instead, we decide to select a random sample of $n$ infants that are *representative of* this large group and use the birthweights $x_1, \ldots, x_n$ from this sample to help us in estimating $\mu$ and $\sigma^2$. What do we mean by a random sample?    ∎

**Definition 6.1**

A **random sample** is a sample chosen such that each member of the group to be studied is equally likely to be chosen.    ∎

**Definition 6.2**

The **reference**, or **study**, population is the group that we wish to study. The random sample is selected from the study population.    ∎

In practice, we rarely have an opportunity to enumerate each member of the reference population, and we must make the assumption that the sample selected has all the properties of a random sample without formally being a random sample.

In Example 6.8 the reference population is finite and well defined and *could* be enumerated if necessary. In many instances the reference population is effectively infinite and is not well defined.

*Example 6.9*    **Cancer** Suppose we wish to estimate the 5-year survival rate of women who are initially diagnosed as having breast cancer at the ages of 45–54 and who are treated with the surgical procedure of radical mastectomy at this time. Our reference population is all women who have ever had a first diagnosis of breast cancer in the past when they were 45–54 years old or who ever will have such a diagnosis in the future when they are 45–54 years old and who receive radical mastectomies.    ∎

This population is effectively infinite. We cannot formally enumerate the population and thus cannot select a truly random sample from it. However, we again will assume that the sample we have selected behaves as if it were a random sample.

In this text we will assume that all reference populations discussed are **effectively infinite**, although, as in Example 6.8, many of them are actually very large but finite. This assumption implies that it is either impossible or impractical to enumerate the whole population and that we must infer any statistical properties of the population from small finite samples of size *n*. Sampling theory is the special branch of statistics that treats statistical inference for finite populations and is beyond the scope of this text. See reference [1] for a good treatment of this subject.

# ■ 6.3 RANDOM NUMBER TABLES

In this section we discuss practical methods for selecting random samples from either finite or infinite populations.

*Example 6.10*    **Hypertension** Suppose we wish to study how effective a hypertension treatment program is in controlling the blood pressure of its participants. We are given a roster of all 1000 participants in the program but, due to limited resources, we can only survey 20 people. We would like the 20 people chosen to be a random sample from the population of all participants in the program. How should we select this random sample?    ∎

In practice we would probably use a table of random numbers to select this sample.

---
**Definition 6.3**
---

A **random number** (or **random digit**) is a random variable $X$ that takes on the values 0, 1, 2, ..., 9 with equal probability. Thus,

$$Pr(X = 0) = Pr(X = 1) = \cdots = Pr(X = 9) = \tfrac{1}{10}$$    ∎

## Definition 6.4

A **random number table** is a collection of digits that satisfies the following two properties:

*1*. Each digit 0, 1, 2, . . . , 9 is equally likely to occur.
*2*. The value of any particular digit is independent of the value of any other digit in the table.  ∎

Table 4 in the appendix consists of 1000 random digits.

**Example 6.11**

Suppose that a 5 appears as a digit in a random number table. Does this mean that 5's are more likely to occur in the next few digits in the table?

**Solution**

No. Each digit either after or before the 5 is still equally likely to be any of the digits 0, 1, 2, . . . , 9.  ∎

In practice, computer programs generate large quantities of random digits that approximately satisfy the conditions in Definition 6.4. Thus, the numbers in random number tables are sometimes referred to as **pseudorandom numbers**, since they are simulated to satisfy the properties in Definition 6.4.

**Example 6.12**

*Hypertension*  How can we use the random digits in Table 4 to select 20 random participants in the hypertension treatment program in Example 6.10?

**Solution**

We must compile a roster of the 1000 participants and assign them numbers from 000 to 999. Perhaps an alphabetical list of the participants already exists, which would make this task easy. We then would select 20 groups of three digits starting at any position in the random number table. Thus, if we start at the first row of Table 4, we have the numbers listed in Table 6.1.

Therefore, our random sample would consist of the persons numbered 329, 242, . . . , 373 in the alphabetical list. In this particular case there were no repeats in the 20 three-digit numbers selected. If there had been repeats, then we would have selected more three-digit numbers until 20 different numbers were selected.  ∎

**Example 6.13**

*Diabetes*  Suppose we wish to conduct a clinical trial of a new treatment for diabetes and compare the new treatment with standard insulin therapy. We want to conduct a small study of this type on 10 patients: 5 patients are randomly assigned to the new therapy and 5 are assigned to insulin therapy. How can we use the table of random numbers to make the assignments?

**Table 6.1**
*20 random participants chosen from 1000 participants in the hypertension treatment program*

| First 3 rows of random number table | | | | Actual random numbers chosen | | | | |
|---|---|---|---|---|---|---|---|---|
| 32924 | 22324 | 18125 | 09077 | 329 | 242 | 232 | 418 | 125 |
| 54632 | 90374 | 94143 | 49295 | 090 | 775 | 463 | 290 | 374 |
| 88720 | 43035 | 97081 | 83373 | 941 | 434 | 929 | 588 | 720 |
|  |  |  |  | 430 | 359 | 708 | 183 | 373 |

**Table 6.2**

Sample of birthweights (oz) obtained from 1000 consecutive deliveries at Boston City Hospital

| Range | 0 | 1 | 2 | 3 | 4 | 5 | 6 | 7 | 8 | 9 | 10 | 11 | 12 | 13 | 14 | 15 | 16 | 17 | 18 | 19 |
|---|---|---|---|---|---|---|---|---|---|---|---|---|---|---|---|---|---|---|---|---|
| 000–019 | 116 | 124 | 119 | 100 | 127 | 103 | 140 | 82 | 107 | 132 | 100 | 92 | 76 | 129 | 138 | 128 | 115 | 133 | 70 | 121 |
| 020–039 | 114 | 114 | 121 | 107 | 120 | 123 | 83 | 96 | 116 | 110 | 71 | 86 | 136 | 118 | 120 | 110 | 107 | 157 | 89 | 71 |
| 040–059 | 98 | 105 | 106 | 52 | 123 | 101 | 111 | 130 | 129 | 94 | 124 | 127 | 128 | 112 | 83 | 95 | 118 | 115 | 86 | 120 |
| 060–079 | 106 | 115 | 100 | 107 | 131 | 114 | 121 | 110 | 115 | 93 | 116 | 76 | 138 | 126 | 143 | 93 | 121 | 135 | 81 | 135 |
| 080–099 | 108 | 152 | 127 | 118 | 110 | 115 | 109 | 133 | 116 | 129 | 118 | 126 | 137 | 110 | 32 | 139 | 132 | 110 | 140 | 119 |
| 100–119 | 109 | 108 | 103 | 88 | 87 | 144 | 105 | 138 | 115 | 104 | 129 | 108 | 92 | 100 | 145 | 93 | 115 | 85 | 124 | 123 |
| 120–139 | 141 | 96 | 146 | 115 | 124 | 113 | 98 | 110 | 153 | 165 | 140 | 132 | 79 | 101 | 127 | 137 | 129 | 144 | 126 | 155 |
| 140–159 | 120 | 128 | 119 | 108 | 113 | 93 | 144 | 124 | 89 | 126 | 87 | 120 | 99 | 60 | 115 | 86 | 143 | 97 | 106 | 148 |
| 160–179 | 113 | 135 | 117 | 129 | 120 | 117 | 92 | 118 | 80 | 132 | 121 | 119 | 57 | 126 | 126 | 77 | 135 | 130 | 102 | 107 |
| 180–199 | 115 | 135 | 112 | 121 | 89 | 135 | 127 | 115 | 133 | 64 | 91 | 126 | 78 | 85 | 106 | 94 | 122 | 111 | 109 | 89 |
| 200–219 | 99 | 118 | 104 | 102 | 94 | 113 | 124 | 118 | 104 | 124 | 133 | 80 | 117 | 112 | 112 | 112 | 102 | 118 | 107 | 104 |
| 220–239 | 90 | 113 | 132 | 122 | 89 | 111 | 118 | 108 | 148 | 103 | 112 | 128 | 86 | 111 | 140 | 126 | 143 | 120 | 124 | 110 |
| 240–259 | 142 | 92 | 132 | 128 | 97 | 132 | 99 | 131 | 120 | 106 | 115 | 101 | 130 | 120 | 130 | 89 | 107 | 152 | 90 | 116 |
| 260–279 | 106 | 111 | 120 | 198 | 123 | 152 | 135 | 83 | 107 | 55 | 131 | 108 | 100 | 104 | 112 | 121 | 102 | 114 | 102 | 101 |
| 280–299 | 118 | 114 | 112 | 133 | 139 | 113 | 77 | 109 | 142 | 144 | 114 | 117 | 97 | 96 | 93 | 120 | 149 | 107 | 107 | 117 |
| 300–319 | 93 | 103 | 121 | 118 | 110 | 89 | 127 | 100 | 156 | 106 | 122 | 105 | 92 | 128 | 124 | 125 | 118 | 113 | 110 | 149 |
| 320–339 | 98 | 98 | 141 | 131 | 92 | 141 | 110 | 134 | 90 | 88 | 111 | 137 | 67 | 95 | 102 | 75 | 108 | 118 | 99 | 79 |
| 340–359 | 110 | 124 | 122 | 104 | 133 | 98 | 108 | 125 | 106 | 128 | 132 | 95 | 114 | 67 | 134 | 136 | 138 | 122 | 103 | 113 |
| 360–379 | 142 | 121 | 125 | 111 | 97 | 127 | 117 | 122 | 120 | 80 | 114 | 126 | 103 | 98 | 108 | 100 | 106 | 98 | 116 | 109 |
| 380–399 | 98 | 97 | 129 | 114 | 102 | 128 | 107 | 119 | 84 | 117 | 119 | 128 | 121 | 113 | 128 | 111 | 112 | 120 | 122 | 91 |
| 400–419 | 117 | 100 | 108 | 101 | 144 | 104 | 110 | 146 | 117 | 107 | 126 | 120 | 104 | 129 | 147 | 111 | 106 | 138 | 97 | 90 |
| 420–439 | 120 | 117 | 94 | 116 | 119 | 108 | 109 | 106 | 134 | 121 | 125 | 105 | 177 | 109 | 109 | 109 | 79 | 118 | 92 | 103 |
| 440–459 | 110 | 95 | 111 | 144 | 130 | 83 | 93 | 81 | 116 | 115 | 131 | 135 | 116 | 97 | 108 | 103 | 134 | 140 | 72 | 112 |
| 460–479 | 101 | 111 | 129 | 128 | 108 | 90 | 113 | 99 | 103 | 41 | 129 | 104 | 144 | 124 | 70 | 106 | 118 | 99 | 85 | 93 |
| 480–499 | 100 | 105 | 104 | 113 | 106 | 88 | 102 | 125 | 132 | 123 | 160 | 100 | 128 | 131 | 49 | 102 | 110 | 106 | 96 | 116 |
| 500–519 | 128 | 102 | 124 | 110 | 129 | 102 | 101 | 119 | 101 | 119 | 141 | 112 | 100 | 105 | 155 | 124 | 67 | 94 | 134 | 123 |
| 520–539 | 92 | 56 | 17 | 135 | 141 | 105 | 133 | 118 | 117 | 112 | 87 | 92 | 104 | 104 | 132 | 121 | 118 | 126 | 114 | 90 |
| 540–559 | 109 | 78 | 117 | 165 | 127 | 122 | 108 | 109 | 119 | 98 | 120 | 101 | 96 | 76 | 143 | 83 | 100 | 128 | 124 | 137 |

Table 6.2(cont.)

| Range | 0 | 1 | 2 | 3 | 4 | 5 | 6 | 7 | 8 | 9 | 10 | 11 | 12 | 13 | 14 | 15 | 16 | 17 | 18 | 19 |
|---|---|---|---|---|---|---|---|---|---|---|---|---|---|---|---|---|---|---|---|---|
| 560–579 | 90 | 129 | 89 | 125 | 131 | 118 | 72 | 121 | 91 | 113 | 91 | 137 | 110 | 137 | 111 | 135 | 105 | 88 | 112 | 104 |
| 580–599 | 102 | 122 | 144 | 114 | 120 | 136 | 144 | 98 | 108 | 130 | 119 | 97 | 142 | 115 | 129 | 125 | 109 | 103 | 114 | 106 |
| 600–619 | 109 | 119 | 89 | 98 | 104 | 115 | 99 | 138 | 122 | 91 | 161 | 96 | 138 | 140 | 32 | 132 | 108 | 92 | 118 | 58 |
| 620–639 | 158 | 127 | 121 | 75 | 112 | 121 | 140 | 80 | 125 | 73 | 115 | 120 | 85 | 104 | 95 | 106 | 100 | 87 | 99 | 113 |
| 640–659 | 95 | 146 | 126 | 58 | 64 | 137 | 69 | 90 | 104 | 124 | 120 | 62 | 83 | 96 | 126 | 155 | 133 | 115 | 97 | 105 |
| 660–679 | 117 | 78 | 105 | 99 | 123 | 86 | 126 | 121 | 109 | 97 | 131 | 133 | 125 | 120 | 120 | 97 | 101 | 92 | 111 | 119 |
| 680–699 | 117 | 80 | 145 | 128 | 140 | 97 | 126 | 109 | 113 | 125 | 157 | 97 | 119 | 103 | 102 | 128 | 116 | 96 | 109 | 112 |
| 700–719 | 67 | 121 | 116 | 126 | 106 | 116 | 77 | 119 | 119 | 122 | 109 | 117 | 127 | 114 | 102 | 75 | 88 | 117 | 99 | 136 |
| 720–739 | 127 | 136 | 103 | 97 | 130 | 129 | 128 | 119 | 22 | 109 | 145 | 129 | 96 | 128 | 122 | 115 | 102 | 127 | 109 | 120 |
| 740–759 | 111 | 114 | 115 | 112 | 146 | 100 | 106 | 137 | 48 | 110 | 97 | 103 | 104 | 107 | 123 | 87 | 140 | 89 | 112 | 123 |
| 760–779 | 130 | 123 | 125 | 124 | 135 | 119 | 78 | 125 | 103 | 55 | 69 | 83 | 106 | 130 | 98 | 81 | 92 | 110 | 112 | 104 |
| 780–799 | 118 | 107 | 117 | 123 | 138 | 130 | 100 | 78 | 146 | 137 | 114 | 61 | 132 | 109 | 133 | 132 | 120 | 116 | 133 | 133 |
| 800–819 | 86 | 116 | 101 | 124 | 126 | 94 | 93 | 132 | 126 | 107 | 98 | 102 | 135 | 59 | 137 | 120 | 119 | 106 | 125 | 122 |
| 820–839 | 101 | 119 | 97 | 86 | 105 | 140 | 89 | 139 | 74 | 131 | 118 | 91 | 98 | 121 | 102 | 115 | 115 | 135 | 100 | 90 |
| 840–859 | 110 | 113 | 136 | 140 | 129 | 117 | 117 | 129 | 143 | 88 | 105 | 110 | 123 | 87 | 97 | 99 | 128 | 128 | 110 | 132 |
| 860–879 | 78 | 128 | 126 | 93 | 148 | 121 | 95 | 121 | 127 | 80 | 109 | 105 | 136 | 141 | 103 | 95 | 140 | 115 | 118 | 117 |
| 880–899 | 114 | 109 | 144 | 119 | 127 | 116 | 103 | 144 | 117 | 131 | 74 | 109 | 117 | 100 | 103 | 123 | 93 | 107 | 113 | 144 |
| 900–919 | 99 | 170 | 97 | 135 | 115 | 89 | 120 | 106 | 141 | 137 | 107 | 132 | 132 | 58 | 113 | 102 | 120 | 98 | 104 | 108 |
| 920–939 | 85 | 115 | 108 | 89 | 88 | 126 | 122 | 107 | 68 | 121 | 113 | 116 | 94 | 85 | 93 | 132 | 146 | 98 | 132 | 104 |
| 940–959 | 102 | 116 | 108 | 107 | 121 | 132 | 105 | 114 | 107 | 121 | 101 | 110 | 137 | 122 | 102 | 125 | 104 | 124 | 121 | 111 |
| 960–979 | 101 | 93 | 93 | 88 | 72 | 142 | 118 | 157 | 121 | 58 | 92 | 114 | 104 | 119 | 91 | 52 | 110 | 116 | 100 | 147 |
| 980–999 | 114 | 99 | 123 | 97 | 79 | 81 | 146 | 92 | 126 | 122 | 72 | 153 | 97 | 89 | 100 | 104 | 124 | 83 | 81 | 129 |

142

**Solution**

We number the prospective patients from 0 to 9 and select five unique random digits from some arbitrary position in the random number table (e.g., from the 28th row). The first five unique digits are 6, 9, 4, 3, 7. Thus, we will assign the patients numbered 3, 4, 6, 7, 9 to the new therapy and the remaining patients (numbered 0, 1, 2, 5, 8) to standard insulin therapy. In some studies the prospective patients are not known in advance and are recruited over time. In this case if we identify 00 with the first patient recruited, 01 with the second patient recruited, ..., and 09 with the tenth patient recruited, then we would assign the new therapy to the fourth $(3 + 1)$, fifth $(4 + 1)$, seventh $(6 + 1)$, eighth $(7 + 1)$, and tenth $(9 + 1)$ patients recruited and the standard therapy to the first $(0 + 1)$, second $(1 + 1)$, third $(2 + 1)$, sixth $(5 + 1)$, and ninth $(8 + 1)$ patients recruited. ∎

**Example 6.14**

**Obstetrics** We have enumerated the birthweights from 1000 consecutive deliveries at Boston City Hospital (serving a low-income population) in Table 6.2. For the purpose of this example, let us consider this population as effectively infinite. Suppose we wish to draw 5

**Table 6.3**

*17th and 18th rows of the random number table (Table 4)*

| | | | |
|---|---|---|---|
| 41871 | 17566 | 61200 | 15994 |
| 25758 | 04625 | 43226 | 32986 |

| | | |
|---|---|---|
| 1st 3-digit no. = 418 | Range = 400–419, birthweight = 97 oz | Column = 418 − 400 = 18 |
| 2nd 3-digit no. = 711 | Range = 700 − 719, birthweight = 117 oz | Column = 711 − 700 = 11 |
| 3rd 3-digit no. = 756 | Range = 740–759, birthweight = 140 oz | Column = 756 − 740 = 16 |

**Table 6.4**

*Five random samples of size 10 from the population of infants whose birthweights (in ounces) appear in Table 6.2*

| | Sample | | | | |
|---|---|---|---|---|---|
| Individual | 1 | 2 | 3 | 4 | 5 |
| 1 | 97 | 177 | 97 | 101 | 137 |
| 2 | 117 | 198 | 125 | 114 | 118 |
| 3 | 140 | 107 | 62 | 79 | 78 |
| 4 | 78 | 99 | 120 | 120 | 129 |
| 5 | 99 | 104 | 132 | 115 | 87 |
| 6 | 148 | 121 | 135 | 117 | 110 |
| 7 | 108 | 148 | 118 | 106 | 106 |
| 8 | 135 | 133 | 137 | 86 | 116 |
| 9 | 126 | 126 | 126 | 110 | 140 |
| 10 | 121 | 115 | 118 | 119 | 98 |
| $\bar{x}$ | 116.90 | 132.80 | 117.00 | 106.70 | 111.90 |
| $s$ | 21.70 | 32.62 | 22.44 | 14.13 | 20.46 |

random samples of size 10 from this population using the random numbers in Table 4. How can we select these samples?

*Solution*    We can start anywhere in the table. We arbitrarily choose to start in the 17th row of the table and read groups of three digits from left to right. The random numbers will thus range from 000 to 999. Suppose the three-digit random number selected is *y*. We then find the appropriate row in Table 6.2 by finding the range of numbers within which *y* falls and the appropriate column by subtracting the lower end of the range from *y*. For example, let us refer to the 17th and 18th rows of the random number table, which are reproduced in Table 6.3.

The random number selection process continues until we have 5 sets of 10 numbers, as shown in Table 6.4.    ∎

# ■ 6.4 ESTIMATION OF THE MEAN OF A DISTRIBUTION

Now we understand the meaning of a random sample from a population and have explored some practical methods for selecting such samples using a random number table. The question remains as to how to use a specific random sample $x_1, \ldots, x_n$ to estimate $\mu$ and $\sigma^2$, the mean and variance of the underlying distribution. We will focus on estimating the mean in this section and the variance in Section 6.5.

## ☐ 6.4.1 Point Estimation

A natural estimator to use for estimating the population mean $\mu$ is the sample mean

$$\bar{x} = \sum_{i=1}^{n} \frac{x_i}{n}$$

What are the properties of $\bar{x}$ that make it a desirable estimator of $\mu$? Suppose we forget about our particular sample for the moment and consider the set of all possible samples of size *n* that could have been selected from the population. The values of $\bar{x}$ in each of these samples will, in general, be different. Let us denote these values by $\bar{x}_1, \bar{x}_2$, and so forth. The key conceptual point in this instance is to forget about our sample as a unique entity and to consider it instead as representative of all possible samples of size *n* that could have been drawn from the population. Stated another way, we forget about the specific value obtained for $\bar{x}$ from our sample. Instead, we regard $\bar{x}$ as a single realization of a random variable over all possible samples of size *n* that could have been selected from the population.

**Definition 6.5**

The **sampling distribution** of $\bar{x}$ is the distribution of values of $\bar{x}$ over all possible samples of size *n* that could have been selected from the reference population.

In Figure 6.1 we provide an example of such a sampling distribution. This example consists of a frequency distribution of the sample mean from 200 randomly selected samples of size 10 drawn from the distribution of 1000 birthweights given in Table 6.2, as generated by the Statistical Analysis System procedure PROC CHART.

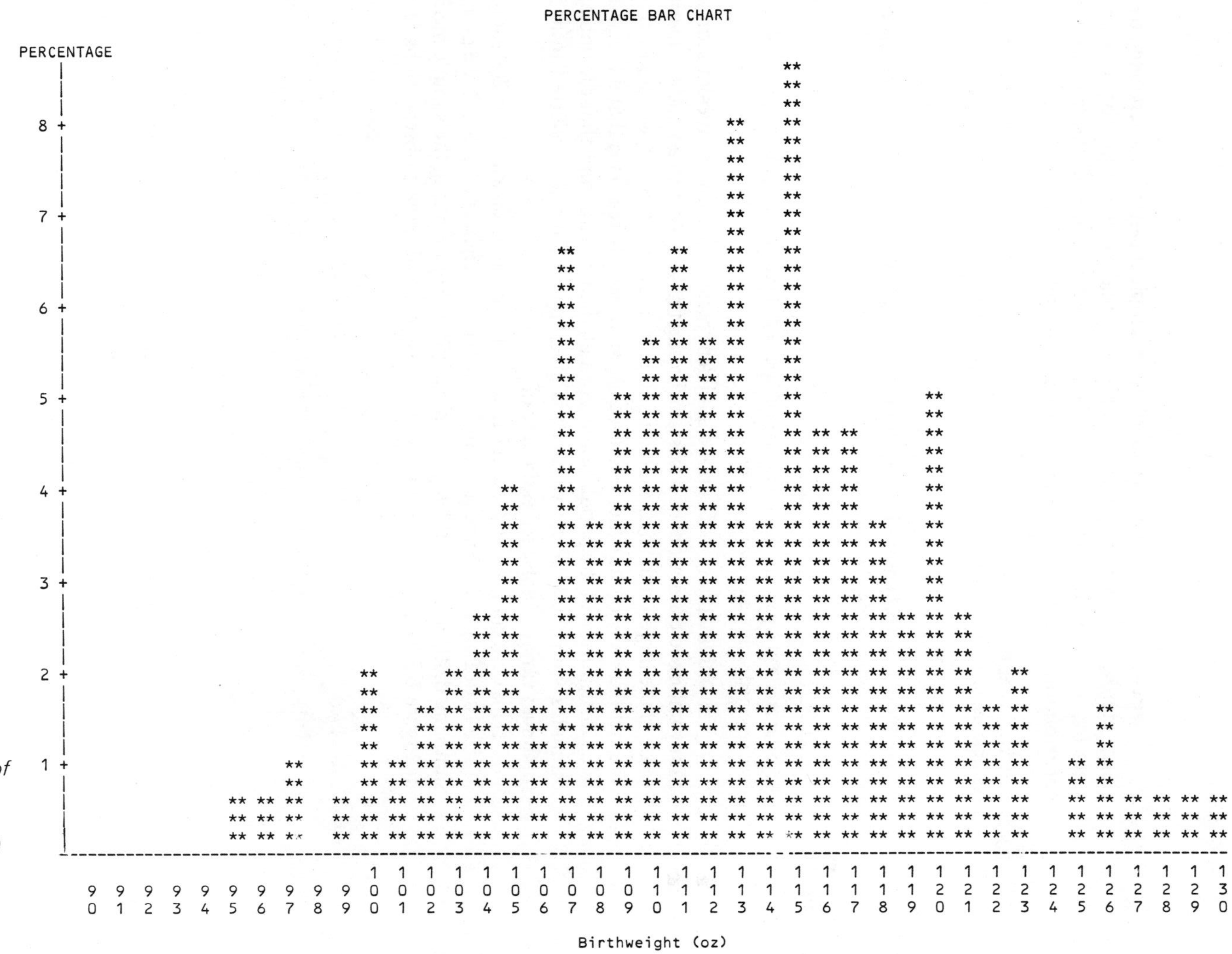

PERCENTAGE BAR CHART

PERCENTAGE

8 +

7 +

6 +

5 +

4 +

3 +

2 +

1 +

Birthweight (oz)

**Figure 6.1**
Sampling
distribution of x̄
over 200 samples of
size 10 selected
from the
population of 1000
birthweights
given in Table 6.2
(100 =
100.0–100.9, etc.)

We can show that the average of these sample means ($\bar{x}$'s) when taken over a large number of samples of size $n$ will approximate $\mu$ as the number of samples selected becomes large. In other words, the expected value of $\bar{x}$ over its sampling distribution is equal to $\mu$. We summarize this result as follows:

| 6.1 |
|---|

Let $x_1, \ldots, x_n$ be a random sample drawn from some population with mean $\mu$. Then for the sample mean $\bar{x}$, $E(\bar{x}) = \mu$.

Note that **(6.1)** holds for any population regardless of its underlying distribution. In other words, $\bar{x}$ is an unbiased estimator of $\mu$.

| Definition 6.6 |
|---|

An **estimator** $e$ of a parameter $\mu$ is unbiased if $E(e) = \mu$. This means that the average value of $e$ over repeated samples of size $n$ will be $\mu$. ∎

The unbiasedness of $\bar{x}$ is not a sufficient reason to use $\bar{x}$ as an estimator of $\mu$. Many unbiased estimators of $\mu$ exist, including the sample median and the average value of the largest and smallest data points in a sample. Why do we choose to use $\bar{x}$ rather than any of the other unbiased estimators? The reason is that if the underlying distribution of the population is normal, then we can show that the unbiased estimator with the smallest variance is given by $\bar{x}$. Thus, $\bar{x}$ is referred to as the **minimum variance unbiased estimator** of $\mu$.

This concept is illustrated in Figure 6.2(a) through (c), where for 200 samples of size 10 drawn from the population of 1000 birthweights in Table 6.2, we plot the sampling distribution of the sample mean ($\bar{x}$) in Figure 6.2(a), the sample median in Figure 6.2(b), and the average of the smallest and largest observations in the

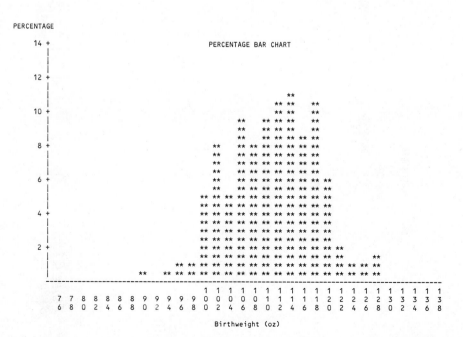

**Figure 6.2(a)**
*Sampling distribution of the sample mean ($\bar{x}$) over 200 samples of size 10 selected from the population of 1000 birthweights given in Table 6.2 (100 = 100.0–101.9, etc.)*

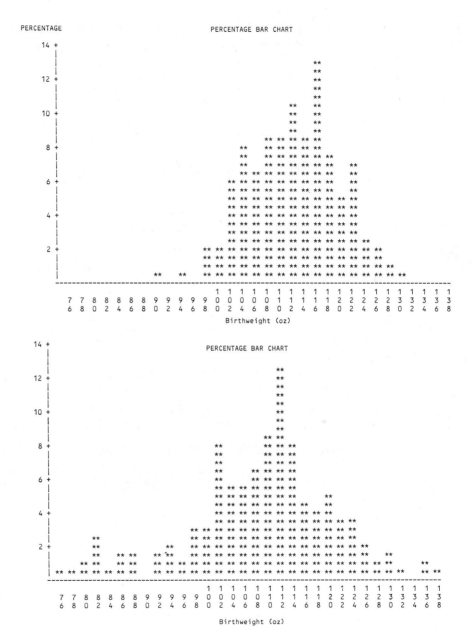

**Figure 6.2(b)**
Sampling
distribution of the
sample median over
200 samples of size
10 selected from the
population of 1000
birthweights given
in Table 6.2 (100 =
100.0–101.9, etc.)

**Figure 6.2(c)**
Sampling
distribution of the
average of the
smallest and largest
observations in each
sample for 200
samples of size 10
selected from the
population of 1000
birthweights given
in Table 6.2 (100 =
100.0–101.9, etc.)

sample in Figure 6.2(c). Note that the variability of the distribution of sample means is slightly smaller than that of the sample median and considerably smaller than that of the average of the smallest and largest observations.

## ☐ 6.4.2 Standard Error of the Mean

From **(6.1)** we see that $\bar{x}$ will be an unbiased estimator for any sample size $n$. Why then do we prefer to estimate parameters from large samples rather than from small samples? The intuitive reason is that the larger the sample size, the more accurate an estimator $\bar{x}$ will be.

**Example 6.15**

**Obstetrics**  Consider Table 6.4. Notice that the 50 individual birthweights range from 62 to 198 oz and have a sample standard deviation of 23.79 oz. The 5 sample means range from 106.7 to 132.8 oz and have a sample standard deviation of 9.77 oz. Thus, the sample means based on 10 observations are less variable from sample to sample than are the individual observations, which can be considered as sample means from samples of size 1.  ∎

Indeed, we would expect that the sample means from repeated samples of size 100 would be less variable than those from samples of size 10. We can show that this is true. By definition we have

$$Var(\bar{x}) = \left(\frac{1}{n^2}\right) Var\left(\sum_{i=1}^{n} x_i\right)$$

Now, if we have sample points $x_1, \ldots, x_n$ drawn independently from the same population, then we can show that

$$Var\left(\sum_{i=1}^{n} x_i\right) = \sum_{i=1}^{n} Var(x_i)$$

Thus,

$$Var(\bar{x}) = \left(\frac{1}{n^2}\right) \sum_{i=1}^{n} Var(x_i)$$

However, by definition $Var(x_i) = \sigma^2$. Therefore,

$$Var(\bar{x}) = (1/n^2)(\sigma^2 + \sigma^2 + \cdots + \sigma^2) = (1/n^2)(n\sigma^2) = \sigma^2/n$$

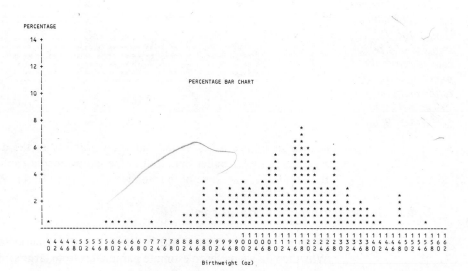

**Figure 6.3(a)**
*Illustration of the standard error of the mean (n = 1) (100 = 100.0–101.9, etc.)*

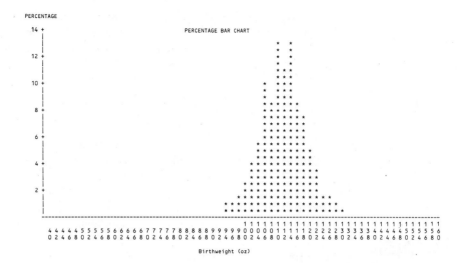

**Figure 6.3(b)**
*Illustration of the standard error of the mean (n = 10) (100 = 100.0–101.9, etc.)*

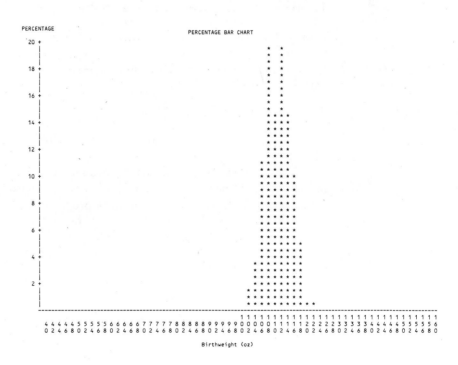

**Figure 6.3(c)**
*Illustration of the standard error of the mean (n = 30) (100 = 100.0–101.9, etc.)*

Since the standard deviation (sd) $= \sqrt{\text{variance}}$, $\text{sd}(\bar{x}) = \sigma/\sqrt{n} \equiv$ **standard error of the mean** (abbreviated to sem). We have the following summary:

6.2 Let $x_1, \ldots, x_n$ be a sample from a population with underlying mean $\mu$ and variance $\sigma^2$. The set of sample means in repeated samples of size $n$ from this population has variance $\sigma^2/n$. The standard deviation of this set of sample means is thus $\sigma/\sqrt{n}$ and is referred to as the **standard error of the mean** (sem) or the **standard error**.

Note that the standard error is *not* the standard deviation of an individual observation $x_i$ but rather of the sample mean $\bar{x}$. The standard error of the mean is illustrated in Figure 6.3(a) through (c). In Figure 6.3(a) we plot the frequency distribution of the sample mean for 200 samples of size 1 drawn from the collection of birthweights in Table 6.2. We plot similar frequency distributions of 200 sample means from samples of size 10 in Figure 6.3(b) and from samples of size 30 in Figure 6.3(c). Notice that the spread of the frequency distribution in Figure 6.3(a) corresponding to $n = 1$ is much larger than the spread of the frequency distribution in Figure 6.3(b) corresponding to $n = 10$. Furthermore, the spread of the frequency distribution in Figure 6.3(b) corresponding to $n = 10$ is much larger than the spread of the frequency distribution in Figure 6.3(c) corresponding to $n = 30$.

In practice we will rarely know the population variance $\sigma^2$. We will see in a later section that a reasonable estimator for the population variance $\sigma^2$ is the sample variance $s^2$, which leads to the following definition:

**Definition 6.7**

The **standard error of the mean** (sem), or the **standard error**, is estimated by $s/\sqrt{n}$. It represents the estimated standard deviation obtained from a set of sample means from repeated samples of size $n$ from a population with underlying variance $\sigma^2$.    ∎

**Example 6.16**    **Obstetrics**  Compute the standard error of the mean for the third sample of birthweights in Table 6.4.

**Solution**    The standard error of the mean is given by

$$s/\sqrt{n} = 22.44/\sqrt{10} = 7.10$$    ∎

The standard error is a quantitative measure of the variability of sample means obtained from repeated samples of size $n$ drawn from the same population. Notice that the standard error is directly proportional to both $1/\sqrt{n}$ and to the population standard deviation of an individual observation ($\sigma$). It justifies why we are concerned with sample size in assessing the accuracy of our estimate $\bar{x}$ of the unknown population mean $\mu$. The reason why we would prefer to estimate $\mu$ from a sample size of 400 rather than a sample of size 100 is that the standard error from the first sample will be $\frac{1}{2}$ as large as in the second sample. Thus, we should have a more accurate estimate of $\mu$. Notice that the accuracy of our estimate is also affected by the underlying variance $\sigma^2$ of individual observations from our population, a quantity which is unrelated to the sample size $n$.

**Example 6.17**    **Gynecology**   Suppose that a woman wishes to estimate her exact day of ovulation for contraceptive purposes. A theory exists that at the time of ovulation the body temperature rises by an amount from 0.5°F to 1.0°F. Thus, changes in body temperature can be used to guess the day of ovulation. Therefore, to use this method, we need a good estimate of basal body temperature during a period when ovulation is definitely not occurring. Suppose that for this purpose a woman measures her body temperature on awakening on the first 10 days after menstruation and obtains the following data: 97.2°, 96.8°, 97.4°, 97.4°, 97.3°, 97.0°, 97.1°, 97.3°, 97.2°, 97.3°. What is the best estimate of her underlying basal body temperature ($\mu$) and how accurate is this estimate?

**Solution**     Her best estimate of underlying body temperature during the nonovulation period ($\mu$) is given by

$$\bar{x} = (97.2 + 96.8 + \cdots + 97.3)/10 = 97.20°$$

The standard error of this estimate is given by

$$s/\sqrt{10} = 0.189/\sqrt{10} = 0.060°$$

We will show in our work on confidence intervals in Section 6.4.6 that for many underlying distributions of temperature, we can be fairly certain that the true mean basal temperature $\mu$ is within two standard errors of $\bar{x}$ or within $97.20° \pm 2(0.06)° \approx (97.1°–97.3°)$. Thus, if the temperature is elevated by at least 0.5° above this range on a given day, then it might indicate that the woman was ovulating, and for contraceptive purposes intercourse should not be attempted on that day. ∎

## ☐ 6.4.3 Central Limit Theorem

If the underlying distribution is normal, then we can show that the sample mean will itself be normally distributed with mean $\mu$ and variance $\sigma^2/n$. In other words, $\bar{x} \sim N(\mu, \sigma^2/n)$. If the underlying distribution is *not* normal, we would also like to make some statement about the sampling distribution of the sample mean. This statement is given by the following theorem:

---

**6.3**     **Central Limit Theorem**

Let $x_1, \ldots, x_n$ be a sample from some population with mean $\mu$ and variance $\sigma^2$. Then for large $n$, $\bar{x} \sim N(\mu, \sigma^2/n)$ even if the underlying distribution of individual observations in the population is not normal. (We use $\sim$ to represent approximately distributed.)

---

This theorem is very important because many of the distributions we will encounter in practice are not normal. In such cases we can use the central limit theorem to perform statistical inference based on the approximate normality of the sample mean and not worry about the nonnormality of the distribution of individual observations.

**Example 6.18**     **Obstetrics**   We illustrate the central limit theorem by plotting, in Figure 6.4(a), the sampling distribution of mean birthweights obtained by drawing 200 random samples of size 1 from the collection of birthweights in Table 6.2. We plot similar sampling distributions of sample means from samples of size 5 in Figure 6.4(b) and samples of size 10 in Figure 6.4(c). Notice that the distribution of individual birthweights (i.e., sample means from samples of size 1) is slightly skewed to the left. However, the distribution of sample means becomes increasingly bell shaped as the sample size increases to 5 in Figure 6.4(b) and 10 in Figure 6.4(c). ∎

**Example 6.19**     **Cardiovascular Disease**   Serum cholesterol is an important risk factor for cardiovascular disease. Its distribution tends to be skewed to the right with a few people with very high values, as is shown in Figure 6.5. However, we can perform hypothesis tests based on mean serum cholesterol over moderate samples of people, since from the central limit theorem the distribution of means will be normal even if the underlying distribution of individual measurements is not. ∎

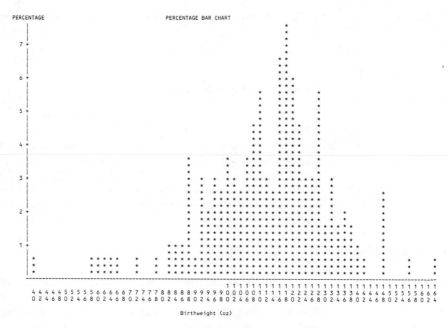

**Figure 6.4(a)**
*Illustration of the central limit theorem (n = 1) (100 = 100.0–101.9, etc.)*

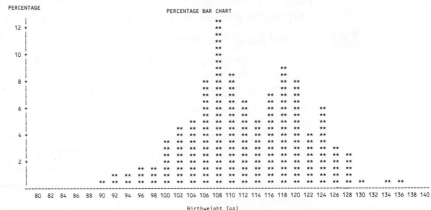

**Figure 6.4(b)**
*Illustration of the central limit theorem (n = 5) (100 = 100.0–101.9, etc.)*

**Example 6.20**    **Obstetrics** Compute the probability that the mean birthweight from a sample of 10 infants drawn from the Boston City Hospital population in Table 6.2 will fall between 98.0 and 126.0 oz (i.e., $98 \leqslant \bar{x} < 126$) if the mean birthweight for the 1000 birthweights from the Boston City Hospital population is 112.0 oz with a standard deviation of 20.6 oz.

**Solution**    We will apply the central limit theorem and assume that $\bar{x}$ follows a normal distribution with mean $\mu = 112.0$ oz and standard deviation $\sigma/\sqrt{n} = 20.6/\sqrt{10} = 6.51$ oz. It follows that

$$Pr(98.0 \leqslant \bar{x} < 126.0) = \Phi\left(\frac{126.0 - 112.0}{6.51}\right) - \Phi\left(\frac{98.0 - 112.0}{6.51}\right)$$

$$= \Phi(2.15) - \Phi(-2.15)$$

$$= \Phi(2.15) - [1 - \Phi(2.15)]$$

$$= 2\Phi(2.15) - 1$$

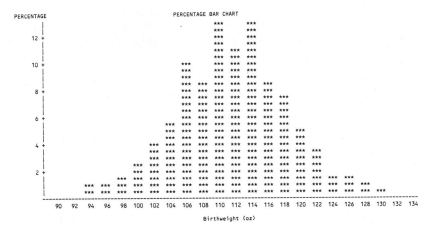

PERCENTAGE BAR CHART

Birthweight (oz)

**Figure 6.4(c)**
*Illustration of the central limit theorem (n = 10) (100 = 100.0–101.9, etc.)*

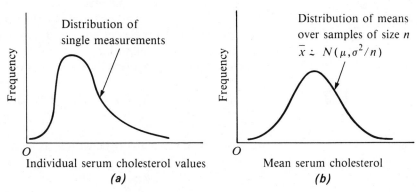

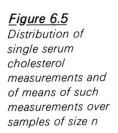

**Figure 6.5**
*Distribution of single serum cholesterol measurements and of means of such measurements over samples of size n*

We refer to Table 3 in the appendix and obtain

$$Pr(98.0 \leqslant \bar{x} < 126.0) = 2(0.9842) - 1.0$$

$$= 0.968$$

Thus, we would expect 96.8% of the samples of size 10 to have mean birthweights between 98 and 126 oz if the central limit theorem holds. We can check this value by referring to Figure 6.2(a). We note that within a specific column four rows of *'s correspond to 2% of the distribution. Thus, for each column a row of *'s corresponds to 0.5% of the distribution. Furthermore, the 90 column corresponds to the birthweight interval 90.0–91.9, the 92 column to 92.0–93.9, and so forth. We note that one column of *'s is in the 90 column, one in the 94 column, two in the 96 column, three in the 128 column, and two in the 126 column. Thus, 4 rows of stars (4 × 0.5% = 2% of the distribution) are less than 98.0 oz, and 5 rows of stars (5 × 0.5% = 2.5% of the distribution) are greater than or equal to 126.0 oz. It follows that 100% − 4.5% = 95.5% of the distribution is actually between 98 and 126 oz. This value corresponds well to the 96.8% predicted by the central limit theorem, showing that the central limit theorem holds well for averages from samples of size 10 drawn from this population. ∎

## ☐ 6.4.4 Interval Estimation—Known Variance

We have been discussing the rationale for why $\bar{x}$ is used to estimate the mean of a distribution and have given a measure of variability of this estimate, namely, the standard error. These statements hold for any underlying distribution. However, we frequently wish to obtain an interval containing the mean as well as a best estimate of its precise value. Our interval estimates will, in contrast, hold exactly if the underlying distribution is normal and only approximately if the underlying distribution is not normal, as stated in the central limit theorem.

*Example 6.21* | **Obstetrics** Suppose we have drawn the first sample of 10 birthweights given in Table 6.4. Our best estimate of the population mean $\mu$ would be the sample mean $\bar{x} = 116.9$ oz. Although 116.9 oz is our best estimate of $\mu$, we still are not certain that $\mu$ is 116.9 oz. Indeed, if we had drawn the second sample of 10 birthweights, we would have used a point estimate of 132.8 oz. Our point estimate would certainly have a different meaning for us if we were quite certain in some sense that $\mu$ was within 1 oz of 116.9 rather than within 5 oz. ∎

We have assumed previously that the distribution of birthweights in Table 6.2 was normal with mean $\mu$ and variance $\sigma^2$. It follows from our previous discussion of the properties of the sample mean that $\bar{x} \sim N(\mu, \sigma^2/n)$. Thus, if $\mu$ and $\sigma^2$ were known, then the behavior of the set of sample means over a large number of samples of size $n$ would be precisely known. In particular, we can say that 95% of all such sample means will fall within the interval $(\mu - 1.96\sigma/\sqrt{n}, \mu + 1.96\sigma/\sqrt{n})$. This statement can be written alternatively as follows:

$$Pr(\mu - 1.96\sigma/\sqrt{n} < \bar{x} < \mu + 1.96\sigma/\sqrt{n}) = 0.95$$

The inequality in **(6.4)** can actually be written as a set of two inequalities,

$$\mu - 1.96\sigma/\sqrt{n} < \bar{x} \quad \text{and} \quad \bar{x} < \mu + 1.96\sigma/\sqrt{n}$$

Suppose we add $1.96\sigma/\sqrt{n}$ to both sides of the first inequality and subtract $1.96\sigma/\sqrt{n}$ from both sides of the second inequality. We then obtain the inequalities

$$\mu < \bar{x} + 1.96\sigma/\sqrt{n} \quad \text{and} \quad \bar{x} - 1.96\sigma/\sqrt{n} < \mu$$

Thus, **(6.4)** can be rewritten in the following form:

$$Pr(\bar{x} - 1.96\sigma/\sqrt{n} < \mu < \bar{x} + 1.96\sigma/\sqrt{n}) = 0.95$$

**Definition 6.8**

We define a **95% confidence interval (CI)** for $\mu$ when $\sigma^2$ is known by

$$(\bar{x} - 1.96\sigma/\sqrt{n}, \ \bar{x} + 1.96\sigma/\sqrt{n})$$ ∎

We may be puzzled at this point as to what the confidence interval means. The parameter $\mu$ is a fixed unknown constant. How can we state that the probability that it lies within some specific interval is 95%? The key point to understand is that the boundaries of the interval depend on the sample points chosen (or more precisely, on the sample mean) and will vary from sample to sample.

Furthermore, *95% of such intervals that could be constructed from repeated samples of size n* will contain the parameter $\mu$.

*Example 6.22*     **Obstetrics**  Let us consider the 5 samples of size 10 from the population of birthweights as shown in Table 6.4. Let us assume that $\sigma$ is known to be 20. The interval

$$(\bar{x} - 1.96\sigma/\sqrt{n}, \ \bar{x} + 1.96\sigma/\sqrt{n}) = \left( \bar{x} - \frac{1.96(20)}{\sqrt{10}}, \ \bar{x} + \frac{1.96(20)}{\sqrt{10}} \right)$$

$$= (\bar{x} - 12.4, \ \bar{x} + 12.4)$$

would be different for each sample and is given in Figure 6.6. We have also drawn in a dashed line to represent an imaginary value for $\mu$. The idea is that over a large number of hypothetical samples of size 10, 95% of such intervals will contain the parameter $\mu$. Any one interval from a particular sample *may* or *may not* contain the parameter $\mu$. For example, in Figure 6.6 the first, third, fourth, and fifth intervals contain the parameter $\mu$, whereas the second interval does not.

Therefore, we cannot say that there is a 95% chance that the parameter $\mu$ will fall within a particular 95% CI. However, we can say the following:

Over the collection of all 95% confidence intervals that could be constructed from repeated samples of size *n*, 95% will contain the parameter $\mu$.

In any event the length of the confidence interval gives us some idea of the precision of our point estimate $\bar{x}$. In this particular case the length of each of the confidence intervals is about 25 oz, which should make us very uneasy about the precision of our point estimate $\bar{x}$ and implies that we need a larger sample size to get a more precise estimate of $\mu$.  ∎

*Example 6.23*     **Gynecology**  Compute a 95% CI for the underlying mean basal body temperature using the data in Example 6.17, assuming that the standard deviation is 0.2°.

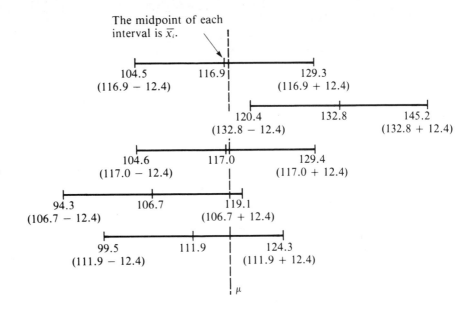

**Figure 6.6**
*A collection of 95% confidence intervals for the mean $\mu$ as computed from repeated samples of size 10 (see Table 6.4) from the population of birthweights given in Table 6.2*

**Solution**    The 95% CI is given by

$$\bar{x} \pm 1.96\sigma/\sqrt{n} = 97.2° \pm 1.96(0.2)/\sqrt{10}$$

$$= 97.2° \pm 0.12°$$

$$= (97.08°, 97.32°) \qquad \blacksquare$$

We are frequently interested in obtaining confidence intervals with levels of confidence other than 95%. In particular, we would like to develop confidence intervals with confidence level $100\% \times (1 - \alpha)$ for any arbitrary $\alpha$. This interval can be developed in the same way as the 95% confidence interval in **(6.5)**.

**Definition 6.9**

We define a $100\% \times (1 - \alpha)$ **confidence interval for** $\mu$ by the interval

$$(\bar{x} - z_{1-\alpha/2}\sigma/\sqrt{n}, \bar{x} + z_{1-\alpha/2}\sigma/\sqrt{n})$$

where $z_{1-\alpha/2}$ equals the upper $\alpha/2$ percentile of a $N(0, 1)$ distribution. $\qquad \blacksquare$

**Example 6.24**    Suppose we have drawn the first sample in Table 6.4. Compute a 99% CI for the underlying mean birthweight, assuming that $\sigma = 20$.

**Solution**    This value is given by

$$(116.9 - z_{.995}(20)/\sqrt{10}, 116.9 + z_{.995}(20)/\sqrt{10})$$

From Table 3 we see that $z_{.995} = 2.576$, and therefore the 99% CI is

$$(116.9 - 2.576(20)/\sqrt{10}, 116.9 + 2.576(20)/\sqrt{10}) = (100.6, 133.2) \qquad \blacksquare$$

Notice that the 99% confidence interval (100.6, 133.2) computed in Example 6.24 is wider than the corresponding 95% confidence interval (104.5, 129.3) computed for the first sample in Figure 6.6. The rationale for this difference is that the higher the level of confidence desired that $\mu$ lies within an interval, the wider the confidence interval must be. Indeed, for 95% confidence intervals the length was $2(1.96)\sigma/\sqrt{n}$; for 99% confidence intervals the length was $2(2.576)\sigma/\sqrt{n}$. In general, the length of the $100\% \times (1 - \alpha)$ confidence interval is given by

$$2z_{1-\alpha/2}\sigma/\sqrt{n}$$

Therefore, we can see that the length of a confidence interval is governed by three variables: $n, \sigma, \alpha$.

The length of a *100%* × *(1 − α) confidence interval* equals

$$2z_{1-\alpha/2}\sigma/\sqrt{n}$$

and is determined by $n, \sigma$, and $\alpha$.

*n.* As the *sample size (n) increases*, the *length* of the confidence interval *decreases*.

$\sigma$. As the *standard deviation* ($\sigma$), which reflects the variability of individual observations, *increases*, the *length* of the confidence interval *increases*.

$\alpha$. As the confidence desired increases ($\alpha$ *decreases*), the length of the confidence interval *increases*.

*Example 6.25*

**Gynecology** Compute a 95% CI for the underlying mean basal body temperature using the data in Example 6.17, assuming that the number of days sampled is 100 rather than 10 and the standard deviation = 0.2°.

*Solution*

The 95% CI is given by

$$97.2° \pm 1.96(0.2)/\sqrt{100} = 97.2° \pm 1.96(0.2)/10 = 97.2° \pm 0.04°$$

$$= (97.16°,\ 97.24°)$$

Notice how this interval is much narrower than the corresponding interval (97.08°, 97.32°) based on a sample of 10 days given in Example 6.23. ∎

*Example 6.26*

Compute a 95% CI for the underlying mean basal temperature using the data in Example 6.17, assuming that the standard deviation of basal body temperature is 0.4° rather than 0.2° with a sample size of 10.

*Solution*

The 95% CI is given by

$$97.2° \pm 1.96(0.4)/\sqrt{10} = 97.2° \pm 0.25° = (96.95°,\ 97.45°)$$

Notice how this interval is much wider than the corresponding interval (97.08°, 97.32°) based on a standard deviation of 0.2° with a sample size of 10. ∎

Usually, only $n$ and $\alpha$ are under our control. $\sigma$ is a function of the type of variable we are studying.

We have utilized confidence intervals mainly as descriptive tools for the purpose of *characterizing the precision* with which we can estimate the parameters of a distribution. Another use for confidence intervals is in *making decisions* on the basis of our data.

*Example 6.27*

**Cardiovascular Disease, Pediatrics** Suppose we know from large studies that the mean cholesterol level in children ages 2–14 is 175 mg%/ml and the standard deviation is 30 mg%/ml. We wish to see if there is a familial aggregation of cholesterol levels. Specifically, we identify a group of fathers who have had a heart attack and who presumably have high cholesterol levels and measure the cholesterol levels of their offspring within the 2–14 age range.

Suppose we find that the mean cholesterol level in a group of 100 of such children is 207.3 mg%/ml. Is this value sufficiently far from 175 mg%/ml for us to believe that the underlying mean cholesterol level in the population of all children selected in this way is greater than 175 mg%/ml?

*Solution*

One approach would be to construct a 95% confidence interval for $\mu$ on the basis of our sample data. We then could make the following decision: If the interval contains 175 mg%/ml, then we cannot say that the underlying mean for this group is any greater than the mean for all children (175) and we would decide that there is no demonstrated familial aggregation of cholesterol levels. If the confidence interval does not contain 175, then we would conclude that the true underlying mean for this group is greater than 175 and therefore there is a demonstrated familial aggregation of cholesterol levels.

The confidence interval in this case is given by

$$[207.3 - z_{.975}(30)/\sqrt{100}, \ 207.3 + z_{.975}(30)/\sqrt{100}]$$

$$= [207.3 - 1.96(30)/10, \ 207.3 + 1.96(30)/10]$$

$$= (201.4, \ 213.2)$$

Clearly, 175 is far from the lower boundary of the interval, and we thus conclude that there is familial aggregation of cholesterol. ∎

## □ 6.4.5 t Distribution

In the previous section we discussed the problem of constructing confidence intervals for the mean of a normal distribution when the variance is known. This situation is somewhat artificial, since the population variance is seldom known when dealing with actual data. Our first step in constructing confidence intervals in the previous section was to assume that if the individual observations come from an underlying normal distribution with mean $\mu$ and variance $\sigma^2$, then the quantity $(\bar{x} - \mu)/(\sigma/\sqrt{n}) \sim N(0, 1)$. Since we do not know $\sigma$, it is reasonable to estimate $\sigma$ by the sample standard deviation $s$ and to try to construct confidence intervals using the quantity $(\bar{x} - \mu)/(s/\sqrt{n})$. The problem is that this quantity is no longer normally distributed.

This problem was first solved in 1908 by a statistician named William Gossett. For his entire professional life, Gossett worked for the Guinness Brewery in Great Britain. He chose to identify himself by the pseudonym "Student," and thus the distribution of $(\bar{x} - \mu)/(s/\sqrt{n})$ is sometimes referred to as **Student's t distribution**. Gossett found that the shape of the distribution depended on the sample size $n$. Thus, the $t$ distribution is not a unique distribution but is instead a family of distributions indexed by a parameter referred to as the **degrees of freedom** $(df)$* of the distribution.

---

**6.6** If

$$x_1, \ldots, x_n \sim N(\mu, \sigma^2)$$

then $(\bar{x} - \mu)/(s/\sqrt{n})$ is distributed as a $t$ distribution with $(n - 1)$ degrees of freedom $(df)$.

---

Once again, Student's $t$ distribution is not a unique distribution but is a family of distributions indexed by the degrees of freedom $d$. We sometimes refer to the $t$ distribution with $d$ degrees of freedom as the $t_d$ distribution.

**Definition 6.10**

The *pth percentile of a t distribution with d degrees of freedom* is denoted by $t_{d,p}$, that is,

$$Pr(t_d < t_{d,p}) \equiv p$$ ∎

*Degrees of freedom appears in this text as both $df$ and d.f.

**Example 6.28**

What does $t_{20,.95}$ mean?

**Solution**

$t_{20,.95}$ is the 95th percentile or the upper 5th percentile of a $t$ distribution with 20 degrees of freedom. ∎

It is of interest to compare a $t$ distribution with $d$ degrees of freedom with an $N(0, 1)$ distribution. The density functions corresponding to these distributions are depicted in Figure 6.7.

Notice that the $t$ distribution is symmetric about 0 but is more spread out than the $N(0, 1)$ distribution. We can show that for any $\alpha$, $t_{d,1-\alpha}$ is always larger than the corresponding percentile for a $N(0, 1)$ distribution ($z_{1-\alpha}$). This relationship is depicted in Figure 6.7. However, as $d$ becomes large, the $t$ distribution converges to a $N(0, 1)$ distribution. An explanation for this convergence is that for finite samples the sample variance ($s^2$) is an approximation to the population variance ($\sigma^2$). This approximation gives the statistic $(\bar{x} - \mu)/(s/\sqrt{n})$ more variability than the corresponding statistic $(\bar{x} - \mu)/(\sigma/\sqrt{n})$. As $n$ becomes large, this approximation gets better and $s^2$ will converge to $\sigma^2$ exactly. The two distributions thus get more and more alike as $n$ becomes large. The upper 2.5th percentile of the $t$ distribution for various degrees of freedom and the corresponding percentile for the normal distribution are given in Table 6.5 and are depicted in Figure 6.8.

The difference between the $t$ distribution and the normal distribution is greatest for very small values of $n$ ($n < 30$). For most applications we can probably assume that a $t$ distribution is approximately normal if the number of degrees of freedom is greater than 60, although an exact $t$ table is always preferable if available. Table 5 in the appendix gives the percentage points of the $t$ distribution for various degrees of freedom. The degrees of freedom are given in the first column of the table, and the percentiles are given across the first row. The $p$th percentile of a $t$ distribution with $d$ degrees of freedom is found by reading across the row marked $d$ and reading down the column marked $p$.

**Figure 6.7**
*Comparison of Student's t distribution with d degrees of freedom with a N(0, 1) distribution*

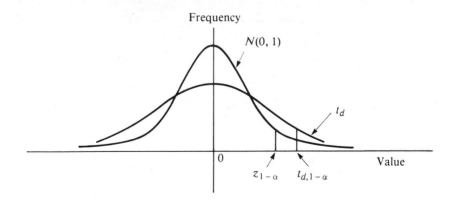

**Table 6.5**
*Comparison of the 97.5th percentile of the t distribution and the normal distribution*

| $d$ | $t_{d,.975}$ | $z_{.975}$ | $d$ | $t_{d,.975}$ | $z_{.975}$ |
|---|---|---|---|---|---|
| 4 | 2.776 | 1.960 | 60 | 2.000 | 1.960 |
| 9 | 2.262 | 1.960 | ∞ | 1.960 | 1.960 |
| 29 | 2.045 | 1.960 | | | |

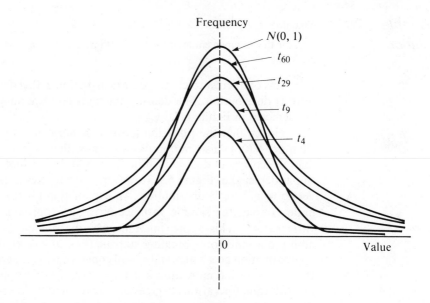

**Figure 6.8**
Comparison of
various t
distributions with
different degrees
of freedom with a
N(0, 1) distribution

*Example 6.29*    Find the upper 5th percentile of a $t$ distribution with 23 $df$.

*Solution*    We wish to find $t_{23,.95}$, which is given in row 23 and column 0.95 of the table and is 1.714.  ∎

## ☐ 6.4.6  Interval Estimation—Unknown Variance

6.7    If we use similar logic to that given in Section 6.4.4, then we can show that a $100\% \times (1 - \alpha)$ *confidence interval for the mean μ of a normal distribution with unknown variance* is given by

$$(\bar{x} - t_{n-1,1-\alpha/2}s/\sqrt{n}, \ \bar{x} + t_{n-1,1-\alpha/2}s/\sqrt{n})$$

*Example 6.30*    **Obstetrics** Now let us consider the birthweight data from the first sample in Table 6.4. Compute a 95% confidence interval for $\mu$ if we do not assume that the variance is known.

*Solution*    If we do not assume that the variance is known, then a 95% confidence interval for $\mu$ is given as follows:

$$[116.90 - t_{9,.975}(21.70)/\sqrt{10}, \ 116.90 + t_{9,.975}(21.70)/\sqrt{10}]$$

$$= [116.90 - 2.262(21.70)/\sqrt{10}, \ 116.90 + 2.262(21.70)/\sqrt{10}]$$

$$= (101.38, 132.42)$$    ∎

Generally, confidence intervals based on the $t$ distribution (unknown variance) will be longer than confidence intervals based on the normal distribution (known variance). However, this principle does not always apply, since for a particular sample the sample variance $s^2$ may be considerably less than the population variance $\sigma^2$.

# ■ 6.5 ESTIMATION OF THE VARIANCE OF A DISTRIBUTION

## □ 6.5.1 Point Estimation

We saw in Chapter 2 that the sample variance was defined as

$$s^2 = \frac{1}{n-1} \sum_{i=1}^{n} (x_i - \bar{x})^2$$

This definition is somewhat counterintuitive, since we would expect that the denominator should be $n$ rather than $n - 1$. We now give a more formal justification for this definition. If we consider our sample $x_1, \ldots, x_n$ as coming from some population with mean $\mu$ and variance $\sigma^2$, then how can we estimate the unknown population variance $\sigma^2$ from our sample? We are aided in this decision by the following principle:

| 6.8 | Let $x_1, \ldots, x_n$ be a sample from some population with mean $\mu$ and variance $\sigma^2$. The **sample variance $s^2$ is an unbiased estimator** of $\sigma^2$ over all possible samples of size $n$ that could have been drawn from this population; that is, $E(s^2) = \sigma^2$. |

Therefore, if we select repeated samples of size $n$ from the population, as was done in Table 6.4, and compute the sample variance $s^2$ from each sample, then the average of these sample variances over a large number of such samples of size $n$ will be the population variance $\sigma^2$. This statement holds for any underlying distribution.

*Example 6.31*    **Gynecology**   Estimate the variance of the distribution of basal body temperatures using the data in Example 6.17.

*Solution*    We have

$$s^2 = \frac{1}{9} \sum_{i=1}^{n} (x_i - \bar{x})^2$$

which is an unbiased estimator of $\sigma^2$.                                                         ■

Note that the intuitive estimator for $\sigma^2$ with $n$ in the denominator rather than $n - 1$, that is,

$$\frac{1}{n} \sum_{i=1}^{n} (x_i - \bar{x})^2$$

will tend to underestimate the underlying variance $\sigma^2$ by a factor of $(n - 1)/n$. This factor is considerable for small samples but tends to be negligible for large samples.

## □ 6.5.2 The Chi-Square Distribution

We discussed the problem of interval estimation of the mean of a normal distribution in Sections 6.4.4 and 6.4.6. We often want to obtain interval estimates of the variance as well. Once again, as was the case for the mean, the interval estimates will hold exactly only if the underlying distribution is normal. The interval estimates will perform much more poorly for the variance than for the mean if the underlying distribution is not normal and should be used with caution in this case.

*Example 6.32*    **Hypertension**  A new machine has been produced, called an arteriosonde machine, that "prints" blood pressure recordings on a tape so that the measurements can be read rather than heard. A major argument for using such a machine is that the variability of measurements obtained by different observers on the same person will be lower than with a standard blood pressure cuff.

Suppose we have the data presented in Table 6.6, consisting of systolic blood pressure measurements obtained on 10 persons and read by 2 observers. We will use the difference $d_i$ between the first and second observer to assess interobserver variability. In particular, if we assume that the underlying distribution of these differences is normal with mean $\mu$ and variance $\sigma^2$, then it is of primary interest to estimate $\sigma^2$. The higher $\sigma^2$ is, the higher the interobserver variability.

We have shown previously that an unbiased estimate of the variance $\sigma^2$ is given by the sample variance $s^2$. In this case,

$$s^2 = \sum_{i=1}^{n}(d_i - \bar{d})^2/9 = \left[\sum_{i=1}^{n}d_i^2 - \left(\sum_{i=1}^{n}d_i\right)^2\Big/10\right]\Big/9$$

$$= \frac{[(-6)^2 + (3)^2 + \cdots + (-2)^2] - [(-6) + (3) + \cdots + (-2)]^2/10}{9} = 8.178$$

How can we obtain an interval estimate for $\sigma^2$?    ∎

To obtain an interval estimate for $\sigma^2$ we must introduce a new family of distributions, called chi-square ($\chi^2$) distributions, to enable us to find the sampling distribution of $s^2$ from sample to sample.

*Table 6.6*
*Systolic blood pressure measurements (mm Hg) from an arteriosonde machine obtained from 10 persons and read by two observers*

|  | Observer | | |
| Person (i) | 1 | 2 | Difference ($d_i$) |
| --- | --- | --- | --- |
| 1 | 194 | 200 | −6 |
| 2 | 126 | 123 | +3 |
| 3 | 130 | 128 | +2 |
| 4 | 98 | 101 | −3 |
| 5 | 136 | 135 | +1 |
| 6 | 145 | 145 | 0 |
| 7 | 110 | 111 | −1 |
| 8 | 108 | 107 | +1 |
| 9 | 102 | 99 | +3 |
| 10 | 126 | 128 | −2 |

**Definition 6.11**

If

$$G = \sum_{i=1}^{n} x_i^2 \quad \text{where} \quad x_1, \ldots, x_n \sim N(0, 1),$$

then $G$ is said to follow a **chi-square distribution with $n$ degrees of freedom ($df$)**. The distribution is often denoted by $\chi_n^2$. ∎

The chi-square distribution is actually a family of distributions indexed by the parameter $n$ referred to, again, as the degrees of freedom, as was the case for the $t$ distribution. Unlike the $t$ distribution, which is always symmetric about 0 for any degrees of freedom, the chi-square distribution only takes on positive values and is generally skewed to the right, except for very large $n$ ($n \geqslant 100$), where the distribution becomes more symmetric. The general shape of these distributions is indicated in Figure 6.9.

For $n = 1, 2$, the distribution has a mode at 0. For $n \geqslant 3$, the distribution has a mode greater than 0 and is skewed to the right. We can show that the expected value of a $\chi_n^2$ distribution is $n$ and the variance is $2n$. For large $n$ ($n \geqslant 100$), the distribution tends to be roughly symmetric and can be approximated by a normal distribution with mean $n$ and variance $2n$.

**Definition 6.12**

We denote the **$p$th percentile of a $\chi_n^2$ distribution by $\chi_{n,p}^2$**, where $Pr(\chi_n^2 < \chi_{n,p}^2) \equiv p$. These percentiles are depicted in Figure 6.10 and appear in Table 6 in the appendix. ∎

Table 6 is constructed similarly to the $t$-table (Table 5), with the degrees of freedom ($d$) indexed in the first column and the percentile ($p$) indexed in the first row. The principal difference between the two tables is that both *lower* ($p \leqslant 0.5$) and *upper* ($p > 0.5$) percentiles are given for the chi-square distribution, whereas only upper percentiles are given for the $t$ distribution. The $t$ distribution is symmetric about 0, and therefore any lower percentile can be obtained as the negative of the corresponding upper percentile. Because the chi-square distribution is,

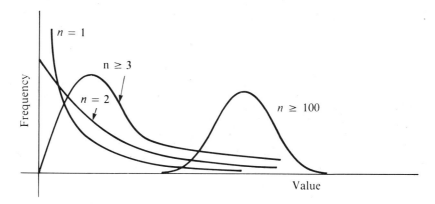

*Figure 6.9*
*General shape of various $\chi^2$ distributions with $n$ df*

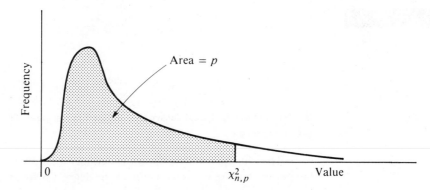

**Figure 6.10**
Graphical display of
the percentiles of a
$\chi_n^2$ distribution

in general, a skewed distribution, there is no simple relationship between the upper and lower percentiles.

*Example 6.33*    Find the upper and lower 2.5th percentile of a chi-square distribution with 10 *df*.

*Solution*    According to Table 6, the upper and lower percentiles are given by

$$\chi_{10,.975}^2 = 20.48 \quad \text{and} \quad \chi_{10,.025}^2 = 3.25$$

respectively.                                                                                                                 ∎

## ☐ *6.5.3  Interval Estimation*

To obtain an interval estimate of $\sigma^2$, we wish to find the sampling distribution of $s^2$. Suppose we assume that $x_1, \ldots, x_n \sim N(\mu, \sigma^2)$. Then, we can show that

6.9

$$s^2 \sim \frac{\sigma^2 \chi_{n-1}^2}{(n-1)}$$

Thus, from **(6.9)** we see that $s^2$ follows a chi-square distribution with $n - 1$ *df* multiplied by the constant $\sigma^2/(n - 1)$. We can now use manipulations similar to those given in Section 6.4.4 to obtain a $100\% \times (1 - \alpha)$ confidence interval for $\sigma^2$ as follows:

6.10

A *$100\% \times (1 - \alpha)$ confidence interval for $\sigma^2$ is given by*

$$[(n - 1)s^2/\chi_{n-1,1-\alpha/2}^2, (n - 1)s^2/\chi_{n-1,\alpha/2}^2]$$

*Example 6.34*    **Hypertension** We now return to the specific data set in Example 6.32. Suppose we wish to construct a 95% confidence interval for the interobserver variability as defined by $\sigma^2$.

*Solution*    Since there are 10 persons and $s^2 = 8.178$, the required interval is given by

$$(9s^2/\chi_{9,.975}^2, 9s^2/\chi_{9,.025}^2) = [9(8.178)/19.02, 9(8.178)/2.70]$$

$$= (3.87, 27.26)$$

Similarly, a 95% confidence interval for $\sigma$ is given by $(\sqrt{3.87}, \sqrt{27.26}) = (1.97, 5.22)$. Notice that the confidence interval for $\sigma^2$ is *not* symmetric about $s^2 = 8.178$, in contrast to the confidence intervals for $\mu$, which *were* symmetric about $\bar{x}$. This characteristic is common in confidence intervals for the variance.

The utility of the confidence interval for $\sigma^2$ for decision-making purposes might be achieved if we had a good estimate of the interobserver variability of blood pressure readings from a standard cuff. For example, suppose we know from previous work that if two people are listening to blood pressure recordings from a standard cuff, then the interobserver variability as measured by the variance of the set of differences between the readings of the two observers is 35. This value is outside the range of the 95% confidence interval for $\sigma^2$ (3.87, 27.26), and we thus conclude that the interobserver variability is decreased by using an arteriosonde machine. Alternatively, if this prior variance were 15, then we could not say that the variances obtained from using the two methods are different. ∎

# 6.6 ESTIMATION FOR THE BINOMIAL DISTRIBUTION

## ☐ 6.6.1 Point Estimation

Now we will discuss point estimation for the parameter $p$ of a binomial distribution.

*Example 6.35*    *Cancer* Let us consider the problem of the estimation of the prevalence of malignant melanoma in 45–54-year-old women in the United States. Suppose that we select a random sample of 5000 women from this age group and find that 28 have the disease. Let the random variable $X$ for each of the 5000 women be 1 if a woman has the disease and 0 if she does not. Suppose that the prevalence rate of the disease in this age group is $p$. How can we estimate $p$? ∎

**Definition 6.13**

Let $X_i$ be a random variable that takes on the value 1 with probability $p$ and the value 0 with probability $q = 1 - p$. This type of random variable is defined as a **Bernoulli trial.** ∎

We know from the definition of an expected value that $E(X_i) = 1(p) + 0(q)$ $= p$ and that $E(X_i^2) = 1^2(p) + 0^2(q) = p$. Therefore,

$$Var(X_i) = E(X_i^2) - [E(X_i)]^2 = p - p^2 = p(1 - p) = pq$$

Let us now consider the random variable

$$X = \sum_{i=1}^{n} X_i$$

In Example 6.35 this random variable simply represents the number of cases of malignant melanoma among $n$ women. We have

$$E(X) = E\left(\sum_{i=1}^{n} X_i\right) = p + p + \cdots + p = np$$

and

$$Var(X) = Var\left(\sum_{i=1}^{n} X_i\right) = pq + pq + \cdots + pq = npq$$

We note that $X$ can also be looked at as a binomial random variable with parameters $n$ and $p$, since it represents the number of events in $n$ trials.

Finally, let us consider the random variable $\hat{p}$ = sample proportion of events. In our example, $\hat{p}$ = proportion of women with malignant melanoma. Thus,

$$\hat{p} = \frac{1}{n}\sum_{i=1}^{n} X_i = \bar{x}$$

Since $\hat{p}$ is a sample mean, the results of **(6.1)** apply and we see that $E(\hat{p}) = E(X_i) \equiv \mu = p$. Furthermore, from **(6.2)** it follows that

$$Var(\hat{p}) = \sigma^2/n = pq/n \quad \text{and} \quad se(\hat{p}) = \sqrt{pq/n}$$

Thus, for any sample of size $n$, the sample proportion $\hat{p}$ is an unbiased estimator of the population proportion $p$. The standard error of this proportion is given exactly by $\sqrt{pq/n}$ and is estimated by $\sqrt{\hat{p}\hat{q}/n}$. These principles can be summarized as follows:

**6.11** | **Point Estimation of the Binomial Parameter p**

Let $X$ be a binomial random variable with parameters $n$ and $p$. An unbiased estimate of $p$ is given by the sample proportion of events $\hat{p}$. Its standard error is given exactly by $\sqrt{pq/n}$ and is estimated by $\sqrt{\hat{p}\hat{q}/n}$.

*Example 6.36*

*Solution*

Estimate the prevalence of malignant melanoma in Example 6.35 and give its standard error.

Our best estimate of the prevalence rate of malignant melanoma among 45–54-year-old women is $28/5000 = 0.0056$. Its estimated standard error is

$$\sqrt{(0.0056)(0.9944)/5000} = 0.0011$$ ∎

### ☐ 6.6.2 *Interval Estimation—Normal Theory Methods*

We discussed the point estimation of the parameter $p$ of a binomial distribution in Section 6.6.1. How can we obtain an **interval estimate** of the parameter $p$?

*Example 6.37*

*Cancer* Suppose we are interested in estimating the prevalence rate of breast cancer among 50–54-year-old women whose mothers have had breast cancer. Suppose that in a random sample of 10,000 such women, we find that 400 have had breast cancer at some point in their lives. We have shown that the best point estimate of the prevalence rate $p$ is given by the sample proportion $\hat{p} = 400/10,000 = 0.040$. How can we obtain an interval estimate of the parameter $p$? (See the solution in Example 6.38 on the following page.) ∎

We will assume that the normal approximation to the binomial distribution is valid—whereby the number of events $X$ observed out of $n$ women will be approximately normally distributed with mean $np$ and variance $npq$ or, correspondingly, the proportion of women with events $= \hat{p} = X/n$ is normally distributed with mean $p$ and variance $pq/n$.

We can actually justify the normal approximation on the basis of the central limit theorem. Indeed, in the previous section we showed that $\hat{p}$ could be represented as an average of $n$ Bernoulli trials, each of which has mean $p$ and variance $pq$. Thus, for large $n$, from the central limit theorem, we can see that $\hat{p} = \bar{x}$ is normally distributed with mean $\mu = p$ and variance $\sigma^2/n = pq/n$ or

**6.12**

$$\hat{p} \sim N(p, pq/n)$$

Alternatively, since the number of successes in $n$ Bernoulli trials $= X = n\hat{p}$ (which is the same as a binomial random variable with parameters $n$ and $p$), if we multiply **(6.12)** by $n$, we have

**6.13**

$$X \sim N(np, npq)$$

This formulation is indeed the same as that for the normal approximation to the binomial distribution, as was given in Chapter 5. How large should $n$ be before we can use this approximation? In Chapter 5 we said that the normal approximation to the binomial distribution is valid if $npq \geqslant 5$. However, in Chapter 5 we assumed that $p$ was known, whereas here we assume that it is unknown. Thus, we shall estimate $p$ by $\hat{p}$ and $q$ by $\hat{q} = 1 - \hat{p}$ and will apply the normal approximation to the binomial if $n\hat{p}\hat{q} \geqslant 5$. Therefore, the results of this section should only be used in this case. An approximate $100\% \times (1 - \alpha)$ confidence interval for $p$ can now be derived from **(6.12)** using methods similar to those given in Section 6.4.4. This derivation can be summarized as follows:

**6.14**    *Normal Theory Method for Obtaining a Confidence Interval for the Binomial Parameter p*

We can show that an approximate $100\% \times (1 - \alpha)$ confidence interval for the binomial parameter $p$ based on the normal approximation to the binomial distribution is given by

$$\left(\hat{p} - z_{1-\alpha/2}\sqrt{\hat{p}\hat{q}/n}, \ \hat{p} + z_{1-\alpha/2}\sqrt{\hat{p}\hat{q}/n}\right)$$

This method of interval estimation should only be used if $n\hat{p}\hat{q} \geqslant 5$.

*Example 6.38*    *Cancer* Using the data in Example 6.37, derive a 95% confidence interval for the prevalence rate of breast cancer among 50–54-year-old women whose mothers have had breast cancer.

*Solution*    We have

$$\hat{p} = 0.040 \qquad \alpha = 0.05 \qquad z_{1-\alpha/2} = 1.96 \qquad n = 10,000$$

Therefore, an approximate 95% confidence interval is given by

$$[0.040 - 1.96\sqrt{(0.04)(0.96)/10{,}000}, \; 0.040 + 1.96\sqrt{(0.04)(0.96)/10{,}000}]$$

$$= (0.040 - 0.004, \; 0.040 + 0.004) = (0.036, 0.044)$$

Suppose we know that the prevalence rate of breast cancer among all 50–54-year-old American women is 2%. Since 2% does *not* fall in the preceding interval, we can be quite confident that the underlying rate for the group of women whose mothers have had breast cancer is higher than the rate in the general population.    ∎

## ☐ 6.6.3 Interval Estimation—Exact Methods

The question remains as to how to obtain a confidence interval for the binomial parameter $p$ when either the normal approximation to the binomial distribution is not valid or when a more exact confidence interval is desired.

*Example 6.39*    *Cancer, Nutrition*  Suppose we want to estimate the rate of bladder cancer in rats that have been fed a diet high in saccharin. We feed this diet to 20 rats and find that 2 develop bladder cancer. In this case our best point estimate of $p$ is $\hat{p} = \frac{2}{20} = 0.1$. However, since

$$n\hat{p}\hat{q} = 20(2/20)(18/20) = 1.8 < 5$$

we cannot use the normal approximation to the binomial distribution and thus cannot use normal theory methods for obtaining confidence intervals. How can we obtain an interval estimate in this case?    ∎

We will present a small sample method for obtaining confidence limits.

**6.15**  **Exact Method for Obtaining a Confidence Interval for the Binomial Parameter p**

An exact $100\% \times (1 - \alpha)$ confidence interval for the binomial parameter $p$ that is always valid is given by $(p_1, p_2)$, where $p_1, p_2$ satisfy the equations

$$Pr(X \geq x \mid p = p_1) = \frac{\alpha}{2} = \sum_{k=x}^{n} \binom{n}{k} p_1^{k}(1 - p_1)^{n-k}$$

$$Pr(X \leq x \mid p = p_2) = \frac{\alpha}{2} = \sum_{k=0}^{x} \binom{n}{k} p_2^{k}(1 - p_2)^{n-k}$$

The main problem with using this method is the difficulty in computing expressions such as

$$\sum_{k=0}^{x} \binom{n}{k} p^{k}(1 - p)^{n-k}$$

Fortunately, special tables exist for the evaluation of such expressions, one of which is given in Table 7 in the appendix. This table can be used as follows:

| 6.16 | **Exact Confidence Limits for Binomial Proportions** |
|---|---|

*1*. The sample size ($n$) is given along each curve. Two curves should correspond to a given sample size. One curve is used to obtain the lower confidence limit and the other to obtain the upper confidence limit.

*2*. If $0 \leqslant \hat{p} \leqslant 0.5$, then

(a) Refer to the lower horizontal axis and find the point corresponding to $\hat{p}$.

(b) Draw a line perpendicular to the horizontal axis and find the two points where this line intersects the two curves identified in *1*.

(c) Read across to the left vertical axis; the smaller value corresponds to the lower confidence limit and the larger value to the upper confidence limit.

*3*. If $0.5 < \hat{p} \leqslant 1.0$, then

(a) Refer to the upper horizontal axis and find the point corresponding to $\hat{p}$.

(b) Draw a line perpendicular to the horizontal axis and find the two points where this line intersects the two curves identified in *1*.

(c) Read across to the right vertical axis; the smaller value corresponds to the lower confidence limit and the larger value to the upper confidence limit.

---

*Example 6.40*

**Cancer** Derive an exact 95% confidence interval from the rat bladder cancer data given in Example 6.39.

*Solution*

We refer to Table 7, $\alpha = 0.05$, and identify the two curves with $n = 20$. Since $\hat{p} = 0.1 \leqslant 0.5$, we refer to the lower horizontal axis and draw a vertical line at 0.10 until it intersects the two curves marked $n = 20$. We then read across to the left vertical axis and find the confidence limits of 0.01 and 0.32. Thus, the exact 95% confidence interval $= (0.01, 0.32)$. Notice that this confidence interval is *not* symmetric about $\hat{p} = 0.10$. ∎

*Example 6.41*

**Cardiovascular Disease** Suppose that as part of a program for counseling patients with many risk factors for heart disease, 100 smokers are identified. Of this group, 10 give up smoking for at least 1 month. After a 1-year follow-up, 6 of the 10 patients are found to have taken up smoking again. We refer to the proportion of ex-smokers who start smoking again as the *recidivism rate*. Derive a 99% confidence interval for the recidivism rate.

*Solution*

We must use exact binomial confidence limits, since

$$n\hat{p}\hat{q} = 10(0.6)(0.4) = 2.4 < 5$$

We refer to the upper horizontal axis of the chart marked $\alpha = 0.01$ in Table 7 and note the point $\hat{p} = 0.60$. We then follow the vertical scale at 0.60 until it intersects the two curves marked $n = 10$. We then read across to the right vertical axis and find the confidence limits of 0.19 and 0.92. Thus, the exact 99% confidence interval $= (0.19, 0.92)$.

# ■ 6.7 ONE-SIDED CONFIDENCE INTERVALS

In all our previous work on interval estimation, we have been describing what are known as *two-sided confidence intervals*. Frequently, the following type of problem occurs.

*Example 6.42*    **Cancer** A standard treatment exists for a certain type of cancer, and the patients receiving the treatment have a 5-year survival rate of 30%. A new treatment is proposed that has some unknown survival rate $p$. We would only be interested in using the new treatment if it were better than the standard treatment. Suppose that 40 out of 100 patients who receive the new treatment survive for 5 years. Can we say that the new treatment is better than the standard treatment? ∎

One way to assess these data is to construct a one-sided confidence interval, where we are interested in only *one* bound of the interval, in this case the lower bound.

---

**6.17**    **Upper One-Sided Confidence Interval for the Binomial Parameter p—Normal Theory Method**

An **upper one-sided $100\% \times (1 - \alpha)$ confidence interval** is of the form $p > p_1$ such that

$$Pr(p > p_1) = 1 - \alpha$$

If we assume that the normal approximation to the binomial holds true, then we can show that this confidence interval is given approximately by

$$p > \hat{p} - z_{1-\alpha}\sqrt{\hat{p}\hat{q}/n}$$

This interval estimator should only be used if $n\hat{p}\hat{q} \geqslant 5$.

---

Notice that we use $z_{1-\alpha}$ in constructing one-sided intervals, whereas we used $z_{1-\alpha/2}$ in constructing two-sided intervals.

*Example 6.43*    Suppose we desire a 95% confidence interval for a binomial parameter $p$. What percentile of the normal distribution should be used for a one-sided interval? a two-sided interval?

*Solution*    For $\alpha = 0.05$, we use

$$z_{1-.05} = z_{.95} = 1.645$$

for a one-sided interval and

$$z_{1-.05/2} = z_{.975} = 1.96$$

for a two-sided interval. ∎

*Example 6.44*    **Cancer** Construct an upper one-sided 95% confidence interval for the survival rate based on the cancer treatment data in Example 6.42.

*Solution*    We first check that $n\hat{p}\hat{q} = 100(0.4)(0.6) = 24 \geqslant 5$. The confidence interval is then given by

$$Pr[p > 0.40 - z_{.95}\sqrt{(0.4)(0.6)/100}] = 0.95$$

$$Pr[p > 0.40 - 1.645(0.049)] = 0.95$$

$$Pr(p > 0.319) = 0.95$$

Since 0.30 is not within the given interval, we would conclude that the new treatment is better than the standard treatment.                                                              ∎

If we were interested in 5-year death rates rather than survival rates, then a one-sided interval of the form $Pr(p < p_2) = 1 - \alpha$ would be appropriate, since we would only be interested in the new treatment if its death rate were lower than that of the standard treatment.

### 6.18 Lower One-Sided Confidence Interval for the Binomial Parameter p—Normal Theory Method

The interval $p < p_2$ such that

$$Pr(p < p_2) = 1 - \alpha$$

is referred to as a **lower one-sided $100\% \times (1 - \alpha)$ confidence interval** and is given approximately by

$$p < \hat{p} + z_{1-\alpha}\sqrt{\hat{p}\hat{q}/n}$$

*Example 6.45*     **Cancer** Compute a lower one-sided 95% confidence interval for the death rate using the cancer treatment data in Example 6.42.

*Solution*     We have that $\hat{p} = 0.6$. Thus, the 95% confidence interval is given by

$$Pr[p < 0.6 + 1.645\sqrt{(0.6)(0.4)/100}] = 0.95$$

$$Pr[p < 0.6 + 1.645(0.049)] = 0.95$$

$$Pr(p < 0.681) = 0.95$$

Since 70% is not within this interval, we can conclude that the new treatment has a lower death rate than the old treatment does.                                                              ∎

We can use similar methods to obtain one-sided confidence intervals for the mean and variance of a normal distribution and for the binomial parameter $p$ using exact methods.

## ■ 6.8 SUMMARY

In this chapter we introduced the concept of a **sampling distribution**. This concept is crucial to understanding the principles of statistical inference. The fundamental idea is to forget about our sample as a unique entity; instead, regard it as a **random sample** from all possible samples of size $n$ that could have been drawn from the population under study. Using this concept, we showed that $\bar{x}$ is an **unbiased estimator** of the population mean $\mu$; that is, the average of all sample means over all possible samples of size $n$ that could have been drawn will equal the population mean. Furthermore, if our population follows a normal distribution, then $\bar{x}$ has minimum variance among all possible unbiased estimators and is thus referred to as a **minimum variance unbiased estimator** of $\mu$. Finally, if our population follows a normal distribution, then $\bar{x}$ will also follow a normal distribution. However, even if our population is not normal, the sample mean will still follow a normal distribution for a sufficiently large sample size. This very important idea, which justifies many of the hypothesis tests we will study in the remainder of this book, is called the **central limit theorem**.

We then introduced the idea of an **interval estimate** (or **confidence interval**). Specifically, a 95% confidence interval is defined as an interval that will contain the true parameter for 95% of all samples that could have been obtained from the reference population. We applied the preceding principles of point and interval estimation to

(a) estimating the mean $\mu$ of a normal distribution when the variance was known

(b) estimating the mean $\mu$ of a normal distribution when the variance was unknown

(c) estimating the variance $\sigma^2$ of a normal distribution

(d) estimating the parameter $p$ of a binomial distribution

We introduced the *t* and **chi-square** distributions to obtain interval estimates for (b) and (c), respectively.

In Chapters 7 through 10, we will continue our discussion of statistical inference, focusing on testing of hypotheses rather than on parameter estimation. In this regard some parallels between inference from the points of view of hypothesis testing and confidence intervals will be discussed.

# *P*roblems

Suppose we wish to construct a list of treatment assignments for patients entering a study comparing different treatments for duodenal ulcer.

**6.1** If we anticipate that 20 patients will be entered in the study and will use 2 treatments, then construct a list of random treatment assignments starting in the 28th row of the random number table (Table 4).

**6.2** Count the number of persons assigned to each treatment group. How does this number compare with the expected number in each group?

**6.3** Suppose we change our minds and decide to enroll 40 patients and use 4 treatment groups. Start at the 12th row of the random number table and construct the list of random treatment assignments referred to in Problem 6.1.

**6.4** Answer Problem 6.2 for the list of treatment assignments derived in Problem 6.3.

*Pulmonary Disease*

The data in Table 6.7 were presented concerning the mean triceps skin fold thickness in a group of normal men and a group of men with chronic airflow limitation [2].

**6.5** What is the standard error of the mean for each group?

**Table 6.7** *Triceps skin fold thickness in normal men and men with chronic airflow limitation*

| Group | Mean | sd | n |
|---|---|---|---|
| Normal | 1.35 | 0.5 | 40 |
| Chronic airflow limitation | 0.92 | 0.4 | 32 |

(Reprinted with permission of *Chest* **85(6)**: 585–595, 1984.)

**6.6** Suppose we assume that the central limit theorem is applicable. What does it mean in this context?

### Cardiology

The data in Table 6.8 on left ventricular ejection fraction (LVEF) were collected from a group of 27 patients with acute dilated cardiomyopathy [3].

**Table 6.8** *Left ventricular ejection fraction (LVEF) for 27 patients with acute dilated cardiomyopathy*

| Patient number | LVEF | Patient number | LVEF |
|---|---|---|---|
| 1 | 0.19 | 15 | 0.24 |
| 2 | 0.24 | 16 | 0.18 |
| 3 | 0.17 | 17 | 0.22 |
| 4 | 0.40 | 18 | 0.23 |
| 5 | 0.40 | 19 | 0.14 |
| 6 | 0.23 | 20 | 0.14 |
| 7 | 0.20 | 21 | 0.30 |
| 8 | 0.20 | 22 | 0.07 |
| 9 | 0.30 | 23 | 0.12 |
| 10 | 0.19 | 24 | 0.13 |
| 11 | 0.24 | 25 | 0.17 |
| 12 | 0.32 | 26 | 0.24 |
| 13 | 0.32 | 27 | 0.19 |
| 14 | 0.28 | | |

*Note:* $\sum x_i = 6.05, \sum x_i^2 = 1.522.$
(Reprinted with permission of the *New England Journal of Medicine* **312(14)**: 885–890, 1985.)

**6.7** Calculate the standard deviation of LVEF for these patients.

**6.8** Calculate the standard error of the mean for LVEF.

**6.9** What is the difference in interpretation between standard deviation and standard error in this case?

**6.10** What does the central limit theorem mean in this context?

**6.11** Find the upper 1st percentile of a $t$ distribution with 16 d.f.

**6.12** Find the lower 10th percentile of a $t$ distribution with 28 d.f.

**6.13** Find the upper 2.5th percentile of a $t$ distribution with 7 d.f.

**6.14** Assuming that the standard deviation is known to be 0.1, compute a 95% confidence interval for the true mean LVEF for patients with acute dilated cardiomyopathy based on the data in Table 6.8.

**6.15** Answer Problem 6.14 without assuming that the standard deviation is known.

**6.16** Assuming that the standard deviation is known to be 6.0, compute a 95% confidence interval for the mean duration of hospitalization using the data in Table 2.11 (p. 37).

**6.17** Compute a 95% confidence interval for the mean duration of hospitalization without assuming that the standard deviation is known.

**6.18** Answer Problem 6.17 for a 90% confidence interval.

**6.19** What is the relationship between your answers to Problems 6.17 and 6.18?

**6.20** What is the upper 10th percentile of a chi-square distribution with 5 d.f.?

**6.21** What is the upper 1st percentile of a chi-square distribution with 3 d.f.?

**6.22** What are the upper and lower 2.5th percentiles for a chi-square distribution with 2 d.f.? What notation do we use to denote these percentiles?

**6.23** What are the upper and lower 2.5 percentiles for a chi-square distribution with 140 d.f.?

**6.24** What is the best point estimate of the variance of LVEF in Table 6.8?

**6.25** Construct a 95% confidence interval for the variance of LVEF in Table 6.8.

**6.26** Using the data in Table 2.10 (p. 36), construct a 99% confidence interval for the variance of total heart weight for left heart disease males.

**6.27** Using the data in Table 2.10 (p. 36), answer Problem 6.26 for normal males.

### Gynecology

In a recent study 89 of 283 women with primary tubal infertility (cases) and 640 of 3833 control women reported ever having used an IUD [4].

**6.28** What is the best point estimate of the rate of IUD use among case and control women, respectively?

**6.29** Provide a 95% confidence interval for the estimates in Problem 6.28.

Refer to the data in Table 2.11 (p. 37). Let us regard this hospital as typical of Pennsylvania hospitals.

**6.30** What is the best point estimate of the percentage

of males among persons discharged from Pennsylvania hospitals?

**6.31** What is the standard error of the estimate obtained in Problem 6.30?

**6.32** Provide a 95% confidence interval for the percentage of males among persons discharged from Pennsylvania hospitals.

**6.33** What is the best point estimate of the percentage of discharged patients 10 years of age and older who received antibiotics while in the hospital?

**6.34** Using the normal approximation method, provide a 95% confidence interval for the estimate in Problem 6.33.

**6.35** Answer Problem 6.34 using the exact method.

**6.36** Compare your results in Problems 6.34 and 6.35.

**6.37** What is the best point estimate of the percentage of discharged patients, exclusive of women of child-bearing age (ages 18–45), who received a bacterial culture while in the hospital?

**6.38** Provide a 95% confidence interval corresponding to the estimate in Problem 6.37.

**6.39** Answer Problem 6.38 for a 99% confidence interval.

*Cardiology*
Suppose a drug to relieve anginal pain is effective within 8 hours in 30% of 100 patients studied.

**6.40** Derive an upper one-sided 95% confidence interval for the percentage of patients who could get pain relief from the drug within 8 hours.

**6.41** Suppose that if the patients are untreated, 15% will be free from pain within 8 hours. If we assume that the drug either benefits the patients or has no effect at all, then what is your opinion on the effectiveness of the drug?

Suppose that in the same study 20% of the patients become pain-free within 4 hours of administration of the drug.

**6.42** Derive an upper one-sided confidence interval for the percentage of patients who could get pain relief from the drug within 4 hours.

**6.43** Suppose 10% of untreated patients will be pain-free within 4 hours. If we assume that the drug either benefits the patients or has no effect at all, then what is your opinion on the effectiveness of the drug?

*Obstetrics*
A new drug therapy is proposed for the prevention of low-birthweight deliveries. A pilot study undertaken, using the drug on 20 pregnant women, found that the mean birthweight in this group is 3500 g with a standard deviation of 500 g.

**6.44** What is the standard error of the mean in this case?

**6.45** What is the difference in interpretation between the standard deviation and standard error in this case (in words)?

*Hypertension*
In an effort to detect hypertension in young children, blood pressure measurements were taken on 30 children aged 5–6 years living in a specific community. For these children the mean diastolic blood pressure was found to be 56.2 mm with standard deviation 7.9 mm. From a nationwide study we know that the mean diastolic blood pressure is 64.2 mm for 5–6-year-old children.

**6.46** Is there evidence that the mean diastolic blood pressure for the children in the study is different from the nationwide average of children of the same age group?

**6.47** Provide a 95% confidence interval for the standard deviation of the diastolic blood pressure of 5–6-year-old children in this community based on the observed 30 children.

*Infectious Disease, Pulmonary Disease, Hospital Epidemiology*
A study was performed to relate reactivity to tuberculin to job activity within a hospital. In particular, Suppose that according to statewide, age-specific rates, 31% of nurses in a hospital are expected to have positive tuberculin skin tests. In the hospital under study, 93 out of 221 nurses are tuberculin positive.

**6.48** Give a 95% confidence interval for the proportion of positive tuberculin skin tests among nurses.

**6.49** How does the nurses' observed rate compare with the expected rate of 31%?

*Opthalmology, Hypertension*
A special study is conducted to test the hypothesis that persons with glaucoma have higher blood pressure than average. In the study 200 persons with glaucoma are recruited with a mean systolic blood pressure of 140 mm and a standard deviation of 25 mm.

**6.50** Construct a 95% confidence interval for the mean systolic blood pressure among persons with glaucoma.

**6.51** If the average systolic blood pressure for persons of comparable age is 130 mm, then is there an association between glaucoma and blood pressure?

*Hypertension*
Hypertensive patients are screened at a neighborhood health clinic and are given methyl dopa, a strong anti-

hypertensive medication for their condition. They are asked to come back 1 week later and have their blood pressures measured again. Suppose the initial and follow-up systolic blood pressures of the patients are given in Table 6.9.

To test the effectiveness of the drug, we want to measure the difference ($D$) between initial and follow-up blood pressures for each person.

_Table 6.9_ Initial and follow-up systolic bp (mm Hg) for hypertensive patients given methyl dopa

| Patient no. | Initial systolic bp | Follow-up systolic bp |
|---|---|---|
| 1 | 200.0 | 188.0 |
| 2 | 194.0 | 212.0 |
| 3 | 236.0 | 186.0 |
| 4 | 163.0 | 150.0 |
| 5 | 240.0 | 200.0 |
| 6 | 225.0 | 222.0 |
| 7 | 203.0 | 190.0 |
| 8 | 180.0 | 154.0 |
| 9 | 177.0 | 180.0 |
| 10 | 240.0 | 225.0 |

_6.52_ What is the mean and sd of $D$?

_6.53_ What is the standard error of the mean?

_6.54_ Suppose we assume that $D$ is normally distributed with unknown mean $\mu$ and known standard deviation $= 20$; that is, $D \sim N(\mu, 400)$. Construct a 95% confidence interval for $\mu$.

_6.55_ Do you have any opinion on the effect of methyl dopa from the results of these 10 patients?

### Venereal Disease
Suppose a clinical trial is conducted to test the efficacy of a new drug spectinomycin in the treatment of gonorrhea for females. Forty-six patients are given a 4-g daily dose of the drug and are seen 1 week later, at which time 6 of the patients still have gonorrhea.

_6.56_ What is the best point estimate for $p$, the probability of a failure with the drug?

_6.57_ What is a 95% confidence interval for $p$?

_6.58_ Suppose we know that penicillin G at a daily dose of 4.8 mega units has a 10% failure rate. What can be said in comparing the two drugs?

### Cancer
Data from American cancer tumor registries suggest

that of all persons with the type of lung cancer where surgery is the recommended therapy, 40% survive for 3 years from the time of diagnosis and 33% survive for 5 years.

_6.59_ Suppose that a group of patients who would have received standard surgery are assigned to a new type of surgery. Of 100 such patients, 55 survive for 3 years and 45 survive for 5 years. Can we say that the new form of surgery is better in any sense than the standard form of surgery?

### Hepatic Disease
Suppose we are experimenting with a group of guinea pigs and inoculate them with a fixed dose of a particular toxin causing liver enlargement. We find that out of 40 guinea pigs, 15 actually have enlarged livers.

_6.60_ What is the best point estimate $p$ of the probability of a guinea pig having an enlarged liver?

_6.61_ What is a two-sided 95% confidence interval for $p$ if we assume that the normal approximation is valid?

_6.62_ Answer Problem 6.61 if we do _not_ assume that the normal approximation is valid.

### Cardiovascular Disease
A recent hypothesis states that vigorous exercise is an effective preventive measure for subsequent cardiovascular death. To test this hypothesis, a sample of 750 men aged 50–75 who report that they jog at least 10 miles per week are ascertained. After 6 years, 64 have died of cardiovascular disease.

_6.63_ Compute a 95% confidence interval for the incidence of cardiovascular death in this group.

_6.64_ If the expected death rate from cardiovascular disease over 6 years in 50–75-year-old men based on large samples is 10%, then can we draw a conclusion concerning this hypothesis from these data?

### Pharmacology
Suppose we wish to estimate the concentration ($\mu g/ml$) of a specific dose of ampicillin in the urine after various periods of time. We recruit 25 volunteers and find that they have a mean concentration of 7.0 $\mu g/ml$ with a standard deviation of 2.0 $\mu g/ml$. Let us assume that the underlying population distribution of concentrations is normally distributed.

_6.65_ Find a 95% confidence interval for the population mean concentration.

_6.66_ Find a 99% confidence interval for the population variance of the concentrations.

_6.67_ How large a sample would be needed to ensure that

the length of the confidence interval in Problem 6.65 is 0.5 $\mu$g/ml if we assume that the sample standard deviation remains at 2.0 $\mu$g/ml?

### Cardiovascular Disease

A group of 50 men under the age of 55 with a prior history of myocardial infarction are put on a strict vegetarian diet as part of an experimental program. After 5 years, 2 men from the group have died.

**6.68** What is the best point estimate of the 5-year mortality rate in this group of men?

**6.69** Derive a 95% confidence interval for the 5-year mortality rate.

**6.70** Suppose that from a large sample of men under age 55 with a prior history of myocardial infarction, we know that the 5-year mortality rate is 18%. How does the observed mortality rate obtained in Problem 6.68 compare with the large sample rate of 18%?

### Environmental Health

Much discussion has taken place concerning possible health hazards from exposure to anesthetic gases. In one study a group of 525 Michigan nurse anesthetists was ascertained by mail questionnaires and telephone interviews in 1972 to determine the incidence rate of cancer [5]. Of this group 7 women reported having a new malignancy other than skin cancer during 1971.

**6.71** What is the best estimate of the 1971 incidence rate from these data?

**6.72** Provide a 95% confidence interval for the true incidence rate.

A comparison was made between the Michigan report and 1969 cancer incidence rates from the Connecticut tumor registry, where the expected incidence rate was determined to be 402.8 per 100,000.

**6.73** Comment on the comparison between the observed incidence rate and the Connecticut tumor registry data.

### Pulmonary Disease

A spirometric tracing is a standard device used to measure pulmonary function. These tracings represent plots of the volume of air expelled over a 6-second period and tend to look like Figure 6.11. One quantity of interest is the slope at various points along the curve. The slopes are referred to as **flow rates**. A problem that arises is that the flow rates cannot be accurately measured, and some observer error is always introduced. To quantify the observer error, an observer measures the flow at 50% of forced vital capacity (volume as measured at 6 seconds) twice on tracings from 10 different people. A machine called a digitizer can trace the curves automatically and can estimate the flow mechanically. Suppose the digitizer is also used to measure the flow twice on these 10 tracings. The data are given in Table 6.10.

**6.74** Find a 95% confidence interval for the standard deviation of the difference between the first and second replicates using the manual method.

**6.75** Answer Problem 6.74 for the difference between the first and second replicates using the digitizer method.

Suppose we want to compare the variability of the two methods within the same person. Let $x_{i1}$, $x_{i2}$ represent the 2 replicates on the $i$th person using the manual method, and let $y_{i1}$, $y_{i2}$ represent the 2 replicates on the $i$th person using the digitizer method. Let

$$d_i = |x_{i1} - x_{i2}| - |y_{i1} - y_{i2}|$$

Then, $d_i$ is a measure of the difference in variability using the two methods. Let us assume that $d_i$ is normally distributed with mean $\mu_d$ and variance $\sigma_d^2$.

**6.76** Find a 95% confidence interval for $\mu_d$.

**6.77** What is your opinion on the relative variability of the two methods?

### Obstetrics, Serology

A new assay is developed to obtain the concentration of

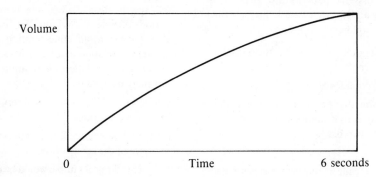

**Figure 6.11**
A typical spirometric tracing

Volume

0                    Time                    6 seconds

M. *Hominis* mycoplasma in the serum of pregnant women. The developers of this assay wish to make a statement as to the variability of their laboratory technique. For this purpose, 10 subsamples of 1 ml each are drawn from a large serum sample from *one* woman, and the assay is performed on each subsample. The concentrations are given as follows: $2^4$, $2^3$, $2^5$, $2^4$, $2^5$, $2^4$, $2^3$, $2^4$, $2^4$, $2^5$.

**6.78** If the concentration is assumed to be normal in the log scale to the base 2, then give the best estimate of the variance of the method from these data.

**6.79** Compute a 95% confidence interval for the variance of the method.

**6.80** If we assume that the point estimate in Problem 6.78 is correct, then what is the probability that a particular assay, when expressed in the log scale to the base 2, is no more than 1.5 log units off from its true value?

**6.81** Answer Problem 6.80 for 2.5 log units.

Turn to the table of random digits (Table 4). Start at the top left. Reading across, record for each of the first 11 sets of 10 consecutive digits (1) the second digit, $X_i$, and (2) the mean of the 10 digits, $Y_i$.

**6.82** Derive the theoretical mean and variance of the distribution of second digits.

**6.83** How do the sample properties of the $X_i$ compare with the results of Problem 6.82?

**6.84** From your answer to Problem 6.82, what should the mean and variance of the $Y_i$ be?

**6.85** How do the actual $Y_i$'s compare with the results of Problem 6.84?

**6.86** Do the actual $Y_i$'s relate to the central limit theorem in any way? Elaborate.

*Hypertension*

Suppose 100 hypertensive persons are given an antihypertensive drug and that the drug is *effective* in 20 of the persons. By *effective*, we mean that their diastolic blood pressure is lowered by at least 10 mm as judged from a repeat measurement 1 week after taking the drug.

**6.87** What is the best point estimate of the probability $p$ of the drug being effective?

**6.88** Suppose we know that 10% of all hypertensive patients who are given a placebo will have their diastolic blood pressure lowered by 10 mm. Can we carry out some procedure to be sure that we are not simply observing the placebo effect?

**6.89** What assumptions have you made to carry out the procedure in Problem 6.88?

Suppose we decide that a better measure of the effectiveness of the drug is the absolute decrease in blood pressure rather than the measure of effectiveness used previously. Let $d_i = x_i - y_i$, $i = 1, \ldots, 100$, where $x_i =$ diastolic blood pressure on the $i$th person before taking the drug and $y_i =$ diastolic blood pressure on the $i$th person 1 week after taking the drug. Suppose that the sample mean of the $d_i$ is $+5.3$ and the sample variance is 144.0.

**6.90** What is the standard error of $d$?

**6.91** What is a 95% confidence interval for the population mean of $d$?

**6.92** Can we make a statement about the effectiveness of the drug?

*Table 6.10* Estimation of flow rates (*l*) at 50% of forced vital capacity by a manual and a digitizer method

| Person | Manual method replicate 1 | Manual method replicate 2 | Digitizer replicate 1 | Digitizer replicate 2 |
|--------|------|------|------|------|
| 1  | 1.80 | 1.84 | 1.82 | 1.83 |
| 2  | 2.01 | 2.09 | 2.05 | 2.04 |
| 3  | 1.63 | 1.52 | 1.62 | 1.60 |
| 4  | 1.54 | 1.49 | 1.49 | 1.45 |
| 5  | 2.21 | 2.36 | 2.32 | 2.36 |
| 6  | 4.16 | 4.08 | 4.21 | 4.27 |
| 7  | 3.02 | 3.07 | 3.08 | 3.09 |
| 8  | 2.75 | 2.80 | 2.78 | 2.79 |
| 9  | 3.03 | 3.04 | 3.06 | 3.05 |
| 10 | 2.68 | 2.71 | 2.70 | 2.70 |

**6.93** What does a 95% confidence interval mean, in words, in this case?

### Bacteriology

Suppose a group of mice are inoculated with a uniform dose of a specific type of bacteria and that all die within 24 days, with the distribution of survival times given in Table 6.11.

**Table 6.11** *Survival time of mice after inoculation with a specific type of bacteria*

| Survival time (days) | No. of mice |
|---|---|
| 10 | 5 |
| 11 | 11 |
| 12 | 29 |
| 13 | 30 |
| 14 | 40 |
| 15 | 51 |
| 16 | 71 |
| 17 | 65 |
| 18 | 48 |
| 19 | 36 |
| 20 | 21 |
| 21 | 12 |
| 22 | 7 |
| 23 | 2 |
| 24 | 1 |

**6.94** Suppose we assume that the underlying distribution of survival times is normal. Estimate the probability $p$ that a mouse will survive for 20 or more days.

**6.95** Suppose we are not willing to assume that the underlying distribution is normal. Estimate the probability $p$ that a mouse will survive for 20 or more days.

**6.96** Compute 95% confidence limits for the parameter estimated in Problem 6.95.

**6.97** Compute 99% confidence limits for the parameter estimated in Problem 6.95.

Draw 6 random samples of size 5 from the data in Table 6.2.

**6.98** Compute the mean birthweight for each of the 6 samples.

**6.99** Compute the standard deviation based on the sample of 6 means.

**6.100** Select the third point from each of the 6 samples and compute the sample standard deviation from this collection of 6 third points.

**6.101** What theoretical relationship should there be between the standard deviation in Problem 6.99 and the standard deviation in Problem 6.100?

**6.102** How do the actual sample results in Problems 6.99 and 6.100 compare?

### Cardiovascular Disease

In Table 2.15 (p. 40) we provided data on serum cholesterol levels of 24 hospital employees before and after they adopted a vegetarian diet.

**6.103** What is your best estimate of the effect of adopting a vegetarian diet on change in serum cholesterol levels?

**6.104** What is the standard error of the estimate given in Problem 6.103?

**6.105** Provide a 95% confidence interval for the estimate given in Problem 6.103.

**6.106** What can you conclude from your results in Problem 6.105?

Some physicians consider only changes of at least 10 mg%/ml (the same units as in Table 2.15) to be clinically significant.

**6.107** Among persons with a clinically significant change in either direction, what is the best estimate of the proportion whose cholesterol levels have declined?

**6.108** Provide a 95% confidence interval for the estimate in Problem 6.107.

**6.109** What can you conclude from your results in Problem 6.108?

### Obstetrics

In Figure 6.4(b) we provided a plot of the sampling distribution of the sample mean from 200 samples of size 5 from the population of 1000 birthweights given in Table 6.2. The mean of the 1000 birthweights in Table 6.2 is 112.0 oz with standard deviation 20.6 oz.

**6.110** If the central limit theorem holds, then what proportion of sample means should fall within 0.5 lb of the population mean (112.0 oz)?

**6.111** Answer Problem 6.110 for 1 lb rather than 0.5 lb.

**6.112** Compare your results in Problems 6.110 and 6.111 with the actual proportion of sample means that fall in these ranges.

**6.113** Do you feel that the central limit theorem is applicable for samples of size 5 from this population?

# References

[1] Cochran, W. G. (1963) *Sampling Techniques*, 2nd ed. (New York: John Wiley).

[2] Arora, N. S. and Rochester, D. F. (1984) "Effect of Chronic Airflow Limitation (CAL) on Sternocleidomastoid Muscle Thickness," *Chest* **85(6)**: 58S–59S.

[3] Dec, G. W. Jr., Palacios, I. F., Fallon, J. T., Aretz, H. T., Mills, J., Lee, D. C. S., and Johnson, R. A. (1985) "Active Myocarditis in the Spectrum of Acute Dilated Cardiomyopathies," *New England Journal of Medicine* **312(14)**: 885–890.

[4] Cramer, D. W., Schiff, I., Schoenbaum, S. C., Gibson, M., Belisle, S., Albrecht, B., Stillman, R. J., Berger, M. J., Wilson, W., Stadel, B. V., and Seibel, M. (1985) "Tubal Infertility and the Intrauterine Device," *New England Journal of Medicine* **312(15)**: 941–947.

[5] Corbett, T. H., Cornell, R. G., Leiding, K., and Endres, J. L. (1973) "Incidence of Cancer Among Michigan Nurse-Anesthetists," *Anesthesiology* **38(3)**: 260–263.

# 7
## Hypothesis Testing: One-Sample Inference

## ■ 7.1 INTRODUCTION

In Chapter 6 we were concerned with methods of point and interval estimation for parameters of various distributions. However, we often have a preconceived ideas as to what these parameters should be and we wish to test whether the data conform with our ideas.

*Example 7.1*

*Pediatrics, Genetics* A current area of research interest is the familial aggregation of cardiovascular risk factors in general and lipid levels in particular. Suppose we know that the "average" cholesterol level in children is 175 mg%/ml. We identify a group of men who have died from heart disease within the past year and measure the cholesterol levels of their offspring. We would like to consider two hypotheses:

1. The average cholesterol level of these children is 175 mg%/ml.
2. The average cholesterol level of these children is greater than 175 mg%/ml.  ■

We will formulate this type of question in a hypothesis testing framework by specifying two hypotheses—a null and an alternative hypothesis. We then will compare the relative probabilities of these two hypotheses. We could say in Example 7.1 that the null hypothesis is that the average cholesterol level of the children is 175 mg%/ml and the alternative hypothesis is that the average cholesterol level of the children is greater than 175 mg%/ml.

Why is hypothesis testing so important? Hypothesis testing provides a framework for making decisions on an *objective* basis by weighing the relative probabilities of different hypotheses rather than on a *subjective* basis by simply looking at the data. People can form different opinions by looking at data, but a hypothesis test provides a uniform decision-making criterion that will be consistent for all people.

In this chapter we develop some of the basic concepts of hypothesis testing and apply them to one-sample problems of statistical inference. In a **one-sample**

**problem** we specify hypotheses about a single distribution; in a **two-sample problem** we compare two different distributions.

# ■ 7.2  GENERAL CONCEPTS

*Example 7.2*    **Obstetrics**  Suppose we wish to test the hypothesis that mothers with a low socioeconomic status (SES) deliver babies whose birthweights are in some sense lower than "normal." To test this hypothesis, we obtain a list of birthweights from 100 consecutive, full-term, live-born deliveries from the maternity ward of a hospital in a low-SES area. We find that the mean birthweight ($\bar{x}$) is 115 oz with a sample standard deviation ($s$) of 24 oz. Suppose we know from large nationwide surveys based on millions of deliveries that the mean birthweight in the United States is 120 oz with a standard deviation of 25 oz. *Can we actually say that the underlying mean birthweight from this hospital is lower than the national average?*    ■

Let us assume that the 100 birthweights from our hospital come from an underlying normal distribution with unknown mean $\mu$ and known standard deviation $\sigma = 25$. We could use the methods of Section 6.7 to construct a 95% lower one-sided confidence interval for $\mu$ based on our sample data, that is, an interval of the form $\mu < c$. If this interval contains 120 oz (i.e., if $c \geqslant 120$), then we would be content with the hypothesis that our birthweights are not different from the national average. If it does not contain 120 oz ($c < 120$), then we would accept the hypothesis that our birthweights tend to be lower than the national average.

Another way of looking at this problem is in terms of hypothesis testing. In particular, the hypotheses under consideration can be formulated in terms of null and alternative hypotheses, which can be defined as follows:

*Definition 7.1*

We define the **null hypothesis**, which we denote by $H_0$, as the hypothesis that is to be tested. We define the **alternative hypothesis**, which we denote by $H_1$, as the hypothesis that in some sense contradicts the null hypothesis.    ■

*Example 7.3*    **Obstetrics**  In Example 7.2 the null hypothesis ($H_0$) is the hypothesis that the mean birthweight in our hospital ($\mu$) is equal to the mean birthweight in the United States ($\mu_0$). This is the hypothesis that we wish to test. The alternative hypothesis ($H_1$) is the hypothesis that the mean birthweight in our hospital ($\mu$) is less than the mean birthweight in the United States ($\mu_0$). We wish to compare the relative probabilities of these two hypotheses.    ■

We also assume that the standard deviation is known to be 25 ($\sigma_0$) and that the underlying distribution is normal under either hypothesis. We can write these hypotheses more succinctly in the following form:

**7.1**
$$H_0: \mu = \mu_0, \quad \sigma = \sigma_0 \quad \text{vs.} \quad H_1: \mu < \mu_0, \quad \sigma = \sigma_0$$

Suppose that our only possible decisions are whether $H_0$ is true or $H_1$ is true. Actually, for ease of notation all outcomes in a hypothesis-testing situation generally refer to the null hypothesis. Hence, if we decide that $H_0$ is true, then we will say that we *accept* $H_0$. If we decide that $H_1$ is true, then we will state that $H_0$ is not true or, equivalently, that we *reject* $H_0$. Thus, the four possible outcomes that can occur are:

*1*. We accept $H_0$, and $H_0$ is in fact true.

*2*. We accept $H_0$, and $H_1$ is in fact true.

*3*. We reject $H_0$, and $H_0$ is in fact true.

*4*. We reject $H_0$, and $H_1$ is in fact true.

These four possibilities are depicted in Table 7.1.

**Table 7.1**
*Four possible outcomes in hypothesis testing*

|  |  | $H_0$ | $H_1$ |
|---|---|---|---|
| **Decision** | Accept $H_0$ | $H_0$ is true and we accept $H_0$ | $H_1$ is true and we accept $H_0$ |
|  | Reject $H_0$ | $H_0$ is true and we reject $H_0$ | $H_1$ is true and we reject $H_0$ |

If $H_0$ is true and we accept $H_0$ or if $H_1$ is true and we reject $H_0$, then we have made the correct decision. If $H_0$ is true and we reject $H_0$ or if $H_1$ is true and we accept $H_0$, then we have made an *error*. The two types of errors are generally treated differently.

**Definition 7.2**

The probability of a **type I error** is the probability of rejecting the null hypothesis given that $H_0$ is in fact true.    ■

**Definition 7.3**

The probability of a **type II error** is the probability of accepting the null hypothesis given that $H_1$ is in fact true. This probability is a function of $\mu$.    ■

*Example 7.4*    **Obstetrics**  In the context of the birthweight data in Example 7.2, a type I error would be the probability of deciding that the mean birthweight in our hospital was less than 120 oz when in fact it was 120 oz. A type II error would be the probability of deciding that the mean birthweight was 120 oz when in fact it was less than 120 oz.    ■

*Example 7.5*    **Cardiovascular Disease, Pediatrics**  What are the type I and type II errors for the cholesterol data in Example 7.1?

*Solution*    The type I error is the probability of deciding that the offspring of men who have died from heart disease have an average cholesterol greater than 175 mg%/ml when in fact their average cholesterol level is 175. The type II error is the probability of deciding that the offspring have normal cholesterol levels when in fact their cholesterol levels are above average.    ■

Making type I and type II errors often results in monetary and nonmonetary costs.

*Example 7.6*    **Obstetrics**  If we consider the birthweight data in Example 7.2, then we might use these data to decide if a special care nursery for low-birthweight babies is needed in this hospital. If $H_1$

were true, that is, if the birthweights in our hospital did tend to be lower than the national average, then the hospital might be justified in having its own special care nursery. If $H_0$ were true and the mean birthweight was no different from the U.S. average, then the hospital probably need not have such a nursery. If we make a type I error, then in real terms we recommend that a special care nursery is needed with all the extra costs involved when in fact it is not needed. If we make a type II error, then we decide not to fund a special care nursery when in fact it is needed. The nonmonetary cost of this decision is that some low-birthweight babies may not survive without the unique equipment in a special care nursery. ∎

**Definition 7.4**

The probability of a type I error is usually denoted by $\alpha$ and is commonly referred to as the **significance level** of a test. ∎

**Definition 7.5**

The probability of a type II error is usually denoted by $\beta$. ∎

**Definition 7.6**

The **power** of a test is defined as

$$1 - \beta = 1 - \text{probability of a type II error} \qquad ∎$$

Our general aim in hypothesis testing is to use statistical tests that make $\alpha$ and $\beta$ as small as possible. This goal requires compromise, since making $\alpha$ small involves rejecting the null hypothesis less often, whereas making $\beta$ small involves accepting the null hypothesis less often. These actions are contradictory. Instead, our general strategy will be to fix $\alpha$ at some specific level, for example, 0.10, 0.05, 0.01, . . . , and to use the test that minimizes $\beta$ or, equivalently, maximizes the power.

# ∎ 7.3 ONE-SAMPLE TEST FOR THE MEAN OF A NORMAL DISTRIBUTION WITH KNOWN VARIANCE: ONE-SIDED ALTERNATIVES

We will now develop the appropriate hypothesis test for the birthweight data given in Example 7.2. The statistical model in this case is that the birthweights come from a normal distribution with mean $\mu$ and variance $\sigma^2$. We assume that $\sigma^2$ is known to be 625 and we wish to test the null hypothesis $H_0$ that $\mu = 120$ oz vs. the alternative hypothesis $H_1$ that $\mu < 120$ oz. Suppose we select a more specific alternative, namely, $H_1$: $\mu = \mu_1 = 110$ oz. We will show that the nature of the best test does not depend on the value chosen for $\mu_1$ provided that $\mu_1$ is less than 120 oz. We will also fix the $\alpha$ level at 0.05 for concreteness.

*Example 7.7*

We could use a very simple test by referring to the table of random digits in Table 4. Suppose we select two digits from this table and reject the null hypothesis if these two digits are between 00 and 04 inclusive and accept the null hypothesis if these two digits are between 05 and 99. Clearly, from the properties of the random number table, the type I error of this test $= \alpha =$

$Pr$(rejecting the null hypothesis|$H_0$ true) = $Pr$(drawing two random digits between 00 and 04) = $\frac{5}{100}$ = 0.05. Thus, the proposed test satisfies the $\alpha$ level criterion given previously. The problem with this test is that it has very low power. Indeed, the power of the test = $Pr$(rejecting the null hypothesis|$H_1$ true) = $Pr$(drawing two random digits between 00 and 04) = $\frac{5}{100}$ = 0.05.

We note that the outcome of the test has nothing to do with the sample birthweights drawn. We will reject $H_0$ just as often when the sample mean birthweight ($\bar{x}$) is 110 oz as when it is 120 oz. Thus, this test must be very poor, since we would expect to reject $H_0$ with near certainty if $\bar{x}$ is sufficiently small and would expect to never reject $H_0$ if $\bar{x}$ is sufficiently large.  ∎

We can show that the best (most powerful) test in this situation is based on the sample mean ($\bar{x}$). If $\bar{x}$ is sufficiently smaller than $\mu_0$, then we reject $H_0$; otherwise, we accept $H_0$. This test is reasonable, since if $H_0$ is true, then the most likely values of $\bar{x}$ will tend to cluster around $\mu_0$, whereas if $H_1$ is true, the most likely values of $\bar{x}$ will tend to cluster around $\mu_1$. The distributions of $\bar{x}$ under $H_0$ and $H_1$ are depicted in Figure 7.1.

Note that if $H_0$ is true, the distribution of $\bar{x}$ is depicted by the right-hand curve in Figure 7.1, whereby small values of $\bar{x}$ are unlikely. Similarly, if $H_1$ is true, then the distribution of $\bar{x}$ is depicted by the left-hand curve in Figure 7.1, whereby large values of $\bar{x}$ are unlikely. These distributions demonstrate why we wish to reject $H_0$ for small values of $\bar{x}$ and accept $H_0$ for large values of $\bar{x}$.

### Definition 7.7

We define the **acceptance region** as the range of values of $\bar{x}$ for which we accept $H_0$.  ∎

### Definition 7.8

We define the **rejection region** as the range of values of $\bar{x}$ for which we reject $H_0$.  ∎

We note that for the birthweight data in Example 7.2, the rejection region consists of small values of $\bar{x}$ because the underlying mean under the alternative hypothesis ($\mu_1$) is less than the underlying mean under the null hypothesis. This type of test is referred to as a one-tailed test.

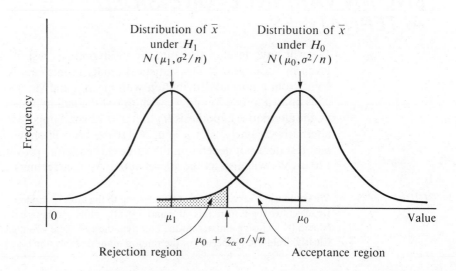

__Figure 7.1__
*The distribution of $\bar{x}$ under the null ($H_0$) and alternative ($H_1$) hypotheses*

We define a **one-tailed test** as a test where the values of the parameter under study (in this case $\mu$) under the alternative hypothesis are allowed to be either greater than or less than the values of the parameter under the null hypothesis ($\mu_0$) *but not both.* ∎

*Example 7.8*

*Cardiovascular Disease, Pediatrics* The hypotheses for the cholesterol data presented in Example 7.1 are $H_0: \mu = \mu_0$ vs. $H_1: \mu > \mu_0$, where $\mu$ is the true mean cholesterol level for children of men who have died from heart disease. This test is also one tailed, since the alternative mean is only allowed to be greater than the null mean. ∎

How small should $\bar{x}$ be for us to reject $H_0$? We can settle this issue by recalling that the significance level of the test is set at $\alpha$. Suppose that we reject $H_0$ for all values of $\bar{x} < c$ and accept $H_0$ otherwise. We wish to select $c$ such that

7.2

$$\alpha = Pr(\text{type I error}|H_0) = Pr[\bar{x} < c|\bar{x} \sim N(\mu_0, \sigma^2/n)]$$

$$= \Phi[(c - \mu_0)/(\sigma/\sqrt{n})]$$

Thus, using the $z$ notation for the percentiles of a normal distribution developed in Chapter 5, we have

7.3

$$z_\alpha = (c - \mu_0)/(\sigma/\sqrt{n})$$

If we multiply both sides of **(7.3)** by $\sigma/\sqrt{n}$ and add $\mu_0$, we have

7.4

$$c = \mu_0 + z_\alpha \sigma/\sqrt{n}$$

Thus, our test takes on the following form:

7.5 *One-Sample Test for the Mean of a Normal Distribution with Known Variance (Alternative Mean < Null Mean)*

If we wish to test the hypothesis

$$H_0: \mu = \mu_0, \quad \sigma = \sigma_0 \qquad \text{vs.} \qquad H_1: \mu < \mu_0, \quad \sigma = \sigma_0$$

with a significance level of $\alpha$, then the best (most powerful) test is based on $\bar{x}$: if

$$\bar{x} < \mu_0 + z_\alpha \sigma/\sqrt{n}$$

then we reject $H_0$; if

$$\bar{x} \geq \mu_0 + z_\alpha \sigma/\sqrt{n}$$

then we accept $H_0$.

The acceptance and rejection regions for the birthweight data in Example 7.2 are depicted in Figure 7.1.

We can show that for a given $\alpha$ level, this test maximizes the power or, equivalently, minimizes the type II error.

**Example 7.9**    **Obstetrics** If we use an $\alpha$ level of 0.05 for the birthweight data in Example 7.2, then $z_\alpha = -1.645$ and we would reject $H_0$ if $\bar{x} < 120 - 1.645(25)/10$ or if $\bar{x} < 120 - 4.11 = 115.89$. We would accept $H_0$ if $\bar{x} \geqslant 115.89$. Thus, our rejection region is $\bar{x} < 115.89$ and our acceptance region is $\bar{x} \geqslant 115.89$. We would reject $H_0$ in this case, since $\bar{x}$ was in fact 115 oz. If, instead, we use an $\alpha$ level of 0.01 rather than 0.05, we would reject $H_0$ if

$$\bar{x} < 120 + z_{.01}(25)/10 = 120 - 2.326(25)/10 = 120 - 5.82 = 114.18$$

and accept $H_0$ if $\bar{x} \geqslant 114.18$. In other words, our rejection region is $\bar{x} < 114.18$ and our acceptance region is $\bar{x} \geqslant 114.18$. Since $\bar{x} = 115$ oz, we would accept $H_0$ in this case.    ∎

How do we know what level of $\alpha$ to use? The actual $\alpha$ level used should depend on the relative importance of type I and type II errors, since the smaller we make $\alpha$ the larger $\beta$ becomes. Most people feel uncomfortable with $\alpha$ levels that are much greater than 0.05. Traditionally, an $\alpha$ level of exactly 0.05 is used most frequently.

In general, we could perform a number of significance tests at different $\alpha$ levels, as we have done in Example 7.9, and note whether we would accept or reject $H_0$ in each instance. This can be somewhat tedious and is unnecessary since, instead, we can effectively perform significance tests *at all* $\alpha$ *levels* by obtaining the *p*-value for the test.

**Definition 7.10**

The **_p_-value** is defined for any hypothesis test as the $\alpha$ level at which we would be indifferent to accepting or rejecting $H_0$ given the sample data at hand. That is, the *p*-value is the $\alpha$ level at which the given value of the statistic (such as $\bar{x}$) would be on the borderline between the acceptance and rejection regions.    ∎

According to our test criterion in **(7.5)**, if we use a significance level of $p$, then we would reject $H_0$ if $\bar{x} < \mu_0 + z_p \sigma/\sqrt{n}$ and accept $H_0$ if $\bar{x} \geqslant \mu_0 + z_p \sigma/\sqrt{n}$. Hence, we would be indifferent to accepting or rejecting $H_0$ if $\bar{x} = \mu_0 + z_p \sigma/\sqrt{n}$. If we subtract $\mu_0$ from both sides of the equation and divide by $\sigma/\sqrt{n}$, we obtain

**7.6**
$$z_p = (\bar{x} - \mu_0)/(\sigma/\sqrt{n})$$

or, alternatively,

**7.7**
$$p = \Phi[(\bar{x} - \mu_0)/(\sigma/\sqrt{n})]$$

The *p*-value can be depicted graphically as the area under a $N(\mu_0, \sigma^2/n)$ curve to the left of the sample value $\bar{x}$, as is shown in Figure 7.2.

**Example 7.10**    **Obstetrics** Compute the *p*-value for the birthweight data given in Example 7.2.

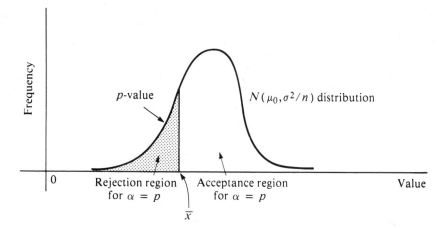

**Figure 7.2**
*Graphical display
of a p-value*

**Solution**

From **(7.7)** we have that the *p*-value is given by

$$\Phi\left[\frac{(115 - 120)}{(25/10)}\right] = \Phi(-2.0) = 0.023$$

∎

**Example 7.11**

**Cardiology** A topic of recent clinical interest is the possibility of using drugs to reduce infarct size in those patients who have had a myocardial infarction within the past 24 hours. Suppose we know that in untreated patients the mean infarct size is 25 $(ck - g - EQ/m^2)$ with a standard deviation of 10. Furthermore, in 8 patients treated with drug, the mean infarct size is 16. Is the drug effective in reducing infarct size?

**Solution**

Our hypotheses are $H_0$: $\mu = 25$, $\sigma = 10$ vs. $H_1$: $\mu < 25$, $\sigma = 10$. We compute the *p*-value using **(7.7)** as follows:

$$p = \Phi\left[\frac{(16 - 25)}{(10/\sqrt{8})}\right] = \Phi(-2.55)$$

$$= 1 - \Phi(2.55)$$

$$= 1 - 0.9946$$

$$\approx 0.005$$

Thus, we reject $H_0$ and conclude that the drug reduces infarct size (all other things being equal). ∎

An alternative definition of a *p*-value that will be useful in other hypothesis-testing problems is given as follows:

**Definition 7.10(a)**

The **p-value** can also be thought of as *the probability of obtaining a result as extreme as or more extreme than the actual sample value obtained given that the null hypothesis is true.* ∎

We know that under the null hypothesis, $\bar{x} \sim N(\mu_0, \sigma^2/n)$. Hence, the probability of obtaining a sample mean that is no larger than $\bar{x}$ under the null hypothesis is $\Phi[(\bar{x} - \mu_0)/(\sigma/\sqrt{n})] = p$-value, as shown in Figure 7.2.

The importance of the *p*-value is that by its very definition all significance tests where the $\alpha$ level is $<p$ will result in accepting $H_0$, whereas all significance tests where the $\alpha$ level is $>p$ will result in rejecting $H_0$. Hence, the *p*-value tells us *exactly* how significant our results are without performing repeated significance tests at different $\alpha$ levels. A question that is typically asked is how small should the *p*-value be for one's results to be considered statistically significant. Although this question has no definite answer, we present some commonly used criteria as follows:

**7.8**    *Guidelines for Judging the Significance of a P-value*

If    $0.01 \leqslant p < 0.05$,    then the results are *significant*.

If    $0.001 \leqslant p < 0.01$,    then the results are *highly significant*.

If       $p < 0.001$,    then the results are *very highly significant*.

If       $p > 0.05$,    then the results are considered *not statistically significant* (sometimes denoted by NS).

However,

If    $0.05 \leqslant p < 0.10$,    then a *trend toward statistical significance* is sometimes noted.

Authors frequently make no distinction as to the exact *p*-value beyond giving ranges of the type shown here, since whether the *p*-value is 0.024 or 0.016 is thought to be unimportant. Other authors give an exact *p*-value even for results that are not statistically significant so that the reader can appreciate how close to statistical significance the results have come. These different approaches lead to the following general principle:

**7.9**    *Determination of Significance Results from Hypothesis Tests*

We can use either of the following methods to establish whether results from hypothesis tests are statistically significant:

*1*. We can compute our test statistic $\bar{x}$ and compare it with the critical value $c$ at an $\alpha$ level of 0.05. Specifically, if we are testing $H_0: \mu = \mu_0$ vs. $H_1: \mu < \mu_0$ and $\bar{x} < c = \mu_0 + z_{.05}\sigma/\sqrt{n}$, then we reject $H_0$ and declare our results to be *statistically significant* (i.e., $p < 0.05$). Otherwise, we accept $H_0$ and declare our results to be *not statistically significant* (i.e., $p \geqslant 0.05$).

*2*. We can compute the exact *p*-value, and if $p < 0.05$, then we reject $H_0$ and declare our results to be *statistically significant*. Otherwise, if $p \geqslant 0.05$, then we accept $H_0$ and declare our results to be *not statistically significant*.

Thus, these two approaches are equivalent regarding the determination of statistical significance (i.e., whether $p < 0.05$ or $p \geqslant 0.05$). The second approach is somewhat more precise in that it yields an exact *p*-value. However, this precision may be unnecessary in many practical situations. The two approaches in **(7.9)** can also be used to determine statistical significance in other hypothesis-testing problems.

**Example 7.12**  ***Obstetrics***  Assess the statistical significance of the birthweight data given in Example 7.2.

**Solution**  Since the *p*-value is 0.023, we would consider the results statistically significant and conclude that the true birthweight is significantly lower in our hospital than in the general population.

**Example 7.13**  ***Cardiology***  Assess the significance of the infarct size data in Example 7.11.

**Solution**  The *p*-value = 0.005, and thus the results are highly significant.  ∎

In writing up the results of a study, we should distinguish between scientific and statistical significance, since the two terms do not necessarily coincide. The results of a study can be statistically significant but still not be scientifically important. This situation would occur if a small difference was found to be statistically significant because of a large sample size. Conversely, some statistically insignificant results can be important and lend encouragement to the performance of larger studies to confirm the findings.

**Example 7.14**  ***Obstetrics***  Suppose the mean birthweight in Example 7.2 was 119 oz based on a sample of size 10,000. Assess the results of the study.

**Solution**  The *p*-value would be given by

$$\Phi\left(\frac{119 - 120}{25/\sqrt{10,000}}\right) = \Phi(-4.00) < 0.001$$

The results are thus very highly significant but are clearly not very important because of the small difference in mean birthweight (1 oz) between this hospital and the national average.  ∎

**Example 7.15**  ***Obstetrics***  Suppose that the mean birthweight in Example 7.2 was 110 oz based on a sample size of 10. Assess the results of the study.

**Solution**  The *p*-value would be given by

$$\Phi\left(\frac{110 - 120}{25/\sqrt{10}}\right) = \Phi(-1.26) = 1 - \Phi(1.26) = 1 - 0.8962 \approx 0.104$$

These results are not statistically significant but could be important if confirmed by a larger sample.  ∎

Our test criterion in **(7.5)** was based on an alternative hypothesis that $\mu < \mu_0$. In many situations we wish to use an alternative hypothesis that $\mu > \mu_0$. In this case we would want to reject $H_0$ if $\bar{x}$ were large and accept $H_0$ if $\bar{x}$ were small. Using similar arguments to those given in this section, we can show that the best test is given as follows:

**7.10**  **One-Sample Test for the Mean of a Normal Distribution with Known Variance (Alternative Mean > Null Mean)**

If we wish to test the hypothesis

$$H_0: \mu = \mu_0, \quad \sigma = \sigma_0 \qquad \text{vs.} \qquad H_1: \mu > \mu_0, \quad \sigma = \sigma_0$$

with a significance level of $\alpha$, then the best test is based on $\bar{x}$: If

$$\bar{x} > \mu_0 + z_{1-\alpha}\sigma/\sqrt{n}, \qquad \text{then we reject } H_0$$

If

$$\bar{x} \leqslant \mu_0 + z_{1-\alpha}\sigma/\sqrt{n}, \qquad \text{then we accept } H_0$$

The *p*-value for this test is given by

$$p = 1 - \Phi[(\bar{x} - \mu_0)/(\sigma/\sqrt{n})]$$

The acceptance and rejection regions for this test are depicted in Figure 7.3.

---

*Example 7.16*     ***Cardiovascular Disease, Pediatrics*** Suppose that the mean cholesterol level of 10 children in Example 7.1 is $200 \, \text{mg}\%/\text{ml}$ and the standard deviation is assumed to be $50 \, \text{mg}\%/\text{ml}$. Test the hypothesis that the mean cholesterol level is higher in this group than in the general population.

*Solution*     We test the hypothesis

$$H_0: \mu = 175, \quad \sigma = 50 \qquad \text{vs.} \qquad H_1: \mu > 175, \quad \sigma = 50$$

using an $\alpha$ level of 0.05. We reject $H_0$ if

$$\bar{x} > 175 + z_{.95}(50)/\sqrt{10} = 175 + 1.645(50)/\sqrt{10}$$

$$= 175 + 26.01$$

$$= 201.01$$

and we accept $H_0$ otherwise. Since $\bar{x} = 200 < 201.01$, we accept $H_0$. We could also compute an

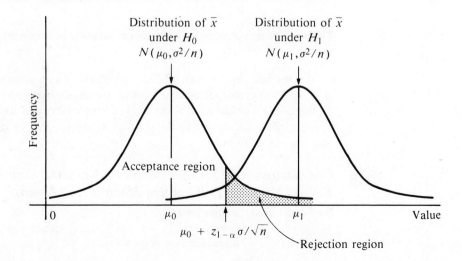

*Figure 7.3*
*Acceptance and rejection regions for the one-sample normal test when the alternative mean ($\mu_1 > $ null mean ($\mu_0$)*

exact *p*-value, which is given by

$$p = 1 - \Phi[(200 - 175)/(50/\sqrt{10})]$$

$$= 1 - \Phi(25/15.811)$$

$$= 1 - \Phi(1.58)$$

$$= 1 - 0.9429$$

$$\approx 0.057$$

Since $p > 0.05$, we conclude that our results are not statistically significant, and we accept the null hypothesis that the mean cholesterol level of these children is no different from that of the average child. ∎

# ■ 7.4 ONE-SAMPLE NORMAL TEST: TWO-SIDED ALTERNATIVES

In the previous section we assumed that the alternative hypothesis was in a *specific direction* relative to the null hypothesis.

*Example 7.17*    **Obstetrics**    In Example 7.2 we assumed that birthweights of infants from a low-SES hospital were either the same or lower than average. In Example 7.1 we assumed that cholesterol levels of children of men who died from heart disease were either the same or higher than average. ∎

In many instances this *prior knowledge* is unavailable. If the null hypothesis is not true, then we have no idea in which direction the alternative mean will fall.

*Example 7.18*    **Cardiovascular Disease**  Suppose that we wish to compare fasting serum cholesterol levels in persons over 21 living in a group of islands in the South Pacific with typical levels found in the United States. Suppose we assume that levels in adults over 21 in the United States are approximately normally distributed with mean 190 mg/dl and standard deviation 40 mg/dl. We have no idea what the relative levels of serum cholesterol are on the islands as compared with the United States. We will assume that the levels on the islands are normally distributed with some unknown mean $\mu$ and standard deviation 40. Hence, we wish to test the null hypothesis: $H_0$: $\mu = \mu_0 = 190$, $\sigma^2 = 1600$ vs. the alternative hypothesis $H_1$: $\mu \neq \mu_0$, $\sigma^2 = 1600$. We perform blood tests on 100 adults from the islands and find that the mean level ($\bar{x}$) is 181.52 mg/dl. What can we conclude on the basis of this evidence? ∎

The type of alternative given in Example 7.18 is known as a *two-sided* alternative, since the alternative mean can be either less than or greater than the null mean.

**Definition 7.11**

We define a **two-tailed test** as a test where the values of the parameter being studied (in this case $\mu$) under the alternative hypothesis are allowed to be either *greater than or less than* the values of the parameter under the null hypothesis ($\mu_0$). ∎

We can show that the best test here depends on the sample mean $\bar{x}$, as it did in the one-sided situation developed in Section 7.3. We showed in **(7.5)** that to test the hypotheses $H_0: \mu = \mu_0$ vs. $H_1: \mu < \mu_0$, the best test was of the form: reject $H_0$ if $\bar{x} < c$ and accept $H_0$ if $\bar{x} \geqslant c$, where $c = \mu_0 + z_\alpha \sigma/\sqrt{n}$. This test is clearly only appropriate for alternatives on one side of the null mean, namely, $\mu < \mu_0$. We also showed in **(7.10)** that to test the hypothesis

$$H_0: \mu = \mu_0 \quad \text{vs.} \quad H_1: \mu > \mu_0$$

the best test was correspondingly of the form: reject $H_0$ if $\bar{x} > c = \mu_0 + z_{1-\alpha}\sigma/\sqrt{n}$ and accept $H_0$ if $\bar{x} \leqslant c$.

---

■ A reasonable decision rule to test for alternatives on *either* side of the null mean is to *reject $H_0$ if $\bar{x}$ is either too small or too large*. Another way of stating this rule is that we will reject $H_0$ if $\bar{x}$ is either $<c_1$ or $>c_2$ for some constants $c_1, c_2$ and accept $H_0$ if $c_1 \leqslant \bar{x} \leqslant c_2$.

---

The question remains as to what are appropriate values for $c_1$ and $c_2$. These values are again determined by the type I error $(\alpha)$. We wish to choose $c_1, c_2$ such that

**7.11**
$$Pr(\text{reject } H_0|H_0 \text{ true}) = Pr(\bar{x} < c_1 \text{ or } \bar{x} > c_2|H_0 \text{ true})$$

$$= Pr(\bar{x} < c_1|H_0 \text{ true}) + Pr(\bar{x} > c_2|H_0 \text{ true}) = \alpha$$

We arbitrarily assign half of the type I error to each of the probabilities on the left-hand side of **(7.11)**. Thus, we wish to find $c_1, c_2$ such that

**7.12**
$$Pr(\bar{x} < c_1|H_0 \text{ true}) = Pr(\bar{x} > c_2|H_0 \text{ true}) = \alpha/2$$

Using a similar argument to that given in the one-sided case, we can show that

$$c_1 = \mu_0 - z_{1-\alpha/2}\sigma/\sqrt{n}$$

$$c_2 = \mu_0 + z_{1-\alpha/2}\sigma/\sqrt{n}$$

This test procedure can be summarized as follows:

**7.13** ### One-Sample Test for the Mean of a Normal Distribution with Known Variance (Two-Sided Alternative)

If we wish to test the hypothesis $H_0: \mu = \mu_0, \sigma = \sigma_0$ vs. $H_1: \mu \neq \mu_0, \sigma = \sigma_0$ with a significance level of $\alpha$, then the best test is based on $\bar{x}$: If

$$\bar{x} < \mu_0 - z_{1-\alpha/2}\sigma/\sqrt{n} \quad \text{or} \quad \bar{x} > \mu_0 + z_{1-\alpha/2}\sigma/\sqrt{n}$$

then we reject $H_0$. If

$$\mu_0 - z_{1-\alpha/2}\sigma/\sqrt{n} \leqslant \bar{x} \leqslant \mu_0 + z_{1-\alpha/2}\sigma/\sqrt{n}$$

then we accept $H_0$.

The acceptance and rejection regions for this test are depicted in Figure 7.4.

*Example 7.19*      **Cardiovascular Disease**  Test the hypothesis that cholesterol levels of adults living in the South Pacific are different from those in the United States using the data in Example 7.18.

*Solution*      We compute $c_1, c_2$ as follows:

$$c_1 = 190 - z_{.975}(40)/\sqrt{100} = 190 - 1.96(4) = 182.16$$

$$c_2 = 190 + 1.96(4) = 197.84$$

Since $\bar{x} = 181.52 < c_1$, we would reject the null hypothesis in favor of the alternative hypothesis that the underlying mean cholesterol level is different from 190. ∎

Alternatively, we might want to compute a *p*-value as we did in the one-sided case. The *p*-value is again defined as the $\alpha$ level at which we would be indifferent to accepting or rejecting $H_0$. We will compute the *p*-value in two different ways, depending on whether $\bar{x}$ is less than or greater than $\mu_0$, since in the former instance we would compare $\bar{x}$ with $c_1$ and in the latter instance we would compare $\bar{x}$ with $c_2$. If we use a similar argument to that given for the one-sided case in Section 7.3, then we have the following *p*-value:

**7.14**  **P-value for the One-Sample Test for the Mean of a Normal Distribution with Known Variance (Two-Sided Alternative)**

$$p = \begin{cases} 2\Phi[(\bar{x} - \mu_0)/(\sigma/\sqrt{n})] & \text{if } \bar{x} \leqslant \mu_0 \\ 2\{1 - \Phi[(\bar{x} - \mu_0)/(\sigma/\sqrt{n})]\} & \text{if } \bar{x} > \mu_0 \end{cases}$$

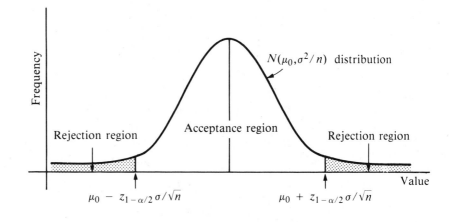

*Figure 7.4*
*One-sample test for the mean of a normal distribution with known variance (two-sided alternative)*

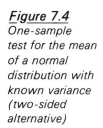

Thus, in words: If $\bar{x} \leqslant \mu_0$, then $p = 2$ times the area under a $N(\mu_0, \sigma^2/n)$ curve to the left of $\bar{x}$; if $\bar{x} > \mu_0$, then $p = 2$ times the area under a $N(\mu_0, \sigma^2/n)$ curve to the right of $\bar{x}$. Another way to interpret the $p$-value is given as follows:

> The **$p$-value** is the probability under the null hypothesis of obtaining a sample mean as extreme as or more extreme than the observed sample mean, where, because we are using a two-sided alternative hypothesis, extremeness is measured as the **absolute value** of the difference between $\bar{x}$ and $\mu_0$.

Hence, if $\bar{x} \leqslant \mu_0$, the $p$-value is the area to the left of $\bar{x}$ plus the area to the right of $\mu_0 + (\mu_0 - \bar{x}) = 2\mu_0 - \bar{x}$ under a $N(\mu_0, \sigma^2/n)$ curve.

However, this area simply amounts to twice the left-hand tail area, since the normal curve is symmetric about $\mu_0$. Similarly, if $\bar{x} > \mu_0$, then the $p$-value is the area to the right of $\bar{x}$ plus the area to the left of $\mu_0 - (\bar{x} - \mu_0) = 2\mu_0 - \bar{x}$ under a $N(\mu_0, \sigma^2/n)$ curve = twice the right-hand tail area.

These areas are illustrated in Figure 7.5.

**Example 7.20**    *Cardiovascular Disease*  Compute the $p$-value for the hypothesis test in Example 7.19.

**Solution**    Since $\bar{x} = 181.52 < 190$, the $p$-value for the test would be twice the left-hand tail area or

$$p = 2 \times \Phi[(181.52 - 190)/(40/10)] = 2 \times \Phi(-8.48/4) = 2 \times \Phi(-2.12)$$

$$= 2 \times [1 - \Phi(2.12)]$$

$$= 2(1 - 0.983) = 0.034$$

Hence, the results are statistically significant with a $p$-value of 0.034. ∎

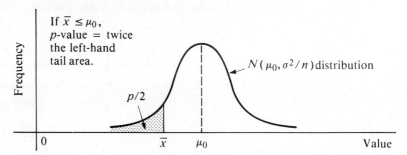

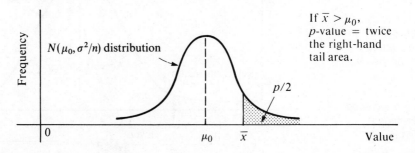

**Figure 7.5**
*Illustration of the p-value for a one-sample test for the mean of a normal distribution with known variance (two-sided alternative)*

When is a one-sided test more appropriate than a two-sided test? Generally, the sample mean falls in the expected direction from $\mu_0$ and it is *easier* to reject $H_0$ using a one-sided test than using a two-sided test. Indeed, with the data in Example 7.18, the *one-sided p-value* to test $H_0: \mu = \mu_0$ vs. $H_1: \mu < \mu_0$ would be

$$p = \Phi\left[ (\bar{x} - \mu_0) \Big/ \left(\frac{\sigma}{\sqrt{n}}\right) \right] = \frac{1}{2}(0.034) = 0.017$$

$$= \frac{1}{2}\text{(two-sided } p\text{-value)}$$

Generally, a two-sided test is always appropriate, since then there can be no question about the conclusions. However, in certain situations only alternatives on one side of the null mean are of interest or are possible, and in this case a one-sided test is better because it has more power than its two-sided counterpart.

**Example 7.21**    *Hypertension*  Suppose we are testing the efficacy of a drug to reduce blood pressure. We will assume that the change in blood pressure (baseline blood pressure minus follow-up blood pressure) is normally distributed with mean $\mu$ and variance $\sigma^2$. An appropriate hypothesis test might be $H_0: \mu = 0$ vs. $H_1: \mu > 0$, since we are only interested in the drug if it reduces the level of blood pressure, not if it raises it.  ■

## ■ 7.5 ONE-SAMPLE t TEST

We have assumed in the previous sections of this chapter that the variance of our underlying distribution was known.

**Example 7.22**    *Obstetrics, Cardiovascular Disease*  We assumed that the null distribution of birth-weights in Example 7.2 and of cholesterol levels in Example 7.18 was the same, respectively, as distributions from much larger populations whose means and variances were known.  ■

This type of information is usually unavailable. Even if it is available, its applicability to our study population is always questionable. Therefore, *we usually have to assume that the underlying variance of our population is unknown.* How then should we conduct our hypothesis tests?

It still makes good sense to base our significance tests on $\bar{x}$. In the two-sided normal test in **(7.13)**, we chose $c_1$ and $c_2$ such that $Pr(\bar{x} < c_1) = Pr(\bar{x} > c_2) = \alpha/2$ and rejected $H_0$ if either $\bar{x} < c_1$ or $\bar{x} > c_2$ and accepted $H_0$ if $c_1 \leqslant \bar{x} \leqslant c_2$. We showed that if $\sigma$ is known, then, because $(\bar{x} - \mu_0)/(\sigma/\sqrt{n})$ is distributed as a $N(0, 1)$ random variable under $H_0$, we can derive $c_1$ and $c_2$ as $\mu_0 - z_{1-\alpha/2}\sigma/\sqrt{n}$ and $\mu_0 + z_{1-\alpha/2}\sigma/\sqrt{n}$, respectively. However, if $\sigma$ is unknown, $c_1$ and $c_2$ cannot be derived in this manner. We know from Section 6.4.5 that if we estimate $\sigma$ by $s$, then under the null hypothesis the random variable $(\bar{x} - \mu_0)/(s/\sqrt{n})$ follows a $t$ distribution with $n - 1$ degrees of freedom. Hence, we have

**7.15**
$$Pr\left[ \frac{(\bar{x} - \mu_0)}{(s/\sqrt{n})} < t_{n-1,\alpha/2} \right] = Pr\left[ \frac{(\bar{x} - \mu_0)}{(s/\sqrt{n})} > t_{n-1,1-\alpha/2} \right] = \alpha/2$$

by the definition of the percentiles of a $t$ distribution. We multiply each inequality in **(7.15)** by $s/\sqrt{n}$ and add $\mu_0$ as follows:

$$Pr(\bar{x} < \mu_0 + t_{n-1,\alpha/2}s/\sqrt{n}) = Pr(\bar{x} > \mu_0 + t_{n-1,1-\alpha/2}s/\sqrt{n}) = \alpha/2$$

Therefore,

**7.16**
$$c_1 = \mu_0 + t_{n-1,\alpha/2}s/\sqrt{n} = \mu_0 - t_{n-1,1-\alpha/2}s/\sqrt{n}$$
$$c_2 = \mu_0 + t_{n-1,1-\alpha/2}s/\sqrt{n}$$

This test can be summarized as follows:

**7.17** ### One-Sample t Test (Two-Sided Alternative)

To test the hypothesis

$$H_0: \mu = \mu_0 \quad \text{vs.} \quad H_1: \mu \neq \mu_0$$

with significance level $\alpha$ assuming that $\sigma^2$ is the same under both hypotheses and is unknown, then the best test is based on $\bar{x}$: If

$$\bar{x} < \mu_0 - t_{n-1,1-\alpha/2}s/\sqrt{n} \quad \text{or} \quad \bar{x} > \mu_0 + t_{n-1,1-\alpha/2}s/\sqrt{n}$$

then we reject $H_0$. If

$$\mu_0 - t_{n-1,1-\alpha/2}s/\sqrt{n} \leqslant \bar{x} \leqslant \mu_0 + t_{n-1,1-\alpha/2}s/\sqrt{n}$$

then we accept $H_0$.

The acceptance and rejection regions for this test are illustrated in Figure 7.6.

We may also wish to compute a $p$-value for this test. The computation of the $p$-value will again depend on whether $\bar{x}$ is greater or less than $\mu_0$. We can show that the $p$-value is given as shown in **(7.18)**.

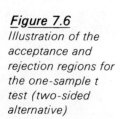

**Figure 7.6**
*Illustration of the acceptance and rejection regions for the one-sample t test (two-sided alternative)*

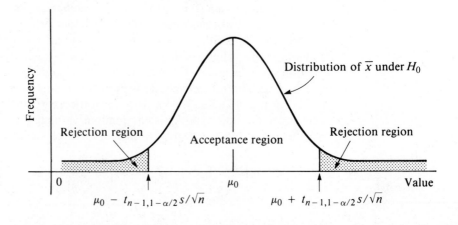

| 7.18 | **P-value for a One-Sample t Test for the Mean of a Normal Distribution (Two-Sided Alternative)** |

If $\bar{x} < \mu_0$,

$$p = 2 \times [\text{area to the left of } (\bar{x} - \mu_0)/(s/\sqrt{n}) \text{ under a } t_{n-1} \text{ distribution}]$$

If $\bar{x} \geq \mu_0$,

$$p = 2 \times [\text{area to the right of } (\bar{x} - \mu_0)/(s/\sqrt{n}) \text{ under a } t_{n-1} \text{ distribution}]$$

This definition is similar to that of a *p*-value for a two-sided test when the variance is known, given in **(7.14)**, except that the $t_{n-1}$ distribution takes the place of a $N(0, 1)$ distribution. It again corresponds to the probability of getting a sample mean as extreme as or more extreme than the one obtained, relative to $\mu_0$. The computation of the *p*-value is illustrated in Figure 7.7.

Note that if *n* is large ($n > 120$) and we substitute *s* for $\sigma$, then the one-sample normal test given in **(7.13)** and **(7.14)** will be virtually the same as the one-sample *t* test given in **(7.17)** and **(7.18)**. In this case we will get very similar results

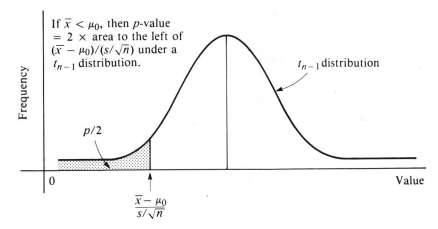

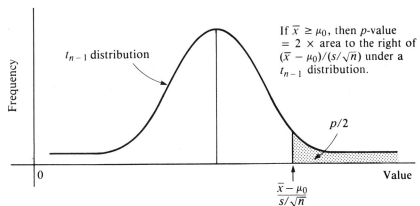

**Figure 7.7**
*Computation of the p-value for a one-sample t test (two-sided alternative)*

using either test. If a computer is unavailable, then the one-sample normal test might be preferable, since the percentiles of the normal distribution are given in more detail in Table 3 in the appendix than are the percentiles of the $t$ distribution in Table 5, and we can thus obtain more precise $p$-values.

## ☐ 7.5.1 Interpolation for the t Table

One problem that we will have in implementing the one-sample $t$ test in (7.17) is that tables are in general not as complete for the $t$ distribution as for the $N(0, 1)$ distribution. We have tables of the $N(0, 1)$ distribution in Table 3, which, for any argument $(x)$ from 0.00 to 3.99 in intervals of 0.01, give various tail areas associated with the normal distribution. An equivalent table for the $t$ distribution would require a comparable amount of information for each number of degrees of freedom, which would be very unwieldy. Instead, in Table 5 we have only selected percentiles of the $t_d$ distribution for various values of $d$. We thus cannot compute exact $p$-values but can only specify a range within which the $p$-value lies.

*Example 7.23*   Suppose that the $t$ value $= (\bar{x} - \mu_0)/(s/\sqrt{n})$ is $-2.42$ with a sample size of 8. Evaluate the $p$-value.

*Solution*   If we refer to Table 5 under the row for 7 degrees of freedom, we see that $t_{7,.975} = 2.365$, whereas $t_{7,.99} = 2.998$. Hence, since the $t$ distribution is symmetric about 0, we know that the area to the left of $-2.42 =$ the area to the right of $+2.42 = p/2$. Furthermore, since $2.365 < 2.42 < 2.998$, we know that $0.01 < p/2 < 0.025$ or $0.02 < p < 0.05$, and the results are statistically significant.   ∎

*Example 7.24*   Suppose that $(\bar{x} - \mu_0)/(s/\sqrt{n}) = 1.425$ based on a sample of size 14. Evaluate the $p$-value.
*Solution*   Since

$$t_{13,.90} = 1.350 \quad \text{and} \quad t_{13,.95} = 1.771$$

and $1.350 < 1.425 < 1.771$, we have $0.05 < p/2 < 0.10$ or $0.1 < p < 0.2$, and the results are not statistically significant.   ∎

*Example 7.25*   **Occupational Medicine, Pulmonary Disease**   Occupational medicine is a relatively new field in medicine, whereby specific health hazards are identified for particular occupations. One topic of recent interest is the effect of fire fighting on pulmonary function. Suppose we identify a group of 25–34-year-old male fire fighters and measure the change in their pulmonary function over a 5-year period. We find that over 5 years, 26 fire fighters have a mean decline in forced expiratory volume (FEV), which is the volume of air expelled in 1 second, of 0.27 liter with a sample standard deviation of 0.32 liter. Can we draw any conclusions about the occupational exposure if the expected change over 5 years is 0.10 liter in normal males in this age group?

*Solution*   We will use a two-sided test, since pulmonary function of fire fighters may decline either more than expected because of their occupational exposure or less than expected because of their likelihood of being healthier than the general population (they must initially pass a rigorous physical examination). We will assume that the decline in FEV is normally distributed with mean $\mu$ and variance $\sigma^2$. We will use a one-sample $t$ test, since $\sigma^2$ is unknown.

We wish to test $H_0: \mu = 0.10$ vs. $H_1: \mu \neq 0.10$. We compute the test statistic

$$\lambda = \frac{(\bar{x} - \mu_0)}{(s/\sqrt{n})} = \frac{(0.27 - 0.10)}{(0.32/\sqrt{26})} = \frac{0.17}{0.063} = 2.70$$

Under $H_0$, $\lambda$ follows a $t$ distribution with 25 degrees of freedom. Referring to Table 5, we see that $t_{25,.99} = 2.485$, $t_{25,.995} = 2.787$ and therefore our $p$-value is between $2(1 - 0.995) = 0.01$ and $2(1 - 0.99) = 0.02$. Our results are statistically significant with $0.01 < p < 0.02$, and we conclude that the pulmonary function of fire fighters declines significantly faster than the typical 25–34-year-old male. ∎

If we wish to obtain a more precise $p$-value, then we must use a computer program that can evaluate areas under the $t$ distribution for any specified degrees of freedom. We have used the HP-41C $t$ distribution program to evaluate the exact $p$-value. The program computes the left-hand tail area, which is given by 0.994 in this case. We subtract this value from 1 to obtain the right-hand tail area and then multiply by 2 to obtain a $p$-value of 0.012. The details are shown in Table 7.2.

*Table 7.2*

*Computation of the exact p-value for the pulmonary function data in Example 7.25 using a one-sample t test with the HP-41C t distribution program*

```
                           XEQ "T"          (a)   Degrees of freedom
                 25.00000000  XEQ A
      (a)   V=25.00000000                   (b)   λ

      (b)          2.700000000  XEQ C       (c)   Left-hand tail area
      (c)   P=0.993870881
                                            (d)   Exact two-sided p-value
                                CHS
              1.000000000        +
              2.000000000        *
      (d)     0.012258239       ***
```

Another problem that we have in implementing the one-sample $t$ test is that not all degrees of freedom are given in the table. How do we use **(7.17)** and **(7.18)** if our degrees of freedom are between two listed degrees of freedom? If a computer is unavailable, then a simple approximate rule that is often used in this case is to interpolate the percentiles of a $t$ distribution using **harmonic interpolation**, which is given as follows:

**7.19** ### Interpolation for the t Table

If we wish to compute $t_{d,p}$ and only $t_{d_1,p}$ and $t_{d_2,p}$ are available in the $t$ table, where $d_1 < d < d_2$, then a good approximation is given by

$$t_{d,p} \approx \frac{w_1 t_{d_1,p} + w_2 t_{d_2,p}}{w_1 + w_2} \quad \text{where } w_1 = \frac{1}{d} - \frac{1}{d_2}, \; w_2 = \frac{1}{d_1} - \frac{1}{d}$$

*Example 7.26*     Evaluate the 97.5th percentile of a $t$ distribution with 99 degrees of freedom.

*Solution*          We want to compute $t_{99,.975}$. If we refer to Table 5, we see that 99 degrees of freedom is not listed in the table, but 60 degrees of freedom and 120 degrees of freedom are listed. Therefore, from **(7.19)** we have $d = 99$, $d_1 = 60$, $d_2 = 120$ and therefore

$$t_{99,.975} \approx \frac{(\frac{1}{99} - \frac{1}{120})t_{60,.975} + (\frac{1}{60} - \frac{1}{99})t_{120,.975}}{(\frac{1}{60} - \frac{1}{120})}$$

$$= \frac{(0.0101 - 0.0083)(2.000) + (0.0167 - 0.0101)(1.980)}{(0.0167 - 0.0083)}$$

$$= \frac{(0.0018)(2.000) + (0.0066)(1.980)}{0.0084}$$

$$= \frac{18(2.000) + 66(1.980)}{84}$$

$$= 1.984 \qquad ■$$

*Example 7.27*

**Cardiovascular Disease**  Let us refer to the cholesterol data in Example 7.18. Suppose that the sample standard deviation is 48.23 and we *do not* assume that the variance is known. Evaluate the statistical significance of the results.

*Solution*

We wish to test the hypothesis: $H_0: \mu = 190$ vs. $H_1: \mu \neq 190$, where $\sigma^2$ is assumed unknown. We know that the mean cholesterol level in our sample of 100 adults is 181.52 and that the sample standard deviation ($s$) is 48.23. Then, from **(7.18)** we compute the argument

$$(\bar{x} - \mu_0)/(s/\sqrt{n}) = \frac{(181.52 - 190)}{(48.23/\sqrt{100})}$$

$$= -8.48/4.823$$

$$= -1.758$$

Since from Example 7.26 we know that $t_{99,.975} = 1.984$, it follows that $p > 2(0.025) = 0.05$ and our results are not statistically significant (NS). Actually, the interpolation was probably unnecessary in this case, since from Table 5 we see that $t_{120,.975} = 1.980$ and $t_{99,.975} > t_{120,.975} = 1.980 > 1.758$. Thus, $p > 2(0.025) = 0.05$ and our results are again not statistically significant.

Another approach to this problem is to use the critical value method given in **(7.17)**. We will reject $H_0$ if

$$\bar{x} < \mu_0 - t_{n-1,1-\alpha/2}s/\sqrt{n} = 190 - t_{99,.975}(48.23)/\sqrt{100}$$

$$= 190 - 1.984(48.23)/10$$

$$= 190 - 9.57 = 180.43$$

or

$$\bar{x} > \mu_0 + t_{n-1,1-\alpha/2}s/\sqrt{n} = 190 + 9.57$$

$$= 199.57$$

Since $\bar{x} = 181.52 > 180.43$ and $\bar{x} = 181.52 < 199.57$, the results are not statistically significant and $p \geqslant 0.05$. ∎

We have been discussing the two-sided version of the one-sample $t$ test in this section. The test procedure for the one-sided case is similar to the one-sample normal test when the variance is known and can be summarized as follows:

**7.20**    **One-Sample t Test (One-Sided Alternative)**

To test the hypothesis: $H_0: \mu = \mu_0$ vs. $H_1: \mu < \mu_0$ with significance level $\alpha$ assuming that $\sigma^2$ is the same under both hypotheses and is unknown, we proceed as follows: If

$$\bar{x} < \mu_0 - t_{n-1,1-\alpha}s/\sqrt{n}$$

then we reject $H_0$. If

$$\bar{x} \geqslant \mu_0 - t_{n-1,1-\alpha}s/\sqrt{n}$$

then we accept $H_0$. The $p$-value for this test is given by the area to the left of $(\bar{x} - \mu_0)/(s/\sqrt{n})$ under a $t_{n-1}$ distribution.

To test the hypothesis: $H_0: \mu = \mu_0$ vs. $H_1: \mu > \mu_0$ with significance level $\alpha$ assuming that $\sigma^2$ is the same under both hypotheses and is unknown, then the best test is based on $\bar{x}$: If

$$\bar{x} > \mu_0 + t_{n-1,1-\alpha}s/\sqrt{n}$$

then we reject $H_0$. If

$$\bar{x} \leqslant \mu_0 + t_{n-1,1-\alpha}s/\sqrt{n}$$

then we accept $H_0$. The $p$-value for this test is given by the area to the right of $(\bar{x} - \mu_0)/(s/\sqrt{n})$ under a $t_{n-1}$ distribution.

# ■ 7.6 THE POWER OF A TEST

## □ 7.6.1 One-Sided Alternatives

In Section 7.3 we derived the appropriate hypothesis test to test

$$H_0: \mu = \mu_0 \quad \text{vs.} \quad H_1: \mu = \mu_1 < \mu_0$$

where the underlying distribution is assumed to be normal and the population variance is assumed to be known. The best test was based on the sample mean $\bar{x}$. In particular, from **(7.5)** for a type I error of $\alpha$, we reject $H_0$ if $\bar{x} < \mu_0 + z_\alpha\sigma/\sqrt{n}$ and we accept $H_0$ if $\bar{x} \geqslant \mu_0 + z_\alpha\sigma/\sqrt{n}$. The form of the best test *does not depend on the alternative mean chosen* $(\mu_1)$ as long as this mean is less than the null mean $\mu_0$.

Hence, if we were interested in an alternative mean of $\mu_1 = 115$ oz rather than $\mu_1 = 110$ oz, then we would still use the same test procedure. However, what *is* different for the two alternative means is the power of the test $= 1 - Pr$(type II error). We recall from Definition 7.6 that

$$\text{Power} = Pr(\text{rejecting } H_0 | H_0 \text{ false}) = Pr(\bar{x} < \mu_0 + z_\alpha \sigma/\sqrt{n} | \mu = \mu_1)$$

We know that under $H_1$, $\bar{x} \sim N(\mu_1, \sigma^2/n)$. Hence upon standardization of limits, we have

$$\text{Power} = \Phi[(\mu_0 + z_\alpha \sigma/\sqrt{n} - \mu_1)/(\sigma/\sqrt{n})] = \Phi\left[ z_\alpha + \frac{(\mu_0 - \mu_1)}{\sigma}\sqrt{n} \right]$$

This power is depicted graphically in Figure 7.8.

Note that the area to the left of $\mu_0 + z_\alpha \sigma/\sqrt{n}$ under the $H_0$ distribution is the significance level $\alpha$, whereas the area to the left of $\mu_0 + z_\alpha \sigma/\sqrt{n}$ under the $H_1$ distribution is the power $= 1 - \beta$.

Why should we be concerned about power? The power of a test tells us how likely we are to find a significant difference given that the alternative hypothesis is true, that is, given that our true mean $\mu$ is different from the mean under the null hypothesis ($\mu_0$). If the power is too low, then we have little chance of finding a significant difference and we are likely to get nonsignificant results even if real differences exist between the true mean $\mu$ of the group we are studying and the null mean $\mu_0$. An inadequate sample size is almost always the cause of low power.

**Example 7.28**    **Obstetrics**  Compute the power of the test for the birthweight data in Example 7.2 with an alternative mean of 115 oz and $\alpha = 0.05$.

**Solution**    We have $\mu_0 = 120$ oz, $\mu_1 = 115$ oz, $\alpha = 0.05$, $\sigma = 25$, $n = 100$. Thus,

$$\text{Power} \doteq \Phi[z_{.05} + (120 - 115)\sqrt{100}/25] = \Phi[-1.645 + 5(10)/25]$$

$$= \Phi(0.355) = 0.639$$

Therefore, there is about a 64% chance of detecting a significant difference using a 5% significance level with this sample size.    ∎

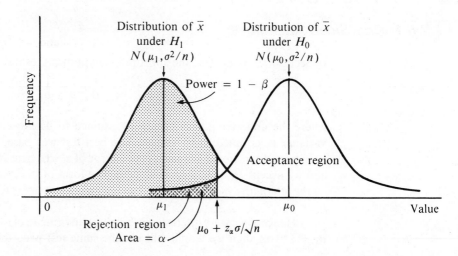

**Figure 7.8**
*Illustration of power for the one-sample test for the mean of a normal distribution with known variance ($\mu_1 < \mu_0$)*

Distribution of $\bar{x}$ under $H_1$  $N(\mu_1, \sigma^2/n)$

Distribution of $\bar{x}$ under $H_0$  $N(\mu_0, \sigma^2/n)$

Power $= 1 - \beta$

Acceptance region

Frequency

0    $\mu_1$    $\mu_0$    Value

Rejection region  Area $= \alpha$

$\mu_0 + z_\alpha \sigma/\sqrt{n}$

We have focused on the situation when $\mu_1 < \mu_0$. We are also interested in power when we wish to test the hypothesis

$$H_0: \mu = \mu_0 \quad \text{vs.} \quad H_1: \mu = \mu_1 > \mu_0$$

as was the case with the cholesterol data in Example 7.1. The best test for this situation was presented in (7.10), where we reject $H_0$ if $\bar{x} > \mu_0 + z_{1-\alpha}\sigma/\sqrt{n}$ and accept $H_0$ if $\bar{x} \leq \mu_0 + z_{1-\alpha}\sigma/\sqrt{n}$. Using a similar argument to that given previously, we can show that the power of this test is given by

$$\Phi\left[ z_\alpha + \frac{(\mu_1 - \mu_0)\sqrt{n}}{\sigma} \right]$$

This power is depicted graphically in Figure 7.9.

*Example 7.29*  **Cardiovascular Disease, Pediatrics** Using a 5% level of significance and a sample of size 10, compute the power of the test for the cholesterol data in Example 7.1 with an alternative mean of 190 mg%/ml.

*Solution*  We have $\mu_0 = 175$, $\mu_1 = 190$, $\alpha = 0.05$, $\sigma = 50$, $n = 10$. Thus,

$$\text{Power} = \Phi[-1.645 + (190 - 175)\sqrt{10}/50]$$

$$= \Phi[-1.645 + 15\sqrt{10}/50]$$

$$= \Phi(-0.70)$$

$$= 1 - \Phi(0.70)$$

$$= 1 - 0.758$$

$$= 0.242$$

Therefore, the chance of finding a significant difference in this case is only 24%. Thus, it is not surprising that we did not find a significant difference in Example 7.16, since our sample size was too small. ∎

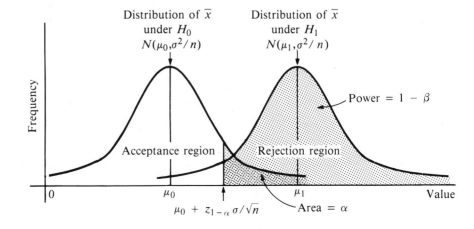

*Figure 7.9*
*Illustration of power for the one-sample test for the mean of a normal distribution with known variance* $(\mu_1 > \mu_0)$

We can summarize the power formulae presented in this section as follows:

**7.21** | **Power for the One-Sample Test for the Mean of a Normal Distribution with Known Variance (One-Sided Alternative)**

The power of the test for the hypothesis

$$H_0: \mu = \mu_0 \quad \text{vs.} \quad H_1: \mu = \mu_1$$

where the underlying distribution is normal and the population variance ($\sigma^2$) is known is given by

$$\Phi[z_\alpha + (\mu_0 - \mu_1)\sqrt{n}/\sigma] \quad \text{if} \quad \mu_1 < \mu_0$$

$$\Phi[z_\alpha + (\mu_1 - \mu_0)\sqrt{n}/\sigma] \quad \text{if} \quad \mu_1 \geq \mu_0$$

Notice from **(7.21)** that the power depends on four factors: $\alpha$, $|\mu_0 - \mu_1|$, $n$, and $\sigma$.

**7.22** | **Factors Affecting the Power**

1. If the *significance level is made smaller* ($\alpha$ decreases), $z_\alpha$ decreases and hence the *power decreases*.

2. If the alternative mean is shifted further away from the null mean ($|\mu_0 - \mu_1|$ *increases*), then the *power increases*.

3. If the standard deviation of an individual observation increases ($\sigma$ *increases*), then the *power decreases*.

4. If the sample size increases ($n$ *increases*), then the *power increases*.

**Example 7.30**

**Cardiovascular Disease, Pediatrics** Compute the power of the test for the cholesterol data in Example 7.1 with a significance level of 0.01 vs. an alternative of 190 mg%/ml.

**Solution**

If $\alpha = 0.01$, then the power is given by

$$\Phi[z_{.01} + (190 - 175)\sqrt{10}/50] = \Phi[-2.326 + 15\sqrt{10}/50]$$

$$= \Phi(-1.38)$$

$$= 1 - \Phi(1.38)$$

$$= 1 - 0.9162$$

$$\approx 8\%$$

which is lower than the power of 24% for $\alpha = 0.05$, as computed in Example 7.29. *What does this mean?* It means that if we lower our $\alpha$ level from 0.05 to 0.01, we pay the price by having a higher $\beta$ error or, equivalently, a lower power, which decreases from 0.24 to 0.08. ∎

**Example 7.31**

**Obstetrics** Compute the power of the test for the birthweight data in Example 7.2 with $\mu_1 = 110$ oz rather than 115 oz.

*Solution*    If $\mu_1 = 110$ oz, then the power is given by

$$\Phi[-1.645 + (120 - 110)10/25] = \Phi(2.355)$$

$$= 0.991 \approx 99\%$$

which is higher than the power of 64%, as computed in Example 7.28 for $\mu_1 = 115$ oz. *What does this mean?* It means that if our alternative mean changes from 115 oz to 110 oz, then our chance of finding a significant difference increases from 64% to 99%. ∎

*Example 7.32*    *Cardiology*  Compute the power of the test for the infarct size data in Example 7.11 with $\sigma = 15$ and $\sigma = 10$ using an alternative mean of 20 ($ck - g - EQ/m^2$).

*Solution*    If $\sigma = 15$, then

$$\text{Power} = \Phi[-1.645 + (25 - 20)\sqrt{8}/15] = \Phi(-0.70)$$

$$= 1 - 0.758$$

$$= 0.242 \approx 24\%$$

whereas if $\sigma = 10$, then

$$\text{Power} = \Phi[-1.645 + (25 - 20)\sqrt{8}/10] = \Phi(-0.23)$$

$$= 1 - \Phi(0.23)$$

$$= 1 - 0.591$$

$$= 0.409 \approx 41\%$$

*What does this mean?* It means that our chance of finding a significant difference declines from 41% to 24% if $\sigma$ increases from 10 to 15. ∎

*Example 7.33*    *Obstetrics*  Assuming a sample size of 10 rather than 100, compute the power for the birthweight data in Example 7.2 with an alternative mean of 115 oz.

*Solution*    We have $\mu_0 = 120$ oz, $\mu_1 = 115$ oz, $\alpha = 0.05$, $\sigma = 25$, and $n = 10$. Thus,

$$\text{Power} = \Phi[z_{.05} + (120 - 115)\sqrt{10}/25] = \Phi(-1.645 + 5\sqrt{10}/25)$$

$$= \Phi(-1.01)$$

$$= 1 - 0.8438$$

$$= 0.156$$

*What does this mean?* It means that we have only a 16% chance of finding a significant difference with a sample size of 10, whereas we had a 64% chance with a sample size of 100. These results imply that if we sampled 10 infants, we would have virtually no chance of finding a significant difference and would almost surely report a false negative result. ∎

For given levels of $\alpha$, $\sigma$, and $n$, we can draw a **power curve** for the power of a test for various alternatives $\mu_1$. We have drawn such a power curve in Figure 7.10 for the birthweight data in Example 7.2.

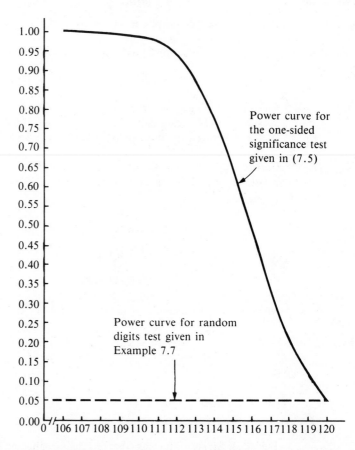

Power curve for the one-sided significance test given in (7.5)

Power curve for random digits test given in Example 7.7

**Figure 7.10**
*Power curve for the
birthweight data in
Example 7.2*

We have also drawn the power curve for the random digits test described in Example 7.7, which is just a straight line parallel to the *x*-axis at 0.05. The point is that the latter power curve is always below the power curve for the test based on the sample mean, since the test we have derived has the most power for a given significance level for any particular alternative $\mu_1$ if the observations are normally distributed.

## □ 7.6.2 Two-Sided Alternatives

The power formula given in **(7.21)** is appropriate for a one-sided significance test at level $\alpha$ for the mean of a normal distribution with known variance. If a two-sided alternative is appropriate, then we replace $\alpha$ by $\alpha/2$ and obtain the following formula:

**7.23** *Power for the One-Sample Test for the Mean of a Normal Distribution with Known Variance (Two-Sided Alternative)*

The power of the test for the hypothesis

$$H_0:\ \mu = \mu_0 \quad \text{vs.} \quad H_1:\ |\mu_1 - \mu_0| = \Delta$$

where the underlying distribution is normal and the population variance ($\sigma^2$) is known, is given by

$$\Phi(z_{\alpha/2} + \Delta\sqrt{n}/\sigma)$$

*Example 7.34*    **Cardiology**  A new drug in the class of calcium channel blockers is to be tested for the treatment of patients with unstable angina, a severe type of angina. We do not know what effect this drug will have on heart rate. Suppose that 20 patients are to be studied and the change in heart rate after 48 hours is known to have a standard deviation of 10 beats per minute. What power would such a study have of detecting a significant difference in heart rate over 48 hours if it is hypothesized that the true change in heart rate from baseline to 48 hours could be 5 beats per minute in either direction?

*Solution*    We use **(7.23)** with $\sigma = 10, \Delta = 5, \alpha = 0.05, n = 20$. We have

$$\text{Power} = \Phi(z_{.05/2} + 5\sqrt{20}/10)$$

$$= \Phi(-1.96 + 2.236)$$

$$= \Phi(0.276)$$

$$= 0.609 \approx 0.61$$

Thus, the study would have a 61% chance of detecting a significant difference.    ■

# ■ 7.7  SAMPLE SIZE DETERMINATION

## ☐ 7.7.1  One-Sided Alternatives

Frequently, for planning purposes we need to have some idea of an appropriate sample size for investigation before a study actually begins. One possible result from making these calculations is that the appropriate sample size is far beyond the financial means of the investigator(s) and the proposed investigation has to be abandoned. Obviously, reaching this conclusion before a study starts is far better than after it is in progress.

What do we actually mean by "the appropriate sample size for investigation"? Suppose we consider the birthweight data discussed in Example 7.2. We are testing the null hypothesis $H_0$: $\mu = \mu_0$ vs. the alternative hypothesis $H_1$: $\mu = \mu_1$, where we assume that the distribution of birthweights is normal in both cases and that the standard deviation $\sigma$ is known. We are presumably going to conduct a test with significance level $\alpha$ and have some idea of what the magnitude of the alternative mean $\mu_1$ is likely to be. If we use the test procedure in **(7.5)**, then we would reject $H_0$ if $\bar{x} < \mu_0 + z_\alpha \sigma/\sqrt{n}$ and accept $H_0$ if $\bar{x} \geq \mu_0 + z_\alpha \sigma/\sqrt{n}$. Suppose the alternative hypothesis is actually true. The investigator should have some idea as to what he or she would like the probability of rejecting $H_0$ to be in this instance. This probability is, of course, nothing other than the power or $1 - \beta$. Typical values for the desired power are 80%, 90%, . . . , and so forth. The problem of determining **sample size** can be summarized as follows: Given that we

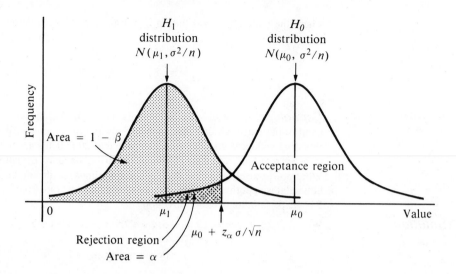

*Figure 7.11*
*Requirements for*
*appropriate sample*
*size*

will conduct a significance test at level $\alpha$ and that we expect the true alternative mean is $\mu_1$, what sample size do we need to be able to detect a significant difference with probability $1 - \beta$? The situation is depicted in Figure 7.11.

In Figure 7.11 we have drawn the underlying distribution of $\bar{x}$ under the null and alternative hypotheses, respectively, and we have identified the actual point $\mu_0 + z_\alpha\sigma/\sqrt{n}$. We will reject $H_0$ if $\bar{x} < \mu_0 + z_\alpha\sigma/\sqrt{n}$. Hence, the area to the left of $\mu_0 + z_\alpha\sigma/\sqrt{n}$ under the rightmost curve is $\alpha$. However, we also want the area to the left of $\mu_0 + z_\alpha\sigma/\sqrt{n}$ under the leftmost curve, which represents the power, to be $1 - \beta$. These requirements will be met if $n$ is made sufficiently large, since the variance of each curve $(\sigma^2/n)$ will decrease as $n$ increases and thus the curves will separate. We can show that the sample size that satisfies our two requirements for $\alpha$ and $1 - \beta$ is $n = \sigma^2(z_{1-\beta} + z_{1-\alpha})^2/(\mu_0 - \mu_1)^2$. Similarly, if we were to test the hypothesis

$$H_0: \mu = \mu_0 \quad \text{vs.} \quad H_1: \mu = \mu_1 > \mu_0$$

as was the case with the cholesterol data in Example 7.1, using a significance level of $\alpha$ and a power of $1 - \beta$, then the same sample size formula would hold. This procedure can be summarized as follows:

### 7.24    *Sample Size Estimation When Testing for the Mean of a Normal Distribution (One-Sided Alternative)*

Suppose we wish to test

$$H_0: \mu = \mu_0 \quad \text{vs.} \quad H_1: \mu = \mu_1$$

where the data are normally distributed with mean $\mu$ and known variance $\sigma^2$. The **sample size** needed to conduct a test with significance level $\alpha$ and probability of detecting a significant difference $= 1 - \beta$ is

$$n = \frac{\sigma^2(z_{1-\beta} + z_{1-\alpha})^2}{|\mu_0 - \mu_1|^2}$$

**Example 7.35**

**Obstetrics**  Let us consider the birthweight data in Example 7.2. Suppose that $\mu_0 = 120$ oz, $\mu_1 = 115$ oz, $\sigma^2 = 625$, $\alpha = 0.05$, $1 - \beta = 0.80$. Compute the appropriate sample size needed to conduct the test.

**Solution**

We have

$$n = \frac{625(z_{.8} + z_{.95})^2}{25}$$

$$= 25(0.84 + 1.645)^2$$

$$= 25(6.175)$$

$$= 154.38$$

Thus, we need a sample size of 155 to have an 80% chance of detecting a significant difference at the 5% level if the alternative mean is 115 oz.  ∎

Notice that the sample size is very sensitive to the alternative mean chosen. We see from **(7.24)** that the sample size is inversely proportional to $|\mu_0 - \mu_1|^2$. Thus, if the distance between the null and alternative means is halved, then the sample size needed is 4 times as large. Similarly, if the distance between the null and alternative means is doubled, then the sample size needed is $\frac{1}{4}$ as large.

**Example 7.36**

**Obstetrics**  Compute the sample size for the birthweight data in Example 7.2 if $\mu_1 = 110$ oz rather than 115 oz.

**Solution**

The required sample size would be $\frac{1}{4}$ as large, since $|\mu_0 - \mu_1|^2 = 100$ rather than 25. Thus, $n = 38.60$, or 39 persons would be needed.  ∎

**Example 7.37**

**Cardiovascular Disease, Pediatrics**  Let us consider the cholesterol data in Example 7.1. Suppose that the null mean is 175 mg%/ml, the alternative mean is 190 mg%/ml, the standard deviation is 50, and we wish to conduct a significance test at the 5% level with a power of 90%. How large a sample size do we need?

**Solution**

We have

$$n = \frac{\sigma^2(z_{1-\beta} + z_{1-\alpha})^2}{|\mu_0 - \mu_1|^2}$$

$$= \frac{(50)^2(z_{.9} + z_{.95})^2}{(190 - 175)^2}$$

$$= \frac{2500(1.28 + 1.645)^2}{15^2}$$

$$= \frac{2500(8.556)}{225}$$

$$= 95.1$$

Thus, we need 96 people to achieve a power of 90% using a 5% significance level. We should not be surprised that we did not find a significant difference with a sample size of 10 in Example 7.16.    ∎

Clearly, the required sample size is related to the following four quantities:

---

**7.25**  **Factors Affecting the Sample Size**

1. The sample size *increases* as $\sigma^2$ *increases*.
2. The sample size *increases* as the significance level is made smaller ($\alpha$ *decreases*).
3. The sample size *increases* as the required *power increases* ($1 - \beta$ *increases*).
4. The sample size *decreases* as the distance between the null and alternative means increases ($|\mu_0 - \mu_1|$ *increases*).

---

*Example 7.38*

**Obstetrics**  What would happen to the sample size estimate in Example 7.35 if $\sigma$ were increased to 30? If $\alpha$ were reduced to 0.01? If the required power were increased to 90%? If the alternative mean were changed to 110 oz (keeping all other parameters the same in each instance)?

*Solution*

From Example 7.35 we see that we need to sample 155 infants to achieve 80% power using a 5% significance level with a null mean of 120 oz, an alternative mean of 115 oz, and a standard deviation of 25 oz.

If $\sigma$ increases to 30, then we need

$$n = (30)^2(z_{.8} + z_{.95})^2/(120 - 115)^2$$

$$= 900(0.84 + 1.645)^2/25$$

$$= 222.3, \text{ or } 223 \text{ infants}$$

If $\alpha$ were reduced to 0.01, then we need

$$n = (25)^2(z_{.8} + z_{.99})^2/(120 - 115)^2$$

$$= 625(0.84 + 2.326)^2/25$$

$$= 250.6, \text{ or } 251 \text{ infants}$$

If $1 - \beta$ were increased to 0.9, then we need

$$n = (25)^2(z_{.9} + z_{.95})^2/(120 - 115)^2$$

$$= 625(1.28 + 1.645)^2/25$$

$$= 213.9, \text{ or } 214 \text{ infants}$$

If $\mu_1$ is decreased to 110 or, equivalently, if $|\mu_0 - \mu_1|$ is increased from 5 to 10, then we need

$$n = (25)^2(z_{.8} + z_{.95})^2/(120 - 110)^2$$

$$= 625(0.84 + 1.645)^2/100$$

$$= 38.6, \text{ or } 39 \text{ infants}$$

Thus, the required sample size increases if $\sigma$ increases, $\alpha$ decreases, or $1 - \beta$ increases, respectively. The required sample size decreases if the distance between the null and alternative means increases. ∎

One question that arises is how to estimate the parameters necessary to compute the sample size. It usually is easy to specify the magnitude of the null mean ($\mu_0$). Similarly, by convention the type I error ($\alpha$) is usually set to 0.05. What the level of the power should be is somewhat less clear, although most investigators seem to feel uncomfortable with powers of less than 0.80. The appropriate values for $\mu_1$ and $\sigma^2$ are usually unknown. The parameters $\mu_1$, $\sigma^2$ may be obtained from previous work, similar experiments, or prior knowledge of the underlying distribution. In the absence of such information, the parameter $\mu_1$ is sometimes estimated by assessing what a *scientifically important difference* $|\mu_0 - \mu_1|$ would be in the context of the problem under study. Conducting a small *pilot study* is sometimes valuable. Such a study is generally inexpensive, and its sole aim is to obtain estimates $\mu_1$ and $\sigma^2$ for the purpose of estimating the sample size needed to conduct the major investigation.

Keep in mind that most sample size estimates are very rough because of the inaccuracy in estimating $\mu_1$ and $\sigma^2$. These estimates are often used merely to check that the proposed sample size of a study is in the vicinity of what is actually needed rather than to identify a precise sample size.

## ☐ 7.7.2 Sample Size Determination (Two-Sided Alternatives)

The sample size formula given in (**7.24**) was appropriate for a one-sided significance test at level $\alpha$ for the mean of a normal distribution with known variance. If we do not know whether the alternative mean ($\mu_1$) is greater or less than the null mean ($\mu_0$), then a two-sided test is appropriate, and the corresponding sample size needed to conduct a study with power $1 - \beta$ is given by

$$n = \frac{\sigma^2(z_{1-\beta} + z_{1-\alpha/2})^2}{|\mu_0 - \mu_1|^2}$$

This procedure can be summarized as follows:

---

**7.26** *Sample Size Estimation When Testing for the Mean of a Normal Distribution (Two-Sided Alternative)*

Suppose we wish to test $H_0: \mu = \mu_0$ vs. $H_1: \mu = \mu_1$, where the data are normally distributed with mean $\mu$ and known variance $\sigma^2$. The **sample size** needed to conduct a two-sided test with significance level $\alpha$ and power $1 - \beta$ is

$$n = \frac{\sigma^2(z_{1-\beta} + z_{1-\alpha/2})^2}{|\mu_0 - \mu_1|^2}$$

---

Note that this sample size is always larger than the corresponding sample size for a one-sided test given in (**7.24**), since $z_{1-\alpha/2}$ is larger than $z_{1-\alpha}$.

*Example 7.39*    *Cardiology*  Let us consider a study of the effect of a calcium channel blocking agent on heart rate for patients with unstable angina, as described in Example 7.34. Suppose we want to have at least 80% power for detecting a significant difference if the effect of the drug is to change heart rate by 5 beats per minute over 48 hours in either direction. How many patients should we enroll in such a study?

*Solution*    We assume that $\alpha = 0.05$ and $\sigma = 10$ beats per minute, as in Example 7.34. We intend to use a two-sided test, since we are not sure in what direction heart rate will change after using the drug. Therefore, we estimate the sample size using the two-sided formulation in **(7.26)**, as follows:

$$n = \frac{\sigma^2(z_{1-\beta} + z_{1-\alpha/2})^2}{|\mu_0 - \mu_1|^2}$$

$$= \frac{10^2(z_{.8} + z_{.975})^2}{5^2}$$

$$= \frac{100(0.84 + 1.96)^2}{25}$$

$$= 4(7.84)$$

$$= 31.36, \text{ or } 32 \text{ patients}$$

Thus, we need to study 32 patients to have at least an 80% chance of finding a significant difference using a two-sided test with $\alpha = 0.05$ if the true mean change in heart rate from using the drug is 5 beats per minute. Note that in Example 7.34 the investigators proposed a study with 20 patients, which would have provided only 61% power for testing the preceding hypothesis.

If the direction of effect of the drug on heart rate were well known, then a one-sided test might be justified. In this case the appropriate sample size could be obtained from the one-sided formulation in **(7.24)**, as follows:

$$n = \frac{\sigma^2(z_{1-\beta} + z_{1-\alpha})^2}{|\mu_0 - \mu_1|^2}$$

$$= \frac{(10)^2(z_{.8} + z_{.95})^2}{5^2}$$

$$= \frac{100(0.84 + 1.645)^2}{25}$$

$$= 4(6.175)$$

$$= 24.7, \text{ or } 25 \text{ patients}$$

Thus, only 25 patients would need to be studied for a one-sided test instead of the 32 patients needed for a two-sided test.    ∎

# ■ 7.8 THE RELATIONSHIP BETWEEN HYPOTHESIS TESTING AND CONFIDENCE INTERVALS

We presented a test procedure in **(7.13)** for testing the hypothesis $H_0: \mu = \mu_0$, $\sigma^2 = \sigma_0^2$ vs. $H_1: \mu \neq \mu_0$, $\sigma^2 = \sigma_0^2$. Similarly, we presented a method in Section 6.4.4 for obtaining a two-sided confidence interval for the parameter $\mu$ of a normal distribution when the variance is assumed known. The relationship between these two procedures can be stated as follows:

**7.27**  **The Relationship Between Hypothesis Testing and Confidence Intervals (Two-Sided Case)**

Suppose we are testing $H_0: \mu = \mu_0, \sigma^2 = \sigma_0^2$ vs. $H_1: \mu \neq \mu_0, \sigma^2 = \sigma_0^2$. We reject $H_0$ with a two-sided level $\alpha$ test if and only if the two-sided $100\% \times (1 - \alpha)$ confidence interval for $\mu$ *does not* contain $\mu_0$. We accept $H_0$ if and only if the two-sided $100\% \times (1 - \alpha)$ confidence interval for $\mu$ *does* contain $\mu_0$. This relationship is illustrated in Figure 7.12.

Suppose that our sample mean $\bar{x}_1$ is in the rejection region. The two-sided $100\% \times (1 - \alpha)$ confidence interval for $\mu$, which ranges from $\bar{x}_1 - z_{1-\alpha/2}\sigma/\sqrt{n}$ to $\bar{x}_1 + z_{1-\alpha/2}\sigma/\sqrt{n}$, *does not* include $\mu_0$ as depicted in the figure. Similarly, the sample mean $\bar{x}_2$ is in the acceptance region, and correspondingly the two-sided $100\% \times (1 - \alpha)$ confidence interval from $\bar{x}_2 - z_{1-\alpha/2}\sigma/\sqrt{n}$ to $\bar{x}_2 + z_{1-\alpha/2}\sigma/\sqrt{n}$ *does* contain $\mu_0$.

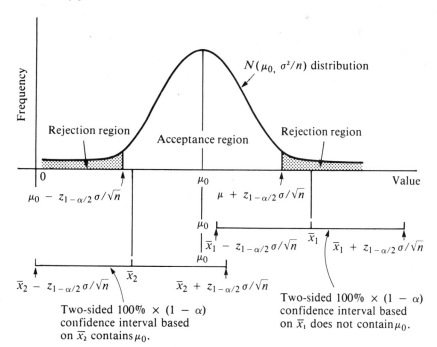

**Figure 7.12**
*The relationship between a two-sided hypothesis test and a two-sided confidence interval*

Hence, this relationship is the rationale for our use of confidence intervals in Chapter 6 to decide on the reasonableness of specific values for the parameter $\mu$. If any specific proposed value $\mu_0$ did not fall in the two-sided $100 \times (1 - \alpha)$ confidence interval for $\mu$, then we said that it was an unlikely value for the parameter $\mu$. Equivalently, we could have tested the hypothesis $H_0: \mu = \mu_0$ vs. $H_1: \mu \neq \mu_0$ and rejected $H_0$ at significance level $\alpha$.

**Example 7.40**    *Cardiovascular Disease* Consider the cholesterol data given in Example 7.18. The two-sided 95% confidence interval for $\mu$ is given by

$$(\bar{x} - z_{1-\alpha/2}\sigma/\sqrt{n}, \, \bar{x} + z_{1-\alpha/2}\sigma/\sqrt{n})$$

$$= \left[ 181.52 - \frac{1.96(40)}{10}, \, 181.52 + \frac{1.96(40)}{10} \right]$$

$$= (181.52 - 7.84, \, 181.52 + 7.84)$$

$$= (173.68, \, 189.36)$$

This 95% confidence interval does *not* contain 190, which corresponds to the statement that the two-sided $p$-value (0.034) as computed in Example 7.20 is less than 0.05.    ∎

**Example 7.41**    *Cardiovascular Disease* Suppose the sample mean for cholesterol was 185 mg/dl for the cholesterol data in Example 7.18. The 95% confidence interval would be

$$(185 - 7.84, \, 185 + 7.84) = (177.16, \, 192.84)$$

which contains the null mean (190). The $p$-value for the hypothesis test would be

$$p = 2 \times \Phi[(185 - 190)/4] = 2 \times \Phi(-1.25)$$

$$= 2[1 - \Phi(1.25)]$$

$$= 2(1 - 0.8944) = 2(0.1056)$$

$$= 0.2112 > 0.05$$

Thus, the conclusions based on the confidence interval and hypothesis-testing approaches are also the same here.    ∎

A similar relationship exists between the one-sided hypothesis test developed in Section 7.3 and a one-sided confidence interval for the parameter $\mu$, which can be stated as follows:

**7.28**    ### The Relationship Between Hypothesis Testing and Confidence Intervals (One-Sided Alternative)

To test the hypothesis

$$H_0: \mu = \mu_0, \quad \sigma^2 = \sigma_0^2 \quad \text{vs.} \quad H_1: \mu < \mu_0, \quad \sigma^2 = \sigma_0^2$$

with significance level $\alpha$, we reject $H_0$ if and only if the lower one-sided $100\% \times (1 - \alpha)$ confidence interval $\mu \leqslant \bar{x} + z_{1-\alpha}\sigma/\sqrt{n}$ *does not contain* $\mu_0$; *we accept* $H_0$ *if this interval does contain* $\mu_0$.

To test the hypothesis

$$H_0: \mu = \mu_0, \quad \sigma^2 = \sigma_0^2 \qquad \text{vs.} \qquad H_1: \mu > \mu_0, \quad \sigma^2 = \sigma_0^2$$

with significance level $\alpha$, we reject $H_0$ if and only if the upper one-sided $100\% \times (1 - \alpha)$ confidence interval $\mu \geqslant \bar{x} - z_{1-\alpha}\sigma/\sqrt{n}$ *does not contain* $\mu_0$; we accept $H_0$ if this interval *does contain* $\mu_0$.

Equivalent confidence interval statements can also be made about any of the other hypothesis tests covered in this text.

Since the hypothesis testing and confidence interval approaches yield the same conclusions, is there any advantage to using one method over the other? The $p$-value from a hypothesis test tells us precisely how statistically significant our results are. However, often results that are statistically significant are in fact not very important in the context of the subject matter, since the actual difference between $\bar{x}$ and $\mu_0$ may not be very large, although the results are statistically significant because of a large sample size. A 95% confidence interval for $\mu$ would give us additional information in this regard, since it would give us a range of values within which $\mu$ is likely to fall. Conversely, the 95% confidence interval does not contain all the information contained in a $p$-value: It does not tell us precisely how significant our results are but merely informs us as to whether or not they are significant at the 5% level. Hence, it is good practice to compute both a $p$-value and a 95% confidence interval for $\mu$.

**Example 7.42**    **Cardiovascular Disease**  Consider the cholesterol data discussed in Examples 7.20 and 7.40. The $p$-value of 0.034 computed in Example 7.20 tells us precisely how significant our results are. The 95% confidence interval for $\mu = (173.68, 189.36)$ computed in Example 7.40 gives us a range of possible values that $\mu$ might assume. The two types of information are complementary.  ∎

# ■ 7.9 ONE-SAMPLE $\chi^2$ TEST FOR THE VARIANCE OF A NORMAL DISTRIBUTION

**Example 7.43**    *Hypertension*  Let us consider the data in Example 6.32 concerning the variability of blood pressure measurements taken on an arteriosonde machine. We were concerned with the difference between measurements taken by two observers on the same person $= d_i = x_{1i} - x_{2i}$, where $x_{1i}$ = the measurement on the $i$th person by the first observer and $x_{2i}$ = the measurement on the $i$th person by the second observer. We will assume that this difference is a good measure of interobserver variability and we wish to compare this variability with comparable data using a standard blood pressure cuff. We have reason to believe that the variability of the arteriosonde machine might be different from that of a standard cuff. Intuitively, the variability of the new method should be lower. However, since the new method is not as widely used, the observers are probably less experienced at using the method, and the variability of the new method could possibly be higher than that of the old method. Thus, we will use a two-sided test to study this question. Suppose we know from previously published work that $\sigma^2 = 35$ for $d_i$ obtained from the standard cuff. We wish to test the hypothesis $H_0: \sigma^2 = \sigma_0^2 = 35$ vs. $H_1: \sigma^2 \neq \sigma_0^2$. How should we perform this test? ∎

We can reasonably base our test on $s^2$, since it is an unbiased estimator of $\sigma^2$. Specifically, if we wish to conduct a two-sided test with significance level $\alpha$, then we wish to find $c_1, c_2$ such that

$$Pr(s^2 \leqslant c_1 | H_0) = Pr(s^2 \geqslant c_2 | H_0) = \alpha/2$$

Using similar methods to those given in Section 6.5.3, we can show that

$$c_1 = \sigma_0^2 \chi_{n-1,\alpha/2}^2 / (n - 1)$$

$$c_2 = \sigma_0^2 \chi_{n-1,1-\alpha/2}^2 / (n - 1)$$

Hence, our test procedure is given as follows:

**7.29** **One-Sample $\chi^2$ Test for the Variance of a Normal Distribution (Two-Sided Alternative)**

If

$$s^2 < \sigma_0^2 \chi_{n-1,\alpha/2}^2 / (n - 1) \qquad \text{or} \qquad s^2 > \sigma_0^2 \chi_{n-1,1-\alpha/2}^2 / (n - 1)$$

then we reject $H_0$. If

$$\sigma_0^2 \chi_{n-1,\alpha/2}^2 / (n - 1) \leqslant s^2 \leqslant \sigma_0^2 \chi_{n-1,1-\alpha/2}^2 / (n - 1)$$

then we accept $H_0$.

The acceptance and rejection regions for this test are depicted in Figure 7.13.

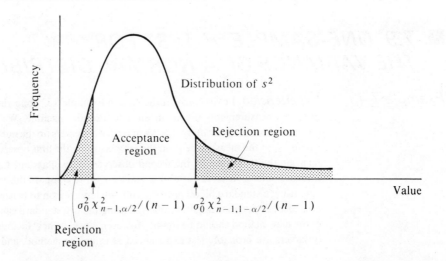

**Figure 7.13**
*Acceptance and rejection regions for the one-sample $\chi^2$ test for the variance of a normal distribution (two-sided alternative)*

Alternatively, if we wish to compute a *p*-value for our experiment, then we wish to find that level of $\alpha$ for which our results are on the margin of being statistically significant. The computation of the *p*-value will again depend on whether $s^2 \leq \sigma_0^2$ or $s^2 > \sigma_0^2$. The rule is given as follows:

---

**7.30** **P-value for a One-Sample χ² Test for the Variance of a Normal Distribution (Two-Sided Alternative)**

If $s^2 \leq \sigma_0^2$,

$$p\text{-value} = 2 \times [\text{area to the left of } (n-1)s^2/\sigma_0^2 \text{ under a } \chi_{n-1}^2 \text{ distribution}]$$

If $s^2 > \sigma_0^2$,

$$p\text{-value} = 2 \times [\text{area to the right of } (n-1)s^2/\sigma_0^2 \text{ under a } \chi_{n-1}^2 \text{ distribution}]$$

These *p*-values are illustrated in Figure 7.14.

---

_Example 7.44_     **Hypertension** Assess the statistical significance of the arteriosonde machine data in Example 7.43.

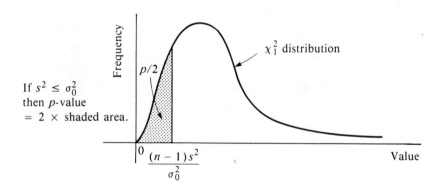

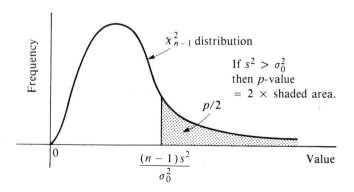

**_Figure 7.14_**
_Illustration of the p-value for a one-sample χ² test for the variance of a normal distribution (two-sided alternative)_

**Solution**

We know from Example 6.32 that $s^2 = 8.178$, $n = 10$. Thus, from (7.29) the critical values are given by

$$c_1 = \sigma_0^2 \chi_{n-1,\alpha/2}^2 / (n-1)$$

$$= 35\chi_{9,.025}^2 / 9$$

$$= 35(2.70)/9$$

$$= 10.50$$

$$c_2 = \sigma_0^2 \chi_{n-1,1-\alpha/2}^2 / (n-1)$$

$$= 35\chi_{9,.975}^2 / 9$$

$$= 35(19.02)/9$$

$$= 73.97$$

Since $s^2 = 8.178 < c_1 = 10.50$, we reject $H_0$ using a two-sided test with $\alpha = 0.05$.

To obtain the $p$-value, we refer to (7.30) and compute the test statistic

$$\lambda = \frac{(n-1)s^2}{\sigma_0^2}$$

$$= 9(8.178)/35$$

$$= 2.103$$

Under $H_0$, $\lambda$ follows a $\chi^2$ distribution with nine degrees of freedom. Thus, since $s^2 = 8.178 < 35 = \sigma_0^2$, we compute the $p$-value as follows:

$$p = 2 \times Pr(\chi_9^2 < 2.103)$$

From Table 4 we see that

$$\chi_{9,.025}^2 = 2.70, \ \chi_{9,.01}^2 = 2.09$$

Thus, since $2.09 < 2.103 < 2.70$, we have $(0.01) < p/2 < (0.025)$ or $0.02 < p < 0.05$.

To obtain the exact $p$-value, we use the HP-41C chi-square distribution program to evaluate areas under the $\chi^2$ distribution. The program computes left-hand tail areas. Thus, we multiply by 2 to obtain the exact two-sided $p$-value $= 0.021$. The details are given in Table 7.3.

Therefore, the results are statistically significant, and we conclude that the inter-observer variance using the arteriosonde machine is significantly different from the inter-

**Table 7.3**
*Computation of the exact p-value for the arteriosonde machine data in Example 7.44 using a one-sample $\chi^2$ test with the HP-41C chi-square distribution program*

```
ΣCHISQD

(a)          9.00   XEQ A        (a)  Degrees of freedom
(b)         2.103   XEQ E
                                 (b)  λ

(c)    0.010267996    ***        (c)  Left-hand tail area
       2.000000000     *
(d)    0.020535992    ***        (d)  Exact two-sided p-value
```

observer variance using the standard cuff. To quantify how different the two variances are, we could obtain a two-sided 95% confidence interval for $\sigma^2$, as was done in Example 6.34. This interval was (3.87, 27.26). Of course, it does not contain 35 because our $p$-value is less than 0.05. ∎

For a one-sided test, we follow a similar procedure.

**7.31** **One-Sample $\chi^2$ Test for the Variance of a Normal Distribution (One-Sided Alternative)**

To test the hypothesis: $H_0: \sigma^2 = \sigma_0^2$ vs. $H_1: \sigma^2 < \sigma_0^2$ with significance level $\alpha$, we proceed as follows: If

$$s^2 < \sigma_0^2 \chi_{n-1,\alpha}^2/(n-1)$$

then we reject $H_0$. If

$$s^2 \geq \sigma_0^2 \chi_{n-1,\alpha}^2/(n-1)$$

then we accept $H_0$. The $p$-value for this test is given by the area to the left of $(n-1)s^2/\sigma_0^2$ under a $\chi_{n-1}^2$ distribution.

To test the hypothesis: $H_0: \sigma^2 = \sigma_0^2$ vs. $H_1: \sigma^2 > \sigma_0^2$ with significance level $\alpha$, we proceed as follows: If

$$s^2 > \sigma_0^2 \chi_{n-1,1-\alpha}^2/(n-1)$$

then we reject $H_0$. If

$$s^2 \leq \sigma_0^2 \chi_{n-1,1-\alpha}^2/(n-1)$$

then we accept $H_0$.

The $p$-value for this test is given by the area to the right of $(n-1)s^2/\sigma_0^2$ under a $\chi_{n-1}^2$ distribution.

# ■ 7.10 ONE-SAMPLE TEST FOR A BINOMIAL PROPORTION

## ☐ 7.10.1 Normal Theory Methods

*Example 7.45*

*Cancer* Let us consider the breast cancer data given in Example 6.37. In that example we were interested in the effect of having a family history of breast cancer on the incidence of breast cancer. Suppose that out of 10,000 50–54-year-old women sampled whose mothers had breast cancer, 400 had breast cancer at some time in their lives. Based on large studies, let us assume that the prevalence rate of breast cancer for American women in this age group is about 2%. The question is, how compatible is our sample rate of 4% with a population rate of 2%?

Another way of asking this question is to restate it in terms of hypothesis testing: If $p$ = incidence rate of breast cancer in 50–54-year-old women whose mothers have had breast cancer, then we wish to test the hypothesis $H_0: p = 0.02 = p_0$ vs. $H_1: p \neq 0.02$. How can we do this? ∎

We will base our significance test on the sample proportion of cases $\hat{p}$. We wish to find $c_1, c_2$ such that we reject $H_0$ if $\hat{p} < c_1$ or $\hat{p} > c_2$ and accept $H_0$ if $c_1 \leqslant \hat{p} \leqslant c_2$. For a given significance level $\alpha$, we must find $c_1, c_2$ such that

**7.32**

$$Pr(\hat{p} < c_1 | H_0) = Pr(\hat{p} > c_2 | H_0) = \alpha/2$$

We will assume that the normal approximation to the binomial distribution is valid. This assumption is reasonable when $np_0q_0 \geqslant 5$. We can then show that **(7.32)** is satisfied by

$$c_1 = p_0 - z_{1-\alpha/2}\sqrt{\frac{p_0q_0}{n}}$$

$$c_2 = p_0 + z_{1-\alpha/2}\sqrt{\frac{p_0q_0}{n}}$$

Thus, our test takes the following form:

**7.33**   ***One-Sample Test for a Binomial Proportion—***
***Normal Theory Method (Two-Sided Alternative)***

If

$$\hat{p} < p_0 - z_{1-\alpha/2}\sqrt{\frac{p_0q_0}{n}} \quad \text{or} \quad \hat{p} > p_0 + z_{1-\alpha/2}\sqrt{\frac{p_0q_0}{n}}$$

then we reject $H_0$. If

$$p_0 - z_{1-\alpha/2}\sqrt{\frac{p_0q_0}{n}} \leqslant \hat{p} \leqslant p_0 + z_{1-\alpha/2}\sqrt{\frac{p_0q_0}{n}}$$

then we accept $H_0$. The acceptance and rejection regions are depicted in Figure 7.15.

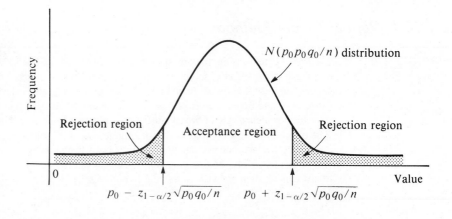

**Figure 7.15**
*Acceptance and rejection regions for the one-sample binomial test— normal theory test (two-sided alternative)*

Alternatively, we could compute a *p*-value by finding the $\alpha$ level at which our results are just statistically significant. The computation of the *p*-value, given as follows, will again depend on whether $\hat{p} \leqslant p_0$ or $\hat{p} > p_0$.

**7.34**   **Computation of the P-value for the One-Sample Binomial Test—Normal Theory Method (Two-Sided Alternative)**

$$p\text{-value} = 2 \times \Phi\left[(\hat{p} - p_0)\Big/ \sqrt{\frac{p_0 q_0}{n}}\right] = \text{twice the area to the left of } \hat{p} \text{ under a } N(p_0, p_0 q_0/n) \text{ curve if } \hat{p} \leqslant p_0$$

$$p\text{-value} = 2 \times \left\{1 - \Phi\left[(\hat{p} - p_0)\Big/ \sqrt{\frac{p_0 q_0}{n}}\right]\right\} = \text{twice the area to the right of } \hat{p} \text{ under a } N(p_0, p_0 q_0/n) \text{ curve if } \hat{p} > p_0$$

The calculation of the *p*-value is illustrated in Figure 7.16.

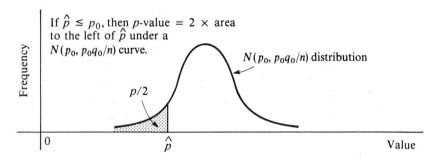

If $\hat{p} \leq p_0$, then *p*-value $= 2 \times$ area to the left of $\hat{p}$ under a $N(p_0, p_0 q_0/n)$ curve.

$N(p_0, p_0 q_0/n)$ distribution

$p/2$

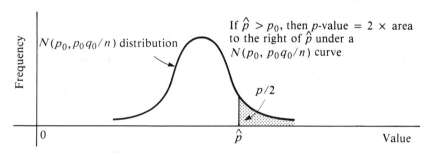

If $\hat{p} > p_0$, then *p*-value $= 2 \times$ area to the right of $\hat{p}$ under a $N(p_0, p_0 q_0/n)$ curve

$N(p_0, p_0 q_0/n)$ distribution

$p/2$

**Figure 7.16**
*Illustration of the p-value for a one-sample binomial test—normal theory method (two-sided alternative)*

These definitions of a *p*-value are again compatible with the idea of a *p*-value as the probability of obtaining results as extreme as or more extreme than the results in our particular sample.

*Example 7.46*   *Cancer* Assess the statistical significance of the data given in Example 7.45.

*Solution*   If we use the critical value method, then we have

$$c_1 = 0.02 - 1.96\sqrt{(0.02)(0.98)/10,000}$$

$$= 0.02 - 0.0027$$

$$= 0.0173$$

$$c_2 = 0.02 + 1.96\sqrt{(0.02)(0.98)/10{,}000}$$

$$= 0.02 + 0.0027$$

$$= 0.0227$$

Since $\hat{p} = 0.04 > c_2$, we can reject $H_0$ using a two-sided test with $\alpha = 0.05$. To use the $p$-value method, we note that $\hat{p} = 0.04 > p_0 = 0.02$. Hence, the $p$-value is given by

$$p = 2 \times \left\{ 1 - \Phi\left[ \frac{0.04 - 0.02}{\sqrt{(0.02)(0.98)/10{,}000}} \right] \right\}$$

$$= 2 \times \left\{ 1 - \Phi\left[ \frac{0.02}{0.0014} \right] \right\}$$

$$= 2 \times [1 - \Phi(14.29)] < 0.001$$

Thus, the results are very highly significant.    ∎

## ☐ 7.10.2  Exact Methods

The test procedure presented in **(7.33)** to test the hypothesis $H_0$: $p = p_0$ vs. $H_1$: $p \ne p_0$ depends on the assumption that the normal approximation to the binomial distribution is valid. This assumption will only be true if $np_0q_0 \geqslant 5$. How can we test the preceding hypothesis if this criterion is not satisfied?

Our approach will be to base our test on *exact* binomial probabilities. In particular, let $X$ be a binomial random variable with parameters $n$ and $p_0$ and let $\hat{p} = x/n$, where $x$ is the observed number of events. We compute the $p$-value as follows:

  **Computation of the P-value for the One-Sample Binomial Test— Exact Method (Two-Sided Alternative)**

If $\hat{p} \leqslant p_0$,

$$p = 2 \times Pr(X \leqslant x) = 2 \sum_{k=0}^{x} \binom{n}{k} p_0^k (1 - p_0)^{n-k}$$

If $\hat{p} > p_0$,

$$p = 2 \times Pr(X \geqslant x) = 2 \sum_{k=x}^{n} \binom{n}{k} p_0^k (1 - p_0)^{n-k}$$

The computation of the $p$-value is depicted in Figure 7.17.

In either case the $p$-value corresponds to the sum of the probabilities of all events that are as extreme as or more extreme than the sample result obtained.

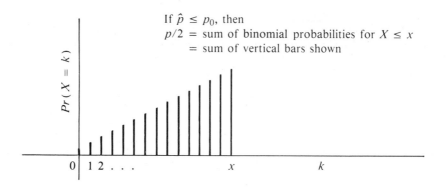

If $\hat{p} \leq p_0$, then
$p/2 = $ sum of binomial probabilities for $X \leq x$
$= $ sum of vertical bars shown

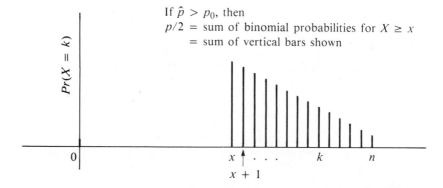

If $\hat{p} > p_0$, then
$p/2 = $ sum of binomial probabilities for $X \geq x$
$= $ sum of vertical bars shown

**Figure 7.17**

*Illustration of the p-value for a one-sample binomial test— exact method (two-sided alternative)*

**Example 7.47**   *Occupational Medicine, Cancer* A widely publicized discussion has recently taken place regarding the safety of those who work at or live in close proximity to nuclear power plants. One possible health hazard due to radiation exposure is an excess of cancer deaths among those exposed. One problem with studying this question is that the number of deaths attributable to either cancer in general or specific types of cancer is small, and reaching statistically significant conclusions is difficult, except after long periods of follow-up. An alternative approach is to perform a *proportional mortality study*, whereby the proportion of deaths attributed to a specific cause in an exposed group is compared with the corresponding proportion in a large population. Suppose, for example, that 13 deaths have occurred among 55–64-year-old male workers in a nuclear power plant over the years 1960–1961 and that the cause of death was cancer in 5 of them. Let us assume, based on vital statistics reports, that approximately 20% of all deaths in 1960 can be attributed to some form of cancer [1]. Is this result significant?

**Solution**   We wish to test the hypothesis $H_0: p = 0.20$ vs. $H_1: p \neq 0.20$, where $p = $ probability that the cause of death was cancer in nuclear power workers. We cannot use the normal approximation to the binomial, since

$$np_0q_0 = 13(0.2)(0.8) = 2.1 < 5$$

However, we can use the exact procedure in (**7.35**). We have

$$\hat{p} = \frac{5}{13} = 0.38 > 0.20$$

Therefore,

$$p = 2 \sum_{k=5}^{13} \binom{13}{k} (0.2)^k (0.8)^{13-k} = 2 \times \left[ 1 - \sum_{k=0}^{4} \binom{13}{k} (0.2)^k (0.8)^{13-k} \right]$$

From Table 1 we have

$$Pr(0) = 0.0550$$
$$Pr(1) = 0.1787$$
$$Pr(2) = 0.2680$$
$$Pr(3) = 0.2457$$
$$Pr(4) = 0.1535$$

Therefore,

$$p = 2 \times [1 - (0.0550 + 0.1787 + 0.2680 + 0.2457 + 0.1535)]$$
$$= 2 \times (1 - 0.9009)$$
$$= 0.198$$

In summary, the results are *not* statistically significant and we cannot attribute an excess cancer proportional mortality to the nuclear power plant workers. ∎

## ☐ 7.10.3 Power and Sample Size Estimation

We can also consider the power of the one-sample binomial test using the large sample test procedure given in Section 7.10.1. Suppose that we are conducting a one-tailed test at level $\alpha$, where $p = p_0$ under the null hypothesis. We can show that under the alternative hypothesis of $p = p_1$, the power is given by the following formula:

---

**7.36** | **Power for the One-Sample Binomial Test (One-Sided Alternative)**

The **power** of the one-sample binomial test for the hypothesis

$$H_0\colon p = p_0 \quad \text{vs.} \quad H_1\colon p = p_1$$

is given by

$$\Phi\left[ \sqrt{\frac{p_0 q_0}{p_1 q_1}} \left( z_\alpha + \frac{|p_1 - p_0|\sqrt{n}}{\sqrt{p_0 q_0}} \right) \right]$$

---

*Example 7.48*   *Cancer*   Suppose we wish to test the hypothesis that women with a sister history of breast cancer are at higher risk of developing breast cancer themselves. Suppose we assume, as in Example 7.45, that the prevalence rate of breast cancer is 2% among 50–54-year-old American women, whereas it is 5% among women with a sister history. We propose to interview 500

50–54-year-old women with a sister history of the disease. What is the power of such a study assuming that we conduct a one-sided test with $\alpha = 0.05$?

*Solution*  We have $\alpha = 0.05$, $p_0 = 0.02$, $p_1 = 0.05$, $n = 500$. The power is given by **(7.36)** as follows:

$$\text{Power} = \Phi\left[\sqrt{\frac{(0.02)(0.98)}{(0.05)(0.95)}}\left(z_{.05} + \frac{0.03\sqrt{500}}{\sqrt{0.02(0.98)}}\right)\right]$$

$$= \Phi[(0.642)(-1.645 + 4.792)]$$

$$= \Phi(2.020)$$

$$= 0.978$$

Thus, we should have a 97.8% chance of finding a significant difference if the true rate of breast cancer among women with a sister history is 2.5 times as high as that of typical 50–54-year-old women.  ∎

Similarly, we can consider the issue of what is an appropriate sample size if we intend to use the one-sample binomial test for a given $\alpha$, $p_0$, $p_1$, and power. The sample size is given by the following formula:

---

**7.37** | **Sample Size Estimation for the One-Sample Binomial Test (One-Sided Alternative)**

Suppose we wish to test $H_0: p = p_0$ vs. $H_1: p = p_1$. The sample size needed to conduct a one-sided test with significance level $\alpha$ and power $1 - \beta$ is

$$n = \frac{p_0 q_0 \left(z_{1-\alpha} + z_{1-\beta}\sqrt{\frac{p_1 q_1}{p_0 q_0}}\right)^2}{|p_1 - p_0|^2}$$

---

*Example 7.49*  **Cancer** How many women should be interviewed in the study proposed in Example 7.48 to achieve 90% power if we intend to use a one-sided significance test with $\alpha = 0.05$?

*Solution*  We have $\alpha = 0.05$, $1 - \beta = 0.90$, $p_0 = 0.02$, $p_1 = 0.05$. The sample size is given by **(7.37)** as follows:

$$n = \frac{(0.02)(0.98)\left[z_{.95} + z_{.90}\sqrt{\frac{(0.05)(0.95)}{(0.02)(0.98)}}\right]^2}{(0.03)^2}$$

$$= \frac{(0.0196)[1.645 + 1.28(1.557)]^2}{0.0009}$$

$$= \frac{(0.0196)(13.235)}{0.0009}$$

$$= 288.2, \text{ or } 289 \text{ women}$$

Thus, we need to interview 289 women to have a 90% chance of detecting a significant difference using a one-sided test with $\alpha = 0.05$ if the true rate of breast cancer among women with a sister history is 2.5 times as high as that of a typical 50–54-year-old woman.  ∎

Note that if we wish to perform a two-sided test rather than a one-sided test at level $\alpha$, then we substitute $\alpha/2$ for $\alpha$ in the power formula in **(7.36)** and the sample size formula in **(7.37)**.

## ☐ *7.10.4 The Standardized Mortality Ratio*

*Example 7.50*    *Occupational Health* Many studies have looked at possible health hazards of rubber workers. In one such study a group of 8418 white male workers ages 40–84 (either active or retired) on January 1, 1964, were followed for 10 years for various mortality outcomes [2]. Their mortality rates were then compared with U.S. white male mortality rates in 1968. In one of the reported findings, 21 deaths due to bladder cancer were observed compared with 18.1 deaths expected from U.S. mortality rates. Is this difference significant?    ∎

One problem with this type of study is that workers of different ages in 1964 have very different mortality risks over time. Thus the test procedures in **(7.33)** and **(7.35)**, which assume a constant *p* for all persons in the sample, are not applicable. However, we can generalize these procedures to take account of the different mortality risks of different individuals. Let

$O$ = total observed number of deaths for members of the study population

$p_i$ = probability of death for the *i*th individual

Under the null hypothesis that the death rates for the study population are the same as those for the general U.S. population, the expected number of events $E$ is given by

$$E = \sum_{i=1}^{n} p_i$$

**Definition 7.12**

The **standardized mortality ratio (SMR)** is defined by $100\% \times O/E = 100\% \times$ the observed number of deaths in the study population divided by the expected number of deaths in the study population under the assumption that the mortality rates for the study population are the same as those for the general population. For nonfatal conditions the standardized mortality ratio is sometimes known as the **standardized morbidity ratio**.    ∎

Thus,

If SMR > 100%, there is an excess risk in the study population relative to the general population.

If SMR < 100%, there is a reduced risk in the study population relative to the general population.

If SMR = 100%, there is neither an excess nor a deficit of risk in the study population relative to the general population.

*Example 7.51*    *Occupational Health* What is the standardized mortality ratio for bladder cancer using the data in Example 7.50?

**Solution**     We have SMR = 100% × 21/18.1 = 116%.     ∎

We will base our significance test on the SMR. If the SMR is far from 100%, then we will reject $H_0$; otherwise, we will accept $H_0$. We need to compute $var$(SMR) under $H_0$. We can show that under $H_0$ $var$(SMR/100) approximately equals $1/E$. This result leads to the following test procedure:

**7.38**   **Generalized One-Sample Binomial Test (Large-Sample Test)**

To test the hypothesis $H_0$: SMR = 100 vs. $H_1$: SMR ≠ 100,

1. We compute

$$O = \text{observed number of deaths in the study population}$$

$$E = \text{expected number of deaths in the study population} = \sum p_i$$

where $p_i$ is the probability of death for the $i$th member of the study population under $H_0$, that is, under the assumption that the general population death rates apply to the study population.

$$\text{SMR} = 100\% \times O/E$$

2. We compute the test statistic

$$\lambda = \frac{(O - E)^2}{E} = E \times \left(\frac{\text{SMR}}{100} - 1\right)^2 \sim \chi_1^2 \text{ under } H_0$$

3. For a significance test at level $\alpha$, we reject $H_0$ if

$$\lambda > \chi_{1,1-\alpha}^2$$

and we accept $H_0$ if

$$\lambda \leq \chi_{1,1-\alpha}^2$$

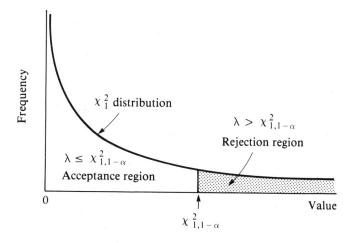

**Figure 7.18**
*Acceptance and rejection regions for the generalized one-sample binomial test (large-sample test)*

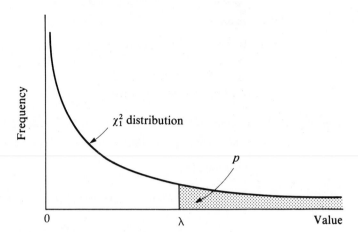

**Figure 7.19**
*Computation of the p-values for the generalized one-sample binomial test (large-sample test)*

**4.** The exact *p*-value is given by

$$Pr(\chi_1^2 > \lambda)$$

**5.** We should only use this test if $E \geqslant 5$.

The acceptance and rejection regions for this test are depicted in Figure 7.18. The computation of the exact *p*-value is given in Figure 7.19.

---

*Example 7.52*

**Occupational Health**  Assess the statistical significance of the bladder cancer data in Example 7.50.

*Solution*

We have $O = 21$, $E = 18.1$, SMR $= 116$. Therefore, we have the test statistic

$$\lambda = \frac{(21 - 18.1)^2}{18.1} \quad \text{or} \quad 18.1 \times (1.16 - 1)^2$$

$$= \frac{8.41}{18.1}$$

$$= 0.46 \sim \chi_1^2 \text{ under } H_0$$

Since $\chi^2_{1,.95} = 3.84 > \lambda$, $p > 0.05$ and we accept $H_0$. Furthermore, from Table 6 we note that $\chi^2_{1,.50} = 0.45$, $\chi^2_{1,.75} = 1.32$, and $0.45 < \lambda < 1.32$. Thus, $1 - 0.75 < p < 1 - 0.50$, or $0.25 < p < 0.50$. Therefore, the rubber workers in this plant do not have a significantly increased or decreased risk of bladder cancer relative to the general population.    ∎

In many applications involving the SMR, the expected number of events will be less than 5. In these cases the large-sample test procedure in **(7.38)** is not applicable, and the following small-sample test procedure should be used:

**7.39**    **Generalized One-Sample Binomial Test (Small-Sample Test)**

To test the hypothesis $H_0$: SMR $= 100$ vs. $H_1$: SMR $\neq 100$,

     *1.* We compute

$$O = \text{observed number of events in the study population}$$

$$E = \text{expected number of events in the study population} = \sum p_i$$

where $p_i$ is the probability of death for the *i*th member of the study population under $H_0$, that is, under the assumption that the general population death rates apply to the study population.

     *2.* The observed number of deaths ($O$) will follow a Poisson distribution with parameter $E$. Thus, the exact *p*-value is given by

$$2 \times \sum_{k=0}^{O} \frac{e^{-E} E^k}{k!} \qquad \text{if } O < E$$

$$2 \times \left( 1 - \sum_{k=0}^{O-1} \frac{e^{-E} E^k}{k!} \right) \qquad \text{if } O \geq E$$

These computations are depicted in Figure 7.20.

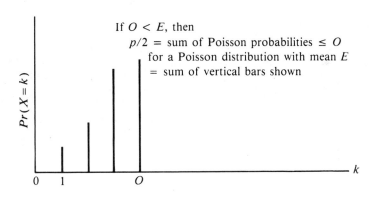

If $O < E$, then
$p/2$ = sum of Poisson probabilities $\leq O$
     for a Poisson distribution with mean $E$
     = sum of vertical bars shown

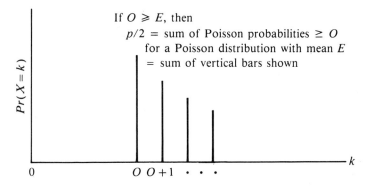

If $O \geq E$, then
$p/2$ = sum of Poisson probabilities $\geq O$
     for a Poisson distribution with mean $E$
     = sum of vertical bars shown

*Figure 7.20*
*Computation of the*
*exact p-value for*
*the generalized*
*one-sample*
*binomial test*
*(small-sample case)*

_Example 7.53_     **Occupational Health**  The observed number of deaths due to Hodgkin's disease in the sample in Example 7.50 was 4 with SMR = 123. Test for the significance of these findings.

_Solution_          We have

$$E = 100 \times \frac{O}{SMR}$$

$$= 100 \times \frac{4}{123}$$

$$= 3.3 < 5.0$$

Thus, we must use the small-sample procedure in **(7.39)**. Since $O \geqslant E$, we have

$$p = 2 \times \left[ 1 - \sum_{k=0}^{3} \frac{e^{-3.3}(3.3)^k}{k!} \right]$$

From the recursion rule for the Poisson distribution, we have

$$Pr(0) = e^{-3.3} = 0.0369$$

$$Pr(1) = \frac{3.3}{1} \times 0.0369 = 0.1218$$

$$Pr(2) = \frac{3.3}{2} \times 0.1218 = 0.2010$$

$$Pr(3) = \frac{3.3}{3} \times 0.2010 = 0.2211$$

Thus

$$p = 2 \times [1 - (0.0369 + 0.1218 + 0.2010 + 0.2211)]$$

$$= 2 \times (1 - 0.5808)$$

$$= 0.838$$

Thus there is no significant excess or deficit of Hodgkin's disease in this population.     ∎

# ■ 7.11  SUMMARY

In this chapter we introduced some of the fundamental ideas of hypothesis testing. these concepts included (a) specification of the **null ($H_0$)** and **alternative ($H_1$)** hypotheses; (b) **type I error ($\alpha$), type II error ($\beta$)**, and **power** of a hypothesis test; (c) the **p-value** of a hypothesis test, which indicates the $\alpha$ level at which we would be indifferent between accepting and rejecting $H_0$; and (d) the distinction between **one-sided** and **two-sided** tests. We also discussed methods for estimating the appropriate **sample size** for a proposed study as determined by the prespecified null and alternative hypotheses and the type I and type II errors.

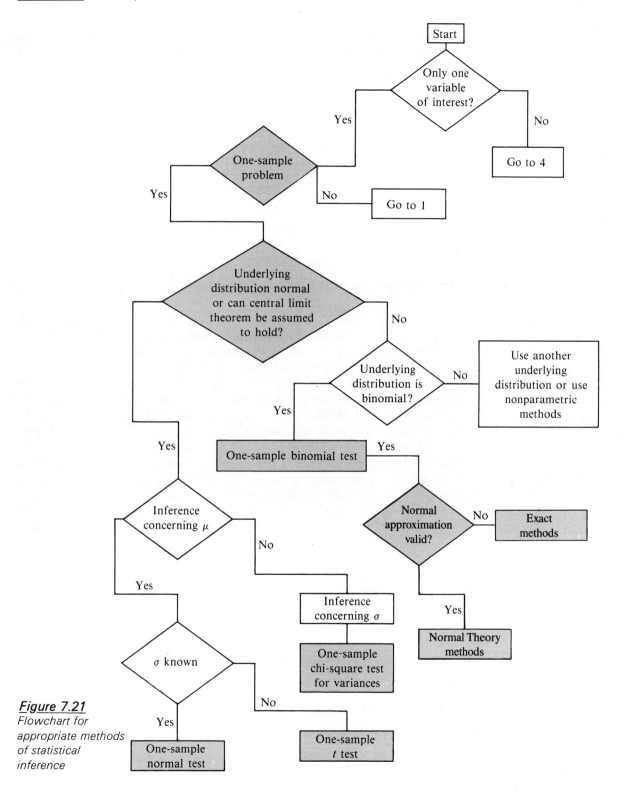

_**Figure 7.21**_
_Flowchart for_
_appropriate methods_
_of statistical_
_inference_

We applied these general concepts to several **one-sample** hypothesis-testing situations concerning:

1. The mean of a normal distribution with known variance **(the one-sample normal test)**
2. The mean of a normal distribution with unknown variance **(the one-sample *t* test)**
3. The variance of a normal distribution **(the one-sample chi-square test)**
4. The parameter $p$ of a binomial distribution **(the one-sample binomial test)**

We showed that each of the hypothesis tests could be conducted in one of two ways:

1. By specifying **critical values** to determine the **acceptance** and **rejection regions**
2. By computing ***p*-values**

These methods were shown to be equivalent in the sense that they yield the same inferences regarding the acceptance and rejection of the null hypothesis.

Finally, we explored the relationship between the **hypothesis-testing methods** in this chapter and the **confidence interval methods** in Chapter 6. We showed that the inferences we can draw from using these methods are the same.

We will be covering many hypothesis tests in this book and have provided a **flowchart** at the back of the book to help clarify the decision process in selecting the appropriate test. We can use the flowchart to choose the proper test by answering a series of yes/no questions. The specific hypothesis tests covered in this chapter have been shaded in an excerpt from the flowchart shown in Figure 7.21. For example, if we are interested in performing hypothesis tests concerning the mean of a normal distribution with known variance, then, beginning at the start box of the flowchart, we would answer *yes* to each of the following questions: (a) only one variable of interest? (b) one-sample problem? (c) underlying distribution normal? (d) inference concerning $\mu$? (e) $\sigma$ known? The flowchart leads us to the box on the lower left of the figure, indicating that we should use the one-sample normal test.

We will extend our study of hypothesis testing in the next chapter to the situation where we are interested in comparing two different samples. This topic corresponds to the answer *yes* to (a) only one variable of interest? and *no* to (b) one-sample problem?

# *P*roblems

*Nutrition*

As part of a dietary instruction program, 10 25–34-year-old males adopted a vegetarian diet for a 1-month period. During the diet, the average daily intake of linoleic acid was 13 g.

**7.1** If the average daily intake among 25–34-year-old males in the general population is 15 g with standard deviation 4 g, then, using a significance level of 0.05, test the hypothesis that the intake of linoleic acid in this group is lower than that in the general population.

**7.2** Compute a *p*-value for the hypothesis test in Problem 7.1.

As part of the same program, 8 25–34-year-old females report an average daily intake of saturated fat of 11 g.

**7.3** If the average daily intake of saturated fat among 25–34-year-old females in the general population is 24 g with standard deviation 11 g, then, using a significance level of 0.01, test the hypothesis that the intake of saturated fat in this group is lower than that in the general population.

**7.4** Compute a _p_-value for the hypothesis test in Problem 7.3.

**7.5** What is the relationship between your answers to Problems 7.3 and 7.4?

Suppose we are uncertain what effect a vegetarian diet will have on the level of linoleic acid intake in Problem 7.1.

**7.6** What are the null and alternative hypotheses in this case?

**7.7** Compare the mean level of linoleic acid in this vegetarian population with that of the general population under the hypotheses in Problem 7.6. Report a _p_-value.

### Infectious Disease
The mean serum creatinine level measured in 12 patients 24 hours after they received a newly proposed antibiotic was 1.2 mg/dl.

**7.8** If the mean and standard deviation of serum creatinine in the general population are 1.0 and 0.4 mg/dl, respectively, then, using a significance level of 0.05, test if the mean serum creatinine level in this group is different from that of the general population.

**7.9** What is the _p_-value for the test?

**7.10** Suppose $\dfrac{\bar{x} - \mu_0}{s/\sqrt{n}} = 2.73$ and we are performing a one-sample _t_ test based on 20 subjects. What is the two-tailed _p_-value?

**7.11** Suppose $\dfrac{\bar{x} - \mu_0}{s/\sqrt{n}} = -1.52$ and we are performing a one-sample _t_ test based on 7 subjects. What is the two-tailed _p_-value?

**7.12** What is the approximate 95th percentile of a _t_ distribution with 35 _df_ (i.e., $t_{35,.95}$)?

**7.13** What is the approximate 99th percentile of a _t_ distribution with 75 _df_?

**7.14** Suppose the sample standard deviation of linoleic acid is 6 g in Problem 7.7. If we do not assume that the standard deviation for the vegetarian population is known, then perform the hypothesis test for the hypotheses in Problem 7.6. Report a _p_-value.

**7.15** Suppose the sample standard deviation of serum creatinine in Problem 7.8 is 0.6 mg/dl. If we do not assume that the standard deviation of serum creatinine is known, then perform the hypothesis test in Problem 7.8. Report a _p_-value.

**7.16** Suppose a larger study is planned with 50 patients to be enrolled. If the alternative mean is 1.2 mg/dl and the standard deviation is 0.4 mg/dl, then what is the power of such a study using a one-sided test with $\alpha = 0.05$?

**7.17** Answer Problem 7.16 if a two-sided test is used.

**7.18** How large of a study would be needed in Problem 7.16 to achieve 80% power?

**7.19** How large of a study would be needed in Problem 7.17 to achieve 80% power?

**7.20** Answer Problem 7.19 for 90% power.

### Diabetes
Plasma glucose levels are used to determine the presence of diabetes. Suppose the mean $\log_e$ plasma glucose concentration (mg/dl) in 35–44 year olds is 4.86 with standard deviation 0.54. We plan to do a study of 100 sedentary persons in this age group to test if they have a higher or lower level of plasma glucose than the general population.

**7.21** If the expected difference is 0.10 $\log_e$ units, then what is the power of such a study if a two-sided test is to be used with $\alpha = 0.05$?

**7.22** Answer Problem 7.21 if the expected difference is 0.20 $\log_e$ units.

**7.23** How many persons would need to be studied to have 80% power under the assumptions in Problem 7.21?

**7.24** Compute a lower one-sided 95% confidence interval for the true mean intake of linoleic acid in the vegetarian population depicted in Problem 7.1. Assume that the standard deviations of the vegetarian population and the general population are the same.

**7.25** How does your answer to Problem 7.24 relate to your answer to Problem 7.1?

**7.26** Compute a two-sided 95% confidence interval for the true mean serum creatinine level in Problem 7.8. (Assume that the standard deviation is known to be 0.4 mg/dl.)

**7.27** How does your answer to Problem 7.26 relate to your answer to Problem 7.8?

### Nutrition

A food frequency questionnaire was mailed to 20 subjects to assess the intake of various food groups. The sample standard deviation of vitamin C intake over the 20 persons was 15 (exclusive of vitamin C supplements). Suppose we know from using an in-person diet interview method in a large previous study that the standard deviation is 20.

**7.28** What hypotheses can be used to test if there are any differences between the standard deviations of the two methods?

**7.29** Perform the test described in Problem 7.28 and report a *p*-value.

The sample standard deviation for $\log_e$ (vitamin A intake) exclusive of supplements based on the 20 persons using the food frequency questionnaire was 0.016. Suppose the standard deviation from the diet interview method is known to be 0.020 based on a large previous study.

**7.30** Test the hypothesis that the variances using the two methods are the same. Use the critical value method with $\alpha = 0.05$.

**7.31** Report a *p*-value corresponding to the test in Problem 7.30.

### Cardiovascular Disease

Suppose the incidence rate of MI per year was 5 per 1000 among 45–54-year-old males in 1960. To look at changes in incidence over time, 5000 45–54-year-old men were followed for 1 year starting in 1980. Fifteen new cases of MI were found.

**7.32** Using the critical value method with $\alpha = 0.05$, test the hypothesis that incidence rates of MI have changed from 1960 to 1980.

**7.33** Report a *p*-value to correspond to your answer to Problem 7.32.

Suppose that 25% of MI cases in 1960 died within 24 hours. This proportion is called the 24-hour case fatality rate.

**7.34** Of the 15 new MI cases in the preceding study, 5 died within 24 hours. Test if the 24-hour case fatality rate has changed from 1960 to 1980.

**7.35** Suppose we eventually plan to accumulate 50 MI cases during the period 1980–1985. Assume that the 24-hour case fatality rate is truly 20% during this period. How much power would such a study have in distinguishing between case fatality rates in 1960 and 1980–1985 if we plan to conduct a two-sided test with significance level 0.05?

**7.36** How large a sample do we need in Problem 7.35 to achieve 90% power?

### Occupational Health

Suppose that 28 cancer deaths are noted among workers exposed to asbestos in a building materials plant from 1971–1980. Only 20.5 cancer deaths are expected from statewide cancer mortality rates.

**7.37** What is the estimated SMR for total cancer mortality?

**7.38** Is there a significant excess or deficit of total cancer deaths among these workers?

In the same group of workers, 7 deaths due to leukemia are noted. Only 4.5 are expected from statewide rates.

**7.39** What is the estimated SMR for leukemia?

**7.40** Is there a significant excess or deficit of leukemia deaths among these workers?

### Ophthalmology

Suppose the distribution of systolic blood pressures in the general population is normal with a mean of 130 mm and a standard deviation of 20 mm. In a special subgroup of 85 persons with glaucoma, we find that the mean systolic blood pressure is 135 mm with a standard deviation of 22 mm.

**7.41** Assuming that the standard deviation of the glaucoma patients is the same as that of the general population, test for an association between glaucoma and high blood pressure.

**7.42** Answer Problem 7.41 without making the assumption concerning the standard deviation.

### Cancer

**7.43** Suppose we identify fifty 50–54-year-old women who have both a mother *and* a sister with a history of breast cancer. Five of these women themselves have developed breast cancer at some time in their lives. If we assume that the expected prevalence rate of breast cancer in women whose mothers have had breast cancer is 4%, then does having a sister with the disease add to the risk?

## Occupational Health

**7.44** Suppose it is known that the average life expectancy of a 50-year-old man in 1945 was 18.5 years. Twenty men aged 50 who have been working for at least 20 years in a potentially hazardous industry were ascertained in 1945. Upon follow-up in 1985 all the men have died, with an average lifetime of 16.2 years and a standard deviation of 7.3 years since 1945. If we assume that the life expectancy of 50-year-old men is approximately normally distributed, test if the underlying life expectancy for workers in this industry is shorter than for comparably aged men in the general population.

## Obstetrics

**7.45** The proportion of multiple deliveries (twins) in the United States is approximately 1 in 90. This proportion is thought to be affected by a number of factors, including age, race, and parity. To test the effect of age, hospital records are abstracted. Of 538 deliveries for women under 20, 2 were found to have resulted in multiple deliveries. What can we say about the effect of age on multiple deliveries?

## Cancer

**7.46** An area of current interest in cancer epidemiology is the possible role of oral contraceptives (OC's) in the development of breast cancer. Suppose that in a group of 1000 premenopausal women ages 40–49 who are current users of OC's, 15 subsequently develop breast cancer over the next 5 years. If the expected incidence of breast cancer in this group is 1.2% based on national incidence rates, then test the hypothesis that there is an association between current OC use and the subsequent development of breast cancer.

## Obstetrics

Erythromycin is a drug that has been proposed to possibly lower the risk of a premature delivery. A related area of interest is its association with the incidence of side effects during pregnancy. Suppose we assume that 30% of all pregnant women complain of nausea between the 24th and 28th week of pregnancy. Furthermore, suppose that of 200 women who are taking erythromycin regularly during this period, 110 complain of nausea.

**7.47** Test the hypothesis that the incidence rate of nausea for the erythromycin group is the same as that for a typical pregnant woman.

## Cancer

A group of investigators wishes to explore the relationship between the use of hair dyes and the development of breast cancer in females. A group of 1000 beauticians 40–49 years of age is identified and followed for 5 years. After 5 years, 20 new cases of breast cancer occurred. Let us assume breast cancer incidence over this time period for an average American woman in this age group is $\frac{7}{1000}$. We wish to test the hypothesis that use of hair dyes increases the risk of breast cancer.

**7.48** Is a one-sided or two-sided test appropriate here?

**7.49** Test the hypothesis.

## Epidemiology

One hundred volunteers agree to participate in a clinical trial involving a dietary intervention. The investigators want to check how representative this sample is of the general population. One interesting finding is that 10 of the volunteers are current cigarette smokers.

**7.50** If we assume that 30% of the general population of adults are current smokers, then state the hypotheses needed to test whether the volunteer group is representative of the general population regarding cigarette smoking.

**7.51** Carry out the test described in Problem 7.50 and report a *p*-value.

## Obstetrics

Let us assume that the distribution of birthweights in the general population is normal with mean 120 oz and standard deviation 20 oz. We wish to test a drug that, when administered to mothers in the prenatal period, will reduce the number of low-birthweight infants. We anticipate that the mean birthweight of the infants whose mothers are on the drug will be $\frac{1}{2}$ lb heavier than that for the general newborn population.

**7.52** How large a sample do we need to have an 80% chance of finding a significant difference if we use a one-sided test with significance level 0.05?

**7.53** Answer Problem 7.52 for a 90% chance.

## Cardiovascular Disease, Nutrition

Much discussion has appeared in the medical literature in recent years on the role of diet in the development of heart disease. The serum cholesterol levels of a group of persons who eat a primarily macrobiotic diet are measured. Among 24 persons aged 20–39, the mean cholesterol level was found to be 175 mg/dl with a standard deviation of 35 mg/dl.

**7.54** If the mean cholesterol level in the general population in this age group is 230 mg/dl and the distribution is assumed to be normal, then test the hypothesis that the group of persons on a macrobiotic diet has choles-terol levels different from those of the general population.

**7.55** Compute a 95% confidence interval for the true mean cholesterol level in this group.

**7.56** What type of complementary information is pro-vided by the hypothesis test and confidence interval in this case?

### Renal Disease

The level of serum creatinine in the blood is considered a good indicator of the presence or absence of kidney disease. Normal persons generally have low concentra-tions of serum creatinine, whereas diseased persons have high concentrations. Suppose we desire to look at the relation between analgesic abuse and kidney disorder. In particular, suppose we look at 15 persons working in a factory who are known to be "analgesic abusers" (i.e., they take more than 10 pills per day) and we measure their creatinine levels. The creatinine levels are

$$0.9, 1.1, 1.6, 2.0, 0.8,$$

$$0.7, 1.4, 1.2, 1.5, 0.8,$$

$$1.0, 1.1, 1.4, 2.2, 1.4$$

**7.57** If we assume that creatinine levels for normal persons are normally distributed with mean 1.0 and standard deviation 0.40, then can we make any comment about the levels for analgesic abusers via some statistical test?

**7.58** Suppose we are skeptical about assuming that the standard deviation is known. Can we test the validity of this assumption?

**7.59** If we do not want to assume that the standard deviation is known, then answer the question in Problem 7.57 in some other way.

### Cardiovascular Disease

High cholesterol levels have for some time been suspected as predictors of future heart attacks. The problem is that other factors such as age, smoking, body weight, family history, and so forth enter into the picture, and the dif-ferent factors are difficult to separate out. Suppose we isolate a group of 100 men who have "high" cholesterol levels and can predict, on the basis of other factors, that 10% of these men will have a heart attack in the next 5 years.

**7.60** Suppose that the incidence rate of heart attacks in the next 5 years in this group is 13%. Is this finding indica-tive of anything about cholesterol?

**7.61** Suppose we had 1000 men instead of 100 men and also found an incidence rate of 13%. Is this finding indica-tive of anything about cholesterol?

**7.62** How large a sample would we need to have an 80% chance of finding a significant difference if the true rate of heart disease in this group is 13%?

### Otolaryngology

Otitis media is an extremely common disease of the middle ear in children under 2 years of age. It can cause prolonged hearing loss during this period and may result in subsequent defects in speech and language. Suppose we wish to design a study to test the latter hypothesis and we set up a study group consisting of children with 3 or more episodes of otitis media in the first 2 years of life. We have no idea what the size of the effect will be. Thus, we set up a pilot study with 20 cases, whereby we find that 5 of the cases have speech and language defects at age 3.

**7.63** If we regard this experience as representative of what would occur in a large study and if we *know* that 15% of all normal children have speech and language defects by age 3, then how large of a study group is needed to have an 80% chance of detecting a significant dif-ference using a one-sided test at the 5% level?

**7.64** Suppose we can only recruit 50 cases for the study group. How likely are we to find a significant difference if the true proportion of affected children with speech and language defects at age 3 is the same as that in the pilot study?

### Hypertension

A pilot study of a new antihypertensive agent is per-formed for the purpose of planning a larger study. Five patients who have a mean diastolic blood pressure of at least 95 mm Hg are recruited for the study and are kept on the agent for a 1-month period. After 1 month the observed mean decline in diastolic blood pressure in these 5 patients is 4.8 mm Hg with a standard deviation of 9 mm Hg.

**7.65** If $\mu_d$ = true mean difference in diastolic pressure between baseline and 1 month, then how many patients would be needed to have a 90% chance of detecting a significant difference using a one-tailed test with a significance level of 5%? Assume that the true mean and standard deviation of the blood pressure difference was the same as that observed in the pilot study.

**7.66** Suppose we conduct a study of the preceding hypothesis based on 20 subjects. What is the probability that we will be able to reject $H_0$ using a one-sided test at the 5% level if the true mean and standard deviation of the blood pressure difference is the same as that in the pilot study?

## Hypertension

Suppose we are interested in investigating the effect of race on level of blood pressure. A study was conducted in Evans County, Georgia, comparing the mean level of blood pressure among whites and blacks for different age-sex groups [3]. The mean and standard deviation of systolic blood pressure among 25–34-year-old white males are reported as 128.6 mm Hg and 11.1 mm Hg, respectively, based on a large sample.

7.67 Suppose the mean bp of 38 25–34-year-old black males is reported as 135.7 mm Hg. If the standard deviation of white males is assumed to hold for black males as well, then test if the underlying mean systolic blood pressures are the same in the two groups.

7.68 The actual reported standard deviation among 25–34-year-old black males is 12.5 mm Hg. Test the hypothesis that the underlying variance of blood pressure for white and black males is the same.

7.69 Suppose the actual underlying mean for black males is 135 mm Hg. What is the power of the test in Problem 7.67 in this case if we assume that the standard deviations for white males and black males are the same?

Suppose we do *not* assume that the standard deviation of 11.1 mm Hg is correct for 25–34-year-old black males.

7.70 Test the hypothesis that the underlying mean systolic blood pressures are the same in the two groups.

7.71 Derive a 95% confidence interval for the mean systolic blood pressure for 25–34-year-old black males under the assumptions in Problem 7.70.

7.72 Relate your answers to Problems 7.70 and 7.71.

## Occupational Health

The proportion of deaths due to lung cancer in males aged 15–64 in England and Wales during the period 1970–1972 was 12%. Suppose that of 20 deaths that occur among male workers in this age group who have worked for at least 1 year in a chemical plant, 5 are due to lung cancer. We wish to determine if there is a difference between the proportion of lung cancer deaths in this plant and the proportion in the general population.

7.73 State the hypotheses to be used in answering this question.

7.74 Is a one-sided or two-sided test appropriate here?

7.75 Perform the hypothesis test and report a *p*-value. After reviewing the results from 1 plant, the company decides to expand its study to include results from 3

additional plants. They find that of 90 deaths occurring among 15–64-year-old male workers who have worked for at least 1 year in these 4 plants, 19 are due to lung cancer.

7.76 Answer Problem 7.75 using the data from 4 plants and report a *p*-value.

One criticism of studies of this type is that they are biased because of the "healthy worker" effect. That is, workers in general are healthier than the general population, particularly regarding cardiovascular endpoints, which makes the proportion of deaths due to noncardiovascular causes seem abnormally high.

7.77 If the proportion of deaths due to ischemic heart disease (IHD) is 40% for all 15–64-year-old men in England and Wales, whereas 18 of the preceding 90 deaths are attributed to IHD, then answer Problem 7.76 if deaths due to IHD are *excluded* from the total.

## Epidemiology

Height and weight are often used in epidemiological studies as possible predictors of disease outcomes. If the persons in the study are assessed in a clinic, then heights and weights are usually measured directly. However, if the persons are interviewed at home or by mail, then a person's self-reported height and weight are often used instead. Suppose we conduct a study on 10 people to test the comparability of these two methods. The data for weight are given in Table 7.4.

*Table 7.4* A comparison of self-reported and measured weight (lb) for 10 subjects

| Person number | Self-reported weight | Measured weight | Difference |
|---|---|---|---|
| 1 | 120 | 125 | −5 |
| 2 | 120 | 118 | +2 |
| 3 | 135 | 139 | −4 |
| 4 | 118 | 120 | −2 |
| 5 | 120 | 125 | −5 |
| 6 | 190 | 198 | −8 |
| 7 | 124 | 128 | −4 |
| 8 | 175 | 176 | −1 |
| 9 | 133 | 131 | +2 |
| 10 | 125 | 125 | 0 |

7.78 Should we use a one-sided or two-sided test here?

7.79 Which test procedure should we use to test the preceding hypothesis?

**7.80** Conduct the test mentioned in Problem 7.79 using the critical value method with $\alpha = 0.05$.

**7.81** Compute the *p*-value for the test mentioned in Problem 7.79.

**7.82** Is there evidence of digit preference among the self-reported weights? Specifically, compare the observed proportion of reported weights whose last digit is 0 or 5 with the expected proportion based on chance and report a *p*-value.

### Nutrition

Iron deficiency anemia is an important nutritional health problem in the United States today. A dietary assessment was performed in 51 9–11-year-old male children whose families were below the poverty level. The mean daily iron intake among these children was found to be 12.50 mg with standard deviation 4.75 mg. Suppose that the mean daily iron intake among a large population of 9–11-year-old boys from all income strata is 14.44 mg. We wish to test if the mean iron intake among the low-income group is different from that of the general population.

**7.83** State the hypotheses that can be used to consider this question.

**7.84** Carry out the hypothesis test in Problem 7.83 using the critical value method with an $\alpha$ level of 0.05 and summarize your findings.

**7.85** What is the *p*-value for the test conducted in Problem 7.84?

The standard deviation of daily iron intake in the larger population of 9–11-year-old boys was 5.56 mg. We wish to test if the standard deviation from the low-income group is comparable to that of the general population.

**7.86** State the hypotheses that can be used to answer this question.

**7.87** Carry out the test in Problem 7.86 using the critical value method with an $\alpha$ level of 0.05 and summarize your findings.

**7.88** What is the *p*-value for the test conducted in Problem 7.87?

**7.89** Compute a 95% confidence interval for the underlying variance of daily iron intake in the low-income group. What can you infer from the confidence interval?

**7.90** Compare the inferences you made from the procedures in Problems 7.87, 7.88, and 7.89.

### Hypertension

Suppose we wish to design an experiment to assess the effectiveness of a new drug for treating hypertensive patients. We decide to declare the drug "effective" if the mean diastolic blood pressure of the 50 patients participating in the study drops by at least 2 mm after using the drug daily for 1 month.

Let us set up this study as a hypothesis-testing problem and assume that the population standard deviation of the before-after blood pressure differences is *known* to be 10 mm.

**7.91** If we identify declaring the drug effective with rejecting the null hypothesis, then what is the significance level of the test?

**7.92** Suppose that the underlying population before-after diastolic blood pressure decrease from using this drug is 3 mm. What is the power of the test in Problem 7.91?

### Gynecology

A survey of contraceptive methods conducted by the National Center for Health Statistics in 1965 indicated that among 30–39-year-old, married, nonpregnant women who practiced contraception, 20% used some form of permanent contraception (i.e., either tubal ligation for the women or vasectomy for their spouses). The frequency of use of permanent contraception was suspected to have changed in the next decade. To test this hypothesis, records were selected of 50 women subscribing to a prepaid health plan in 1975 who satisfied the preceding demographic criteria. From the records, 35 of the women were found to have practiced some form of contraception, of whom 10 used the method of permanent contraception. Suppose we wish to test the hypothesis that a change has occurred in the percentage of contraceptors who use permanent contraception, without specifying the direction of the change.

**7.93** Specify the hypotheses needed to perform this test.

**7.94** Use the critical value method to conduct the hypothesis test with an $\alpha$ level of 0.01.

**7.95** What is the exact *p*-value for this test?

The investigators are encouraged by the results of the small study and wish to enlarge the study.

**7.96** How large a sample would be needed to test the preceding hypotheses if the following assumptions hold:

(a) The true rate of permanent contraception among contraceptors is 30%.

(b) Seventy percent of the women use some form of contraception.

(c) We wish to have a 90% chance of finding a significant difference using an $\alpha$ level of 0.05.

# References

[1] *Vital Statistics of the United States*, 1960, Vol. II, Mortality, Part A, Table I.M, Government Printing Office, Washington, DC, 1963.

[2] Andjelkovic, D., Taulbee, J., and Symons, M. (1976) "Mortality Experience of a Cohort of Rubber Workers, 1964–1973," *Journal of Occupational Medicine* **18(6)**: 387–394.

[3] McDonough, J. R., Garrison, G. E., and Hames, C. G. (1967) "Blood Pressure and Hypertensive Disease among Negroes and Whites in Evans County, Georgia," *The Epidemiology of Hypertension*, Stamler, J., Stamler, R., and Pullman, T. N., eds. (New York: Grune and Stratton).

# 8 Hypothesis Testing: Two-Sample Inference

## ■ 8.1 INTRODUCTION

All the tests introduced in Chapter 7 were one-sample tests. We have been comparing the underlying parameters of the population from which our sample is drawn with comparable values from other generally large populations *whose parameters are assumed to be known.*

**Example 8.1**    **Obstetrics**  In our birthweight data in Example 7.2, we compared the underlying mean birthweight in one hospital with the underlying mean birthweight in the United States, *whose value was assumed known.*    ■

A more frequently encountered situation is the two-sample hypothesis-testing problem.

**Definition 8.1**

In a *two-sample* hypothesis-testing problem, we compare the underlying parameters of two different populations, *neither of whose values is assumed known.*    ■

**Example 8.2**    **Cardiovascular Disease, Hypertension**  We might be interested in the relationship between the use of oral contraceptives (OC) and the level of blood pressure (bp) in women. Two different experimental designs can be used to assess this relationship. One method would involve the following design:

**8.1**    *Longitudinal Study*

*1*. Identify a group of nonpregnant, premenopausal women of childbearing age (16–49) from a prepaid health plan who are not currently OC users and measure their bp, which we will refer to as baseline bp.

*2*. Rescreen these women 1 year later to ascertain a subgroup who have remained nonpregnant throughout the year and have become OC users. This subgroup will be the study population.

*3*. Measure the bp of the study population at the follow-up visit.

*4*. Compare the baseline and follow-up bp of the women in the study population to determine the difference between the bp of women when they *were* using the pill at follow-up and when they *were not* using the pill at baseline.

Another method would involve the following design:

## 8.2 Cross-Sectional Study

*1*. Identify both a group of OC users and a group of non-OC users among nonpregnant, premenopausal women of childbearing age (16–49) from a prepaid health plan and measure their bp.

*2*. Compare the bp of the OC users and nonusers.

**Definition 8.2**

The first type of study is called a **longitudinal** or **follow-up study**, since the same group of women are followed *over time*. ∎

**Definition 8.3**

The second type of study is called a **cross-sectional study**, since the women are seen at only one point in time. ∎

There is another important difference between these two designs. The first study represents a *paired sample* design, since the same woman is used as her own control. The second study represents an *independent sample* design, since two completely different groups of women are being compared.

**Definition 8.4**

Two samples are said to be **paired** when each data point of the first sample is matched and is related to a unique data point of the second sample. ∎

*Example 8.3*

The paired samples may represent two sets of measurements on the same people. In this case each person is serving as his or her own control, as is the case in **(8.1)**. The paired samples may also represent measurements on different people who are chosen on an individual basis using matching criteria, such as age and sex, to be very similar to each other. ∎

**Definition 8.5**

Two samples are said to be **independent** when the data points in one sample are unrelated to the data points in the second sample. ∎

*Example 8.4*

The samples in **(8.2)** are completely independent, since the data are obtained from unrelated groups of women. ∎

Which type of study is better in this case? The first type of study is probably more definitive, since most confounding factors that influence blood pressure in women at the first screening will also be present at the second screening and will not influence the comparison of blood pressure levels at the first and second screenings. The second type of study by itself can only be considered suggestive, since other confounding factors may influence blood pressure in the two samples and cause an apparent difference to be found where none is actually present.

For example, OC users are known to be lighter than non-OC users. Since low weight tends to be associated with low bp, OC users' blood pressure levels as a group would appear lower than non-OC users'.

On the other hand, a follow-up study is more expensive to do than a cross-sectional study. Therefore, a cross-sectional study may be the only financially feasible way of doing the study.

In this chapter we will be studying the appropriate methods of hypothesis testing for both the paired-sample and independent-sample situations.

# ■ *8.2 THE PAIRED t TEST*

Suppose we adopt the paired-samples study design given in **(8.1)** and obtain the sample data in Table 8.1. We denote the systolic bp level of the $i$th woman at baseline by $x_{i1}$ and at follow-up by $x_{i2}$.

| 8.3 | We will assume that the systolic bp of the $i$th woman at baseline is normally distributed with mean $\mu_i$ and variance $\sigma^2$ and at follow-up is normally distributed with mean $\mu_i + \Delta$ and variance $\sigma^2$. |

We thus are assuming that the mean difference in bp between follow-up and baseline is $\Delta$, which is constant for all persons. If $\Delta = 0$, then there is no difference between baseline and follow-up bp. If $\Delta > 0$, then the use of OC pills is associated with an increase in bp. If $\Delta < 0$, then the use of OC pills is associated with a decline in bp.

We wish to test the hypothesis $H_0: \Delta = 0$ vs. $H_1: \Delta \neq 0$. How should we do this? Our problem is that we do not know $\mu_i$, and we are assuming, in general, that it is different for each woman. However, let us consider the difference $d_i = x_{i2} - x_{i1}$. From **(8.3)** we know that $d_i$ is normally distributed with mean $\Delta$ and a variance that we shall denote by $\sigma_d^2$. Thus, although bp levels $\mu_i$ are different for

**Table 8.1**
*Systolic blood pressure levels (mm Hg) in 10 women while not using (baseline) and while using (follow-up) oral contraceptives*

| $i$ | Systolic blood pressure level while not using OC's $(x_{i_1})$ | Systolic blood pressure level while using OC's $(x_{i2})$ | $d_i (x_{i_1} - x_{i2})$ |
|---|---|---|---|
| 1 | 115 | 128 | 13 |
| 2 | 112 | 115 | 3 |
| 3 | 107 | 106 | −1 |
| 4 | 119 | 128 | 9 |
| 5 | 115 | 122 | 7 |
| 6 | 138 | 145 | 7 |
| 7 | 126 | 132 | 6 |
| 8 | 105 | 109 | 4 |
| 9 | 104 | 102 | −2 |
| 10 | 115 | 117 | 2 |

each woman, the differences in bp between baseline and follow-up have the same underlying mean ($\Delta$) and variance ($\sigma_d^2$) for each woman. Our hypothesis-testing problem can thus be considered as a *one-sample test based on the differences* ($d_i$). From our work on the one-sample $t$ test in Section 7.5, we know that the best test of the hypothesis: $H_0: \Delta = 0$ vs. $H_1: \Delta \neq 0$, when the variance is unknown, is based on the mean difference

$$\bar{d} = (d_1 + d_2 + \cdots + d_n)/n$$

Specifically, from **(7.17)** for a two-sided level $\alpha$ test, we have the following test procedure, which we refer to as the *paired t test*.

**8.4** **Paired t Test**

We denote the test statistic $\bar{d}/(s_d/\sqrt{n})$ by $\lambda$, where $s_d$ is the sample standard deviation of the observed differences:

$$s_d = \sqrt{\left[\sum_{i=1}^{n} d_i^2 - \left(\sum_{i=1}^{n} d_i\right)^2 \Big/ n\right]\Big/(n-1)}$$

$n$ = number of matched pairs

If

$$\lambda > t_{n-1, 1-\alpha/2} \qquad \text{or} \qquad \lambda < -t_{n-1, 1-\alpha/2}$$

then we reject $H_0$. If

$$-t_{n-1, 1-\alpha/2} \leqslant \lambda \leqslant t_{n-1, 1-\alpha/2}$$

then we accept $H_0$. The acceptance and rejection regions for this test are depicted in Figure 8.1.

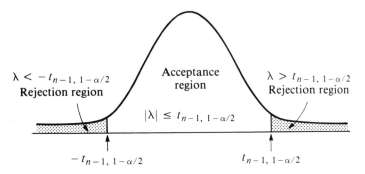

Distribution of $\lambda$ in **(8.4)** under $H_0 = y_{n-1}$ distribution

$\lambda < -t_{n-1, 1-\alpha/2}$
Rejection region

Acceptance region

$\lambda > t_{n-1, 1-\alpha/2}$
Rejection region

$|\lambda| \leq t_{n-1, 1-\alpha/2}$

$-t_{n-1, 1-\alpha/2}$

$t_{n-1, 1-\alpha/2}$

**Figure 8.1**
*Acceptance and rejection regions for the paired t test*

Similarly, we can compute a *p*-value for our test as follows:

**8.5** **Computation of the P-value for the Paired t Test**

If $\lambda < 0$,

$$p = 2 \times [\text{the area to the left of } \lambda = \bar{d}/(s_d/\sqrt{n}) \text{ under a } t_{n-1} \text{ distribution}]$$

If $\lambda \geq 0$,

$$p = 2 \times [\text{the area to the right of } \lambda \text{ under a } t_{n-1} \text{ distribution}]$$

The computation of the $p$-value is illustrated in Figure 8.2.

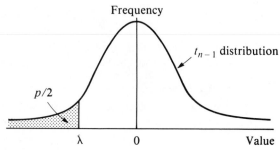

If $\lambda = \bar{d}/(s_d/\sqrt{n}) < 0$, then $p = 2 \times$ (area to the left of $\lambda$ under a $t_{n-1}$ distribution).

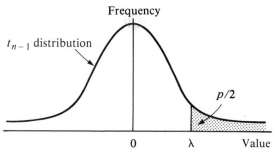

If $\lambda = \bar{d}/(s_d/\sqrt{n}) \geq 0$, then $p = 2 \times$ (area to the right of $\lambda$ under a $t_{n-1}$ distribution).

**Figure 8.2**
*Computation of the
p-value for the
paired t test*

### Example 8.5

*Cardiovascular Disease, Hypertension*  Assess the statistical significance of the OC-bp data given in Table 8.1.

### Solution

We have

$$\bar{d} = (13 + 3 + \cdots + 2)/10 = 4.80$$

$$s_d^2 = \{[(13)^2 + (3)^2 + \cdots + (2)^2] - 10(4.80)^2\}/9 = 20.844$$

$$s_d = \sqrt{20.844} = 4.566$$

$$\lambda = (4.80)/(4.566/\sqrt{10}) = 4.80/1.444 = 3.32$$

We first use the critical value method to perform the significance test. We have $10 - 1 = 9$ degrees of freedom, and from Table 5 we see that $t_{9,.975} = 2.262$. Since $\lambda = 3.32 > 2.262$, it follows from **(8.4)** that we can reject $H_0$ using a two-sided significance test with $\alpha = 0.05$. To compute an approximate $p$-value, we refer to Table 5 and note that $t_{9,.9995} = 4.781$, $t_{9,.995} = 3.250$. Thus, since $3.25 < 3.32 < 4.781$, it follows that $0.0005 < p/2 < 0.005$ or $0.001 < p < 0.01$.

**Table 8.2**
*Use of the SPSS/PC Paired T-TEST program to analyze the blood pressure data in Table 8.1*

```
                          SPSS/PC  Release 1.0


    Paired samples t-test:  FUP      SYS BP WHILE USING OCS
                            BASE     SYS BP WHILE NOT USING OCS

    Variable    Number               Standard   Standard
              of Cases     Mean      Deviation    Error

      FUP         10     120.4000     13.226      4.183
      BASE        10     115.6000     10.309      3.260
```

| (Difference) Mean | Standard Deviation | Standard Error | 2-Tail Corr. Prob. | t Value | Degrees of Freedom | 2-Tail Prob. |
|---|---|---|---|---|---|---|
| 4.8000 | 4.566 | 1.444 | 0.955  0.000 | 3.32 | 9 | 0.009 |

To compute a more exact *p*-value, we must use a computer program. We present the results in Table 8.2 from using the SPSS/PC paired T-TEST program.

The output provides the mean, standard deviation, and standard error for systolic blood pressure at each of the baseline and follow-up visits. In addition, the mean, standard deviation, and standard error of the difference scores are provided along with the paired *t* statistic $= \lambda$ (labeled *t* value), the degrees of freedom, and the two-tailed *p*-value (labeled 2-Tail Prob.). Finally, the **correlation coefficient** between baseline and follow-up blood pressures is given (labeled Corr.) along with a two-tailed *p*-value associated with this correlation. We will discuss the meaning of a correlation coefficient in detail in Chapter 11.

We note from Table 8.2 that the exact two-sided *p*-value = 0.009. Therefore, we can conclude that starting oral contraceptive use is associated with a significant increase in blood pressure. We can quantify the amount of increase by computing a 95% confidence interval for the mean difference. A 95% confidence interval for the true mean blood pressure change is given by

$$\bar{d} \pm t_{n-1,.975} \, s_d/\sqrt{n} = 4.80 \pm t_{9,.975}(1.444)$$

$$= 4.80 \pm 2.262(1.444) = 4.80 \pm 3.27$$

$$= (1.53, 8.07)$$

Thus, the expected amount of change is between 1.5 and 8 mm.  ∎

Example 8.5 is a classic example of a paired study, since each woman is used as her own control. In many other paired studies, different people are used for the two groups, but they are matched individually on the basis of specific matching characteristics.

*Example 8.6*

***Family Planning, Gynecology*** A topic of recent clinical interest is the effect of different contraceptive methods on fertility. In particular, suppose we wish to compare how long it takes users of oral contraceptives and diaphragms, respectively, to become pregnant after stopping contraception. We form a study group of 20 oral contraceptive users and find diaphragm users who match each OC user in age (within 5 years), race, parity (number of previous pregnancies), and socioeconomic status (SES). We compute the differences in time to fertility between previous OC and diaphragm users and find that the mean difference $\bar{d}$ (OC minus diaphragm) in time to fertility is 4 months with a standard deviation ($s_d$) of 8 months. What can we conclude from these data?

**Solution**

We will perform the paired $t$ test. We have

$$\lambda = \bar{d}/(s_d/\sqrt{n}) = 4/(8/\sqrt{20}) = 4/1.789 = 2.24 \sim t_{19}$$

under $H_0$. If we refer to Table 5, we find that

$$t_{19,.975} = 2.093 \quad \text{and} \quad t_{19,.99} = 2.539$$

Then, since $2.093 < 2.24 < 2.539$, it follows that $0.01 < p/2 < 0.025$ or $0.02 < p < 0.05$. Therefore, previous OC users take a significantly longer time to become pregnant than do previous diaphragm users.    ∎

# ■ 8.3 TWO-SAMPLE t TEST FOR INDEPENDENT SAMPLES WITH EQUAL VARIANCES

We will now discuss the question posed in Example 8.2, assuming we are doing the cross-sectional study defined in **(8.2)** rather than the longitudinal study defined in **(8.1)**.

*Example 8.7*

*Cardiovascular Disease, Hypertension* Suppose we select a random sample of 8 women from the group of 35–39-year-old nonpregnant premenopausal OC users in our prepaid health plan who have mean systolic blood pressure of 132.86 mm and sample standard deviation of 15.34 mm. We also select a random sample of 21 women from the group of 35–39-year-old nonpregnant premenopausal non-OC users in our prepaid health plan who have mean systolic blood pressure of 127.44 mm and sample standard deviation of 18.23 mm. What can we say about the underlying mean difference in blood pressure between the two populations?    ∎

We will assume that the blood pressure in the first group is normally distributed with mean $\mu_1$ and variance $\sigma_1^2$ and in the second group is normally distributed with mean $\mu_2$ and variance $\sigma_2^2$. We wish to test the hypothesis $H_0: \mu_1 = \mu_2$ vs. $H_1: \mu_1 \neq \mu_2$. We will assume in this section that the underlying variances in the two groups are *the same* (i.e., $\sigma_1^2 = \sigma_2^2 = \sigma^2$). We denote the means and variances in the two samples by $\bar{x}_1, \bar{x}_2, s_1^2, s_2^2$, respectively.

It seems reasonable to base our significance test on the difference between the two sample means, $\bar{x}_1 - \bar{x}_2$. If this difference is far from 0, then we will reject $H_0$; otherwise, we will accept $H_0$. Thus, we wish to study the behavior of $\bar{x}_1 - \bar{x}_2$ under $H_0$. We know that $\bar{x}_1$ is normally distributed with mean $\mu_1$ and variance $\sigma^2/n_1$ and that $\bar{x}_2$ is normally distributed with mean $\mu_2$ and variance $\sigma^2/n_2$. Hence since the two samples are independent, we have that $\bar{x}_1 - \bar{x}_2$ is normally distributed with mean $\mu_1 - \mu_2$ and variance $\sigma^2(1/n_1 + 1/n_2)$. In symbols,

**8.6**

$$\bar{x}_1 - \bar{x}_2 \sim N\left[\mu_1 - \mu_2, \sigma^2\left(\frac{1}{n_1} + \frac{1}{n_2}\right)\right]$$

Under $H_0$ we know that $\mu_1 = \mu_2$. Thus, **(8.6)** reduces to

8.7

$$\bar{x}_1 - \bar{x}_2 \sim N\left[0, \sigma^2\left(\frac{1}{n_1} + \frac{1}{n_2}\right)\right]$$

If $\sigma^2$ were known, then we could divide $\bar{x}_1 - \bar{x}_2$ by $\sigma\sqrt{1/n_1 + 1/n_2}$. From **(8.7)**,

8.8

$$\frac{\bar{x}_1 - \bar{x}_2}{\sigma\sqrt{\dfrac{1}{n_1} + \dfrac{1}{n_2}}} \sim N(0, 1)$$

and we could use the test statistic in **(8.8)** as a basis for our hypothesis test. Unfortunately, $\sigma^2$ in general is unknown, and we must estimate it from our data. How can we best estimate $\sigma^2$ in this situation?

From the first and second sample, we have sample variances $s_1^2$, $s_2^2$, respectively, each of which could be used to estimate $\sigma^2$. We could simply use the average of $s_1^2$ and $s_2^2$ as our estimate of $\sigma^2$. However, this average will weight the sample variances equally even if the sample sizes are very different from each other. The sample variances should not be weighted equally, since the sample variance from the larger sample is probably more precise and should be weighted more heavily. We can show that the best estimate of the population variance $\sigma^2$, which we denote by $s^2$, is given by a weighted average of the two sample variances, where the weights are the number of degrees of freedom in each sample.

8.9

The **pooled estimate of the variance** from two independent samples is given by

$$s^2 = \frac{[(n_1 - 1)s_1^2 + (n_2 - 1)s_2^2]}{n_1 + n_2 - 2}$$

In particular, $s^2$ will then have $n_1 - 1$ d.f. from the first sample and $n_2 - 1$ d.f. from the second sample, or

$$(n_1 - 1) + (n_2 - 1) = n_1 + n_2 - 2 \text{ d.f.}$$

overall. We then substitute $s$ for $\sigma$ in **(8.8)**, and the resulting test statistic can then be shown to follow a $t$ distribution with $n_1 + n_2 - 2$ d.f. rather than a $N(0, 1)$ distribution, since $\sigma^2$ is unknown. Thus we will use the following test procedure:

8.10

### Two-Sample t Test for Independent Samples with Equal Variances

Suppose we wish to test the hypothesis $H_0\colon \mu_1 = \mu_2$ vs. $H_1\colon \mu_1 \neq \mu_2$ with a significance level of $\alpha$ for two normally distributed populations, where $\sigma^2$ is assumed to be the same for each population.

We compute the test statistic

$$\lambda = \frac{\bar{x}_1 - \bar{x}_2}{\left(s\sqrt{\dfrac{1}{n_1} + \dfrac{1}{n_2}}\right)}$$

where

$$s = \sqrt{[(n_1 - 1)s_1^2 + (n_2 - 1)s_2^2]/(n_1 + n_2 - 2)}$$

If

$$\lambda > t_{n_1 + n_2 - 2, 1 - \alpha/2} \quad \text{or} \quad \lambda < -t_{n_1 + n_2 - 2, 1 - \alpha/2}$$

then we reject $H_0$. If

$$-t_{n_1 + n_2 - 2, 1 - \alpha/2} \leqslant \lambda \leqslant t_{n_1 + n_2 - 2, 1 - \alpha/2}$$

then we accept $H_0$.

The acceptance and rejection regions for this test are depicted in Figure 8.3.

**Figure 8.3**
*Acceptance and rejection regions for the two-sample t test for independent samples with equal variances*

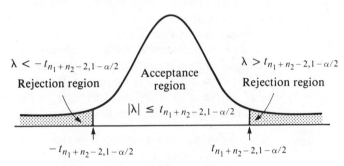

$$\lambda < -t_{n_1 + n_2 - 2, 1 - \alpha/2}$$
Rejection region

Acceptance region

$$\lambda > t_{n_1 + n_2 - 2, 1 - \alpha/2}$$
Rejection region

$$|\lambda| \leqslant t_{n_1 + n_2 - 2, 1 - \alpha/2}$$

$$-t_{n_1 + n_2 - 2, 1 - \alpha/2}$$

$$t_{n_1 + n_2 - 2, 1 - \alpha/2}$$

Distribution of $\lambda$ in **(8.10)** under $H_0 = t_{n_1 + n_2 - 2}$ distribution

Similarly, we can compute a *p*-value for our test as follows:

**8.11**    *Computation of the P-value for the Two-Sample t Test for Independent Samples with Equal Variances*

If $\lambda \leqslant 0$,

$$p = 2 \times \text{area to the left of } \lambda = \frac{\bar{x}_1 - \bar{x}_2}{s\sqrt{1/n_1 + 1/n_2}} \text{ under a } t_{n_1 + n_2 - 2} \text{ distribution}$$

where

$$s = \sqrt{[(n_1 - 1)s_1^2 + (n_2 - 1)s_2^2]/(n_1 + n_2 - 2)}$$

If $\lambda > 0$,

$$p = 2 \times [\text{area to the right of } \lambda \text{ under a } t_{n_1 + n_2 - 2} \text{ distribution}]$$

The computation of the *p*-value is illustrated in Figure 8.4.

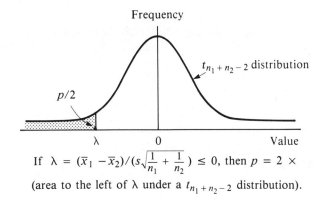

Frequency

$t_{n_1+n_2-2}$ distribution

$p/2$

$\lambda$    0    Value

If $\lambda = (\bar{x}_1 - \bar{x}_2)/(s\sqrt{\frac{1}{n_1} + \frac{1}{n_2}}) \le 0$, then $p = 2 \times$

(area to the left of $\lambda$ under a $t_{n_1+n_2-2}$ distribution).

Frequency

$t_{n_1+n_2-2}$ distribution

$p/2$

0    $\lambda$    Value

If $\lambda = (\bar{x}_1 - \bar{x}_2)/(s\sqrt{\frac{1}{n_1} + \frac{1}{n_2}}) > 0$, then $p = 2 \times$

(area to the right of $\lambda$ under a $t_{n_1+n_2-2}$ distribution).

**Figure 8.4**
*Computation of the p-value for the two-sample t test for independent samples with equal variances*

**Example 8.8**    ***Cardiovascular Disease, Hypertension*** Assess the statistical significance of the data given in Example 8.7.

**Solution**    We first estimate the common variance as follows:

$$s^2 = \frac{7(15.34)^2 + 20(18.23)^2}{27} = \frac{8293.87}{27} = 307.18$$

or $s = 17.527$. We then form the test statistic

$$\lambda = \frac{132.86 - 127.44}{17.527\sqrt{1/8 + 1/21}} = \frac{5.42}{17.527 \times 0.415}$$

$$= \frac{5.42}{7.274} = 0.75$$

If we use the critical value method, then we note that under $H_0$, $\lambda$ comes from a $t_{27}$ distribution. If we refer to Table 5, we see that $t_{27,.975} = 2.052$. Since $-2.052 \le 0.75 \le 2.052$, it follows that we accept $H_0$ using a two-sided test at the 5% level and conclude that the mean blood pressures of the two groups of OC users and non-OC users are not significantly different from each other. In a sense this result shows the superiority of the longitudinal design in Example 8.5. Despite the similarity in the magnitudes of the blood pressure differences between users and nonusers in the two studies, we could detect significant differences in Example 8.5

in contrast to the nonsignificant results that we obtained using the preceding cross-sectional design. The longitudinal design is more efficient because it uses people as their own controls.

To compute an approximate $p$-value, we note from Table 5 that $t_{27,.75} = 0.684$, $t_{27,.80} = 0.855$. Since $0.684 < 0.75 < 0.855$, it follows that $0.2 < p/2 < 0.25$ or $0.4 < p < 0.5$. The exact $p$-value is given by the HP 41-C $t$ distribution program as $2 \times Pr(t_{27} > 0.75) = 2 \times 0.230 = 0.46$. ∎

Using similar methods to those developed in Section 6.4, we can also obtain the following two-sided $100\% \times (1 - \alpha)$ confidence interval for the underlying mean difference $\mu_1 - \mu_2$:

**8.12**    ***Two-Sided $100\% \times (1 - \alpha)$ Confidence Interval for $\mu_1 - \mu_2$***

$$\left( \bar{x}_1 - \bar{x}_2 - t_{n_1 + n_2 - 2, 1 - \alpha/2}\, s \sqrt{\frac{1}{n_1} + \frac{1}{n_2}}, \quad \bar{x}_1 - \bar{x}_2 + t_{n_1 + n_2 - 2, 1 - \alpha/2}\, s \sqrt{\frac{1}{n_1} + \frac{1}{n_2}} \right)$$

*Example 8.9*    ***Cardiovascular Disease, Hypertension*** Compute a 95% confidence interval for the mean difference in blood pressure between the two groups using the data in Example 8.7.

*Solution*    A 95% confidence interval for the underlying mean difference in systolic blood pressure between the population of 35–39-year-old OC users and non-OC users is given by

$$[5.42 - t_{27,.975}(7.274), 5.42 + t_{27,.975}(7.274)]$$

$$= [5.42 - 2.052\,(7.274), 5.42 + 2.052\,(7.274)]$$

$$= (-9.51, 20.35)$$

This interval is rather wide and indicates that we need a much larger sample to accurately assess the mean difference. ∎

*Example 8.10*    ***Environmental Health, Pediatrics*** A topic of recent interest is the short- and long-term health effects of exposure to various agents in the environment. A study was performed by Landrigan et al. to look at the effect of chronic exposure to low levels of lead in children who lived near a lead smelter in El Paso, Texas [1]. A lead absorption group and a control group of children were identified by the amount of lead in blood samples, and various neurological and psychological tests were performed to compare the two groups. In particular, the WISC performance IQ test was performed on 34 children, 5 years of age and older, in the lead absorption group and 36 comparably aged children in the control group. Assess the statistical significance of the IQ test results, which are given in Table 8.3.

*Solution*    We perform the two-sample $t$ test for independent samples with equal variances. We first compute a pooled estimate of the variance as follows:

$$s^2 = [33(13.74)^2 + 35(17.87)^2]/68 = 255.98 \quad \text{or} \quad s = \sqrt{255.98} = 16.00$$

**Table 8.3**
*Results of WISC performance IQ test for exposed and control children*

|                  | Mean   | sd    | n  |
|------------------|--------|-------|----|
| Lead absorption  | 96.44  | 13.74 | 34 |
| Control          | 103.29 | 17.87 | 36 |

(Reprinted with permission of *The Lancet*, March 29, 708–715, 1975.)

Thus we compute the test statistic

$$\lambda = (96.44 - 103.29)/[16.00\sqrt{(1/34) + (1/36)}] = -6.85/3.826 = -1.79$$

which follows a $t$ distribution with $34 + 36 - 2 = 68$ d.f. under $H_0$.

The critical value is given by $t_{68,.975}$, which is not given in Table 5. However, since $t_{60,.975} = 2.000$, $t_{120,.975} = 1.980$, we see that $1.980 <$ critical value $< 2.000$. Since $1.79 = |\lambda| < 1.980 <$ critical value, we can accept $H_0$ using a two-sided test with $\alpha = 0.05$. To compute an approximate $p$-value, we note from Table 5 that $t_{60,.95} = 1.671$. Thus, since $1.671 < 1.79 < 2.000$, it follows that if there were 60 d.f., then $0.025 < p/2 < 0.05$ or $0.05 < p < 0.10$. Similarly, since $t_{120,.95} = 1.658$ and $1.658 < 1.79 < 1.980$, it follows that if there were 120 d.f., then $0.025 < p/2 < 0.05$ or $0.05 < p < 0.10$. Since the results agree for 60 and 120 d.f. and our d.f. (68) is between 60 and 120, we must reach the same conclusion; that is, $0.05 < p < 0.10$. Thus, we see a trend toward statistical significance, but the results are not quite significant using a two-sided test ($0.05 < p < 0.10$).

The exact $p$-value is given by the HP 41-C $t$ distribution program as $2 \times Pr(t_{68} > 1.79)$ $= 2 \times 0.039 = 0.078$. Actually, we can make an argument for using a one-sided test here, since we would only expect the presence of high lead levels to worsen IQ. Thus, we would be testing the hypothesis $H_0: \mu_1 = \mu_2$ vs. $H_1: \mu_1 < \mu_2$, in which case the one-sided $p$-value would be half of the two-sided $p$-value, or 0.039. This is what the authors of the study actually did. ∎

# ■ *8.4 TESTING FOR THE EQUALITY OF TWO VARIANCES*

In the previous section, when we conducted a two-sample $t$ test for independent samples, we assumed that the underlying variances of the two samples were the same. We then proceeded to estimate the common variance using a weighted average of the individual sample variances. In this section we proceed to develop a significance test to validate this assumption.

*Example 8.11*    *Cardiovascular Disease, Pediatrics* Let us consider a problem we have discussed previously, namely, the familial aggregation of cholesterol levels. In particular, suppose we assess cholesterol levels in 100 2–14-year-old children of men who have died from heart disease and find that the mean cholesterol level in this group ($\bar{x}_1$) is 207.3 mg%/ml. Suppose that the sample standard deviation in this group ($s_1$) is 35.6. We previously compared the cholesterol levels in this group of children with the baseline level of 175 mg%/ml, which we assumed was the underlying mean level in children in this age group based on previous large studies.

A better experimental design would be to select a group of control children whose fathers are alive and do not have heart disease and who are similar to the case children and then compare their cholesterol levels with those of the case children. If we identify the case fathers by a search of death records, then we can select control children who live on the same block as the case families but whose fathers have no history of heart disease. We can then measure the cholesterol levels in these children. Suppose we do this procedure and find that among 74 control children, the mean cholesterol level ($\bar{x}_2$) is 193.4 mg%/ml with a sample standard deviation ($s_2$) of 17.3 mg%/ml. We would like to compare the means of these two groups using the two-sample $t$ test for independent samples given in **(8.10)**, but we are hesitant to assume equal variances because the sample variance of the case group is about 4 times as large as that of the control group:

$$(35.6)^2/(17.3)^2 = 4.23$$

What should we do?    ∎

What we need is a significance test to determine if the underlying variances are in fact equal; that is, we wish to test the hypothesis $H_0: \sigma_1^2 = \sigma_2^2$ vs. $H_1: \sigma_1^2 \neq \sigma_2^2$. It seems reasonable to base our significance test on the relative magnitudes of the sample variances $(s_1^2, s_2^2)$. We can show that the best test in this case is based on the ratio of the sample variances $(s_1^2/s_2^2)$ rather than on the difference between the sample variances $(s_1^2 - s_2^2)$. Thus, we would want to reject $H_0$ if the variance ratio is either too large or too small and accept $H_0$ otherwise. To accomplish this end, we need to find the sampling distribution of $s_1^2/s_2^2$ under the null hypothesis.

## □ 8.4.1  The F Distribution

The distribution of the variance ratio $(s_1^2/s_2^2)$ was studied by the statisticians R. A. Fisher and G. Snedecor. It can be shown that the variance ratio follows an **F distribution** under the null hypothesis that $\sigma_1^2 = \sigma_2^2$. There is no unique $F$ distribution but instead a family of $F$ distributions. This family is indexed by two parameters termed the *numerator and denominator degrees of freedom* (d.f.), respectively. Specifically, if the sample sizes of the first and second samples are $n_1$ and $n_2$, respectively, then the variance ratio follows an $F$ distribution with $n_1 - 1$ (numerator d.f.) and $n_2 - 1$ (denominator d.f.), which we denote by $F_{n_1-1, n_2-1}$.

The $F$ distribution is generally positively skewed, with the skewness dependent on the relative magnitudes of the two degrees of freedom. If the numerator degree of freedom is 1, then the distribution has a mode at 0; otherwise, it has a mode at some point greater than 0. This distribution is illustrated in Figure 8.5. Table 8 gives the percentiles of the $F$ distribution.

**Definition 8.6**

We shall denote the **pth percentile of an F distribution** with $d_1$ and $d_2$ degrees of freedom by $F_{d_1, d_2, p}$. Thus

$$Pr(F_{d_1, d_2} \leqslant F_{d_1, d_2, p}) = p$$    ∎

The $F$ table is organized such that the different numerator d.f. $(d_1)$ are listed in the first row, the different denominator d.f. $(d_2)$ are listed in the first column, and the various percentiles $(p)$ are listed in the second column.

**Example 8.12**    Find the upper 1st percentile of an $F$ distribution with 5 and 9 degrees of freedom.

**Solution**    We must find $F_{5,9,.99}$. We look in the 5 column, the 9 row, and the sub row marked 0.99 to obtain

$$F_{5,9,.99} = 6.06$$    ∎

Generally, $F$ distribution tables give only upper percentage points because the symmetry properties of the $F$ distribution make it possible to derive the

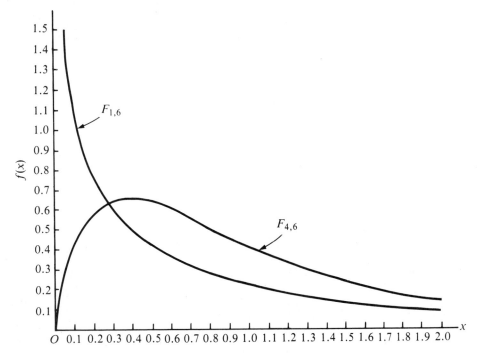

**Figure 8.5**
Probability density
for the F distribution

lower percentage points of any $F$ distribution from the corresponding upper percentage points of an $F$ distribution with the appropriate degrees of freedom. The computation is shown as follows:

### 8.13 Computation of the Lower Percentiles of an F Distribution

The *lower pth percentile* of an $F$ distribution with $d_1$ and $d_2$ d.f. is the reciprocal of the *upper pth percentile* of an $F$ distribution with $d_2$ and $d_1$ d.f. In symbols,

$$F_{d_1, d_2, p} = 1/F_{d_2, d_1, 1-p}$$

Thus, from **(8.13)** we see that the lower $p$th percentile of any $F$ distribution is the same as the inverse of the upper $p$th percentile of an $F$ distribution with the degrees of freedom reversed.

*Example 8.13*  Estimate $F_{6,8,.05}$.

*Solution*  From **(8.13)**,

$$F_{6,8,.05} = 1/F_{8,6,.95} = 1/4.15 = 0.241$$  ∎

### ☐ 8.4.2 Interpolation for the F Table

Frequently, either the numerator d.f. or the denominator d.f. does not appear in the $F$ tables. We then need to estimate percentiles by performing some type of interpolation based on the percentiles given in the table. **Harmonic interpolation** is a useful method of interpolation whereby we interpolate linearly using the inverse of both the numerator and denominator degrees of freedom. This method of interpolation is similar to that presented for the $t$ distribution in Section 7.5.1 and is shown as follows:

**8.14**    *Interpolation for the F Table*

Suppose we wish to estimate the $p$th percentile of an $F$ distribution with $d_1$ and $d_2$ d.f. ($F_{d_1, d_2, p}$), where neither $d_1$ nor $d_2$ appears in the table.

*1.* We find $a_1$ and $b_1$ such that $a_1 \leqslant d_1 \leqslant b_1$, and $a_1$ and $b_1$ are given in the table for the numerator d.f.

*2.* We find $a_2$ and $b_2$ such that $a_2 \leqslant d_2 \leqslant b_2$, and $a_2$ and $b_2$ are given in the table for the denominator d.f.

*3.* We estimate $F_{d_1, a_2, p}$ by

$$F_{d_1, a_2, p} \approx \frac{[(1/d_1) - (1/b_1)]F_{a_1, a_2, p} + [(1/a_1) - (1/d_1)]F_{b_1, a_2, p}}{[(1/a_1) - (1/b_1)]}$$

*4.* We estimate $F_{d_1, b_2, p}$ by

$$F_{d_1, b_2, p} \approx \frac{[(1/d_1) - (1/b_1)]F_{a_1, b_2, p} + [(1/a_1) - (1/d_1)]F_{b_1, b_2, p}}{[(1/a_1) - (1/b_1)]}$$

*5.* We then interpolate linearly in the inverse of the denominator d.f. as follows:

$$F_{d_1, d_2, p} \approx \frac{[(1/d_2) - (1/b_2)]F_{d_1, a_2, p} + [(1/a_2) - (1/d_2)]F_{d_1, b_2, p}}{[(1/a_2) - (1/b_2)]}$$

*Example 8.14*    Estimate the 99.9th percentile of an $F$ distribution with 99 and 73 d.f.

*Solution*    We note that 99 is not listed for the numerator d.f. nor is 73 listed for the denominator d.f. However, 24 and $\infty$ are listed for the numerator d.f., where $24 \leqslant 99 \leqslant \infty$, and 60 and 120 are listed for the denominator d.f., where $60 \leqslant 73 \leqslant 120$. Thus, we set $a_1 = 24$, $b_1 = \infty$, $a_2 = 60$, $b_2 = 120$, $d_1 = 99$, $d_2 = 73$ and apply **(8.14)**. First, we estimate $F_{99, 60, .999}$ as follows, noting that $1/\infty = 0$.

$$F_{99, 60, .999} = \frac{[(1/99) - (1/\infty)]F_{24, 60, .999} + [(1/24) - (1/99)]F_{\infty, 60, .999}}{[(1/24) - (1/\infty)]}$$

$$= \frac{(1/99)(2.69) + [(1/24) - (1/99)](1.89)}{1/24}$$

$$= 0.0868/0.0417 = 2.082$$

Second, we estimate $F_{99, 120, .999}$ as follows:

$$F_{99, 120, .999} = \frac{[(1/99) - (1/\infty)]F_{24, 120, .999} + [(1/24) - (1/99)]F_{\infty, 120, .999}}{[(1/24) - (1/\infty)]}$$

$$= \frac{(1/99)(2.40) + [(1/24) - (1/99)](1.54)}{1/24}$$

$$= 0.0729/0.0417 = 1.748$$

Third, we estimate $F_{99,73,.999}$ as follows:

$$F_{99,73,.999} = \frac{[(1/73) - (1/120)]F_{99,60,.999} + [(1/60) - (1/73)]F_{99,120,.999}}{[(1/60) - (1/120)]}$$

$$= \frac{[(1/73) - (1/120)](2.082) + [(1/60) - (1/73)](1.748)}{[(1/60) - (1/120)]}$$

$$= 0.01636/0.00833 = 1.96 \qquad \blacksquare$$

## ☐ 8.4.3 The F Test

We now return to our significance test for the equality of two variances. We wish to test the hypothesis $H_0: \sigma_1^2 = \sigma_2^2$ vs. $H_1: \sigma_1^2 \neq \sigma_2^2$. We stated that we would base our test on the variance ratio $s_1^2/s_2^2$, which under $H_0$ follows an $F$ distribution with $n_1 - 1$ and $n_2 - 1$ d.f. Since we are conducting a two-sided test, we wish to reject $H_0$ for both small and large values of $s_1^2/s_2^2$. This procedure can be made more specific, as follows:

**8.15**  **F Test for the Equality of Two Variances**

In conducting a test of the hypothesis $H_0: \sigma_1^2 = \sigma_2^2$ vs. $H_1: \sigma_1^2 \neq \sigma_2^2$ with significance level $\alpha$, if

$$\lambda = s_1^2/s_2^2 > F_{n_1-1,n_2-1,1-\alpha/2} \qquad \text{or} \qquad \lambda < F_{n_1-1,n_2-1,\alpha/2}$$

then we reject $H_0$. If

$$F_{n_1-1,n_2-1,\alpha/2} \leqslant \lambda \leqslant F_{n_1-1,n_2-1,1-\alpha/2}$$

then we accept $H_0$. The acceptance and rejection regions for this test are depicted in Figure 8.6.

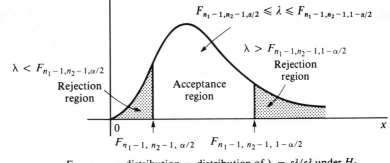

**Figure 8.6**
*Acceptance and rejection regions for the F test for the equality of two variances*

$$F_{n_1-1, n_2-1} \text{ distribution} = \text{distribution of } \lambda = s_1^2/s_2^2 \text{ under } H_0$$

Alternatively, the exact $p$-value is given by:

**8.16**  **Computation of the P-value for the F Test for the Equality of Two Variances**

$$p = 2 \times Pr(F_{n_1-1,n_2-1} > \lambda) \qquad \text{if } \lambda = s_1^2/s_2^2 \geqslant 1$$

$$p = 2 \times Pr(F_{n_1-1,n_2-1} < \lambda) \qquad \text{if } \lambda < 1$$

This computation is illustrated in Figure 8.7.

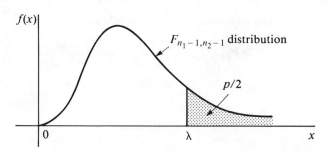

If $\lambda = s_1^2/s_2^2 \geq 1$, then $p = 2 \times$ (area to the right of $\lambda$ under an $F_{n_1-1,\,n_2-1}$ distribution).

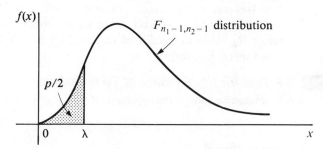

**Figure 8.7**
Computation of the
p-value for the F
test for the equality
of two variances

If $\lambda = s_1^2/s_2^2 < 1$, then $p = 2 \times$ (area to the left of $\lambda$ under an $F_{n_1-1,\,n_2-1}$ distribution).

**Example 8.15**　　**Cardiovascular Disease, Pediatrics**　Test for the equality of the two variances given in Example 8.11.

**Solution**　　We see that

$$\lambda = s_1^2/s_2^2 = (35.6)^2/(17.3)^2 = 4.23$$

Since the two samples have 100 and 74 persons, respectively, we know from **(8.15)** that under $H_0, \lambda \sim F_{99,73}$. Thus, we reject $H_0$ if

$$\lambda > F_{99,73,.975} \quad \text{or} \quad \lambda < F_{99,73,.025}$$

We note from Example 8.14 that $F_{99,73,.999} = 1.96$. Since $\lambda = 4.23 > 1.96$, it follows that $p/2 < 1 - 0.999 = 0.001$ or $p < 0.002$. Thus the two sample variances are significantly different. We cannot use the two-sample $t$ test with equal variances, as given in Section 8.3, since this test depends on the assumption that the variances are equal. ■

We can often compute a satisfactory approximate $p$-value for our test using the d.f. that appear in Table 8, without the need for interpolating. The general rule is to find a numerator ($a_1$) d.f. and denominator ($a_2$) d.f. in the table that are either both less than or both greater than the d.f. we are interested in (say, $d_1, d_2$):

**8.17**　　If $p > 0.50$

$$a_1 \leqslant d_1 \quad \text{and} \quad a_2 \leqslant d_2$$

Then,

$$F_{d_1,d_2,p} \leqslant F_{a_1,a_2,p}$$

Similarly, if

$$a_1 \geqslant d_1 \quad \text{and} \quad a_2 \geqslant d_2$$

then

$$F_{d_1,d_2,p} \geqslant F_{a_1,a_2,p}$$

From **(8.17)**, if $a_1 \leqslant d_1$, $a_2 \leqslant d_2$, and $\lambda = s_1^2/s_2^2 > F_{a_1,a_2,1-\alpha/2}$, then $\lambda > F_{d_1,d_2,1-\alpha/2}$, and we can reject $H_0$ using a two-sided test with significance level $\alpha$. Similarly, if $a_1 \geqslant d_1$, $a_2 \geqslant d_2$, and $\lambda = s_1^2/s_2^2 < F_{a_1,a_2,1-\alpha/2}$, then $\lambda < F_{d_1,d_2,1-\alpha/2}$, and we can accept $H_0$ using a two-sided test with significance level $\alpha$.

**Example 8.16**     Evaluate the significance of the test statistic in Example 8.15 without using interpolation.

**Solution**     We need percentiles for an $F_{99,73}$ distribution, but 99 does not appear under the numerator d.f. and 73 does not appear under the denominator d.f. However, 24 does appear under numerator d.f., and 60 appears under denominator d.f. Thus from **(8.17)**,

$$F_{99,73,.999} \leqslant F_{24,60,.999} = 2.69 < 4.23 = s_1^2/s_2^2 = \lambda$$

Thus, without interpolation we can conclude that $p/2 < 0.001$ or $p < 0.002$ and that the two variances are significantly different.     ∎

A question often asked about the $F$ test is whether or not it makes a difference which sample is selected as the "numerator sample" and which as the "denominator sample." The answer is that it *does not* make a difference, because of the rules for calculating lower percentiles given in **(8.13)**. A variance ratio $> 1$ usually is more convenient, so that we do not need to use **(8.13)**. Thus, the larger variance is usually put in the numerator and the smaller variance in the denominator.

**Example 8.17**     *Cardiovascular Disease, Hypertension*  Using the data in Example 8.7, test whether or not the variance of blood pressure is significantly different among OC users and non-OC users.

**Solution**     We note that the sample standard deviation of blood pressure for the 8 OC users was 15.34 and for the 21 non-OC users was 18.23. Hence the variance ratio is

$$\lambda = (18.23/15.34)^2 = 1.41$$

Under $H_0$, $\lambda$ follows an $F$ distribution with 20 and 7 d.f. We note that from **(8.17)**

$$F_{20,7,.975} \geqslant F_{24,7,.975} = 4.42 > 1.41$$

It follows that $p > 2(0.025) = 0.05$, and the underlying variances of the two samples are not significantly different from each other. Thus we were correct in using the two-sample $t$ test for independent samples with *equal variances* for these data, where we assumed the variances were the same.

Suppose we changed the numerator and denominator samples so that the variance for OC users was in the numerator and the variance for non-OC users was in the denominator. The variance ratio $= \lambda$ would then be $(15.34/18.23)^2 = 1/1.41 = 0.71$. Under $H_0$, $\lambda$ follows an $F_{7,20}$ distribution. Thus, from **(8.15)**, since $\lambda < 1$, we wish to compare 0.71 with $F_{7,20,.025}$ to test for statistical significance at the 5% level. However, from **(8.13)** we have

$$F_{7,20,.025} = 1/F_{20,7,.975} \leqslant 1/F_{24,7,.975} = 1/4.42 = 0.23 < 0.71 = \lambda$$

and it follows that $\lambda$ falls in the acceptance region at the 5% level or $p/2 > 0.025$ or $p > 0.05$. Notice that the arithmetic is equivalent whether we compare 1.41 with 4.42 when the non-OC users were in the numerator or 1/1.41 with 1/4.42 when the OC users were in the numerator. Which sample is placed in the numerator is simply a matter of convenience. ∎

If we wish to compute an exact $p$-value, and/or avoid using the preceding interpolation methods, then we must use a computer program to evaluate the area under the $F$ distribution. We have evaluated the exact $p$-value for Example 8.17 using the HP-41C $F$ distribution program, with the results given in Table 8.4. The program evaluates the right-hand tail area $= Pr(F_{20,7} > 1.41) = 0.335$. Thus, the two-tailed $p$-value $= 2 \times 0.335 = 0.670$.

**Table 8.4**

*Computation of the exact p-value for the blood pressure data in Example 8.17 using the F test for the equality of two variances with the HP-41C F distribution program*

```
                    XEQ "FDIST"
                 20.00000  XEQ A
(a)   V1=20.00000
                  7.00000  XEQ B
(b)   V2=7.00000
(c)               1.41000  XEQ C
                           RUN
(d)   P=0.33516
                  2.00000     *
(e)               0.67031   ***
```

(a)   Numerator degrees of freedom

(b)   Denominator degrees of freedom

(c)   $\lambda$

(d)   Right-hand tail area

(e)   Exact two-tailed p-value

# ■ 8.5 TWO-SAMPLE $t$ TEST FOR INDEPENDENT SAMPLES WITH UNEQUAL VARIANCES

We have presented the $F$ test for the equality of two variances from two independent, normally distributed samples in **(8.15)**. If the two variances *are not* significantly different, then we can use the two-sample $t$ test for independent samples with *equal variances* outlined in Section 8.3. If the two variances *are* significantly different, then we must use a two-sample $t$ test for independent samples with *unequal variances*, which will be presented in this section.

Specifically, we assume that we have two normally distributed samples, where the first sample has mean $\mu_1$ and variance $\sigma_1^2$ and the second sample has mean $\mu_2$ and variance $\sigma_2^2$ ($\sigma_1^2 \neq \sigma_2^2$). We again wish to test the hypothesis $H_0: \mu_1 = \mu_2$ vs. $H_1: \mu_1 \neq \mu_2$. Statisticians refer to this problem as the **Behrens-Fisher problem**.

It still makes sense to base our significance test on the difference between the sample means $\bar{x} - \bar{y}$. Under either hypothesis, $\bar{x}$ is normally distributed with mean $\mu_1$ and variance $\sigma_1^2/n_1$, and $\bar{y}$ is normally distributed with mean $\mu_2$ and variance $\sigma_2^2/n_2$. Hence it follows that

**8.18**

$$\bar{x} - \bar{y} \sim N\left(\mu_1 - \mu_2, \frac{\sigma_1^2}{n_1} + \frac{\sigma_2^2}{n_2}\right)$$

Under $H_0$, $\mu_1 - \mu_2 = 0$. Thus from **(8.18)** we have

**8.19**

$$\bar{x} - \bar{y} \sim N\left(0, \frac{\sigma_1^2}{n_1} + \frac{\sigma_2^2}{n_2}\right)$$

If $\sigma_1^2$ and $\sigma_2^2$ were known, then we could use the test statistic

**8.20**

$$\lambda' = (\bar{x} - \bar{y}) \Bigg/ \sqrt{\frac{\sigma_1^2}{n_1} + \frac{\sigma_2^2}{n_2}}$$

for our significance test, which under $H_0$ would be distributed as a $N(0, 1)$ distribution. However, $\sigma_1^2$ and $\sigma_2^2$ in general are unknown, and we estimate them by $s_1^2$ and $s_2^2$, respectively (i.e., the sample variances in the two samples). Notice that we do not compute a pooled estimate of the variance as we did in **(8.9)**, because the variances $(\sigma_1^2, \sigma_2^2)$ are assumed to be different. If we substitute $s_1^2$ for $\sigma_1^2$ and $s_2^2$ for $\sigma_2^2$ in **(8.20)**, then we obtain the test statistic

**8.21**

$$\lambda = (\bar{x} - \bar{y})/\sqrt{s_1^2/n_1 + s_2^2/n_2}$$

We can show that under $H_0$, $\lambda$ follows a $t$ distribution. The problem is that the appropriate number of degrees of freedom for $\lambda$ depends on $\sigma_1^2, \sigma_2^2, n_1$, and $n_2$. Several approximate solutions have been proposed that yield comparable results. We present the Satterthwaite approximation here, the advantage of which is its easy implementation using the ordinary $t$ tables and the interpolation formula for the $t$ distribution given in **(7.19)** [2].

**8.22** *Two-Sample t Test for Independent Samples with Unequal Variances (Satterthwaite's Method)*

*1.* Compute the test statistic

$$\lambda = \frac{\bar{x} - \bar{y}}{\sqrt{\dfrac{s_1^2}{n_1} + \dfrac{s_2^2}{n_2}}}$$

*2.* Compute the approximate degrees of freedom $d'$, where

$$d' = \frac{(s_1^2/n_1 + s_2^2/n_2)^2}{(s_1^2/n_1)^2/(n_1 - 1) + (s_2^2/n_2)^2/(n_2 - 1)}$$

3. Round $d'$ down to the nearest integer $d''$. If

$$\lambda > t_{d'',1-\alpha/2} \quad \text{or} \quad \lambda < -t_{d'',1-\alpha/2}$$

then we reject $H_0$. If

$$-t_{d'',1-\alpha/2} \leqslant \lambda \leqslant t_{d'',1-\alpha/2}$$

then we accept $H_0$.

The acceptance and rejection regions for this test are illustrated in Figure 8.8.
Similarly, we can compute the exact *p*-value for our hypothesis test as follows:

**8.23** **Computation of the P-value for the Two-Sample Test for Independent Samples with Unequal Variances (Satterthwaite Approximation)**

If

$$\lambda = \frac{\bar{x} - \bar{y}}{\sqrt{\dfrac{s_1^2}{n_1} + \dfrac{s_2^2}{n_2}}} \leqslant 0$$

then

$$p = 2 \times (\text{area to the left of } \lambda \text{ under a } t_{d''} \text{ distribution})$$

If $\lambda > 0$, then

$$p = 2 \times (\text{area to the right of } \lambda \text{ under a } t_{d''} \text{ distribution})$$

The computation of the *p*-value is illustrated in Figure 8.9.

*Example 8.18*

**Cardiovascular Disease, Pediatrics** Let us consider the cholesterol data presented in Example 8.11. Test for the equality of the mean cholesterol levels of the children whose fathers have died from heart disease and whose fathers do not have a history of heart disease.

*Solution*

We have already tested for the equality of the two variances in Example 8.15 and have found them to be significantly different. Thus, we must use the *t* test for unequal variances given in

*Figure 8.8*

*Acceptance and rejection regions for the two-sample t test for independent samples with unequal variances*

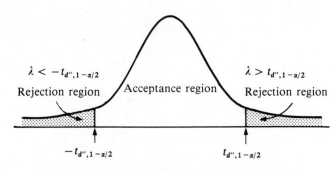

$\lambda < -t_{d'',1-\alpha/2}$    $\lambda > t_{d'',1-\alpha/2}$

Rejection region    Acceptance region    Rejection region

$-t_{d'',1-\alpha/2}$    $t_{d'',1-\alpha/2}$

$t_{d''}$ distribution = distribution of $\lambda$ in **(8.22)** under $H_0$

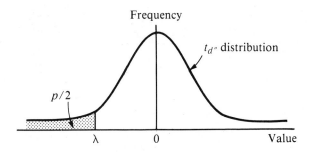

If $\lambda = (\bar{x}_1 - \bar{x}_2)/(\sqrt{s_1^2/n_1 + s_2^2/n_2}) \leqslant 0$,

then $p = 2 \times$ (area to the left of $\lambda$ under a $t_{d''}$ distribution).

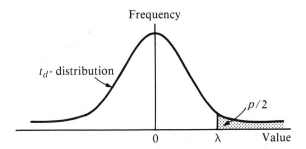

**Figure 8.9**
*Computation of the p-value for the two-sample t test for independent samples with unequal variances*

If $\lambda = (\bar{x}_1 - \bar{x}_2)/(\sqrt{s_1^2/n_1 + s_2^2/n_2}) > 0$,

then $p = 2 \times$ (area to the right of $\lambda$ under a $t_{d''}$ distribution).

**(8.22).** Our test statistic is

$$\lambda = \frac{207.3 - 193.4}{\sqrt{35.6^2/100 + 17.3^2/74}} = \frac{13.9}{4.089} = 3.40$$

We now compute the approximate degrees of freedom. We have

$$d' = \frac{(s_1^2/n_1 + s_2^2/n_2)^2}{(s_1^2/n_1)^2/(n_1 - 1) + (s_2^2/n_2)^2/(n_2 - 1)}$$

$$= \frac{(35.6^2/100 + 17.3^2/74)^2}{(35.6^2/100)^2/99 + (17.3^2/74)^2/73}$$

$$= \frac{(16.718)^2}{1.8465}$$

$$= 151.4$$

Therefore, the approximate degrees of freedom $= d'' = 151$. If we use the critical value method, we note that $\lambda = 3.40 > t_{120,.975} = 1.980 > t_{151,.975}$. Therefore, we can reject $H_0$ using a two-sided test with $\alpha = 0.05$. Furthermore, $\lambda = 3.40 > t_{120,.9995} = 3.373 > t_{151,.9995}$, which implies that the p-value $< 2 \times (1.0 - 0.9995) = 0.001$. We conclude that the cholesterol levels in children of fathers who have died from heart disease is greater than the cholesterol

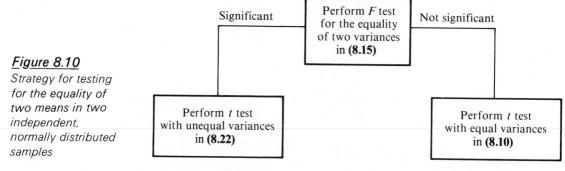

**Figure 8.10**
*Strategy for testing for the equality of two means in two independent, normally distributed samples*

levels in children of fathers without heart disease. It would be of great interest to identify the source of this difference, that is, whether it is due to genetic factors, environmental factors such as diet, or both.    ∎

In this chapter we have presented a number of procedures for the comparison of two means from independent, normally distributed samples. The first step in this process is to test for the equality of the two variances using the $F$ test in **(8.15)**. If this test is not significant, then we use the $t$ test with equal variances; otherwise, we use the $t$ test with unequal variances. This overall strategy is illustrated in Figure 8.10.

**Example 8.19**

*Infectious Disease*  Using the data in Table 2.11, compare the duration of hospitalization among antibiotic users and nonantibiotic users.

**Solution**

We refer to Table 8.5, where the SPSS/PC independent samples T-TEST program was used to analyze these data. We note that among the 7 antibiotic users (ANTIB = 1), the mean duration of hospitalization was 11.57 days with standard deviation 8.81 days; whereas among the 18 nonantibiotic users (ANTIB = 2), the mean duration of hospitalization was 7.44 days with standard deviation 3.70 days. Both the $F$ test and the $t$ test with equal and unequal vari-

**Table 8.5**
*Use of the SPSS/PC independent samples T-TEST program to analyze the association between antibiotic use and duration of hospitalization (raw data presented in Table 2.11)*

```
                            SPSS/PC   Release 1.0

        Independent samples of  ANTIB     received antibiotic

        Group 1:  ANTIB  EQ     1.00          Group 2:  ANTIB  EQ     2.00


        t-test for:  DUR       duration of hospitalization

                         Number              Standard    Standard
                        of Cases    Mean     Deviation     Error

            Group 1        7       11.5714     8.810       3.330
            Group 2       18        7.4444     3.698       0.872
```

| | Pooled Variance Estimate | | | Separate Variance Estimate | | |
|---|---|---|---|---|---|---|
| F    2-Tail<br>Value  Prob. | t<br>Value | Degrees of<br>Freedom | 2-Tail<br>Prob. | t<br>Value | Degrees of<br>Freedom | 2-Tail<br>Prob. |
| 5.68   0.004 | 1.68 | 23 | 0.106 | 1.20 | 6.84 | 0.270 |

ances are displayed in this program. Using Figure 8.10, we note that the first step in comparing the two means is to perform the $F$ test for the equality of two variances in order to decide whether to use the $t$ test with equal or with unequal variances. The $F$ statistic is given in Table 8.5 by $F$ Value $= 5.68$, with $p$-value (labeled 2-Tail Prob.) $= 0.004$. Thus, the variances are significantly different, and we should use a two-sample $t$ test with unequal variances. Therefore, we refer to the output labeled Separate Variance Estimate, where we find that the $t$ statistic [as given in **(8.22)**] is 1.20 with degrees of freedom $d' = 6.84$. The corresponding two-tailed $p$-value (labeled 2-Tail Prob.) $= 0.270$. Thus, there is no significant difference between the mean durations of hospitalization in these two groups.

If the results of the $F$ test had revealed a nonsignificant difference between the variances of the two samples, then we would have used the $t$ test with equal variances, which is provided in the output labeled Pooled Variance Estimate. In this case considerable differences are present in both the test statistics (1.68 vs. 1.20) and the two-tailed $p$-values (0.106 vs. 0.270) resulting from using these two procedures. ∎

Using similar methods to those developed in Section 6.4, we can also show that a two-sided $100\% \times (1 - \alpha)$ confidence interval for the underlying mean difference $\mu_1 - \mu_2$ in the case of unequal variances is given as follows:

**8.24**    ***Two-Sided 100% × (1 − α) Confidence Interval for*** $\mu_1 - \mu_2 (\sigma_1^2 \neq \sigma_2^2)$

$$(\bar{x}_1 - \bar{x}_2 - t_{d'',1-\alpha/2}\sqrt{s_1^2/n_1 + s_2^2/n_2}, \quad \bar{x}_1 - \bar{x}_2 + t_{d'',1-\alpha/2}\sqrt{s_1^2/n_1 + s_2^2/n_2})$$

*Example 8.20*    **Cardiovascular Disease, Pediatrics** Using the data in Table 8.5, compute a 95% confidence interval for the mean difference in duration of hospital stay between patients who do and patients who do not receive antibiotics.

*Solution*    Referring to Table 8.5, we see that the 95% confidence interval is given by

$$[11.571 - 7.444 - t_{6,.975}\sqrt{(8.810)^2/7 + (3.698)^2/18}\,,$$

$$11.571 - 7.444 + t_{6,.975}\sqrt{(8.810)^2/7 + (3.698)^2/18}]$$

$$= [4.127 - 2.447(3.442), 4.127 + 2.447(3.442)]$$

$$= (4.127 - 8.423, 4.127 + 8.423)$$

$$= (-4.30, 12.55)$$

∎

# ■ 8.6 SAMPLE SIZE DETERMINATION FOR COMPARING TWO MEANS

We have presented methods of sample size estimation for the one-sample normal test in Section 7.7. We now present estimates of sample size that are useful in planning studies in which *two* samples are to be compared.

*Example 8.21*    **Cardiovascular Disease, Hypertension** Let us consider the blood pressure data for OC users and non-OC users given in Example 8.7 as a pilot study conducted to obtain parameter estimates to plan for a larger study. Suppose we assume that the true blood pressure distribution of 35–39-year-old OC users is normal with mean $\mu_1$ and variance $\sigma_1^2$. Similarly, for non-OC users we assume that the distribution is normal with mean $\mu_2$ and variance $\sigma_2^2$. We wish to test the hypothesis $H_0: \mu_1 = \mu_2$ vs. $H_1: \mu_1 \neq \mu_2$. How can we estimate the sample size needed for the larger study?  ∎

Suppose we assume that $\sigma_1^2$ and $\sigma_2^2$ are known and we anticipate equal sample sizes in the two groups. If we wish to conduct a two-sided test with significance level $\alpha$ and a power of $1 - \beta$, then we can show that the appropriate sample size for *each* group is as follows:

---

**8.25**   **Sample Size Needed for Comparing the Means of Two Normally Distributed Samples of Equal Size Using a Two-Sided Test with Significance Level $\alpha$ and Power $1 - \beta$**

$$n = \frac{(\sigma_1^2 + \sigma_2^2)(z_{1-\alpha/2} + z_{1-\beta})^2}{\Delta^2} = \text{sample size for each sample}$$

where $\Delta = \mu_2 - \mu_1$. The means and variances of the two respective samples are $(\mu_1, \sigma_1^2)$ and $(\mu_2, \sigma_2^2)$.

---

In words, $n$ is the appropriate sample size in each group to have a probability of $1 - \beta$ of finding a significant difference if the true difference in means between the two groups is $\mu_2 - \mu_1$ based on a two-sided level $\alpha$ significance test.

*Example 8.22*     **Cardiovascular Disease, Hypertension**  Determine the appropriate sample size for the large study proposed in Example 8.21 using a two-sided test with a significance level of 0.05 and a power of 0.80.

*Solution*     We found that

$$\bar{x}_1 = 132.86$$

$$s_1 = 15.34$$

$$\bar{x}_2 = 127.44$$

$$s_2 = 18.23$$

in our small study. If we assume that

$$\mu_1 = \bar{x}_1$$

$$\sigma_1^2 = s_1^2$$

$$\mu_2 = \bar{x}_2$$

$$\sigma_2^2 = s_2^2$$

then ensuring an 80% chance of finding a significant difference using a two-sided significance test with $\alpha = 0.05$ would require a sample size of

$$n = (15.34^2 + 18.23^2)(1.96 + 0.84)^2/(132.86 - 127.44)^2 = 151.5$$

or 152 persons in each group. It is not surprising that we did not find a significant difference with sample sizes of 8 and 21 in the two groups, respectively.  ∎

In many instances we can anticipate an imbalance between the groups and can predict in advance that the number of persons in one group will be $k$ times the number in the other group for some number $k \neq 1$. In this case, where $n_2 = kn_1$, the appropriate sample size in the two groups for achieving a power of $1 - \beta$ using a two-sided level $\alpha$ significance test is given by the following formulas:

**8.26** **Sample Size Needed for Comparing the Means of Two Normally Distributed Samples of Unequal Size Using a Two-Sided Test with Significance Level $\alpha$ and Power $1 - \beta$**

$$n_1 = \frac{(\sigma_1^2 + \sigma_2^2/k)(z_{1-\alpha/2} + z_{1-\beta})^2}{\Delta^2} = \text{sample size of first sample}$$

$$n_2 = \frac{(k\sigma_1^2 + \sigma_2^2)(z_{1-\alpha/2} + z_{1-\beta})^2}{\Delta^2} = \text{sample size of second sample}$$

where $\Delta = \mu_2 - \mu_1$; $(\mu_1, \sigma_1^2)$, $(\mu_2, \sigma_2^2)$ are the means and variances of the two respective samples; and $k = n_2/n_1 = $ projected ratio of the two sample sizes.

*Example 8.23*    **Cardiovascular Disease** Suppose we anticipate 2 times as many non-OC users as OC users entering the study proposed in Example 8.21. Project the required sample size if a two-sided test is used with a 5% significance level and an 80% power is desired.

*Solution*    If we use **(8.26)** with

$$\mu_1 = 132.86$$
$$\sigma_1 = 15.34$$
$$\mu_2 = 127.44$$
$$\sigma_2 = 18.23$$
$$k = 2$$
$$\alpha = 0.05$$
$$1 - \beta = 0.8$$

then, to achieve an 80% power in the study using a two-sided significance test with $\alpha = 0.05$, we need to enroll

$$n_1 = \frac{(15.34^2 + 18.23^2/2)(1.96 + 0.84)^2}{(132.86 - 127.44)^2}$$

$$= 107.1, \text{ or } 108 \text{ OC users}$$

and

$$n_2 = 2(108) = 216 \text{ non-OC users} \qquad \blacksquare$$

If the variances in the *two groups* are *the same*, then we can show that for a given $\alpha$, $\beta$, the smallest total sample size needed is achieved by the *equal sample size allocation rule* in **(8.25)**. Thus in this case, that is, with equal variances, we want to have the sample sizes in the two groups as nearly equal as possible.

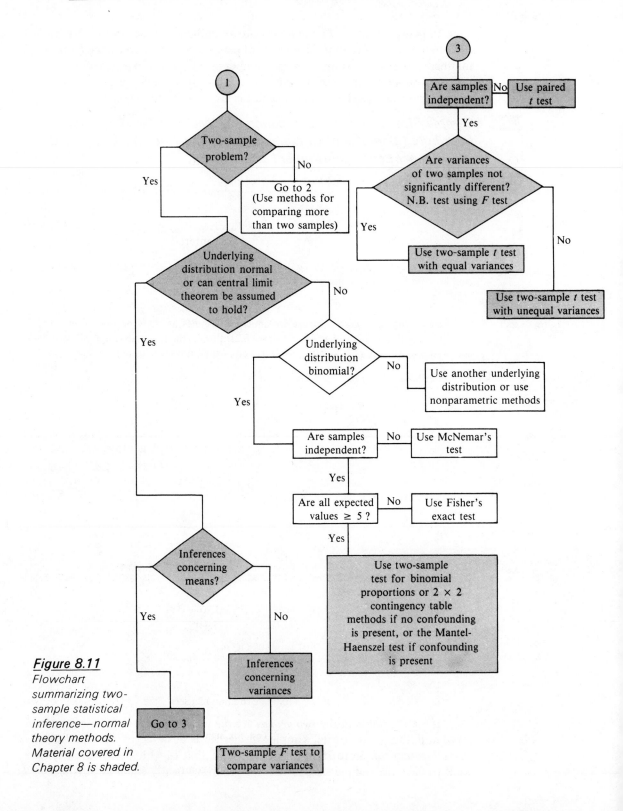

***Figure 8.11***

*Flowchart summarizing two-sample statistical inference—normal theory methods. Material covered in Chapter 8 is shaded.*

Finally, if we intend to perform a one-sided test rather than a two-sided test, then we simply replace $1 - \alpha/2$ by $1 - \alpha$ in the sample size formulas in **(8.25)** and **(8.26)**.

# ■ *8.7 SUMMARY*

In this chapter we studied methods of hypothesis testing for comparing the means and variances of two samples that are assumed to be normally distributed. The basic strategy is outlined in the shaded boxes of the flowchart in Figure 8.11, which is an extract from the larger flowchart in the back of this book. Referring to ① in the upper left, we first note that we are dealing with the case of a two-sample problem in which either the underlying distributions are normal or the central limit theorem can be assumed to hold. If we are interested in comparing the means of the two samples, then we refer to box ③. If our two samples are paired, that is, if each person is used as his or her own control or if the samples consist of different persons who are matched on a one-to-one basis, then the **paired *t* test** is appropriate. If the samples are independent, then we first use the ***F* test for the equality of two variances** to decide whether or not the variances are significantly different. If the variances are not significantly different, then we use the **two-sample *t* test with equal variances**; if the variances are significantly different, then we use the **two-sample *t* test with unequal variances**. If we are only interested in comparing the variances of the two samples, then we need only use the *F* test for comparing variances, as indicated in the lower left of Figure 8.11.

We concluded the chapter by presenting appropriate sample size formulas for planning investigations in which the goal is to compare the means from two finite samples. We will proceed in the next chapter to look at alternative test procedures to those presented in this chapter, when the assumptions of normality are no longer valid. These procedures are called **nonparametric tests** opposed to the **parametric tests** presented in Chapters 7 and 8, where specific assumptions are made about the underlying distributions.

# $P$*roblems* ▬▬▬▬▬▬▬▬▬▬▬▬▬

*Ophthalmology*

In a study of the natural history of retinitis pigmentosa (RP), 94 RP patients were followed for 3 years [3]. Among 90 patients with complete follow-up, the mean $\pm 1$ se of $\log_e$ (visual field loss) over 1, 2, and 3 years was $0.02 \pm 0.04$, $0.08 \pm 0.05$, and $0.14 \pm 0.07$, respectively.

**8.1** What test procedure can be used to test for changes in $\log_e$ (visual field) over any given time period?

**8.2** Implement the procedure in Problem 8.1 to test for significant changes in visual field over 1 year. Report a *p*-value.

**8.3** Answer Problem 8.2 for changes over 2 years.

**8.4** Answer Problem 8.2 for changes over 3 years.

*Cardiovascular Disease*

Twenty volunteers adopt a low-cholesterol diet for a 3-month period. The mean $\pm 1$ sd of changes in serum cholesterol over the 3-month period was $20.0 \pm 35.0$ (mg/dl).

**8.5** Test for significant changes in cholesterol over 3 months.

One important component of cholesterol, which is

widely believed to have a beneficial effect on heart disease, is HDL cholesterol. The mean $\pm 1$ sd of changes in HDL cholesterol over the 3-month period was $3.0 \pm 12.0$ (mg/dl).

**8.6** Test for significant changes in HDL cholesterol over 3 months.

The mean $\pm 1$ sd weight loss over the 3-month period was $5.2 \pm 8.0$ (lb).

**8.7** Test for significant changes in weight over 3 months.

**8.8** Find the upper 5th percentile of an $F$ distribution with 24 and 30 $df$.

**8.9** Find the lower 2.5th percentile of an $F$ distribution with 14 and 7 $df$.

**8.10** Find the upper 5th percentile of an $F$ distribution with 22 and 14 $df$.

**8.11** Find the upper 1st percentile of an $F$ distribution with 22 and 35 $df$.

**8.12** Find the lower 2.5th percentile of an $F$ distribution with 50 and 10 $df$.

**8.13** Suppose we have two samples of sizes 9 and 15 with sample standard deviations of 13.7 and 7.2, respectively. Test if the variances are significantly different in the two samples.

**8.14** Suppose we have two samples of sizes 16 and 12 with sample standard deviations of 12.6 and 6.2, respectively. Test if the variances are significantly different in the two samples.

### Nutrition

The mean $\pm 1$ sd of $\log_e$ [calcium intake (mg)] among 25 12–14-year-old females below the poverty level is $6.56 \pm 0.64$. Similarly, the mean $\pm 1$ sd of $\log_e$ [calcium intake (mg)] among 40 12–14-year-old females above the poverty level is $6.80 \pm 0.76$.

**8.15** Test for a significant difference between the variances of the two groups.

**8.16** What is the appropriate procedure to test for a significant difference in means between the two groups?

**8.17** Implement the procedure in Problem 8.16 using the critical value method.

**8.18** What is the $p$-value corresponding to your answer to Problem 8.17?

**8.19** Compute a 95% confidence interval for the difference in means between the two groups.

Refer to the data in Table 2.11 on page 37.

**8.20** Test for a significant difference in the variances

of the initial white blood count (WBC) between persons who did and persons who did not receive a bacterial culture.

**8.21** What is the appropriate test procedure to test for significant differences in mean WBC between persons who do and persons who do not receive a bacterial culture?

**8.22** Perform the procedure in Problem 8.21 using the critical value method.

**8.23** What is the $p$-value corresponding to your answer to Problem 8.22?

**8.24** Compute a 95% confidence interval for the true difference in mean WBC between the two groups.

### Health Services Administration

A comparison is made of demographic characteristics of patients using fee-for-service practices and prepaid group health plans. Suppose we have the data presented in Table 8.6.

**Table 8.6**  *Characteristics of patients using fee-for-service practices and prepaid group health plans*

| Characteristic | Fee-for-service | | | Prepaid group health plans | | |
|---|---|---|---|---|---|---|
| | Mean | sd | n | Mean | sd | n |
| Age (years) | 58.1 | 6.2 | 57 | 52.6 | 4.3 | 48 |
| Education (years) | 11.8 | 0.7 | 57 | 12.7 | 0.8 | 48 |

**8.25** Test for a significant difference in the variance of age between the two groups.

**8.26** What is the appropriate test to compare the mean ages of the two groups?

**8.27** Perform the test in Problem 8.26 and report a $p$-value.

**8.28** Compute a 95% confidence interval for the mean age difference between the two groups.

**8.29** Answer Problem 8.25 for number of years of education.

**8.30** Answer Problem 8.26 for number of years of education.

**8.31** Answer Problem 8.27 for number of years of education.

**8.32** Answer Problem 8.28 for number of years of education.

Refer to Problem 8.15.

*8.33* Suppose we recruit an equal number of 12–14-year-old girls below and above the poverty level to study differences in mean $\log_e$ (calcium intake). How many girls should we recruit to have an 80% chance of detecting a significant difference using a two-sided test with $\alpha = 0.05$?

*8.34* Answer Problem 8.33 if a one-sided rather than a two-sided test is used.

*8.35* Using a two-sided test with $\alpha = 0.05$, answer Problem 8.33 if we anticipate that 2 girls above the poverty level will be recruited for every girl below the poverty level.

For Problems 8.36 and 8.37, refer to the data on hospital stays displayed in Table 2.11. (page 37).

*8.36* Test whether or not the mean duration of hospitalization is the same among those patients under 50 years old and those patients 50 years old or older.

*8.37* Test whether or not the mean duration of hospitalization is the same among those patients using the medical service and those patients using the surgical service.

## Gynecology

A study was conducted to compare the age at menarche (the age at the first menstrual period) of girls entering the first-year class of a small American private college in the year 1960 with that of girls entering the first-year class of the same college in 1970. This study is in response to reports of differences over time in other countries. Suppose that 30 girls in the 1960 class have a mean age at menarche of 12.78 years with a standard deviation of 0.43 year and 40 girls in the class of 1970 have a mean age at menarche of 12.42 years with a standard deviation of 0.67 year.

*8.38* What are the appropriate null and alternative hypotheses to test whether or not the ages at menarche are comparable in the two groups? Justify your choice of the appropriate hypotheses.

*8.39* Perform the significance test indicated in Problem 8.38 and state your conclusions.

*8.40* What is the advantage of comparing two different classes of the same school as opposed to comparing the 1960 entering class of one school with the 1970 entering class of another school?

## Pathology

Refer to the heart weight data in Table 2.10 (page 36).
*8.41* Test for a significant difference in total heart weight between the diseased and normal groups.

*8.42* Test for a significant difference in body weight between the diseased and normal groups.

## Psychiatry, Renal Disease

Severe anxiety often occurs in patients who must undergo chronic hemodialysis. A set of progressive relaxation exercises were shown on videotape to a group of 38 experimental subjects, while a set of neutral videotapes were shown to a control group of 23 patients who were also on chronic hemodialysis [4]. The results of a psychiatric questionnaire (the State-Trait Anxiety Inventory) are presented in Table 8.7.

**Table 8.7** *Pretest and post-test State-Trait Anxiety means and standard deviations for the experimental and control groups of hemodialysis patients*

|  | Pretest | | | Post-test | | |
|---|---|---|---|---|---|---|
|  | Mean | sd | n | Mean | sd | n |
| Experimental | 37.51 | 10.66 | 38 | 33.42 | 10.18 | 38 |
| Control | 36.42 | 8.59 | 23 | 39.71 | 9.16 | 23 |

A lower score on the test corresponds to less anxiety.
(Reprinted with permission of the *Journal of Chronic Diseases* **35(10)**: 797–802.)

*8.43* Perform a statistical test to compare the experimental and control groups' pretest scores.

*8.44* Perform a statistical test to compare the experimental and control groups' post-test scores.

## Cardiovascular Disease, Pediatrics

A study in Pittsburgh looked at various cardiovascular risk factors in children, as measured at birth and during their first 5 years of life [5]. In particular, heart rate was assessed at birth, 5 months, 15 months, 24 months, and annually thereafter until 5 years of age. Heart rate was

**Table 8.8** *Relationship of heart rate to race among newborns*

| Race | Mean (beats per minute) | sd | n |
|---|---|---|---|
| White | 125 | 11 | 218 |
| Black | 133 | 12 | 156 |

(Reprinted with permission of the *American Journal of Epidemiology* **119(4)**: 554–563.)

related to age, sex, race, and socioeconomic status. The data in Table 8.8 were presented relating heart rate to race among newborns.

8.45 Test for a significant difference in heart rates between white and black newborns.

8.46 Report a p-value for the test performed in Problem 8.45.

### Hypertension

An investigator wishes to determine if sitting upright in a chair vs. lying down on a bed will affect a person's blood pressure. The investigator decides to use each of 10 patients as his or her own control and collects systolic blood pressure data in both the sitting and lying positions as given in Table 8.9.

Table 8.9  Effect of position on level of bp (mmHg)

| Patient | Sitting upright | Lying down |
|---------|-----------------|------------|
| 1 | 142 | 154 |
| 2 | 100 | 106 |
| 3 | 112 | 110 |
| 4 | 92 | 100 |
| 5 | 104 | 112 |
| 6 | 100 | 100 |
| 7 | 108 | 120 |
| 8 | 94 | 90 |
| 9 | 104 | 104 |
| 10 | 98 | 114 |

8.47 What is the distinction between a one-sided and a two-sided hypothesis test in this problem?

8.48 Which hypothesis test is appropriate here? Why?

8.49 Using an $\alpha$ level of 0.05, test the hypothesis that the position affects the level of blood pressure.

8.50 What is the p-value of the preceding test? Compute either the specific p-value or a range within which the p-value lies.

### Pharmacology

One method for assessing the effectiveness of a drug is to note its concentration in blood and/or urine samples at certain periods of time after giving the drug. Suppose we wish to compare the concentrations of two types of aspirin (types A and B) in urine specimens taken from the same person, 1 hour after he or she has taken the drug. Hence we give a specific dosage of either type A or type B aspirin at one time and measure the 1-hour urine concentration. One week later, after the first

aspirin has presumably been cleared from the system, we give the same dosage of the other aspirin to the same person and note the 1-hour urine concentration. Since the order of giving the drugs may affect the results, we use a table of random numbers to decide which of the two types of aspirin to give first. We perform this experiment on 10 people; the results are given in Table 8.10.

Table 8.10  Concentration of aspirin in urine samples

| Person | Aspirin A 1-hour concentration (mg%) | Aspirin B 1-hour concentration (mg%) |
|--------|-------------------------|-------------------------|
| 1 | 15 | 13 |
| 2 | 26 | 20 |
| 3 | 13 | 10 |
| 4 | 28 | 21 |
| 5 | 17 | 17 |
| 6 | 20 | 22 |
| 7 | 7 | 5 |
| 8 | 36 | 30 |
| 9 | 12 | 7 |
| 10 | 18 | 11 |
| Mean | 19.20 | 15.60 |
| sd | 8.63 | 7.78 |

Suppose we wish to test the hypothesis that the concentrations of the two drugs are the same in urine specimens.

8.51 What are the appropriate hypotheses?

8.52 What are the assumptions behind the test used?

8.53 Conduct the test mentioned in Problem 8.51.

8.54 What is the best point estimate of the difference in concentrations between the two drugs?

8.55 What is a 95% confidence interval for the mean difference?

8.56 Suppose we use an $\alpha$ level of 0.05 for the test in Problem 8.53. What is the relationship between the decision reached with the test procedure in Problem 8.53 and the nature of the confidence interval in Problem 8.55?

### Hypertension

Blood pressure measurements taken on the left and right arms of a person are assumed to be comparable. To test this assumption, 10 volunteers are obtained and systolic blood pressure readings are taken simultaneously on both arms by two different observers, Mr. Jones for

**Table 8.11** *Effect of arm on level of blood pressure (mm Hg)*

| Patient | Left arm | Right arm |
|---------|----------|-----------|
| 1 | 130 | 126 |
| 2 | 120 | 124 |
| 3 | 135 | 127 |
| 4 | 100 | 95 |
| 5 | 98 | 102 |
| 6 | 110 | 109 |
| 7 | 123 | 124 |
| 8 | 136 | 132 |
| 9 | 140 | 137 |
| 10 | 155 | 156 |

the left arm and Mr. Smith for the right arm. The data are given in Table 8.11.

**8.57** Assuming that the two observers are comparable, test whether or not the two arms give comparable readings.

**8.58** Suppose we do *not* assume that the two observers are comparable. Can the experiment as it is defined detect differences between the two arms? If not, can you design the experiment differently so as to achieve this aim.

## Nutrition

A hypothesis of current clinical interest is that vitamin C prevents the common cold. A study is organized to test this hypothesis using 20 prisoners as participants. In the study 10 are randomly allocated to receive vitamin C capsules and 10 are randomly allocated to receive placebo capsules. The number of colds over a 12-month period for each participant is given in Table 8.12. We wish to test the hypothesis that vitamin C prevents the common cold.

**8.59** Is a one-sample or two-sample test needed here?

**8.60** Is a one-sided or two-sided test needed here?

**8.61** Which of the following test procedures should be used to test this hypothesis? (More than one may be necessary.)

(a) Paired $t$ test

(b) Two-sample $t$ test with equal variances

(c) Two-sample $t$ test with unequal variances

(d) Two-sample $F$ test

(e) One-sample $t$ test

**8.62** Carry out the test procedure(s) in Problem 8.61 and report a *p*-value.

**8.63** Derive a lower one-sided 95% confidence interval for the mean difference (vitamin C − placebo) in number of colds per year between the two groups.

**8.64** What is the relationship between your answers to Problems 8.62 and 8.63?

**Table 8.12** *Number of colds over a 12-month period for persons taking vitamin C and placebo capsules*

| Vitamin C | | Placebo | | |
|---|---|---|---|---|
| $i$ | $x_{i1}$ | $i$ | $x_{i2}$ | $d_i\,(x_{i1} - x_{i2})$ |
| 1 | 4 | 1 | 7 | −3 |
| 2 | 0 | 2 | 8 | −8 |
| 3 | 3 | 3 | 4 | −1 |
| 4 | 4 | 4 | 6 | −2 |
| 5 | 4 | 5 | 6 | −2 |
| 6 | 3 | 6 | 4 | −1 |
| 7 | 4 | 7 | 6 | −2 |
| 8 | 3 | 8 | 4 | −1 |
| 9 | 2 | 9 | 6 | −4 |
| 10 | 6 | 10 | 6 | 0 |
| $\sum_{i=1}^{10} x_{i1} = 33$ | | $\sum_{i=1}^{10} x_{i2} = 57$ | | $\sum_{i=1}^{10} d_i = -24$ |
| $\sum_{i=1}^{10} x_{i1}^2 = 131$ | | $\sum_{i=1}^{10} x_{i2}^2 = 341$ | | $\sum_{i=1}^{10} d_i^2 = 104$ |

*Table 8.13*
Spherical refraction in the right and left eye

| (i) Person | ($x_i$) Spherical refraction OD (right eye) (diopters) | ($y_i$) Spherical refraction OS (left eye) (diopters) | ($d_i = x_i - y_i$) Difference (OD − OS) |
|---|---|---|---|
| 1 | +1.75 | +2.00 | −0.25 |
| 2 | −4.00 | −4.00 | 0 |
| 3 | −1.25 | −1.00 | −0.25 |
| 4 | +1.00 | +1.00 | 0 |
| 5 | −1.00 | −1.00 | 0 |
| 6 | −0.75 | +0.25 | −1.00 |
| 7 | −2.25 | −2.25 | 0 |
| 8 | +0.25 | +0.25 | 0 |

$\sum_{i=1}^{17} x_i = -27.00$  $\sum_{i=1}^{17} x_i^2 = 180.00$  $\sum_{i=1}^{17} y_i = -23.50$  $\sum_{i=1}^{17} y_i^2 = 129.25$

| (i) Person | ($x_i$) Spherical refraction OD | ($y_i$) Spherical refraction OS | ($d_i = x_i - y_i$) Difference (OD − OS) |
|---|---|---|---|
| 9 | 0 | 0.50 | −0.50 |
| 10 | −1.00 | −1.25 | +0.25 |
| 11 | +0.50 | −1.75 | +2.25 |
| 12 | −8.50 | −5.00 | −3.50 |
| 13 | +0.50 | +0.50 | 0 |
| 14 | −5.25 | −4.75 | −0.50 |
| 15 | −2.25 | −2.50 | +0.25 |
| 16 | −6.50 | −6.25 | −0.25 |
| 17 | +1.75 | +1.75 | 0 |

$\sum_{i=1}^{17} d_i = -3.50$  $\sum_{i=1}^{17} d_i^2 = 19.13$

272

## Ophthalmology

A topic of current interest in ophthalmology is whether or not spherical refraction is different between the left and right eyes. For this purpose refraction is measured in both eyes of 17 people. The data are given in Table 8.13.

**8.65** Is a one-sample or two-sample test needed here?

**8.66** Is a one-sided or two-sided test needed here?

**8.67** Which of the following test procedures is appropriate to use on these data? (More than one may be necessary.)

    (a) Paired $t$ test

    (b) Two-sample $t$ test for independent samples with equal variances

    (c) Two-sample $t$ test for independent samples with unequal variances

    (d) One-sample $t$ test

**8.68** Carry out the hypothesis test in Problem 8.67 and report a $p$-value.

**8.69** Estimate a 90% confidence interval for the mean difference in spherical refraction between the two eyes.

## Pulmonary Disease

A recent study attempted to compare the working environment in offices where smoking was permitted with that in offices where smoking was not permitted [6]. Measurements were made of carbon monoxide (CO) at 1:20 PM in 40 work areas where smoking was permitted and 40 work areas where smoking was not permitted. Where smoking was permitted, the mean CO = 11.6 parts per million (ppm) and the standard deviation CO = 7.3 ppm. Where smoking was not permitted, the mean CO = 6.9 ppm and the standard deviation CO = 2.7 ppm.

**8.70** Test for whether or not the standard deviation of CO is significantly different in the two types of working environments.

**8.71** Test for whether or not the mean CO is significantly different in the two types of working environments.

**872** Does your answer to Problem 8.70 affect your answer to Problem 8.71? If so, in what way?

## Cardiovascular Disease

A study was performed in 1976 to relate the use of oral contraceptives with the levels of various lipid fractions in a group of 163 nonpregnant, premenopausal women ages 21–39. The mean serum cholesterol among 66 current users of oral contraceptives was $201 \pm 37$ (mg%/ml) (mean $\pm$ sd), whereas for 97 nonusers it was $193 \pm 37$.

**8.73** Test for significant differences in cholesterol levels between the two groups.

**8.74** Report a $p$-value based on your hypothesis test in Problem 8.73.

**8.75** Derive a 95% confidence interval for the true mean difference in cholesterol levels between the groups.

**8.76** Suppose we compute the two-tailed $p$-value in Problem 8.74 and obtain 0.03 and compute the two-sided 95% confidence interval in Problem 8.75 and obtain $(-0.6, 7.3)$. Do these two results contradict each other? Why or why not? (N.B. These values are not necessarily the actual results in Problems 8.74 and 8.75.)

## Ophthalmology

A camera has been developed to detect the presence of cataract more accurately. Using this camera, one can characterize the gray level of each point (or pixel) in the lens of a human eye into 256 gradations, where a gray level of 1 represents black and a gray level of 256 represents white. To test the camera, photographs were taken of 6 randomly selected normal eyes and 6 randomly selected cataractous eyes (the two groups consist of different people). The median gray level of each eye was computed over the 10,000+ pixels in the lens. The data are given in Table 8.14.

*Table 8.14* Median gray level for cataractous and normal eyes

| Patient number | Cataractous median gray level | Normal median gray level |
|---|---|---|
| 1 | 161 | 158 |
| 2 | 140 | 182 |
| 3 | 136 | 185 |
| 4 | 171 | 145 |
| 5 | 106 | 167 |
| 6 | 149 | 177 |
| $\bar{x}$ | 143.8 | 169.0 |
| $s$ | 22.7 | 15.4 |

**8.77** What statistical procedure can be used to test if there is a significant difference in the median gray levels between the cataractous and the normal eyes?

**8.78** Carry out the test procedure mentioned in Problem 8.77 and report a $p$-value.

**8.79** Provide a 99% confidence interval for the mean difference in gray levels between cataractous and normal eyes.

### Hypertension

A recent study by the Lipid Research Clinics looked at the relationship between alcohol consumption and level of systolic blood pressure in women not using oral contraceptives [7]. Alcohol consumption was categorized as follows: no alcohol use; $\leqslant 10$ oz per week alcohol consumption; $> 10$ oz per week alcohol consumption. The results for women 30–39 years of age are given in Table 8.15.

**Table 8.15** *Relationship of systolic blood pressure and alcohol consumption in 30–39-year-old women not using oral contraceptives*

| | Systolic blood pressure (mm Hg) | | |
| --- | --- | --- | --- |
| | Mean | sd | n |
| A. No alcohol use | 110.5 | 13.3 | 357 |
| B. $\leqslant 10$ oz per week alcohol consumption | 109.1 | 13.4 | 440 |
| C. $> 10$ oz per week alcohol consumption | 114.5 | 14.9 | 23 |

(Reprinted with permission of the *Journal of Chronic Diseases* **35(4)**: 251–257.)

Suppose we wish to compare the levels of systolic blood pressure of groups A and B and we have no prior information regarding which group has higher blood pressure.

**8.80** Should we use a one-sample or two-sample test here?

**8.81** Should we use a one-sided or two-sided test here?

**8.82** Which test procedure(s) should we use to test the preceding hypotheses?

**8.83** Carry out the test in Problem 8.82 and report a *p*-value.

**8.84** Compute a 95% confidence interval for the mean difference in blood pressure between the two groups.

**8.85** Answer Problem 8.82 for a comparison of groups A and C.

**8.86** Answer Problem 8.83 for a comparison of groups A and C.

**8.87** Answer Problem 8.84 for a comparison of groups A and C.

### Obstetrics

A clinical trial is conducted at the gynecology unit of a major hospital to determine the effectiveness of drug A in preventing premature birth. In the trial 30 pregnant women are to be studied, 15 assigned to a treatment group that will receive drug A and 15 assigned to a control group that will receive a placebo. The patients are to take a fixed dose of each drug on a one-time-only basis between the 24th and 28th weeks of pregnancy. The patients are assigned to groups using a random number table, whereby for every 2 patients eligible for the study, one is assigned randomly to the treatment group and the other to the control group.

**8.88** Suppose *you* are conducting the study. What would be a reasonable way of allocating women to the treatment and control groups?

Suppose the weights of the babies are those given in Table 8.16.

**Table 8.16** *Birthweights in a clinical trial to test a drug for preventing low birthweights*

| Number of pregnant women | Treatment group baby weight (lb) | Control group baby weight (lb) |
| --- | --- | --- |
| 1 | 6.9 | 6.4 |
| 2 | 7.6 | 6.7 |
| 3 | 7.3 | 5.4 |
| 4 | 7.6 | 8.2 |
| 5 | 6.8 | 5.3 |
| 6 | 7.2 | 6.6 |
| 7 | 8.0 | 5.8 |
| 8 | 5.5 | 5.7 |
| 99 | 5.8 | 6.2 |
| 10 | 7.3 | 7.1 |
| 11 | 8.2 | 7.0 |
| 12 | 6.9 | 6.9 |
| 13 | 6.8 | 5.6 |
| 14 | 5.7 | 4.2 |
| 15 | 8.6 | 6.8 |

**8.89** How would you assess the effects of drug A in light of your answer to Problem 8.88? Specifically, would you use a paired or an unpaired analysis and of what type?

**8.90** Perform both a paired and an unpaired analysis of the data. Does the type of analysis affect the assessment of the results?

*8.91* Suppose patient 3 in the control group subsequently moves to another city before giving birth and her child's weight is unknown. Does this event affect the analyses in Problem 8.90?

### Pulmonary Disease

Forced expiratory volume (FEV) is a standard measure of pulmonary function. We would expect that any reasonable measure of pulmonary function would reflect that a person's pulmonary function declines with age after 20. Suppose we test this hypothesis by looking at 10 nonsmoking males ages 35–39, heights 68–72 inches, and measuring their FEV in liters initially and then once again 2 years later. We obtain the data in Table 8.17.

*8.92* What are the appropriate null and alternative hypotheses in this case?

*8.93* In words, what is the meaning of a type I and a type II error here?

*8.94* Carry out the test in Problem 8.92. What are your conclusions?

Another aspect of the preceding study involves looking at the effect of smoking on baseline pulmonary function and on change in pulmonary function over time. We must be careful, since FEV depends on many factors, particularly age and height. Suppose we have a comparable group of 15 men in the same age and height group who are smokers, and we measure their FEV at year 0 and year 2. The data are given in Table 8.18.

*8.95* What are the appropriate null and alternative hypotheses to compare the smokers and nonsmokers at baseline?

**Table 8.17** *Pulmonary function in nonsmokers at two points in time*

| Person | Year 0 FEV (l) | Year 2 FEV (l) | Person | Year 0 FEV (l) | Year 2 FEV (l) |
|--------|--------|--------|--------|--------|--------|
| 1 | 3.22 | 2.95 | 6 | 3.25 | 3.20 |
| 2 | 4.06 | 3.75 | 7 | 4.20 | 3.90 |
| 3 | 3.85 | 4.00 | 8 | 3.05 | 2.76 |
| 4 | 3.50 | 3.42 | 9 | 2.86 | 2.75 |
| 5 | 2.80 | 2.77 | 10 | 3.50 | 3.32 |
|   |      |      | Mean | 3.43 | 3.28 |
|   |      |      | sd | 0.485 | 0.480 |

**Table 8.18** *Pulmonary function in smokers at two points in time*

| Person | FEV year 0 (l) | FEV year 2 (l) | Person | FEV year 0 (l) | FEV year 2 (l) |
|--------|--------|--------|--------|--------|--------|
| 1 | 2.85 | 2.88 | 9 | 2.76 | 3.02 |
| 2 | 3.32 | 3.40 | 10 | 3.00 | 3.08 |
| 3 | 3.01 | 3.02 | 11 | 3.26 | 3.00 |
| 4 | 2.95 | 2.84 | 12 | 2.84 | 3.40 |
| 5 | 2.78 | 2.75 | 13 | 2.50 | 2.59 |
| 6 | 2.86 | 3.20 | 14 | 3.59 | 3.29 |
| 7 | 2.78 | 2.96 | 15 | 3.30 | 3.32 |
| 8 | 2.90 | 2.74 |   |      |      |
|   |      |      | Mean | 2.98 | 3.03 |
|   |      |      | sd | 0.279 | 0.250 |

*8.96* Carry out the procedure(s) necessary to conduct the test in Problem 8.95.

*8.97* Suggest a procedure for testing whether or not the *change* in pulmonary function over 2 years is the same in the two groups.

### Pharmacology

In a pediatric clinic a study is carried out to see how effective aspirin is in reducing temperature. Twelve 5-year-old girls suffering from influenza had their temperatures taken immediately before and 1 hour after administration of aspirin. The results are given in Table 8.19. Suppose we assume normality and want to test the hypothesis that aspirin is reducing the temperature.

**Table 8.19**  *Body temperature (°F) before and after taking aspirin*

| Patient | Before | After |
|---------|--------|-------|
| 1       | 102.4  | 99.6  |
| 2       | 103.2  | 100.1 |
| 3       | 101.9  | 100.2 |
| 4       | 103.0  | 101.1 |
| 5       | 101.2  | 99.8  |
| 6       | 100.7  | 100.2 |
| 7       | 102.5  | 101.0 |
| 8       | 103.1  | 100.1 |
| 9       | 102.8  | 100.7 |
| 10      | 102.3  | 101.1 |
| 11      | 101.9  | 101.3 |
| 12      | 101.4  | 100.2 |

*8.98* What are the null and alternative hypotheses in this situation?

*8.99* In words, what is meant by a type I error in this situation?

*8.100* Suppose we consider the alternative that aspirin reduces the temperature by 1 degree. What is meant by the power of the test against this specific alternative?

*8.101* How would the power in Problem 8.100 change if the alternative were a temperature reduction of 2 degrees?

*8.102* Perform a significance test for the hypotheses in Problem 8.98.

### Hypertension

A study of the relationship between salt intake and blood pressure of infants is in the planning stages. A pilot study is done, comparing 5 1-year-old infants on a high-salt diet with 5 1-year-old infants on a low-salt diet. The results are given in Table 8.20.

**Table 8.20**  *Relationship between salt intake and level of blood pressure*

|                 | High-salt diet | Low-salt diet |
|-----------------|----------------|---------------|
| Mean systolic bp | 90.8          | 87.2          |
| sd systolic bp  | 10.3           | 9.2           |
| $n$             | 5              | 5             |

*8.103* If the means and standard deviations are considered to be true population parameters, then, using a one-sided test with significance level = 0.05, how many infants are needed in each group to have an 80% chance of detecting a significant difference?

*8.104* Suppose it is easier to recruit high-salt-diet infants and the investigators decide to enroll twice as many high-salt-diet infants as low-salt-diet infants. How many infants are needed in each group to have a 90% chance of detecting a significant difference using a one-sided test with an $\alpha$ level of 0.05?

### Pulmonary Disease

A possible important environmental determinant of lung function in children is the level of cigarette smoke in the home. Suppose we study this question by selecting two groups: Group 1 consists of 23 nonsmoking children 5–9 years of age, *both* of whose parents smoke, who have a mean FEV of 2.1 l and sd of 0.7 l; group 2 consists of 20 nonsmoking children of comparable age, *neither* of whose parents smoke, who have a mean FEV of 2.3 l and sd of 0.4 l.

*8.105* What are the appropriate null and alternative hypotheses in this situation?

*8.106* What is the appropriate test procedure for the hypotheses in Problem 8.105?

*8.107* Carry out the test in Problem 8.106 using the critical value method.

*8.108* Provide a 95% confidence interval for the true mean difference in FEV between 5–9-year-old children whose parents smoke and comparable children whose parents do not smoke.

*8.109* If we regard this as a pilot study, then how many children are needed in each group (assuming equal numbers in each group) to have a 95% chance of detecting a significant difference using a two-sided test with $\alpha = 0.05$?

**8.110** Answer the question in Problem 8.109 if the investigators intend to use a one-sided rather than a two-sided test.

# *References*

[1] Landrigan, P. J., Whitworth, R. H., Baloh, R. W., Staehling, N. W., Barthel, W. F., and Rosenblum, B. F. (1975) "Neuropsychological Dysfunction in Children with Chronic Low-Level Lead Absorption," *The Lancet*, March 29: 708–715.

[2] Satterthwaite, F. W. (1946) "An Approximate Distribution of Estimates of Variance Components," *Biometrics Bulletin* **2**: 110–114.

[3] Berson, E. L., Sandberg, M. A., Rosner, B., Birch, D. G., and Hanson, A. H. (1985) "Progression of Retinitis Pigmentosa Over a Three-Year Interval," *American Journal of Ophthalmology* **99**: 246–251.

[4] Alarcon, R. D., Jenkins, C. S., Heestand, D. E., Scott, L. K., and Cantor, L. (1982) "The Effectiveness of Progressive Relaxation in Chronic Hemodialysis Patients," *Journal of Chronic Diseases* **35(10)**: 797–802.

[5] Schachter, J., Kuller, L. H., and Perfetti, C. (1984) "Heart Rate During the First Five Years of Life: Relation to Ethnic Group (Black or White) and to Parental Hypertension," *American Journal of Epidemiology* **119(4)**: 554–563.

[6] White, J. R., and Froeb, H. E. (1980) "Small Airway Dysfunction in Nonsmokers Chronically Exposed to Tobacco Smoke," *New England Journal of Medicine* **302(13)**: 720–723.

[7] Wallace, R. B., Barrett-Connor, E., Criqui, M., Wahl, P., Hoover, J., Hunninghake, D., and Heiss, G. (1982) "Alteration in Blood Pressures Associated with Combined Alcohol and Oral Contraceptive Use—The Lipid Research Clinics Prevalence Study," *Journal of Chronic Diseases* **35(4)**: 251–257.

# 9 Nonparametric Methods

## ■ 9.1 INTRODUCTION

In the previous work in this text, we assumed that our data came from some underlying distribution, such as the normal or binomial, whose general form is known. We then proceeded to develop methods of estimation and hypothesis testing based on these assumptions. This procedure is usually referred to as **parametric statistical inference**, since the parametric form of the distribution is assumed known. If we do not wish to make these assumptions about the shape of the distribution and if the central limit theorem also seems to be inapplicable, then we must use **nonparametric statistical methods**, which make fewer assumptions about the shape of the distribution.

Another assumption we made in our previous work in this text is that common arithmetic can be performed on our data, which is characteristic of *cardinal data*.

**Definition 9.1**

**Cardinal data** are data that are on a scale where common arithmetic is meaningful. ■

**Example 9.1**    Body weight is a cardinal variable because a difference of 6 lb is actually twice as large as 3 lb, that is, the scale of measure is arithmetically meaningful. ■

Another type of data that occurs frequently in medical and biological work but does not satisfy Definition 9.1 is *ordinal data*.

**Definition 9.2**

**Ordinal data** are data that can be ordered but do not have specific numerical values. Thus, common arithmetic *cannot* be performed on ordinal data in a meaningful way. ■

**Example 9.2**    *Ophthalmology* Visual acuity can be measured on an ordinal scale, since we know that 20-20 vision is better than 20-30, which is better than 20-40, . . . , and so on. However, we cannot easily assign a numerical value to each level of visual acuity that all ophthalmologists would agree upon. ∎

*Example 9.3*   In some clinical studies the major outcome variable is the change in a patient's condition after treatment. This variable is often measured on the following five-point scale: 1 = much improved, 2 = slightly improved, 3 = stays the same, 4 = slightly worse, 5 = much worse. This variable is ordinal because the different outcomes 1, 2, 3, 4, 5 are ordered in the sense that condition 1 is better than condition 2, which is better than condition 3, ..., and so on. However, this variable is nonnumeric because we cannot say that the difference between categories 1 and 2 (2 − 1) is the same as the difference between categories 2 and 3 (3 − 2), ..., and so on. If these categories were on an arithmetic scale, the variable would have this property. ∎

Since ordinal variables cannot be given a numerical scale that makes sense, computing means and standard deviations for such data is not meaningful. Therefore, we cannot use any of the methods of estimation and hypothesis testing that have been discussed in Chapters 6 through 8. However, we still are interested in making comparisons between groups for variables such as visual acuity and outcome of treatment, and we can use nonparametric methods for this purpose.

In this chapter we develop the most commonly used nonparametric statistical tests, including the sign test, the Wilcoxon sign rank test, and the Wilcoxon rank sum test.

# ■ 9.2 THE SIGN TEST

## ☐ 9.2.1 Normal Theory Method

*Example 9.4*   **Dermatology** Suppose we wish to compare the effectiveness of two ointments (A, B) in reducing excessive redness in persons who cannot otherwise be exposed to sunlight. We randomly apply ointment A to either the left or right arm and apply ointment B to the corresponding area on the other arm. We then expose the person to 1 hour of sunlight and compare the two arms for degrees of redness. Suppose that we can only make the following qualitive assessments:

*1.* The "A" arm is not as red as the "B" arm.

*2.* The "B" arm is not as red as the "A" arm.

*3.* The arms are equally red.

We find that of 45 people tested with the condition, 22 are better off on the "A" arm, 18 are better off on the "B" arm, and 5 are equally well off on both arms. We wish to decide if this evidence is sufficient to conclude that ointment A is better than ointment B. How can we do this? ∎

Suppose that we were able to measure the degree of redness on a quantitative scale. Let $x_i$ = degree of redness on the "A" arm, $y_i$ = degree of redness on the "B" arm for the $i$th person. We will focus on $d_i = x_i - y_i$ = difference in redness between the "A" and "B" arms and will test the hypothesis $H_0 : \Delta = 0$ vs. $H_1 : \Delta \neq 0$, where $\Delta$ = the population median of the $d_i$ or the 50th percentile of the underlying distribution of the $d_i$.

1. If $\Delta = 0$, then the ointments are equally effective.
2. If $\Delta < 0$, then ointment A is better, since arm "A" is less red than arm "B."
3. If $\Delta > 0$, then ointment B is better, since arm "A" is more red than arm "B."

Notice that we cannot observe the actual $d_i$ but can only observe if $d_i > 0$, $d_i < 0$, or $d_i = 0$. We will exclude the persons for whom $d_i = 0$, since we cannot tell which ointment is better for them. We will base our test on the number of persons $C$ for whom $d_i > 0$ out of the total number of persons $n$ with nonzero $d_i$. This test makes sense, since if $C$ is large, then treatment B is preferred by most people over treatment A, whereas if $C$ is small, then treatment A is preferred over treatment B. We would expect under $H_0$ that $Pr(\text{nonzero } d_i > 0) = \frac{1}{2}$. We will assume that the normal approximation to the binomial is valid. This assumption will be true if

$$npq \geqslant 5 \quad \text{or} \quad n(\tfrac{1}{2})(\tfrac{1}{2}) \geqslant 5$$

or

$$\frac{n}{4} \geqslant 5 \quad \text{or} \quad n \geqslant 20$$

where $n =$ the number of nonzero $d_i$'s.
We can then use the following test procedure for a two-sided level $\alpha$ test, which is referred to as the **sign test**.

### 9.1 *The Sign Test*

If we wish to test the hypothesis $H_0: \Delta = 0$ vs. $H_1: \Delta \neq 0$ and the number of nonzero $d_i$'s $= n \geqslant 20$, then if

$$C > \frac{n}{2} + \frac{1}{2} + z_{1-\alpha/2}\sqrt{n/4} \quad \text{or} \quad C < \frac{n}{2} - \frac{1}{2} - z_{1-\alpha/2}\sqrt{n/4}$$

we reject $H_0$. Otherwise, we accept $H_0$.
The acceptance and rejection regions for this test are depicted in Figure 9.1.

Similarly, the exact $p$-value of the procedure is given by the following computation:

### 9.2 *Computation of the P-value for the Sign Test (Normal Theory Method)*

$$p = 2 \times \left[ 1 - \Phi\left( \frac{C - \frac{n}{2} - 0.5}{\sqrt{n/4}} \right) \right] \quad \text{if } C \geqslant \frac{n}{2}$$

$$p = 2 \times \left[ \Phi\left( \frac{C - \frac{n}{2} + 0.5}{\sqrt{n/4}} \right) \right] \quad \text{if } C < \frac{n}{2}$$

This computation is illustrated in Figure 9.2.

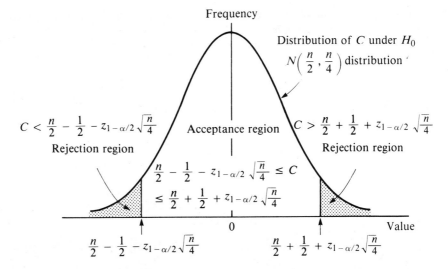

Frequency

Distribution of $C$ under $H_0$

$N\left(\frac{n}{2},\frac{n}{4}\right)$ distribution

$C < \frac{n}{2} - \frac{1}{2} - z_{1-\alpha/2}\sqrt{\frac{n}{4}}$     Acceptance region     $C > \frac{n}{2} + \frac{1}{2} + z_{1-\alpha/2}\sqrt{\frac{n}{4}}$

Rejection region                        Rejection region

$$\frac{n}{2} - \frac{1}{2} - z_{1-\alpha/2}\sqrt{\frac{n}{4}} \le C$$

$$\le \frac{n}{2} + \frac{1}{2} + z_{1-\alpha/2}\sqrt{\frac{n}{4}}$$

0                Value

$$\frac{n}{2} - \frac{1}{2} - z_{1-\alpha/2}\sqrt{\frac{n}{4}} \qquad \frac{n}{2} + \frac{1}{2} + z_{1-\alpha/2}\sqrt{\frac{n}{4}}$$

**Figure 9.1**

*Acceptance and rejection regions for the sign test*

If $C < n/2$, then $p = 2 \times$ area to the left of $\left( C - \frac{n}{2} + \frac{1}{2} \right)\bigg/\sqrt{\frac{n}{4}}$ under a $N(0,1)$ distribution.

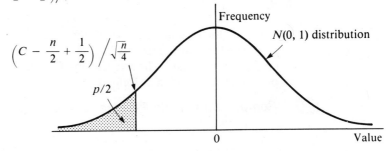

$\left( C - \frac{n}{2} + \frac{1}{2} \right)\bigg/\sqrt{\frac{n}{4}}$

Frequency

$N(0, 1)$ distribution

$p/2$

0               Value

If $C \ge n/2$, then $p = 2 \times$ area to the right of $\left( C - \frac{n}{2} - \frac{1}{2} \right)\bigg/\sqrt{\frac{n}{4}}$ under a $N(0,1)$ distribution.

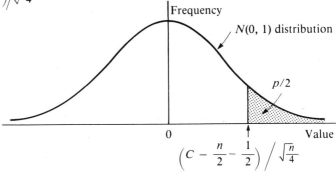

Frequency

$N(0, 1)$ distribution

$p/2$

0               Value

$\left( C - \frac{n}{2} - \frac{1}{2} \right)\bigg/\sqrt{\frac{n}{4}}$

**Figure 9.2**

*Computation of the p-value for the sign test*

This test is called the sign test because it depends only on the sign of the differences and not on their actual magnitude.

*Example 9.5*      **Dermatology** Assess the statistical significance of the skin ointment data in Example 9.4.

**Solution**    In this case we have 40 untied pairs, and $C = 22 \geqslant n/2 = 20$. From **(9.1)** the critical values are given by

$$c_1 = n/2 + 1/2 + z_{1-\alpha/2}\sqrt{n/4}$$
$$= 40/2 + 1/2 + z_{.975}\sqrt{40/4}$$
$$= 20.5 + 1.96(3.162) = 26.7$$

and

$$c_2 = n/2 - 1/2 - z_{1-\alpha/2}\sqrt{n/4}$$
$$= 19.5 - 1.96(3.162) = 13.3$$

Since $13.3 \leqslant C = 22 \leqslant 26.7$, we accept $H_0$ using a two-sided test with $\alpha = 0.05$ and conclude that the ointments are not significantly different in effectiveness. From **(9.2)**, since $C = 22 \geqslant n/2 = 20$, the exact $p$-value is given by

$$p = 2 \times \{1 - \Phi[(22 - 20 - \tfrac{1}{2})/\sqrt{40/4}]\} = 2 \times [1 - \Phi(0.47)] = 2 \times (1 - 0.6808) = 0.638$$

which is not statistically significant. Therefore, we accept $H_0$ that the ointments are equally effective.                                                                    ∎

## □ 9.2.2 Exact Method

If $n < 20$, then we must use exact binomial probabilities rather than the normal approximation to compute the $p$-value. We still want to reject $H_0$ if $C$ is very large or very small. The expressions for the $p$-value based on exact binomial probabilities are given as follows:

**9.3** **Computation of the P-value for the Sign Test (Exact Test)**

If $C \geqslant n/2$,

$$p = 2 \times \sum_{k=C}^{n} \binom{n}{k}\left(\frac{1}{2}\right)^n$$

If $C < n/2$,

$$p = 2 \times \sum_{k=0}^{C} \binom{n}{k}\left(\frac{1}{2}\right)^n$$

This computation is depicted in Figure 9.3.

*Example 9.6*    **Ophthalmology** Suppose we wish to compare two different types of eye drops (A, B) that are intended to prevent redness in persons with hay fever. We randomly give drug A to one eye and drug B to the other eye. The redness is noted at baseline and after 10 minutes by an observer who is not aware of which drug was administered to which eye. We find that for 15 persons with an equal amount of redness in each eye at baseline, after 10 minutes the drug A eye is less red than the drug B eye for 8 persons; the drug B eye is less red than the drug A eye for 2 persons; and the eyes are equally red for 5 persons. Assess the statistical significance of the results.

**Solution**    We base our test on the 10 persons who had a differential response to the two types of eye

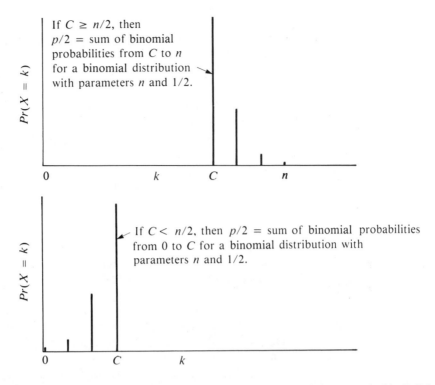

**Figure 9.3**
Computation of the
p-value for the sign
test (exact test)

drops. We note that since $n = 10 < 20$, we cannot use the normal theory method in **(9.2)** but must use the exact method in **(9.3)**. Since $C = 8 > \frac{10}{2} = 5$, we have

$$p = 2 \times \sum_{k=8}^{10} \binom{10}{k}\left(\frac{1}{2}\right)^{10}$$

We refer to the binomial tables (Table 1) using $n = 10$, $p = 0.5$ and note that $Pr(X = 8) = 0.0439$, $Pr(X = 9) = 0.0098$, $Pr(X = 10) = 0.0010$. Thus, $p = 2 \times Pr(X \geq 8) = 2(0.0439 + 0.0098 + 0.0010) = 2 \times 0.0547 = 0.109$, which is not statistically significant. Thus, we accept $H_0$ that the two types of eye drops are equally effective in reducing redness in persons with hay fever. ∎

# ■ 9.3 THE WILCOXON SIGN RANK TEST

*Example 9.7*      **Dermatology** Let us consider the data in Example 9.4 from a different perspective. We assumed that our only assessment was that the degree of sunburn with ointment A was either better or worse than that with ointment B. Suppose that instead we can quantify the degree of burn on a 10-point scale, with 10 being the worst burn and 1 being no burn at all. We can now compute $d_i = x_i - y_i$, where $x_i$ = degree of burn for ointment A and $y_i$ = degree of burn for ointment B. If $d_i$ is positive, then ointment B is doing better than ointment A; if $d_i$ is negative, then ointment A is doing better than ointment B. For example, if $d_i = +5$, then the degree of redness is 5 units greater with the ointment A arm than with the ointment B arm, whereas if $d_i = -3$, then the degree of redness is 3 units less with the ointment A arm than with the ointment B arm. How can we use this additional information to test if the ointments are equally effective? ∎

Suppose we obtain the sample data in Table 9.1. The $f_i$ represent the frequency or the number of people with difference in redness $d_i$ between the ointment A and ointment B arms.

Notice that there is only a slight excess of persons with negative $d_i$, that is, who are better off with ointment A (22), than with positive $d_i$, that is, who are better off with ointment B (18). However, the extent to which the 22 people are better off appears to be far greater than that of the 18 people, since the negative $d_i$ generally have a much greater absolute value than the positive $d_i$. This condition is illustrated in Figure 9.4.

We wish to test the hypothesis $H_0: \Delta = 0$ vs. $H_1: \Delta \neq 0$, where $\Delta$ = median score difference between the ointment A and ointment B arms. If $\Delta < 0$, then ointment A is better, whereas if $\Delta > 0$, then ointment B is better.

Based on Figure 9.4, a seemingly reasonable test of this hypothesis would be to take into account both the magnitude and the sign of the differences $d_i$. A paired $t$ test might be used here, but the problem is that the rating scale is ordinal rather than cardinal. The measurement $d_i = -5$ does not mean that the difference in degree of burn is 5 times as great as $d_i = -1$, but simply that there is a relative ranking of differences in degree of burn, with $-8$ being most favorable to ointment A, $-7$ the next most favorable, ..., and so on. Thus we need a nonparametric test here that is analogous to the paired $t$ test. Such a test is called the **Wilcoxon sign rank test**. It is nonparametric because it is based on the ranks of the observations rather than on their actual values, as is the case for the paired $t$ test.

The first step in performing this test is to compute ranks for each of the observations, as follows:

**9.4**   *Ranking Procedure for the Wilcoxon Sign Rank Test*

*1.* Arrange the differences $d_i$ in order of *absolute value* as has been done in Table 9.1.

*2.* Count the number of differences with the same absolute value.

*3.* Ignore the observations where $d_i = 0$ and rank the remaining observations from 1, for the observation with the lowest absolute value, up to $n$, for the observation with the highest absolute value.

*4.* If there is a group of several observations with the same absolute value, then find the lowest rank in the range $= 1 + R$ and the highest rank in the range $= G + R$, where $R =$ the highest rank used prior to considering this group and $G =$ the number of differences in the *range of ranks* for the group. Assign the *average rank* = (lowest rank in the range + highest rank in the range)/2 as the rank for each difference in the group.

*Example 9.8*   **Dermatology** Compute the ranks for the skin ointment data in Table 9.1.

*Solution*   We first collect the differences with the same absolute value. Fourteen persons have absolute value 1; this group of persons has a rank range from 1–14 and an average rank of $(1 + 14)/2 = 7.5$. The group of 10 persons with absolute value 2 has a rank range from $(1 + 14)$ to $(10 + 14) = 15 - 24$ and an average rank $= (15 + 24)/2 = 19.5, \ldots$, and so on.   ∎

The test is based on the sum of the ranks, or **rank sum** $(R_1)$, for the group of persons with positive $d_i$, that is, the rank sum for persons for whom ointment A does worse than ointment B. A large rank sum indicates that differences in degree of burn in favor of treatment B tend to be larger than those for treatment A, whereas

*Table 9.1*
Difference in degree of redness between ointment A and ointment B arms after 10 minutes of exposure to sunlight

| $|d_i|$ | Negative $d_i$ | $f_i$ | Positive $d_i$ | $f_i$ | Number of persons with same absolute value | Range of ranks | Average rank |
|---|---|---|---|---|---|---|---|
| 10 | −10 | 0 | 10 | 0 | 0 | — | — |
| 9 | −9 | 0 | 9 | 0 | 0 | — | — |
| 8 | −8 | 1 | 8 | 0 | 1 | 40 | 40.0 |
| 7 | −7 | 3 | 7 | 0 | 3 | 37–39 | 38.0 |
| 6 | −6 | 2 | 6 | 0 | 2 | 35–36 | 35.5 |
| 5 | −5 | 2 | 5 | 0 | 2 | 33–34 | 33.5 |
| 4 | −4 | 1 | 4 | 0 | 1 | 32 | 32.0 |
| 3 | −3 | 5 | 3 | 2 | 7 | 25–31 | 28.0 |
| 2 | −2 | 4 | 2 | 6 | 10 | 15–24 | 19.5 |
| 1 | −1 | 4 | 1 | 10 | 14 | 1–14 | 7.5 |
|  |  | 22 |  | 18 |  |  |  |
| 0 | 0 | 5 |  |  |  |  |  |

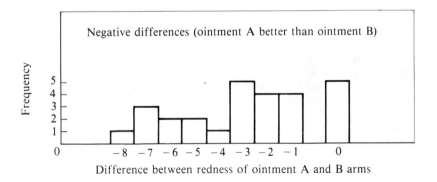

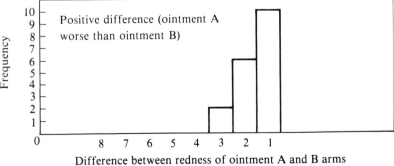

*Figure 9.4*
Bar graph of the differences in redness between the ointment A and ointment B arms for the data in Example 9.7

a small rank sum indicates that differences in degree of burn in favor of treatment A tend to be larger than those for treatment B. We can show that if the null hypothesis is true, then the expected value and variance of the rank sum are given by

$$E(R_1) = n(n + 1)/4, \ Var(R_1) = n(n + 1)(2n + 1)/24$$

where $n$ is the number of nonzero differences.

If the number of nonzero $d_i$'s is $\geq 16$, then a normal approximation can be used for the test procedure. We denote this test procedure as the **Wilcoxon sign rank test**, which is given as follows:

**9.5**   *Wilcoxon Sign Rank Test (Normal Approximation Method— Two-Sided Level $\alpha$ Test)*

*1*. Rank the differences as shown in **(9.4)**.

*2*. Compute the rank sum $R_1$ of the positive differences.

*3a*. Compute

$$T = \left[ \left| R_1 - \frac{n(n + 1)}{4} \right| - \frac{1}{2} \right] \Big/ \sqrt{n(n + 1)(2n + 1)/24}$$

if there *are no ties* (i.e., no groups of differences with the same absolute value).

*3b*. Compute

$$T = \left[ \left| R_1 - \frac{n(n + 1)}{4} \right| - \frac{1}{2} \right] \Big/ \sqrt{n(n + 1)(2n + 1)/24 - \sum_{i=1}^{g} (t_i^3 - t_i)/2}$$

if there *are ties*, where $t_i$ refers to the number of differences with the same absolute value in the $i$th tied group.

*4*. If

$$T > z_{1 - \alpha/2}$$

then reject $H_0$. Otherwise, accept $H_0$.

*5*. The $p$-value for the test is given by

$$p = 2 \times [1 - \Phi(T)]$$

*6*. This test should be used only if the number of nonzero differences $\geq 16$.

The computation of the $p$-value is illustrated in Figure 9.5.

If there are no ties,

$$T = \left[ \left| R_1 - \frac{n(n + 1)}{4} \right| - \frac{1}{2} \right] \Big/ \sqrt{n(n + 1)(2n + 1)/24}$$

If there are ties,

$$T = \left[\left|R_1 - \frac{n(n + 1)}{4}\right| - \frac{1}{2}\right] \Big/ \sqrt{n(n + 1)(2n + 1)/24 - \sum_{i=1}^{g} (t_i^3 - t_i)/2}$$

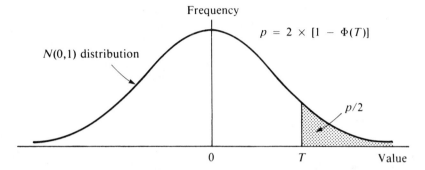

**Figure 9.5**
Computation of
the p-value for the
Wilcoxon sign
rank test

**Example 9.9**

**Solution**

*Dermatology* Perform the Wilcoxon sign rank test for the data in Example 9.7.

Since the number of nonzero differences $(22 + 18 = 40) \geqslant 16$, we can use the normal approximation method in (9.5). We compute the rank sum for the persons with positive $d_i$, that is, where ointment B performs better than ointment A, as follows:

$$R_1 = 10(7.5) + 6(19.5) + 2(28.0) = 75 + 117 + 56 = 248$$

The expected rank sum is given by

$$E(R_1) = 40(41)/4 = 410$$

whereas the variance of the rank sum corrected for ties is given by

$$Var(R_1) = 40(41)(81)/24 - [(14^3 - 14) + (10^3 - 10) + (7^3 - 7) + (1^3 - 1)$$
$$+ (2^3 - 2) + (2^3 - 2) + (3^3 - 3) + (1^3 - 1)]/2$$
$$= 5535 - (2730 + 990 + 336 + 0 + 6 + 6 + 24 + 0)/2$$
$$= 5535 - 4092/2 = 3489$$

Thus, $sd(R_1) = \sqrt{3489} = 59.07$. Therefore, the test statistic $T$ is given by

$$T = (|248 - 410| - \tfrac{1}{2})/59.07 = 161.5/59.07 = 2.73$$

The *p*-value of the test is given by

$$= 2[1 - \Phi(2.73)] = 2 \times (1 - 0.9968) = 0.006$$

We therefore can conclude that there is a significant difference between ointments, with ointment A doing better than ointment B, since the observed rank sum (248) is smaller than the expected rank sum (410). This conclusion is different from our conclusion based on the sign test in Example 9.5, where we found no significant difference between ointments. This result indicates that when the information is available, it is worthwhile to consider both the magnitude and the direction of the difference between treatments, as is done by the sign rank test, rather than just the direction of the difference, as is done by the sign test. ∎

In general, if we base the sign rank test on negative differences rather than positive differences, we will always get the same test statistic and *p*-value. Thus we can arbitrarily compute the rank sum based on either positive or negative differences.

*Example 9.10*    **Dermatology** Perform the Wilcoxon sign rank test for the data in Example 9.7 based on negative rather than positive difference scores.

*Solution*    We note that

$$R_2 = \text{rank sum for negative differences}$$

$$= 4(7.5) + 4(19.5) + 5(28.0) + 1(32.0) + 2(33.5) + 2(35.5) + 3(38.0) + 1(40.0)$$

$$= 572$$

Thus,

$$\left| R_2 - \frac{n(n+1)}{4} \right| - 0.5 = |572 - 410| - 0.5 = 161.5 = \left| R_1 - \frac{n(n+1)}{4} \right| - 0.5$$

Since $Var(R_1) = Var(R_2)$, we see that we get the same test statistic $T = 2.73$ and *p*-value = 0.006 as we did when using positive difference scores.    ■

If the number of pairs with nonzero $d_i \leq 15$, then the normal approximation is no longer valid, and special tables giving significance levels for this test must be used. Such a table is Table 9, which gives upper and lower critical values for $R_1$ for a two-sided test with $\alpha$ levels of 0.10, 0.05, 0.02, and 0.01, respectively. In general, the results are statistically significant at a particular $\alpha$ level only if either $R_1 \leq$ the lower critical value or $R_1 \geq$ the upper critical value for that $\alpha$ level.

*Example 9.11*    Suppose we have 9 untied pairs and a rank sum of 43. Evaluate the statistical significance of the results.

*Solution*    Since $R_1 = 43 \geq 42$, it follows that $p < 0.02$. Since $R_1 = 43 < 44$, it follows that $p \geq 0.01$. Thus we have $0.01 \leq p < 0.02$, and the results are statistically significant.    ■

We have presented an example of the sign rank test with ordinal data. We can apply this test and the other nonparametric tests to cardinal data as well, particularly if the assumption of normality appears to be grossly violated. If the actual distribution turns out to be normal, then the sign rank test has less power than the paired *t* test, which is the penalty we pay.

## ■ 9.4  *THE WILCOXON RANK SUM TEST*

In the previous section we presented a nonparametric analogue to the paired *t* test, namely, the Wilcoxon sign rank test. In this section we present a nonparametric analogue to the *t* test for two independent samples.

*Example 9.12*    **Ophthalmology** Different genetic types of the disease retinitis pigmentosa are thought to have different rates of progression, with the dominant form of the disease progressing the slowest, the recessive form of the disease the next slowest, and the sex-linked form of the disease the quickest. We can test this hypothesis by comparing the visual acuity of persons aged 10–19 who have different genetic types. Suppose we have 25 persons with dominant disease and 30 persons with sex-linked disease. The best corrected visual acuities (that is, with appropriate glasses) in the better eye of these persons are presented in Table 9.2. How can we use these data to see if the median visual acuity is different in the two groups?  ∎

**Table 9.2**
*Comparison of visual acuity in persons aged 10–19 with the dominant and sex-linked form of retinitis pigmentosa*

| Visual acuity | Dominant | Sex-linked | Combined sample | Range of ranks | Average rank |
|---|---|---|---|---|---|
| 20-20 | 5 | 1 | 6 | 1–6 | 3.5 |
| 20-25 | 9 | 5 | 14 | 7–20 | 13.5 |
| 20-30 | 6 | 4 | 10 | 21–30 | 25.5 |
| 20-40 | 3 | 4 | 7 | 31–37 | 34.0 |
| 20-50 | 2 | 8 | 10 | 38–47 | 42.5 |
| 20-60 | 0 | 5 | 5 | 48–52 | 50.0 |
| 20-70 | 0 | 2 | 2 | 53–54 | 53.5 |
| 20-80 | 0 | 1 | 1 | 55 | 55.0 |
| | — | — | | | |
| | 25 | 30 | | | |

We wish to test the hypothesis $H_0: \lambda_D = \lambda_{SL}$ vs. $H_1: \lambda_D \neq \lambda_{SL}$, where $\lambda_D$ and $\lambda_{SL}$ are the median visual acuities in the dominant and sex-linked groups, respectively. We ordinarily would use the two-sample $t$ test for independent samples, discussed in Sections 8.3 and 8.5, for this type of problem. However, visual acuity cannot be given a specific numerical value that all ophthalmologists would agree on. Thus, the $t$ test is inapplicable, and a nonparametric analogue must be used. The nonparametric analogue to the independent samples $t$ test is the **Wilcoxon rank sum test**. This test is nonparametric because it is based on the *ranks* of the individual observations rather than on their actual values, which would be used in the $t$ test. The ranking procedure for this test is given as follows:

**9.6**  **Ranking Procedure for the Wilcoxon Rank Sum Test**

*1.* Combine the data from the two groups and order the values from the lowest to highest, or in the case of visual acuity, from best visual acuity (20-20) to worst visual acuity (20-80).

*2.* Assign ranks to the individual values, with the best visual acuity (20-20) having the lowest rank and the worst visual acuity (20-80) having the highest rank.

*3.* If a group of observations has the same value, then compute the *range of ranks* for the group, as was done for the sign rank test in **(9.4)**, and assign the *average rank* for each observation in the group.

*Example 9.13*    Compute the ranks for the visual acuity data in Table 9.2.

*Solution*    We first collect all persons with the same visual acuity over the two groups, as shown in Table 9.2. There are 6 persons with visual acuity 20-20 who have a rank range of 1–6 and are assigned an average rank of $(1 + 6)/2 = 3.5$. There are 14 persons over the two groups with visual acuity 20-25. The rank range for this group is from $(1 + 6)$ to $(14 + 6) = 7 - 20$. Thus, all persons in this group are assigned the average rank $= (7 + 20)/2 = 13.5$, and similarly for the other groups.    ∎

The test statistic that is used for this test is the sum of the ranks in the first sample $(R_1)$. If this sum is large, then the dominant group has poorer visual acuity than the sex-linked group, whereas if it is small, the dominant group has better visual acuity. If the number of observations in the two groups are $n_1$ and $n_2$, respectively, then the average rank in the combined sample is $(1 + n_1 + n_2)/2$. Thus, under $H_0$, the expected rank sum in the first group $\equiv E(R_1) = n_1 \times$ average rank in the combined sample $= n_1(n_1 + n_2 + 1)/2$. We can show that the variance of $R_1$ under $H_0$ is given by $Var(R_1) = n_1 n_2(n_1 + n_2 + 1)/12$. Furthermore, if the smaller of the two groups is at least 10, then we can show that the distribution of the rank sum $R_1$ is approximately normal. Thus, we have the following test procedure:

**9.7** **Wilcoxon Rank Sum Test (Normal Approximation Method for Two-Sided Level $\alpha$ Test)**

*1.* Rank the observations as shown in **(9.6)**.
*2.* Compute the rank sum $R_1$ in the first sample (the choice of sample is arbitrary).
*3a.* Compute

$$T = \left[ \left| R_1 - \frac{n_1(n_1 + n_2 + 1)}{2} \right| - \frac{1}{2} \right] \Big/ \sqrt{\left( \frac{n_1 n_2}{12} \right)(n_1 + n_2 + 1)}$$

if there *are no ties*.
*3b.* Compute

$$T = \left[ \left| R_1 - \frac{n_1(n_1 + n_2 + 1)}{2} \right| - \frac{1}{2} \right] \Big/ \sqrt{\left( \frac{n_1 n_2}{12} \right)\left[ n_1 + n_2 + 1 - \frac{\sum_{i=1}^{g} t_i(t_i^2 - 1)}{(n_1 + n_2)(n_1 + n_2 - 1)} \right]}$$

if there *are ties*, where $t_i$ refers to the number of observations with the same value in the *i*th tied group.
*4.* If

$$T > z_{1-\alpha/2}$$

then reject $H_0$. Otherwise, accept $H_0$.
*5.* Compute the exact *p*-value by

$$p = 2 \times [1 - \Phi(T)]$$

*6.* This test should be used only if both $n_1$ and $n_2$ are at least 10.

The computation of the *p*-value is illustrated in Figure 9.6.

If there are no ties,

$$T = \left[ \left| R_1 - \frac{n_1(n_1 + n_2 + 1)}{2} \right| - \frac{1}{2} \right] \Big/ \sqrt{\frac{n_1 n_2(n_1 + n_2 + 1)}{12}}$$

If there are ties,

$$T = \left[ \left| R_1 - \frac{n_1(n_1 + n_2 + 1)}{2} \right| - \frac{1}{2} \right] \Big/ \sqrt{\left(\frac{n_1 n_2}{12}\right) \left[ n_1 + n_2 + 1 - \frac{\sum\limits_{i=1}^{g} t_i(t_i^2 - 1)}{(n_1 + n_2)(n_1 + n_2 - 1)} \right]}$$

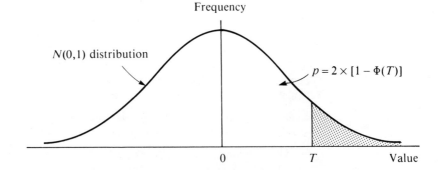

**Figure 9.6**
Computation of
the p-value for the
Wilcoxon rank sum
test

*Example 9.14*

Perform the Wilcoxon rank sum test for the data in Example 9.12.

*Solution*

We first note that the minimum sample size in the two samples is $25 \geqslant 10$ and thus we can use the normal approximation. We note that the rank sum in the dominant group is given by

$$R_1 = 5(3.5) + 9(13.5) + 6(25.5) + 3(34) + 2(42.5)$$

$$= 17.5 + 121.5 + 153 + 102 + 85$$

$$= 479$$

Furthermore,

$$E(R_1) = \frac{25(56)}{2} = 700$$

and $Var(R_1)$ corrected for ties is given by

$$[(25)(30)/12]\{56 - [6(6^2 - 1) + 14(14^2 - 1) + 10(10^2 - 1) + 7(7^2 - 1)$$

$$+ 10(10^2 - 1) + 5(5^2 - 1) + 2(2^2 - 1) + 1(1^2 - 1)]/[55(54)]\}$$

$$= 62.5(56 - 5382/2970)$$

$$= 3386.74$$

Thus, the test statistic $T$ is given by

$$T = \frac{(|479 - 700| - 0.5)}{\sqrt{3386.74}}$$

$$= \frac{220.5}{58.2} = 3.79$$

which follows a $N(0, 1)$ distribution under $H_0$. The p-value of the test is

$$2 \times [1 - \Phi(3.79)] < 0.001$$

Since the observed rank sum in the dominant group (479) is lower than the expected rank sum (700), our conclusion is that the visual acuities of the two groups are significantly different: The dominant group has better visual acuity than the sex-linked group.                              ∎

If either sample size is less than 10, the normal approximation is not valid, and we must use a table of exact significance levels. Table 10 gives upper and lower critical values for the rank sum in the first of two samples ($T$) for a two-sided test with α levels of 0.10, 0.05, 0.02, and 0.01, respectively. In general, the results are statistically significant at a particular α level only if either $T \leqslant T_l$ = the lower critical value or $T \geqslant T_r$ = the upper critical value for that α level.

*Example 9.15*

Suppose we have two samples of size 8 and 15, with a rank sum of 73 in the sample size of 8. Evaluate the statistical significance of the results.

*Solution*

We refer to $n_1 = 8$, $n_2 = 15$, $\alpha = 0.05$ and find that $T_l = 65$, $T_r = 127$. Since $T = 73 > 65$, $T < 127$, the results are not statistically significant using a two-sided test at the 5% level.    ∎

The Wilcoxon rank sum test is also sometimes referred to in the literature as the **Mann–Whitney $U$ test**. The test statistic for the Mann–Whitney $U$ test is based on the number of pairs of observations $(x_i, y_j)$, one from each sample, such that $x_i < y_j$. We can show that the Mann–Whitney $U$ test and the Wilcoxon rank sum test are completely equivalent, since we obtain exactly the same p-value by applying either test. Therefore, choosing which test to use is a matter of convenience.

Because ranking all the observations in a large sample is tedious, a computer program is useful in performing the Wilcoxon rank sum test. We have implemented the SPSS/PC Wilcoxon rank sum test procedure on the dataset in Table 9.2 and have displayed the results in Table 9.3.

The average ranks in the dominant and sex-linked groups are listed first. Both the Mann–Whitney $U$ statistic (labeled U) = 154 and the Wilcoxon rank sum test statistic (labeled W) = 479 are given in the output. The test statistic

*Table 9.3*
*SPSS/PC Wilcoxon rank sum test program used on the data in Table 9.2.*

```
                              SPSS/PC   Release 1.0

  - - - - - Mann-Whitney U - Wilcoxon Rank Sum W Test

        VA          VISUAL ACUITY
     BY DDX         GENETIC TYPE


     Mean Rank    Cases

        19.16        25  DDX = 1.00  DOMINANT
        35.37        30  DDX = 2.00  SEX-LINKED
                     —
                     55  Total

                                    Corrected for Ties
        U            W            Z       2-tailed P
      154.0        479.0       -3.7975     0.0001
```

(labeled Z) $= -3.7975$ and the two-tailed $p$-value $= 0.0001 < 0.001$ are also given. The test statistic differs slightly from that computed in Example 9.14, since the program does not correct for continuity; that is, $|Z| = |479 - 700|/58.2 = 3.80$, whereas $T = (|479 - 700| - 0.5)/58.2 = 3.79$. The difference is minor in this case.

Finally, a necessary condition for the strict validity of the rank sum test is that the underlying distributions being compared must be continuous. However, McNeil has investigated the use of this test in comparing discrete distributions and has found only small losses in power when applying this test to grouped data from normal distributions, as compared with the actual ungrouped observations from such distributions [1]. He concludes that the rank sum test is approximately valid in this case, with the appropriate provision for ties as given in **(9.7)**.

The tests covered in this chapter, the material on rank correlation in Chapter 11, and the Kruskal-Wallis test in Chapter 12 are among the most basic of nonparametric tests. Hollander and Wolfe provide a more comprehensive treatment of nonparametric statistics [2].

# ■ *9.5 SUMMARY*

In this chapter we presented some of the most widely used nonparametric statistical tests corresponding to the parametric procedures in Chapter 8. The key advantage of nonparametric methods is that we can relax the assumptions of normality that we made in previous chapters when such assumptions are unreasonable. One drawback of nonparametric procedures is that we lose some power relative to using a parametric procedure (such as a $t$ test) if the data truly follow a normal distribution or if the central limit theorem is applicable. Also, the data typically have to be expressed in terms of ranks, a scale that some researchers find difficult to understand compared with maintaining the raw data in their original scale.

The specific procedures we covered include the **sign test**, the **Wilcoxon sign rank test**, and the **Wilcoxon rank sum test**. Both the sign test and the sign rank test are nonparametric analogues to the paired $t$ test. For the **sign test** we need only determine whether one member of a matched pair has a higher or lower score than the other member of the pair. For the **sign rank test** we use the magnitude of the difference score (expressed in the form of a rank) as well as its direction in performing the significance test. Furthermore, the **Wilcoxon rank sum test** (also known as the Mann-Whitney $U$ test) is an analogue to the two-sample $t$ test for independent samples, in which we replace the actual values by rank scores. Finally, we will introduce other nonparametric procedures in Chapters 11 and 12 as analogues to correlation methods and the analysis of variance.

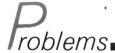 *roblems*

*Ophthalmology*

Suppose an ophthalmologist reviews fundus photographs of 30 patients with macular degeneration both before and 3 months after receiving a laser treatment. To assess the efficacy of treatment, each patient is rated as improved, remained the same, or declined.

*9.1* If 20 patients improved, 7 declined, and 3 remained the same, then assess whether or not patients undergoing this treatment are showing significant change from baseline to 3 months afterward. Report a *p*-value.

Suppose that the patients are divided into two groups according to initial visual acuity (VA). Of the 14 patients with VA of 20/40 or better, 8 improved, 5 declined, and 1 stayed the same. Of the 16 patients with VA worse than 20/40, 12 improved, 2 declined, and 2 stayed the same.

*9.2* Assess the results in the subgroup of patients with VA of 20/40 or better.

*9.3* Assess the results in the subgroup of patients with VA worse than 20/40.

*Dentistry*
In a study 28 adults with mild periodontal disease are assessed before and 6 months after the implementation of a dental education program intended to promote better oral hygiene. After 6 months periodontal status improved in 15 persons, declined in 8 persons, and remained the same in 5 persons.

*9.4* Assess the impact of the program statistically (use a two-sided test).

*Diabetes*
An experiment was conducted to study responses to different methods of taking insulin in patients with type I diabetes. The percentages of glycosolated hemoglobin initially and 3 months after taking insulin by nasal spray are given in Table 9.4 [3].

*Table 9.4* *Percentages of glycosolated hemoglobin before and 3 months after taking insulin by nasal spray*

| Patient number | Before | 3 months after |
|:---:|:---:|:---:|
| 1 | 11.0 | 10.2 |
| 2 | 7.7 | 7.9 |
| 3 | 5.9 | 6.5 |
| 4 | 9.5 | 10.4 |
| 5 | 8.7 | 8.8 |
| 6 | 8.6 | 9.0 |
| 7 | 11.0 | 9.5 |
| 8 | 6.9 | 7.6 |

(Reprinted with permission of the *New England Journal of Medicine* **312**(17): 1078–1084, 1985.)

*9.5* Perform a *t* test to compare the percentages of glycosolated hemoglobin before and 3 months after treatment.

*9.6* Suppose we do not wish to assume normality. Perform a nonparametric test corresponding to the *t* test in Problem 9.5.

*9.7* Compare your results in Problems 9.5 and 9.6.

*Dentistry*
Refer to Problem 9.4. Suppose that patients are graded on the degree of change in periodontal status on a 7-point scale, with $+3$ indicating the greatest improvement, 0 indicating no change, and $-3$ indicating the greatest decline. The data are given in Table 9.5.

*Table 9.5* *Degree of change in periodontal status*

| Change score | Number of persons |
|:---:|:---:|
| $+3$ | 4 |
| $+2$ | 5 |
| $+1$ | 6 |
| 0 | 5 |
| $-1$ | 4 |
| $-2$ | 2 |
| $-3$ | 2 |

*9.8* What nonparametric test can be used to determine whether or not a significant change in periodontal status has occurred over time?

*9.9* Implement the procedure in Problem 9.8 and report a *p*-value.

*9.10* Suppose we wish to use the Wilcoxon sign rank test and have a rank sum of 27 based on 7 untied pairs. Evaluate the significance of the results.

*9.11* Answer Problem 9.10 for a rank sum of 65 based on 13 untied pairs.

*9.12* Answer Problem 9.10 for a rank sum of 90 with 15 untied pairs.

*9.13* Suppose we have two samples of sizes 6 and 7, with a rank sum of 58 in the sample of size 6. Using the Wilcoxon rank sum test, evaluate the significance of the results.

*9.14* Answer Problem 9.13 for two samples of sizes 7 and 10, with a rank sum of 47 in the sample of size 7.

*9.15* Answer Problem 9.13 for two samples of sizes 12 and 15, with a rank sum of 220 in the sample of size 12 (assume that there are no ties).

Refer to Table 2.10 (page 36).

*9.16* Suppose we do not wish to assume normality. What nonparametric test can be used to compare total heart weight of males with left heart disease with that of normal males?

**9.17** Implement the test in Problem 9.16 and report a *p*-value.

### Obstetrics
**9.18** Reanalyze the data in Table 8.16 (page 274) using nonparametric methods. Assume the samples are unpaired.

**9.19** Would such methods be preferable to parametric methods in analyzing the data? Why or why not?

### Cardiology
Propranolol is a standard drug given to ease the pain of patients with episodes of unstable angina. A new drug for the treatment of this disease is tested on 30 pairs of patients who are matched on a one-to-one basis according to age, sex, and clinical condition and are assessed as to the severity of their pain. Suppose that in 15 pairs of patients, the patient with the new drug has less pain; in 10 pairs of patients, the patient with propranolol has less pain; and in 5 pairs of patients, the pain is about the same with the two drugs.

**9.20** What is the appropriate test to use here?

**9.21** Perform the test in Problem 9.20 and report a *p*-value.

### Health Services Administration
Suppose we wish to compare the length of stay in the hospital for patients with the same diagnosis at two different hospitals. We have the following results:

| First hospital | 21, 10, 32, 60, 8, 44, 29, 5, 13, 26, 33 |
|---|---|
| Second hospital | 86, 27, 10, 68, 87, 76, 125, 60, 35, 73, 96, 44, 238 |

**9.22** Why might a *t* test not be very useful in this case?

**9.23** Carry out a nonparametric procedure for testing the hypothesis that the lengths of stay are comparable in the two hospitals.

### Ophthalmology
Table 8.14 presents data giving the median gray levels in the lens of the human eye for 6 cataractous and 6 normal persons (page 273).

**9.24** What nonparametric test could be used to compare the median gray levels of normal and cataractous eyes?

**9.25** Carry out the test in Problem 9.24 and report a *p*-value.

### Infectious Disease
The distribution of white blood count is typically positively skewed, and assumptions of normality are usually not valid.

**9.26** If we wish to compare the white blood counts of patients on the medical and surgical services in Table 2.11 (page 37) and do not wish to assume normality, then what test can we use?

**9.27** Perform the test in Problem 9.26 and report a *p*-value.

### Psychiatry
Suppose we are conducting a study of the effectiveness of lithium therapy for manic-depressive patients. The study is carried out at two different centers, and we wish to determine if the patient populations are comparable at baseline. We administer a self-rating questionnaire to the prospective patients at the two different centers about their general psychological well-being, in which the outcome measure is a four-category scale as follows: (1) = feel good; (2) = usually feel good, once in a while feel nervous; (3) = feel nervous half the time; (4) = usually feel nervous. Suppose the data at the two different centers are as follows:

| Center 1 | 3, 4, 1, 1, 3, 2, 3, 4, 4, 3, 2, 4, 4, 4 |
|---|---|
| Center 2 | 1, 2, 1, 3, 2, 4, 1, 2, 1, 3, 1, 2, 2, 2, 1, 3 |

**9.28** What type of data does this type of scale represent?

**9.29** Why might a parametric test not be useful with this type of data?

**9.30** Assess if there is any significant difference in the responses of the two patient populations using a nonparametric test.

### Sports Medicine
Many tennis players develop acute lateral epicondylitis whereby they experience acute elbow pain (tennis elbow). A variety of nonsurgical treatments are used for this condition, including rest, heat, and anti-inflammatory agents. A clinical trial was set up to compare the effects of the anti-inflammatory agent ibuprofen (Motrin) with those of a placebo in the treatment of tennis elbow. Patients were given 400 mg of ibuprofen orally or an identical looking placebo 4 times per day and were evaluated after 3 weeks of treatment. Patients subjectively rated their pain as (1) worse, (2) unchanged, (3) slightly improved, (4) moderately improved, (5) mostly improved, and (6) completely improved. The results are given in Table 9.6.

**Table 9.6** *A comparison of pain during maximal activity after 3 weeks of therapy with Motrin and placebo as compared with baseline*

| Treatment group | Total | Worse | Unchanged | Slightly improved | Moderately improved | Mostly improved | Completely improved |
|---|---|---|---|---|---|---|---|
| Motrin | 43 | 0 | 14 | 7 | 10 | 10 | 2 |
| Placebo | 44 | 5 | 20 | 11 | 3 | 5 | 0 |

**9.31** If we regard all levels of improvement as equivalent, then what test can be used to assess whether or not patients on Motrin have improved over the 3-week period?

**9.32** Perform the test in Problem 9.31 and report a *p*-value.

**9.33** Perform the same test as in Problem 9.32 for patients on placebo and report a *p*-value.

Suppose we differentiate between levels of improvement using the scale in Table 9.6.

**9.34** What tests can be used to compare the degree of improvement between Motrin and placebo?

**9.35** Perform the test in Problem 9.34 and report a *p*-value.

**9.36** What conclusions can you draw from your results in Problems 9.32, 9.33, and 9.35?

**Otolaryngology, Pediatrics**

A common symptom of otitis media in young children is the prolonged presence of fluid in the middle ear, known as *middle ear effusion*. The presence of fluid may result in temporary hearing loss and interfere with normal learning skills in the first 2 years of life. One hypothesis is that babies who are breast-fed for at least 1 month build up some immunity against the effects of the disease and have less prolonged effusion than do bottle-fed babies. A small study of 24 pairs of babies is set up, where the babies are matched on a one-to-one basis according to age, sex, socioeconomic status, and type of medications taken. One member of the matched pair is a breast-fed baby whereas the other member is a bottle-fed baby. The outcome variable is the duration of middle ear effusion after the first episode of otitis media. The results are given in Table 9.7.

**9.37** What are the hypotheses being tested here?

**Table 9.7** *Duration of middle ear effusion in breast-fed and bottle-fed babies*

| Pair number | Duration of effusion in breast-fed baby (days) | Duration of effusion in bottle-fed baby (days) | Pair number | Duration of effusion in breast-fed baby (days) | Duration of effusion in bottle-fed baby (days) |
|---|---|---|---|---|---|
| 1 | 20 | 18 | 13 | 52 | 39 |
| 2 | 11 | 35 | 14 | 14 | 15 |
| 3 | 3 | 7 | 15 | 12 | 21 |
| 4 | 24 | 182 | 16 | 30 | 28 |
| 5 | 7 | 6 | 17 | 7 | 8 |
| 6 | 28 | 33 | 18 | 15 | 27 |
| 7 | 58 | 223 | 19 | 65 | 77 |
| 8 | 7 | 7 | 20 | 10 | 12 |
| 9 | 39 | 57 | 21 | 7 | 8 |
| 10 | 17 | 76 | 22 | 19 | 16 |
| 11 | 17 | 186 | 23 | 34 | 28 |
| 12 | 12 | 29 | 24 | 25 | 20 |

**9.38** Why might a nonparametric test be useful in testing the hypotheses?

**9.39** Which nonparametric test should be used here?

**9.40** Test the hypothesis that the duration of effusion is less prolonged among breast-fed babies than among bottle-fed babies using a nonparametric test.

### Psychiatry

Much attention has been given in recent years to the role of transcendental meditation in improving health, particularly in lowering blood pressure. One hypothesis that emerges from this work is that transcendental meditation might also be useful in treating psychiatric patients with symptoms of anxiety. Suppose that a protocol of meditational therapy is administered once per day to 20 patients with anxiety. The patients are given a psychiatric exam at baseline and at a follow-up exam 2 months later. The degree of improvement is rated on a 10-point scale, with 1 indicating the most improvement and 10 the least improvement. Similarly, 26 comparably affected patients with anxiety are given standard psychotherapy and are asked to come back 2 months later for a follow-up exam. The results are given in Table 9.8.

**9.41** Why might a parametric test not be useful here?

**Table 9.8** *Degree of improvement in patients with anxiety who are treated with transcendental meditation or psychotherapy*

| Meditation | | Psychotherapy | |
|---|---|---|---|
| $d^*$ | $f$† | $d^*$ | $f$† |
| 1 | 3 | 1 | 0 |
| 2 | 4 | 2 | 2 |
| 3 | 7 | 3 | 5 |
| 4 | 3 | 4 | 3 |
| 5 | 2 | 5 | 8 |
| 6 | 1 | 6 | 4 |
| 7 | 0 | 7 | 2 |
| 8 | 0 | 8 | 1 |
| 9 | 0 | 9 | 1 |
| 10 | 0 | 10 | 0 |
| | 20 | | 26 |

\* $d$ = degree of improvement
† $f$ = frequency

**9.42** What nonparametric test should be used to analyze these data?

**9.43** Compare the degree of improvement in the two groups using the test in Problem 9.42.

### Hypertension

Unsaturated fatty acids in the diet favorably affect several risk factors for cardiovascular disease. The principal dietary polyunsaturated fat is linoleic acid. To test the effects of dietary supplements of linoleic acid on blood pressure, 17 adults consumed 23 g/day of safflower oil, high in linoleic acid, for 4 weeks. Blood pressure measurements were taken at baseline (before ingestion of oil) and 1 month later, with the mean values over several readings at each visit given in Table 9.9.

**9.44** What parametric test could be used to test for the effect of linoleic acid on blood pressure?

**9.45** Perform the test in Problem 9.44 and report a *p*-value.

**9.46** What nonparametric test could be used to test for the effect of linoleic acid on blood pressure?

**9.47** Perform the test in Problem 9.46 and report a *p*-value.

**9.48** Compare your results in Problems 9.45 and 9.47 and discuss which method you feel is appropriate here.

### Ophthalmology

A new drug is developed to relieve the ocular symptoms of hay fever. The drug is composed of two components A and B: the former is supposed to relieve itching of the eye and the latter is supposed to prevent redness; the combination is supposed to relieve both itching and redness. Federal regulations require that each component should be proven effective both separately and in combination. Three experiments are performed on a group of 25 patients with hay fever. In the first experiment drug A is administered to a randomly selected eye and a placebo is administered to the other eye, and the change from baseline is noted for each eye. The data are given in Table 9.10. A plus sign represents more improvement in the drug-treated eye; a minus sign represents more improvement in the placebo-treated eye; 0 represents equal improvement in both eyes.

**9.49** Why might a nonparametric statistical test be useful in comparing drug A with placebo for this experiment?

**9.50** Why was it important to administer the placebo to the second eye of the same person rather than to a different group of people with hay fever?

**9.51** What nonparametric statistical test would you use

**Table 9.9**   Effect of linoleic acid on systolic blood pressure

| Subject | Baseline blood pressure | 1-month blood pressure | Baseline minus 1-month blood pressure |
|---|---|---|---|
| 1 | 119.67 | 117.33 | 2.34 |
| 2 | 100.00 | 98.78 | 1.22 |
| 3 | 123.56 | 123.83 | −0.27 |
| 4 | 109.89 | 107.67 | 2.22 |
| 5 | 96.22 | 95.67 | 0.55 |
| 6 | 133.33 | 128.89 | 4.44 |
| 7 | 115.78 | 113.22 | 2.56 |
| 8 | 126.39 | 121.56 | 4.83 |
| 9 | 122.78 | 126.33 | −3.55 |
| 10 | 117.44 | 110.39 | 7.05 |
| 11 | 111.33 | 107.00 | 4.33 |
| 12 | 117.33 | 108.44 | 8.89 |
| 13 | 120.67 | 117.00 | 3.67 |
| 14 | 131.67 | 126.89 | 4.78 |
| 15 | 92.39 | 93.06 | −0.67 |
| 16 | 134.44 | 126.67 | 7.77 |
| 17 | 108.67 | 108.67 | 0.00 |

**Table 9.10** Comparison of drug A vs. placebo for the relief of redness and itching in hay fever patients

| Subject | Redness | Itching | Subject | Redness | Itching |
|---|---|---|---|---|---|
| 1 | 0 | + | 13 | + | + |
| 2 | 0 | + | 14 | 0 | 0 |
| 3 | − | − | 15 | 0 | 0 |
| 4 | + | − | 16 | − | 0 |
| 5 | 0 | + | 17 | − | + |
| 6 | + | + | 18 | − | 0 |
| 7 | + | + | 19 | 0 | 0 |
| 8 | − | 0 | 20 | − | + |
| 9 | − | + | 21 | − | 0 |
| 10 | 0 | − | 22 | − | + |
| 11 | + | + | 23 | 0 | 0 |
| 12 | 0 | + | 24 | − | 0 |
|  |  |  | 25 | − | 0 |

to compare drug A with placebo for redness or itching? Why?

**9.52** Compare redness in the drug A and placebo eyes and report a *p*-value.

**9.53** Compare itching in the drug A and placebo eyes and report a *p*-value.

In the second experiment drug **B** is administered to a randomly selected eye and a placebo is administered to the other eye. The data are given in Table 9.11.

**9.54** Compare redness in drug B and placebo eyes and report a *p*-value.

**Table 9.11**  _Comparison of drug B vs. placebo for the relief of redness and itching in hay fever patients_

| Subject | Redness | Itching | Subject | Redness | Itching |
|---------|---------|---------|---------|---------|---------|
| 1 | + | − | 13 | + | 0 |
| 2 | + | − | 14 | + | 0 |
| 3 | + | + | 15 | + | 0 |
| 4 | + | + | 16 | 0 | 0 |
| 5 | + | + | 17 | + | − |
| 6 | 0 | − | 18 | + | − |
| 7 | + | 0 | 19 | + | + |
| 8 | + | + | 20 | + | + |
| 9 | + | 0 | 21 | + | 0 |
| 10 | 0 | 0 | 22 | + | 0 |
| 11 | + | − | 23 | + | 0 |
| 12 | + | + | 24 | + | 0 |
|    |   |   | 25 | + | 0 |

**9.55** Compare itching in drug B and placebo eyes and report a _p_-value.

In the third experiment the combination of drugs A and B is administered to a randomly selected eye and a placebo is administered to the other eye. The data are given in Table 9.12.

**9.56** Compare redness in the combination and placebo eyes and report a _p_-value.

**9.57** Compare itching in the combination and placebo eyes and report a _p_-value.

**9.58** Summarize the results of the three experiments as concisely as possible.

### Hypertension

An instrument that is in fairly common use in blood pressure epidemiology is the random zero device, whereby the zero point of the machine is randomly set with each use and the observer is not aware of the actual level of blood pressure at the time of measurement. This instrument is intended to reduce observer bias. Before using such a machine, it is important to

**Table 9.12**  _Comparison of combination of drugs A and B vs. placebo for the relief of redness and itching in hay fever patients_

| Subject | Redness | Itching | Subject | Redness | Itching |
|---------|---------|---------|---------|---------|---------|
| 1 | + | + | 13 | + | + |
| 2 | + | 0 | 14 | + | 0 |
| 3 | + | + | 15 | + | 0 |
| 4 | + | + | 16 | + | + |
| 5 | + | + | 17 | + | + |
| 6 | + | − | 18 | + | + |
| 7 | + | + | 19 | 0 | + |
| 8 | + | 0 | 20 | 0 | + |
| 9 | + | + | 21 | + | 0 |
| 10 | + | + | 22 | + | 0 |
| 11 | + | − | 23 | + | 0 |
| 12 | + | − | 24 | + | 0 |
|    |   |   | 25 | + | + |

check that readings are, on the average, comparable to those of a standard cuff. For this purpose, two measurements were made on 20 children with both the standard cuff and the random zero machine. The mean blood pressures for the two readings are given in Table 9.13. Suppose observers are reluctant to assume that the distribution of blood pressure is normal.

**9.59** Which nonparametric test should be used to test the hypothesis that the two machines are comparable?

**9.60** Conduct the test recommended in Problem 9.59.

Another aspect of the same study is to compare the variability of blood pressure with each method. This comparison is achieved by measuring $|x_1 - x_2|$ for each method (i.e., the absolute difference between first and second readings) and comparing the absolute differences between machines. The data are given in Table 9.14. The observers are reluctant to assume that the distributions are normal.

**9.61** Which nonparametric test should be used to test the hypothesis that the variability of the two machines is comparable?

**9.62** Conduct the test recommended in Problem 9.61.

**Table 9.13** *Comparison of mean blood pressure with the standard cuff and the random zero machine (mm Hg)*

| Person (i) | Mean systolic bp (standard cuff) | Mean systolic bp (random zero) | Person (i) | Mean systolic bp (standard cuff) | Mean systolic bp (random zero) |
|---|---|---|---|---|---|
| 1 | 79 | 84 | 11 | 98 | 97 |
| 2 | 112 | 99 | 12 | 103 | 103 |
| 3 | 103 | 92 | 13 | 105 | 107 |
| 4 | 104 | 103 | 14 | 117 | 120 |
| 5 | 94 | 94 | 15 | 94 | 94 |
| 6 | 106 | 106 | 16 | 88 | 87 |
| 7 | 103 | 97 | 17 | 101 | 97 |
| 8 | 97 | 108 | 18 | 98 | 93 |
| 9 | 88 | 77 | 19 | 91 | 87 |
| 10 | 113 | 94 | 20 | 105 | 104 |

**Table 9.14** *Comparison of variability of blood pressure with the standard cuff and the random zero machine*

| Person (i) | Absolute difference, standard cuff ($a_s$) | Absolute difference, random zero ($a_r$) | Person (i) | Absolute difference, standard cuff ($a_s$) | Absolute difference, random zero ($a_r$) |
|---|---|---|---|---|---|
| 1 | 2 | 12 | 11 | 0 | 6 |
| 2 | 4 | 6 | 12 | 2 | 6 |
| 3 | 6 | 0 | 13 | 6 | 6 |
| 4 | 4 | 2 | 14 | 2 | 4 |
| 5 | 8 | 4 | 15 | 8 | 8 |
| 6 | 4 | 4 | 16 | 0 | 2 |
| 7 | 2 | 6 | 17 | 6 | 6 |
| 8 | 2 | 8 | 18 | 4 | 6 |
| 9 | 4 | 2 | 19 | 2 | 14 |
| 10 | 2 | 4 | 20 | 2 | 4 |

# References

[1] McNeil, D. R. (1967) "Efficiency Loss Due to Grouping in Distribution Free Tests," *Journal of the American Statistical Association* **62**: 954–965.

[2] Hollander, M. and Wolfe, D. (1973) *Nonparametric Statistical Methods* (New York: John Wiley).

[3] Salzman, R., Manson, J. E., Griffing, G. T., Kimmerle, R., Ruderman, N., McCall, A., Stoltz, E. I., Mullin, C., Small, D., Armstrong, J., and Melby, J. C. (1985) "Intranasal Aerosolized Insulin: Mixed-Meal Studies and Long Term Use in Type I Diabetes," *New England Journal of Medicine* **312(17)**: 1078–1084.

# 10 Hypothesis Testing: Categorical Data

## ■ 10.1 INTRODUCTION

In Chapters 7 and 8 we presented the basic methods of hypothesis testing for continuous data. We assumed that for each of the tests our data came from an underlying normal distribution and we proceeded to develop appropriate inference procedures based on this assumption. In Chapter 9 we relaxed the assumption of normality and developed alternative nonparametric tests that did not depend on the underlying distribution of the data.

If the variable under study is not continuous but is instead classified into categories, then the methods of Chapters 7 and 8 are not applicable, and different methods of inference should be used. We will consider the following types of problems in this chapter.

*Example 10.1*    *Cancer* Suppose we are interested in the association between the use of oral contraceptives (OC use) and the 1-year incidence of cervical cancer from January 1, 1978, to January 1, 1979. We classify women who are disease free on January 1, 1978, into two OC-use categories as of that date: ever users and never users. We are interested in whether or not the proportion of women who develop cervical cancer is different between ever users and never users. Hence we have a two-sample problem comparing two binomial proportions, and we cannot use the *t* test methodology of Chapter 8 because our outcome variable, "the development of cervical cancer," is a discrete variable with two categories (yes/no), not a continuous variable. ■

*Example 10.2*    *Cancer* Suppose we subdivide oral contraceptive users in Example 10.1 into "heavy" users, who have used the pill for 5 years or more, and "light" users, who have used the pill for less than 5 years. We may be interested in comparing 1-year cervical cancer incidence rates among heavy users, light users, and nonusers. In this problem we are comparing *three* binomial proportions, and again, the methods of Chapter 8 are not applicable. ■

*Example 10.3*    *Infectious Disease* We have discussed the fitting of a probability model based on the Poisson distribution to the random variable defined by the annual number of deaths due to polio in the United States during the period 1968–1976, as given in Table 4.7. We are interested in developing a general procedure for testing the goodness of fit of this and other probability models based on actual sample data. ■

In this chapter we will develop methods of hypothesis testing for comparing two or more binomial proportions. We also will develop methods for testing the goodness of fit of a previously specified probability model to actual data.

# ■ *10.2 TWO-SAMPLE TEST FOR BINOMIAL PROPORTIONS*

*Example 10.4*  *Cancer* A hypothesis has been proposed that breast cancer in women is caused in part by events that occur between the age at menarche (i.e., the age when menstruation begins) and the age at first childbirth. In particular, the hypothesis states that the risk of breast cancer increases as the length of this time interval increases. If this theory is correct, then an important risk factor is age at first birth. This theory would explain in part why breast cancer incidence seems to be higher for women in the upper socioeconomic groups, since they tend to have their children relatively late.

An international study was set up to test this hypothesis [1]. Breast cancer cases were identified among women in selected hospitals in the United States, Greece, Yugoslavia, Brazil, Taiwan, and Japan. Controls were chosen from women of comparable age who were in the hospital at the same time as the cases but who did *not* have breast cancer. All women were asked about their age at first birth.

We will arbitrarily divide women with at least one birth into two categories: (1) women whose age at first birth was $\leqslant 29$ and (2) women whose age at first birth was $\geqslant 30$. We find the following results among women with at least one birth: 683 out of 3220 (21.2%) women with breast cancer (case women) and 1498 out of 10,245 (14.6%) women without breast cancer (control women) had an age at first birth $\geqslant 30$. How can we assess whether this difference is significant or is simply due to chance? ■

Let $p_1$ = probability that the age at first birth is $\geqslant 30$ in case women with at least one birth and $p_2$ = probability that the age at first birth is $\geqslant 30$ in control women with at least one birth. The question is whether or not the underlying probability of having an age at first birth of $\geqslant 30$ is different in the two groups. This problem is equivalent to testing the hypothesis $H_0: p_1 = p_2 = p$ vs. $H_1: p_1 \neq p_2$ for some constant $p$.

We will present two approaches for testing the hypothesis. One approach uses normal theory methods similar to those developed in Chapter 8, which we will discuss in Section 10.2.1. A second approach uses contingency table methods and will be discussed in Section 10.2.2. These two approaches can be shown to be *equivalent* in that they always yield the same $p$-values, and which one is used is a matter of convenience.

## ☐ *10.2.1 Normal Theory Method*

It is reasonable to base our significance test on the difference between the sample proportions $(\hat{p}_1 - \hat{p}_2)$. If this difference is either very large or very small, then we would reject $H_0$; otherwise, we would accept $H_0$. We will assume that our samples are large enough so that the *normal approximation to the binomial distribution is valid*. Then under $H_0$, $\hat{p}_1$ is normally distributed with mean $p$ and variance $pq/n_1$, and $\hat{p}_2$ is normally distributed with mean $p$ and variance $pq/n_2$. Therefore, since the samples are independent, we have that $\hat{p}_1 - \hat{p}_2$ is normally distributed with mean 0 and variance

$$\frac{pq}{n_1} + \frac{pq}{n_2} = pq\left(\frac{1}{n_1} + \frac{1}{n_2}\right)$$

If we divide by the standard deviation

$$\sqrt{pq\left(\frac{1}{n_1} + \frac{1}{n_2}\right)}$$

then under $H_0$,

**10.1**
$$\lambda = (\hat{p}_1 - \hat{p}_2)/\sqrt{pq(1/n_1 + 1/n_2)} \sim N(0, 1)$$

Our problem again is that $p$ and $q$ are unknown, and thus we cannot compute the denominator of $\lambda$ unless we find some estimate for $p$. We can show that the best estimator for $p$ is based on a weighted average of the sample proportions $\hat{p}_1$, $\hat{p}_2$. This weighted average, which we refer to as $\hat{p}$, is given by

**10.2**
$$\hat{p} = \frac{n_1\hat{p}_1 + n_2\hat{p}_2}{n_1 + n_2} = \frac{x_1 + x_2}{n_1 + n_2}$$

where $x_1 = $ observed number of events in the first sample and $x_2 = $ observed number of events in the second sample. This estimate makes intuitive sense, since each of the sample proportions is weighted by the number of people in the sample. Thus, if we substitute our estimate $\hat{p}$ in **(10.2)** for $p$ in **(10.1)**, then we have the following test procedure:

**10.3** ### Two-Sample Test for Binomial Proportions (Normal Theory Test)

If we wish to test the hypothesis $H_0$: $p_1 = p_2$ vs. $H_1$: $p_1 \neq p_2$, where the proportions are obtained from two independent samples, then:

*1.* We compute the test statistic

$$\lambda = \frac{\hat{p}_1 - \hat{p}_2}{\sqrt{\hat{p}\hat{q}\left(\frac{1}{n_1} + \frac{1}{n_2}\right)}}$$

where

$$\hat{p} = (n_1\hat{p}_1 + n_2\hat{p}_2)/(n_1 + n_2), \quad \hat{q} = 1 - \hat{p}$$
$$= (x_1 + x_2)/(n_1 + n_2)$$

and $x_1$, $x_2$ are the number of events in the first and second samples, respectively.

2. For a two-sided level $\alpha$ test, if

$$\lambda > z_{1-\alpha/2} \quad \text{or} \quad \lambda < z_{\alpha/2}$$

then we reject $H_0$; if

$$z_{\alpha/2} \leqslant \lambda \leqslant z_{1-\alpha/2}$$

then we accept $H_0$.

3. The exact $p$-value for this test is given by

$$p = 2[1 - \Phi(\lambda)] \quad \text{if } \lambda \geqslant 0$$
$$= 2\Phi(\lambda) \quad \text{if } \lambda < 0$$

*4.* This test should be used only when the normal approximation to the binomial distribution is valid for each of the two samples, that is, when $n_1 \hat{p} \hat{q} \geqslant 5$ and $n_2 \hat{p} \hat{q} \geqslant 5$.

The acceptance and rejection regions for this test are depicted in Figure 10.1. Similarly, the computation of the exact $p$-value is illustrated in Figure 10.2.

---

*Example 10.5*

*Cancer* Assess the statistical significance of the results from the international study in Example 10.4.

*Solution*

We note from the study that the sample proportion of case women whose age at first birth was $\geqslant 30$ is $683/3220 = 0.212 = \hat{p}_1$ and that the sample proportion of control women whose age at first birth was $\geqslant 30$ is $1498/10{,}245 = 0.146 = \hat{p}_2$. To compute the test statistic $\lambda$ in **(10.3)**, we need to compute the estimated common proportion $\hat{p}$, which is given by

$$\hat{p} = (683 + 1498)/(3220 + 10{,}245)$$
$$= 2181/13{,}465 = 0.162$$
$$\hat{q} = 1 - 0.162 = 0.838$$

$$\lambda = \frac{\hat{p}_1 - \hat{p}_2}{\sqrt{\hat{p}\hat{q}\,(1/n_1 + 1/n_2)}}, \quad \text{where } \hat{p} = \frac{n_1\hat{p}_1 + n_2\hat{p}_2}{n_1 + n_2}, \; \hat{q} = 1 - \hat{p}$$

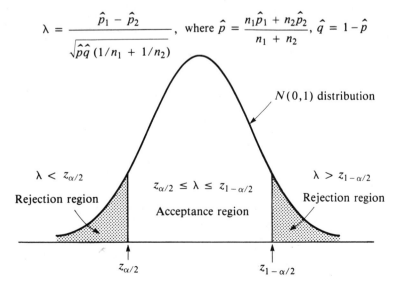

$N(0,1)$ distribution

*Figure 10.1*
Acceptance and
rejection regions
for the two-sample
test for binomial
proportions (normal
theory test)

$\lambda < z_{\alpha/2}$

Rejection region

$z_{\alpha/2} \leq \lambda \leq z_{1-\alpha/2}$

Acceptance region

$\lambda > z_{1-\alpha/2}$

Rejection region

$z_{\alpha/2}$

$z_{1-\alpha/2}$

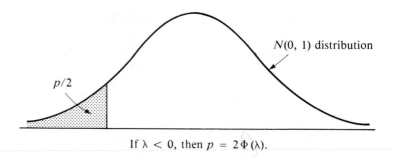

$$\text{If } \lambda < 0, \text{ then } p = 2\Phi(\lambda).$$

**_Figure 10.2_**
*Computation of the
exact p-value for
the two-sample test
for binomial
proportions (normal
theory test)*

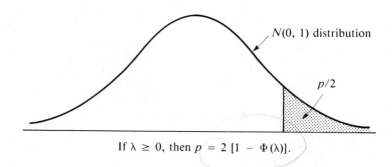

$$\text{If } \lambda \geq 0, \text{ then } p = 2[1 - \Phi(\lambda)].$$

We note that

$$n_1 \hat{p}\hat{q} = 3220(0.162)(0.838) = 437.1 \geq 5$$

and

$$n_2 \hat{p}\hat{q} = 10{,}245(0.162)(0.838) = 1390.8 \geq 5$$

Thus, we can use the test in **(10.3)**.
     The test statistic is given by

$$\lambda = (0.212 - 0.146)\Big/ \sqrt{(0.162)(0.838)\left(\frac{1}{3220} + \frac{1}{10{,}245}\right)}$$

$$= 0.0660/0.00744 = 8.9$$

Since $\lambda > 0$, the p-value $= 2 \times [1 - \Phi(8.9)] < 0.001$, and the results are extremely significant. Therefore, we can conclude that women with breast cancer are significantly more likely to have had their children after the age of 30 than are comparable women without breast cancer.    ■

*Example 10.6*    **Obstetrics** A subject of recent research in obstetrics is the medical management of women who go into labor prematurely, which we will define as labor occurring between 20 and 36 weeks of pregnancy. Premature labor is undesirable because infants born prematurely have a higher rate of infant mortality and morbidity. Terbutaline is a drug that is effectively used to arrest labor and prolong the duration of the pregnancy beyond 36 weeks. However, it sometimes has undesirable cardiovascular and metabolic side effects, such as tremors and hyperglycemia, which limit its use for some women. Another possibility is to give terbutaline in combination with another drug (metoprolol), which would neutralize these side effects.

However, before using this combination therapy, we want to compare its effectiveness in prolonging pregnancy with that of terbutaline alone. Suppose that we set up a clinical trial to compare the effectiveness of the two therapies, where the outcome is whether the pregnancy lasts beyond 36 weeks. We find that in 200 patients treated with terbutaline alone, 130 have a pregnancy lasting more than 36 weeks, whereas in 200 patients treated with terbutaline and metoprolol, 120 have a pregnancy lasting more than 36 weeks. Assess the significance of these results.

**Solution**     We wish to test the hypothesis $H_0: p_1 = p_2$ vs. $H_1: p_1 \neq p_2$, where $p_1$ = probability that a pregnancy lasts more than 36 weeks in the terbutaline group and $p_2$ = probability that a pregnancy will last more than 36 weeks in the terbutaline and metoprolol group. We have

$$n_1 = n_2 = 200$$

$$\hat{p} = (130 + 120)/400 = 0.625$$

We note that

$$n_1 \hat{p}\hat{q} = n_2 \hat{p}\hat{q} = 200(0.625)(0.375) = 46.9 \geqslant 5$$

Therefore, we can use the test procedure in **(10.3)**.
Thus, we compute the test statistic in **(10.3)** as follows:

$$\lambda = (\hat{p}_1 - \hat{p}_2) \Big/ \sqrt{\hat{p}\hat{q}\left(\frac{1}{n_1} + \frac{1}{n_2}\right)} = (0.65 - 0.6) \Big/ \sqrt{(0.625)(0.375)\left(\frac{1}{200} + \frac{1}{200}\right)}$$

$$= 0.05/\sqrt{0.002344} = 0.05/0.0484 = 1.03$$

Therefore, there is no significant difference between the effectiveness of the two therapies. To compute the *p*-value, we note that $\lambda \geqslant 0$. Thus,

$$p = 2 \times [1 - \Phi(1.03)] = 2(1 - 0.8485) = 0.303$$

We conclude that the combination therapy can be used instead of terbutaline alone to prolong pregnancy, since the two treatments have equal efficacy and the combination therapy has fewer side effects. ∎

## ☐ 10.2.2  Contingency Table Method

$Q \times 1.03 = 0.8485$

$Q = 0.8485/1.03$

We now pursue the same test posed in Section 10.2.1 but from a different perspective.

**Example 10.7**     *Cancer* Suppose we classify all women with at least one birth in the international study in Example 10.4 as either cases or controls and with age at first birth either $\leqslant 29$ or $\geqslant 30$. We can display the four possible combinations, as shown in Table 10.1.

We display the case/control status along the rows of the table and the age at first birth group down the columns of the table. Hence, each woman falls into one of the four boxes, or *cells*, of the table. In particular, we have 683 women with breast cancer whose age at first birth is $\geqslant 30$; 2537 women with breast cancer whose age at first birth is $\leqslant 29$; 1498 control women whose age at first birth is $\geqslant 30$; and 8747 control women whose age at first birth is $\leqslant 29$. Furthermore, we can total the number of units in each row and column and display them in the margins of the table. Thus, we see that there are 3220 case women $(683 + 2537)$; 10,245 control women $(1498 + 8747)$; 2181 women with age at first birth $\geqslant 30$ $(683 + 1498)$; and

**Table 10.1**

*Data for the international study in Example 10.4 comparing age at first birth in breast cancer cases with comparable controls*

|  | Age at first birth | | |
|---|---|---|---|
| Case/control status | ⩾30 | ⩾29 | Total |
| Case | 683 | 2537 | 3220 |
| Control | 1498 | 8747 | 10,245 |
| Total | 2181 | 11,284 | 13,465 |

(Reprinted with permission of *WHO Bulletin* **43**: 209–221, 1970)

11,284 women with age at first birth ⩽29 (2537 + 8747). These sums are referred to as **row margins** and **column margins,** respectively. Finally, we can display the total number of units = 13,465 in the lower-right-hand corner of the table, which can be obtained either by summing the four cells (683 + 2537 + 1498 + 8747) or by summing the row margins (3220 + 10,245) or the column margins (2181 + 11,284). This sum is sometimes referred to as the **grand total**. ∎

Table 10.1 is called a **2 × 2 contingency table** because of the two groups for case/control status and the two groups for age at first birth status.

**Definition 10.1**

A **2 × 2 contingency table** is a table composed of two rows and two columns. It is an appropriate way to display data that can be classified by two different variables, *each* of which has only two possible outcomes. One variable is arbitrarily assigned to the rows and the other to the columns. Each of the four *cells* represents the number of units with a specific value for each of the two variables. The cells are sometimes referred to by number, with the (1, 1) cell being the cell in the first row and first column, the (1, 2) cell being the cell in the first row and second column, the (2, 1) cell being the cell in the second row and first column, and the (2,2) cell being the cell in the second row and second column. The observed number of units in the four cells is likewise referred to as $O_{11}$, $O_{12}$, $O_{21}$, and $O_{22}$, respectively. Furthermore, it is customary to total

1. The number of units in each row and display them in the right margins, which are referred to as **row margins**

2. The number of units in each column and display them in the bottom margins, which are referred to as **column margins**

3. The total number of units in the columns and the rows in the four cells, which is displayed in the lower-right-hand corner of the table and is referred to as the **grand total**

**Example 10.8**    *Obstetrics* Display the premature labor data in Example 10.6 in the form of a 2 × 2 contingency table.

**Solution**    We let the rows of the table represent the treatment group, with the first row representing the terbutaline group and the second row representing the terbutaline and metoprolol group. We let the columns of the table represent the duration of pregnancy, with the first column representing pregnancies lasting >36 weeks and the second column representing pregnancies lasting ⩽36 weeks. We have 200 women on terbutaline alone, of whom 130 had pregnancies lasting >36 weeks and 70 had pregnancies lasting ⩽36 weeks. We have 200 women on ter-

**Table 10.2**
*2 × 2 contingency table for the premature labor data in Example 10.6*

| Treatment group | Duration of pregnancy | | Total |
|---|---|---|---|
| | *>36 weeks* | *≤36 weeks* | |
| Terbutaline | 130 | 70 | 200 |
| Terbutaline and metoprolol | 120 | 80 | 200 |
| Total | 250 | 150 | 400 |

butaline and metoprolol, of whom 120 had pregnancies lasting > 36 weeks and 80 had pregnancies lasting ≤ 36 weeks. Thus, our contingency table should look like Table 10.2.

Note that two different sampling designs lend themselves to a contingency table framework. In the breast cancer data in Example 10.4, we have two independent samples (i.e., case women and control women) and we want to compare the proportion of women in each group who have first birth at a late age. Similarly, in the premature labor data in Example 10.6, we have two independent samples of women assigned to different treatment groups, and we wish to compare the proportion of women in each group with a favorable outcome (i.e., a pregnancy lasting > 36 weeks). In both instances we want to test whether or not the proportions are the same in the two independent samples. This test is referred to as a **test for homogeneity of binomial proportions**. Another possible sampling design from which contingency tables arise is in testing for the independence of two characteristics in the same sample when neither characteristic is particularly appropriate as a denominator.

*Example 10.9*

*Nutrition* The food frequency questionnaire is widely used to measure dietary intake. A person specifies the number of servings consumed per week of each of many different food items. The total nutrient composition is then calculated from the specific dietary components of each food item. One way to judge how well a questionnaire measures dietary intake is by its reproducibility. To assess reproducibility we distribute the questionnaire at two different points in time to 50 persons and compare the reported nutrient intake from the two questionnaires. Suppose we quantify dietary cholesterol on each questionnaire as high if > 300 mg/day and normal otherwise. The contingency table provided in Table 10.3 is a natural way to compare the results of the two surveys. Notice that there is no natural denominator in this example. We simply want to test how closely related the two reported measures of dietary

**Table 10.3**
*A comparison of dietary cholesterol assessed by a food frequency questionnaire at two different points in time*

| First food frequency questionnaire | Second food frequency questionnaire | | Total |
|---|---|---|---|
| | *High* | *Normal* | |
| High | 15 | 5 | 20 |
| Normal | 9 | 21 | 30 |
| Total | 24 | 26 | 50 |

cholesterol are for the same person. This test is referred to as a **test of independence** or a **test of association** between the two characteristics.

Fortunately, we use the same test procedure whether we are performing a test of homogeneity or a test of independence, and we will no longer distinguish between these two sampling designs in this section. ■

## ☐ *10.2.3 Significance Testing Using the Contingency Table Approach*

In Table 10.1 we presented what we will refer to as the **observed contingency table** or the **observed table**. What we need to develop is an **expected table**, which is the contingency table we would expect if there were no relationship between breast cancer and age at first birth, that is, if $H_0: p_1 = p_2 = p$ were true. In this example $p_1$ and $p_2$ are the probabilities (among women with at least one birth) of a breast cancer case and a control, respectively, having a first birth at an age $\geqslant 30$. For this purpose we give a general observed table if there were $x_1$ events out of $n_1$ women with breast cancer and $x_2$ events out of $n_2$ control women, as shown in Table 10.4.

**Table 10.4**
*General contingency table for the international study data in Example 10.4 if (1) of $n_1$ women in the case group, $x_1$ have events, and (2) of $n_2$ women in the control group, $x_2$ have events. (An event here means having an age at first birth $\geqslant 30$.)*

|  | Age at first birth | | |
|---|---|---|---|
| *Case/control status* | $\geqslant 30$ | $\leqslant 29$ | *Total* |
| *Case* | $x_1$ | $n_1 - x_1$ | $n_1$ |
| *Control* | $x_2$ | $n_2 - x_2$ | $n_2$ |
| *Total* | $x_1 + x_2$ | $n_1 + n_2 - (x_1 + x_2)$ | $n_1 + n_2$ |

If $H_0$ were true, then the best estimate of the common proportion $p$ is $\hat{p}$, which is given in **(10.2)** as

$$(n_1 \hat{p}_1 + n_2 \hat{p}_2)/(n_1 + n_2)$$

or, alternatively, as

$$(x_1 + x_2)/(n_1 + n_2)$$

where $x_1$ and $x_2$ are the numbers of events in groups 1 and 2, respectively. Furthermore, under $H_0$ the expected number of units in the (1, 1) cell equals the expected number of women with age at first birth $\geqslant 30$ among women with breast cancer, which is given by

$$n_1 \hat{p} = n_1(x_1 + x_2)/(n_1 + n_2)$$

However, if we refer to Table 10.4, this number is simply the product of the first row margin ($n_1$) multiplied by the first column margin ($x_1 + x_2$), divided by the grand total ($n_1 + n_2$). Similarly, the expected number of units in the (2, 1) cell equals the expected number of women with age at first birth $\geq 30$ among control women:

$$n_2 \hat{p} = n_2(x_1 + x_2)/(n_1 + n_2)$$

which is equal to the product of the second row margin multiplied by the first column margin, divided by the grand total. In general terms we have the following rule:

**10.4** **Computation of Expected Values for 2 × 2 Contingency Tables**

The **expected number of units** in the **(*i,j*) cell**, which is usually denoted by $E_{ij}$, is the product of the ***i*th** row margin multiplied by the ***j*th** column margin, divided by the grand total.

*Example 10.10* *Cancer* Compute the expected table for the breast cancer data in Example 10.4.

*Solution* We refer to Table 10.1, which gives the observed table for these data. The row totals are 3220 and 10,245; the column totals are 2181 and 11,284; and the grand total is 13,465. Thus,

$$E_{11} = \text{expected number of units in the (1, 1) cell}$$
$$= 3220(2181)/13{,}465 = 521.6$$
$$E_{12} = \text{expected number of units in the (1, 2) cell}$$
$$= 3220(11{,}284)/13{,}465 = 2698.4$$
$$E_{21} = \text{expected number of units in the (2, 1) cell}$$
$$= 10{,}245(2181)/13{,}465 = 1659.4$$
$$E_{22} = \text{expected number of units in the (2, 2) cell}$$
$$= 10{,}245(11{,}284)/13{,}465 = 8585.6$$

These expected values are displayed in Table 10.5.

*Table 10.5*
*Expected table for the breast cancer data in Example 10.4*

| | Age at first birth | | |
|---|---|---|---|
| *Case/control status* | $\geq 30$ | $\leq 29$ | *Total* |
| *Case* | 521.6 | 2698.4 | 3220 |
| *Control* | 1659.4 | 8585.6 | 10,245 |
| *Total* | 2181 | 11,284 | 13,465 |

*Example 10.11* *Obstetrics* Compute the expected table for the premature labor data in Example 10.6.

*Solution* We refer to Table 10.2, which gives the observed table for these data. We have

$$E_{11} = 200(250)/400 = 125$$

$$E_{12} = 200(150)/400 = 75$$

$$E_{21} = 200(250)/400 = 125$$

$$E_{22} = 200(150)/400 = 75$$

These expected values are displayed in Table 10.6.

**Table 10.6**

*Expected table for the premature labor data in Example 10.6*

|  | Duration of pregnancy | | |
|---|---|---|---|
| *Treatment group* | *>36 weeks* | *⩽36 weeks* | *Total* |
| *Terbutaline* | 125 | 75 | 200 |
| *Terbutaline and metoprolol* | 125 | 75 | 200 |
| *Total* | 250 | 150 | 400 |

We can show from **(10.4)** that the *total* of the expected number of units in any row or column should be the same as the corresponding observed row or column total. This relationship provides a useful check that the expected values are computed correctly.

**Example 10.12**    Check that the expected values in Table 10.5 are computed correctly.

**Solution**    We have the following information:

1. The total of the expected values in the first row = $E_{11} + E_{12} = 521.6 + 2698.4 = 3220 = $ first row total in the observed table.
2. The total of the expected values in the second row = $E_{21} + E_{22} = 1659.4 + 8585.6 = 10,245 = $ second row total in the observed table.
3. The total of the expected values in the first column = $E_{11} + E_{21} = 521.6 + 1659.4 = 2181 = $ first column total in the observed table.
4. The total of the expected values in the second column = $E_{12} + E_{22} = 2698.4 + 8585.6 = 11,284 = $ second column total in the observed table.

We now wish to compare the observed table in Table 10.1 with the expected table in Table 10.5. If the corresponding cells in these two tables are close, then we will accept $H_0$; if they are sufficiently different, then we will reject $H_0$. How should we decide how different the cells should be for us to reject $H_0$? We can show that the best way of comparing the cells in the two tables is to use the statistic $(O - E)^2/E$, where $O$ and $E$ are the observed and expected number of units, respectively, in a particular cell. In particular, under $H_0$ we can show that the sum of $(O - E)^2/E$ over the four cells in the table approximately follows a chi-square distribution with 1 d.f. We wish to reject $H_0$ only if this sum is large and accept $H_0$ otherwise, since small values of this sum correspond to good agreement between the two tables, whereas large values correspond to poor agreement. We will use this test procedure only when the normal approximation to the binomial distribution is valid. In this setting it can be shown to be approximately true if *no expected value in the table is less than 5.*

Furthermore, we can show that under certain circumstances a version of this test statistic with a *continuity correction* yields more accurate *p*-values than does the uncorrected version when approximated by a chi-square distribution. For the continuity corrected version, we compute the statistic $(|O - E| - \tfrac{1}{2})^2/E$ for each cell rather than $(O - E)^2/E$ and sum the preceding expression over the four cells. This test procedure is referred to as the chi-square test using the Yates correction and is summarized as follows:

**10.5** **Yates Corrected Chi-Square Test for a 2 × 2 Contingency Table**

Suppose we wish to test the hypothesis $H_0: p_1 = p_2$ vs. $H_1: p_1 \neq p_2$ using a contingency table format, where $O_{ij}$ represents the observed number of units in the $(i, j)$ cell and $E_{ij}$ represents the expected number of units in the $(i, j)$ cell.

1. We compute the test statistic

$$T = (|O_{11} - E_{11}| - 0.5)^2/E_{11} + (|O_{12} - E_{12}| - 0.5)^2/E_{12}$$
$$+ (|O_{21} - E_{21}| - 0.5)^2/E_{21} + (|O_{22} - E_{22}| - 0.5)^2/E_{22}$$

which under $H_0$ approximately follows a $\chi_1^2$ distribution.

2. For a level $\alpha$ test, we reject $H_0$ if $T > \chi_{1,1-\alpha}^2$ and accept $H_0$ if $T \leq \chi_{1,1-\alpha}^2$.

3. The exact *p*-value is given by the area to the right of $T$ under a $\chi_1^2$ distribution.

4. We use this test only if none of the four expected values is less than 5.

The acceptance and rejection regions for this test are depicted in Figure 10.3. The computation of the exact *p*-value is illustrated in Figure 10.4.

*Example 10.13*     **Cancer** Assess the breast cancer data in Example 10.4 for statistical significance.

*Solution*     We first must compute the observed and expected tables as given in Tables 10.1 and 10.5, respectively. We check that all expected values in Table 10.5 are at least 5, which is clearly the

*Figure 10.3*
Acceptance and rejection regions for the Yates corrected chi-square test for a 2 × 2 contingency table

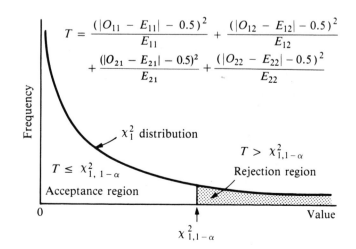

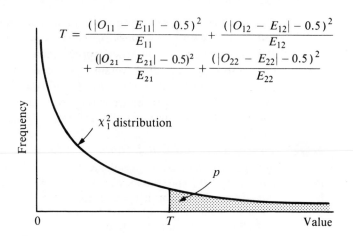

$$T = \frac{(|O_{11} - E_{11}| - 0.5)^2}{E_{11}} + \frac{(|O_{12} - E_{12}| - 0.5)^2}{E_{12}}$$
$$+ \frac{(|O_{21} - E_{21}| - 0.5)^2}{E_{21}} + \frac{(|O_{22} - E_{22}| - 0.5)^2}{E_{22}}$$

**Figure 10.4**
*Computation of the p-value for the Yates corrected chi-square test for a 2 × 2 contingency table*

case. Thus, following **(10.5)**, we have

$$T = \frac{(|683 - 521.6| - 0.5)^2}{521.6} + \frac{(|2537 - 2698.4| - 0.5)^2}{2698.4}$$
$$+ \frac{(|1498 - 1659.4| - 0.5)^2}{1659.4} + \frac{(|8747 - 8585.6| - 0.5)^2}{8585.6}$$
$$= \frac{(160.9)^2}{521.6} + \frac{(160.9)^2}{2698.4} + \frac{(160.9)^2}{1659.4} + \frac{(160.9)^2}{8585.6}$$
$$= 49.633 + 9.594 + 15.601 + 3.015$$
$$= 77.84 \sim \chi_1^2 \text{ under } H_0$$

Since

$$\chi_{1,.999}^2 = 10.83 < 77.84 = T$$

we have

$$p < 1 - 0.999 = 0.001$$

and the results are extremely significant.                                                   ∎

**Example 10.14**   **Obstetrics**   Assess the premature labor data in Example 10.6 for statistical significance.

**Solution**   We must first compute the observed and expected tables as given in Tables 10.2 and 10.6, respectively. We note that the minimum expected value in Table 10.6 is 75, which is $\geqslant 5$. Thus, we can use the test procedure in **(10.5)**. We have

$$T = \frac{(|130 - 125| - 0.5)^2}{125} + \frac{(|70 - 75| - 0.5)^2}{75} + \frac{(|120 - 125| - 0.5)^2}{125} + \frac{(|80 - 75| - 0.5)^2}{75}$$
$$= \frac{(4.5)^2}{125} + \frac{(4.5)^2}{75} + \frac{(4.5)^2}{125} + \frac{(4.5)^2}{75}$$
$$= 0.162 + 0.270 + 0.162 + 0.270$$
$$= 0.86 \sim \chi_1^2 \text{ under } H_0$$

Since

$$\chi^2_{1,.95} = 3.84 > 0.86 = T$$

we see that

$$p > 1 - 0.95 = 0.05$$

and the results are *not* statistically significant. Thus, there is no significant difference between the treatments in terms of prolonging pregnancy. Thus, the combination therapy would be preferable, since it is as effective as terbutaline alone in prolonging pregnancy but has fewer side effects. ∎

We can show that the test procedure in (**10.3**) and the test procedure in (**10.5**) used without continuity correction are equivalent in the sense that they always give the same *p*-values and always result in the same decisions about accepting or rejecting $H_0$. Which test procedure is used is a matter of convenience. Most research workers find the contingency table approach more understandable, and results are more frequently reported in this format in the scientific literature.

At this time statisticians disagree widely about whether or not a continuity correction is needed for the contingency table test in (**10.5**). Generally, *p*-values obtained using the continuity correction are slightly larger. Thus, results obtained are slightly less significant than comparable results obtained without using a continuity correction. However, the difference in results obtained using these two methods should be small for tables based on large sample sizes. I believe that the Yates corrected test statistic is slightly more widely used in the applied literature and therefore I use it in this section.

## ☐ 10.2.4 Short Computational Form for the Yates-Corrected Chi-Square Test for 2 × 2 Contingency Tables

The test statistic $T$ in (**10.5**) has another computational version that is more convenient to use with a hand calculator and does not require the computation of an expected table. In particular:

**10.6** *Short Computational Form for the Yates-Corrected Chi-Square Test for 2 × 2 Contingency Tables*

Suppose we have the 2 × 2 contingency table in Table 10.7. The test statistic $T$ in (**10.5**) can be written in the form

$$T = n\left(|ad - bc| - \frac{n}{2}\right)^2 \Big/ [(a + b)(c + d)(a + c)(b + d)]$$

Thus, the test statistic $T$ depends only on (1) the grand total $n$, (2) the row and column margins $a + b, c + d, a + c, b + d$, and (3) the quantity $ad - bc$. To compute $T$, we proceed as follows:

*1.* Compute

$$\left(|ad - bc| - \frac{n}{2}\right)^2$$

Start with the first column margin and proceed counterclockwise.

2. Divide by each of the two column margins.

3. Multiply by the grand total.

4. Divide by each of the two row margins.

This computation is particularly easy with a hand calculator, since previous products and quotients can be maintained in the display and used for further calculations.

**Table 10.7**

*General contingency table*

| $a$ | $b$ | $a + b$ |
|-----|-----|---------|
| $c$ | $d$ | $c + d$ |
| $a + c$ | $b + d$ | $n = a + b + c + d$ |

**Example 10.15**

**Nutrition** Compute the chi-square statistic for the nutrition data in Example 10.9 using the short computational form in **(10.6)**.

**Solution**

From Table 10.3 we have

$$a = 15 \quad b = 5 \quad c = 9 \quad d = 21 \quad n = 50$$

Furthermore, the smallest expected value $= (24 \times 20)/50 = 9.6 \geqslant 5$. Thus, it is valid to use the chi-square test. We follow the approach in **(10.6)** as follows:

1. We compute

$$\left( |ad - bc| - \frac{n}{2} \right)^2 = \left[ |15 \times 21 - 5 \times 9| - \frac{50}{2} \right]^2$$

$$= (270 - 25)^2$$

$$= 245^2 = 60{,}025$$

2. We divide the result in step 1 (60,025) by each of the two column margins (24 and 26), thus obtaining 96.194.

3. We multiply the result in step 2 (96.194) by the grand total (50), thus obtaining 4809.70.

4. We divide the result in step 3 (4809.70) by each of the two row margins (20 and 30), thus obtaining 8.02.

Since the critical value $= \chi^2_{1,.95} = 3.84$ and $T = 8.02 > 3.84$, the results are statistically significant. To obtain a range for the *p*-value, we note from the chi-square table that $\chi^2_{1,.995} = 7.88$, $\chi^2_{1,.999} = 10.83$, and thus, since $7.88 < 8.02 < 10.83$, we have $0.001 < p < 0.005$.

We have also analyzed these data using the SPSS/PC CROSSTABS program, as shown in Table 10.8. The program prints out the cell counts, the row and column totals and percentages, and the grand total. Furthermore, it prints out the minimum expected frequency (min E.F. $= 9.6$), and it is noted that there are no expected frequencies $<5$. Finally, the significance test is performed using both the Yates corrected chi-square test (chi-square $= 8.02$, $df = 1$, *p*-value $= 0.0046$) and the uncorrected chi-square test (chi-square $= 9.74$, $df = 1$, *p*-value $= 0.0018$).

**Table 10.8**
*Use of SPSS/PC CROSSTABS program to analyze the nutrition data in Table 10.3*

```
                              SPSS/PC   Release 1.0

      Crosstabulation:      CHOL1     1ST FOOD FREQUENCY QUESTIONNAIRE
                        By CHOL2     2ND FOOD FREQUENCY QUESTIONNAIRE


                  Count |HIGH    | NORMAL  |
           CHOL2->       |        |         |       Row
                         |   1.00 |    2.00 |     Total
           CHOL1         |        |         |
                    1.00 |    15  |     5   |      20
             HIGH        |        |         |     40.0

                    2.00 |     9  |    21   |      30
             NORMAL      |        |         |     60.0

                 Column      24       26         50
                 Total      48.0     52.0      100.0


      Chi-Square     D.F.      Significance      Min E.F.     Cells with E.F.< 5
      ----------     ----      ------------      --------     ------------------

         8.01616      1          0.0046           9.600            None
         9.73558      1          0.0018        ( Before Yates Correction )

      Number of Missing Observations =        0
```

The results show a highly significant association between dietary cholesterol intake reported by the same person at two different points in time, which gives us confidence in the reproducibility of our instrument. We will discuss the issue of reproducibility for discrete data in more detail in Section 11.14. ∎

# ■ *10.3 INTERVAL ESTIMATES FOR BINOMIAL PROPORTIONS*

In Section 10.2 we focused on methods for testing hypotheses concerning two binomial proportions. In many applications we are also interested in interval estimates for either the difference or the ratio between two proportions, in addition to the determination of statistical significance.

## □ *10.3.1 Interval Estimates for the Difference Between Two Proportions*

We note from Section 10.2.1 that if the normal approximation to the binomial distribution is valid, then $p_1 - p_2$ is normally distributed with mean 0 and variance $pq(1/n_1 + 1/n_2)$. As we discussed in Section 10.2, since $p$ is generally unknown, we estimate $p$ by $\hat{p}$ and $q$ by $\hat{q}$. If we use the general method for constructing confidence limits provided in Section 6.4, then a two-sided $100\% \times (1 - \alpha)$ confidence interval for $p_1 - p_2$ is given by

**10.7**

$$[\hat{p}_1 - \hat{p}_2 - z_{1-\alpha/2}\sqrt{\hat{p}\hat{q}(1/n_1 + 1/n_2)},\ \hat{p}_1 - \hat{p}_2 + z_{1-\alpha/2}\sqrt{\hat{p}\hat{q}(1/n_1 + 1/n_2)}]$$

**Example 10.16**    **Obstetrics** Referring to the premature labor data in Table 10.2, compute a 95% confidence interval for the difference in the proportion of women with a successful outcome (i.e., duration of pregnancy $> 36$ weeks) between the two treatment groups.

**Solution**    We have

$\hat{p}_1$ = proportion of women on terbutaline with a duration of pregnancy
   $> 36$ weeks = $\frac{130}{200} = 0.65$

$\hat{p}_2$ = proportion of women on terbutaline and metoprolol with a duration of pregnancy
   $> 36$ weeks = $\frac{120}{200} = 0.60$

Furthermore,

$$\hat{p} = (130 + 120)/(200 + 200) = 0.625$$

$$\hat{q} = 1 - \hat{p} = 1 - 0.625 = 0.375$$

From **(10.7)** the 95% confidence interval for $p_1 - p_2$ is given by

$$[0.65 - 0.60 - z_{.975}\sqrt{\hat{p}\hat{q}(1/n_1 + 1/n_2)},\ 0.65 - 0.60 + z_{.975}\sqrt{\hat{p}\hat{q}(1/n_1 + 1/n_2)}]$$

$$= [0.05 - 1.96\sqrt{(0.625)(0.375)(0.01)},\ 0.05 + 1.96\sqrt{(0.625)(0.375)(0.01)}]$$

$$= (0.05 - 0.095,\ 0.05 + 0.095)$$

$$= (-0.045,\ 0.145)$$    ∎

## ☐ 10.3.2 The Odds Ratio

We can often understand the relationship between proportions more easily in terms of a ratio than in terms of a difference. For this purpose we define the odds in favor of a success as follows:

**Definition 10.2**

If the probability of a success = $p$, then **the odds in favor of success** = $p/(1 - p)$.

If we consider two proportions $p_1$, $p_2$ and compute the odds in favor of success for each proportion, then the ratio of odds, or **odds ratio**, becomes a useful measure for relating the two proportions.

**Definition 10.3**

Let $p_1$, $p_2$ be the probability of success for two populations. The **odds ratio** ($OR$) is defined as

$$OR = \frac{p_1/q_1}{p_2/q_2} = \frac{p_1 q_2}{p_2 q_1}$$

and is estimated by

$$\widehat{OR} = \frac{\hat{p}_1 \hat{q}_2}{\hat{p}_2 \hat{q}_1}$$

Equivalently, if the four cells of the $2 \times 2$ contingency table are labeled by $a, b, c, d$, as they are in

Table 10.7, then

$$\widehat{OR} = \frac{ad}{bc}$$

**Example 10.17**    **Obstetrics**  Using the premature labor data in Table 10.2, compute the odds ratio in favor of a successful outcome for terbutaline therapy vs. that for combination therapy.

**Solution**    We have $\hat{p}_1 = 0.65$, $\hat{q}_1 = 0.35$, $\hat{p}_2 = 0.60$, $\hat{q}_2 = 0.40$. Thus,

$$\widehat{OR} = \frac{(0.65)(0.40)}{(0.60)(0.35)} = \frac{0.260}{0.210} = 1.24$$

We could have also computed $OR$ from the contingency table in Table 10.2, whereby

$$\widehat{OR} = \frac{130 \times 80}{70 \times 120} = 1.24 \qquad \blacksquare$$

If the probability of success is the same in the two groups (i.e., $H_0$ is true), then $OR = 1$. Conversely, odds ratios greater than 1 indicate a greater likelihood of success in the first group than in the second group, whereas odds ratios less than 1 indicate a greater likelihood of success in the second group than in the first group.

In Chapter 3 we introduced a related measure of association called the **relative risk** ($RR$). The relative risk can be expressed as the ratio of the success rates in the two groups or, in symbols, as $p_1/p_2$. Although easily understandable, the relative risk has the disadvantage of being constrained by the denominator probability ($p_2$). For example, if $p_2 = 0.5$, then $RR$ can be no larger than $1/0.5 = 2$; if $p_2 = 0.8$, then $RR$ can be no larger than $1/0.8 = 1.25$. The odds ratio, on the other hand, has no such restriction and can range from 0 to $\infty$, regardless of the denominator probability. This property is particularly advantageous when we wish to combine results over several $2 \times 2$ tables, as we will discuss in Section 10.8. Finally, if the probabilities of success are low (i.e., $p_1$, $p_2$ are small), then $1 - p_1$ and $1 - p_2$ will each be close to 1, and the odds ratio will be approximately the same as the relative risk.

## ☐ 10.3.3 Interval Estimates for the Odds Ratio

Several methods exist for obtaining interval estimates for the odds ratio. The **test-based method** of Miettinen has the advantages of easy implementation and the determination of the significance of results that are always consistent with the chi-square test in **(10.5)**. The method is given as follows:

| 10.8 |
|---|

### *Interval Estimates for the Odds Ratio (Test-Based Method)*

A two-sided $100\% \times (1 - \alpha)$ confidence interval for $OR$ is given by

$$(\widehat{OR}^{1 - \sqrt{\chi_{1,1-\alpha}^2/T}},\ \widehat{OR}^{1 + \sqrt{\chi_{1,1-\alpha}^2/T}}) \qquad \text{if } \widehat{OR} \geq 1$$

$$(\widehat{OR}^{1 + \sqrt{\chi_{1,1-\alpha}^2/T}},\ \widehat{OR}^{1 - \sqrt{\chi_{1,1-\alpha}^2/T}}) \qquad \text{if } \widehat{OR} < 1$$

where $\hat{p}_1$, $\hat{p}_2$ are the estimated probabilities of success in the two samples and

$$\widehat{OR} = \frac{(\hat{p}_1 \hat{q}_2)}{(\hat{p}_2 \hat{q}_1)}$$

$T$ = chi-square statistic in **(10.5)**

Note that if the chi-square statistic is statistically significant at level $\alpha$, then $T > \chi^2_{1,1-\alpha}$ and $1 - \sqrt{\chi^2_{1,1-\alpha}/T} > 0$. Therefore, if $\widehat{OR} > 1$, then the lower confidence limit $> 1.0$, whereas if $\widehat{OR} < 1$, then the upper confidence limit $< 1.0$. In either case the confidence interval will not include 1 (the value under the null hypothesis). By similar logic, if the chi-square statistic is not statistically significant at level $\alpha$, then the confidence interval will always include 1. This relationship is summarized as follows:

**10.9**   **Relationship of the Test-Based Confidence Interval and the Chi-Square Test**

The two-sided $100\% \times (1 - \alpha)$ test-based confidence interval in **(10.8)** will contain 1 (the null value) if the chi-square test statistic in **(10.5)** is not statistically significant at level $\alpha$.

Similarly, the $100\% \times (1 - \alpha)$ test-based confidence interval in **(10.8)** will exclude 1 if the chi-square test statistic in **(10.5)** is statistically significant at level $\alpha$.

*Example 10.18*   **Obstetrics**  Using the premature labor data in Table 10.2, compute a 95% confidence interval for the odds ratio in favor of a duration of pregnancy $> 36$ weeks for the terbutaline group vs. that for the combination group.

*Solution*   We have from Example 10.17 that $\widehat{OR} = 1.24$ and from Example 10.14 that $T = 0.86$. Furthermore, $\chi^2_{1,.95} = 3.84$. Therefore, since $OR > 1$, it follows that

$$c_1 = 1.24^{1 - \sqrt{3.84/0.86}}$$

$$= 1.24^{1 - 2.11}$$

$$= 1.24^{-1.11}$$

$$= 0.79$$

$$c_2 = 1.24^{1 + \sqrt{3.84/0.86}}$$

$$= 1.24^{1 + 2.11}$$

$$= 1.24^{3.11}$$

$$= 1.95$$

Therefore, the 95% confidence interval for $OR = (0.79, 1.95)$. Notice that the confidence interval contains 1, which is consistent with the nonsignificant results of the hypothesis test.    ∎

*Example 10.19*   **Cancer**  Using the international study data in Table 10.1, compute the odds ratio for an age at first birth $\geqslant 30$ for the breast cancer cases compared with that for the controls.

**Solution**    From Table 10.1 we have

$$\widehat{OR} = \frac{683 \times 8747}{2537 \times 1498} = 1.57$$

Furthermore, from Example 10.13, $T = 77.84$. Therefore, from **(10.8)** we have

$$c_1 = 1.57^{1-\sqrt{3.84/77.84}}$$

$$= 1.57^{1-0.22}$$

$$= 1.57^{0.78}$$

$$= 1.42$$

$$c_2 = 1.57^{1+\sqrt{3.84/77.84}}$$

$$= 1.57^{1+0.22}$$

$$= 1.57^{1.22}$$

$$= 1.73$$

Thus, the 95% confidence interval for $OR = (1.42, 1.73)$. Note that the confidence interval does not contain 1 (the value under the null hypothesis), which is consistent with the highly significant chi-square statistic. ∎

**Example 10.20**    **Obstetrics** Suppose the successful outcome in Example 10.18 is changed to premature delivery ($\leqslant 36$ weeks). Compute the odds ratio and the associated 95% confidence interval for terbutaline vs. combination therapy.

**Solution**    If we interchange the first and second columns in Table 10.2, we have

$$a = 70 \quad b = 130 \quad c = 80 \quad d = 120$$

Therefore,

$$\widehat{OR} = \frac{ad}{bc} = \frac{70 \times 120}{130 \times 80} = 0.81$$

Furthermore, we have the same chi-square statistic as that in Example 10.18, that is, $T = 0.86$. Since $\widehat{OR} < 1$, it follows from **(10.8)** that

$$c_1 = 0.81^{1+\sqrt{3.84/0.86}}$$

$$= 0.81^{1+2.11}$$

$$= 0.81^{3.11}$$

$$= 0.52$$

$$c_2 = 0.81^{1-\sqrt{3.84/0.86}}$$

$$= 0.81^{1-2.11}$$

$$= 0.81^{-1.11}$$

$$= 1.26$$

Therefore, the estimated odds ratio = 0.81, with the associated 95% confidence interval = (0.52, 1.26). Once again, the confidence interval contains the value that is under the null hypothesis (1), since the chi-square test statistic was not significant at the 5% level.    ∎

Some statisticians have found that the test-based method is inaccurate if the estimated odds ratio is too far from 1 in either direction. Specifically, this method should be used only if $0.2 \leqslant \widehat{OR} \leqslant 5.0$. If $\widehat{OR}$ is outside this range, then more sophisticated methods should be used for confidence interval estimation. See Kleinbaum, Kupper, and Morgenstern for more details on this subject [2].

# ◼ *10.4 ESTIMATION OF SAMPLE SIZE AND POWER FOR COMPARING TWO BINOMIAL PROPORTIONS*

In Section 8.6 we presented methods for estimating the sample size needed to compare means from two normally distributed populations. We now wish to develop similar methods for estimating the sample size required to compare two proportions.

*Example 10.21*    *Cancer, Nutrition* Suppose we know from Connecticut tumor registry data that the incidence rate of breast cancer over a 1-year period for initially disease-free women ages 45–49 is 150 cases per 100,000 [3]. We wish to study whether or not the ingestion of large doses of vitamin A in tablet form will prevent breast cancer. We set up our study with (1) a control group of 45–49-year-old women who are given placebo pills by mail and are anticipated to have the same disease rate as indicated in the Connecticut tumor registry data and (2) a case group of similarly aged women who are given vitamin A pills by mail and are anticipated to have a 20% reduction in risk. How large a sample do we need if we wish to do a two-sided test with a significance level of 0.05 and a power of 80%?    ∎

We wish to test the hypothesis $H_0: p_1 = p_2$ vs. $H_1: p_1 \neq p_2$. Suppose that we wish to conduct a test with significance level $\alpha$ and power $1 - \beta$ and anticipate that we will have $k$ times as many people in group 2 than in group 1; that is, $n_2 = kn_1$. We can show that the sample size required in each of the two groups to achieve these objectives is given as follows:

**10.10**  *Sample Size Needed to Compare Two Binomial Proportions Using a Two-Sided Test with Significance Level $\alpha$ and Power $1 - \beta$, Where One Sample ($n_2$) Is k Times As Large As the Other Sample ($n_1$)*

$$n_1 = \left[ \sqrt{\bar{p}\bar{q}\left(1 + \frac{1}{k}\right)}\, z_{1-\alpha/2} + \sqrt{p_1 q_1 + \frac{p_2 q_2}{k}}\, z_{1-\beta} \right]^2 \Big/ \Delta^2$$

$$n_2 = kn_1$$

where

$p_1, p_2$ = projected true probabilities of success in the two groups

$q_1, q_2 = 1 - p_1, 1 - p_2$

$\Delta = p_2 - p_1$

$$\bar{p} = \frac{p_1 + kp_2}{1 + k}$$

$$\bar{q} = 1 - \bar{p}$$

**Example 10.22**    **Cancer, Nutrition** Estimate the sample size required for the study proposed in Example 10.21 if an equal sample size is anticipated in each group.

**Solution**    We have

$$p_1 = 150 \text{ per } 100{,}000 \text{ or } 150/10^5 = 0.00150$$

$$q_1 = 1 - 0.00150 = 0.99850$$

$$p_2 = (150 \times 0.8)/10^5 = 120/10^5 = 0.00120$$

$$q_2 = 1 - 0.00120 = 0.99880$$

$$\alpha = 0.05$$

$$1 - \beta = 0.8$$

$$k = 1 \text{ (since } n_1 = n_2 )$$

$$\bar{p} = \frac{0.00150 + 0.00120}{2} = 0.00135$$

$$\bar{q} = 1 - 0.00135 = 0.99865$$

$$z_{1-\alpha/2} = z_{.975} = 1.96$$

$$z_{1-\beta} = z_{.80} = 0.84$$

Thus, referring to **(10.10)**, we have

$$n_1 = \frac{[\sqrt{(0.00135)(0.99865)(1 + 1)}(1.96) + \sqrt{(0.00150)(0.99850) + (0.00120)(0.99880)}(0.84)]^2}{(0.00150 - 0.00120)^2}$$

$$= \frac{[(0.05193)(1.96) + (0.05193)(0.84)]^2}{(0.00030)^2}$$

$$= \frac{(0.14540)^2}{(0.00030)^2}$$

$$= 234.902 = n_2$$

or about 235,000 women in each group.    ∎

If we intend to perform a one-tailed test rather than a two-tailed test, then we simply substitute $\alpha$ for $\alpha/2$ in the sample-size formula in **(10.10)**.

**Example 10.23**    **Cancer, Nutrition** Suppose that in considering the study design proposed in Example 10.21 more carefully, we decide that a one-sided test is really better, since we anticipate that vitamin A consumption will either lower the risk of breast cancer or will have no effect, but will not raise it. Estimate the required sample size for the study proposed in Example 10.21 if an equal sample size is anticipated for each group.

**Solution**    We have the same parameters as in Example 10.22. We use $1 - \alpha = 0.95$ here rather than $1 - \alpha/2 = 0.975$, as was the case in Example 10.21. We have

$$n_1 = \frac{[\sqrt{(0.00135)(0.99865)(2)}(1.645) + \sqrt{(0.00150)(0.99850) + (0.00120)(0.99880)}(0.84)]^2}{(0.00030)^2}$$

$$= \frac{[(0.05193)(1.645) + (0.05193)(0.84)]^2}{(0.00030)^2}$$

$$= \frac{(0.12905)^2}{(0.00030)^2}$$

$$= 185{,}043 = n_2$$

or about 185,000 women in each group.    ∎

Clearly, from the results in Examples 10.22 and 10.23, it would be infeasible to conduct such a large study over a 1-year period. The sample size needed would be reduced considerably if the period of study was lengthened beyond 1 year, since the expected number of events would increase in a multiyear study.

**Example 10.24**    *Obstetrics*  Suppose we consider the premature labor data presented in Example 10.6. We found that 65% of the women who took terbutaline alone and 60% of the women who took terbutaline and metoprolol had a pregnancy lasting greater than 36 weeks. The results of this study were not significant at the 5% level with 200 women in each group. Suppose researchers find that obstetricians are reluctant to enter their patients in the study, since they already regard terbutaline alone as effective therapy and consider it unethical to try the combination therapy. As a compromise, the investigators propose a new clinical trial with (1) a larger sample and (2) twice as many patients randomized to the terbutaline therapy as to the terbutaline and metoprolol therapy. How many patients are needed in each group to have 80% power using a two-sided test with significance level 0.05?

**Solution**    We will assume that

$$p_1 = 0.65$$

$$q_1 = 1 - 0.65 = 0.35$$

$$p_2 = 0.60$$

$$q_2 = 1 - 0.60 = 0.40$$

$$\alpha = 0.05$$

$$1 - \beta = 0.80$$

Furthermore, from the study design we note that $n_2 = 0.5n_1$, since twice as many people are randomized to group 1 as to group 2. From **(10.10)** we have

$$\bar{p} = \frac{0.65 + (0.60)(0.5)}{1.5} = 0.633$$

$$\bar{q} = 1 - 0.633 = 0.367$$

$$z_{1-\alpha/2} = z_{.975} = 1.96$$

$$z_{1-\beta} = z_{.80} = 0.84$$

$$n_1 = \frac{[\sqrt{(0.633)(0.367)(1 + 1/0.5)}(1.96) + \sqrt{(0.65)(0.35) + (0.60)(0.40)/0.5}(0.84)]^2}{(0.65 - 0.60)^2}$$

$$= \frac{[(0.83483)(1.96) + (0.84113)(0.84)]^2}{(0.05)^2}$$

$$= \frac{(2.34282)^2}{(0.05)^2}$$

$$= 2195.5, \text{ or } 2196$$

$$n_2 = 0.5 \times n_1 = 1098$$

Thus, we would need to randomize 2196 persons to the terbutaline group and 1098 persons to the terbutaline and metoprolol group. ∎

In many instances the sample size available for investigation is fixed by practical constraints, and what we desire is an estimate of statistical power with the anticipated available sample size. In other instances, after a study is completed, we want to calculate the power using the sample sizes that were actually used in the study. For these purposes we provide the following estimate of power to test the hypothesis $H_0: p_1 = p_2$ vs. $H_1: p_1 \neq p_2$, with significance level $\alpha$ and sample sizes of $n_1$ and $n_2$ in the two groups.

**10.11** **Power Achieved in Comparing Two Binomial Proportions Using a Two-Sided Test with Significance Level $\alpha$ and Samples of Sizes $n_1$ and $n_2$**

$$\text{Power} = \Phi\left[\frac{\Delta}{\sqrt{p_1 q_1/n_1 + p_2 q_2/n_2}} - z_{1-\alpha/2}\frac{\sqrt{\bar{p}\bar{q}(1/n_1 + 1/n_2)}}{\sqrt{p_1 q_1/n_1 + p_2 q_2/n_2}}\right]$$

where

$p_1, p_2$ = projected true probabilities of success in groups 1, 2, respectively

$q_1, q_2 = 1 - p_1, 1 - p_2$

$\Delta = |p_2 - p_1|$

$\bar{p} = \dfrac{n_1 p_1 + n_2 p_2}{n_1 + n_2}$

$\bar{q} = 1 - \bar{p}$

*Example 10.25* **Otolaryngology** Suppose we plan a study comparing a medical and a surgical treatment for children who have an excessive number of episodes of otitis media (OTM) during the first 3 years of life. We assume success rates of 50% and 70% in the medical and surgical groups, respectively, and can realistically anticipate recruiting 100 patients for each group. We define success as $\leq 1$ episode of OTM in the first 12 months after treatment. How much power does such a study have of detecting a significant difference if a two-sided test is to be used with an $\alpha$ level of 0.05?

**Solution**

We note that $p_1 = 0.5, p_2 = 0.7, q_1 = 0.5, q_2 = 0.3, n_1 = n_2 = 100, \Delta = 0.2, \bar{p} = (0.5 + 0.7)/2 = 0.6, \bar{q} = 0.4, \alpha = 0.05, z_{1-\alpha/2} = z_{.975} = 1.96$. Thus, from **(10.11)** we can compute power as follows:

$$\text{Power} = \Phi\left[\frac{0.2}{\sqrt{[(0.5)(0.5) + (0.7)(0.3)]/100}} - \frac{1.96\sqrt{(0.6)(0.4)(1/100 + 1/100)}}{\sqrt{[(0.5)(0.5) + (0.7)(0.3)]/100}}\right]$$

$$= \Phi\left(\frac{0.2}{0.0678} - 1.96\frac{0.0693}{0.0678}\right)$$

$$= \Phi(2.950 - 2.003)$$

$$= \Phi(0.947) = 0.83$$

Thus, we will have an 83% chance of finding a significant difference using the anticipated sample sizes. ∎

If we use a one-sided test, then we can use **(10.11)** after replacing $z_{1-\alpha/2}$ by $z_{1-\alpha}$.

# ■ *10.5 FISHER'S EXACT TEST*

*Example 10.26*   *Cardiovascular Disease, Nutrition* Suppose we wish to investigate the relationship between high salt intake and the occurrence of death from cardiovascular disease (CVD). We could identify groups of high- and low-salt users and follow them over a long period of time to compare the relative frequency of death from CVD in the two groups. On the other hand, a much less expensive study would involve looking at death records, separating the CVD deaths from the non-CVD deaths, and then asking a close relative (such as a husband or wife) about the dietary habits of the deceased. ∎

The latter type of retrospective study may be impossible to perform for a number of reasons, but if it is possible, it will almost always be less expensive than the former type of prospective study.

**Definition 10.4**

A **prospective study** is a study in which we identify a group of disease-free individuals at one point in time and follow them over a period of time until some of them develop the disease. We then try to relate the development of disease over time to other variables measured at baseline. ∎

**Definition 10.5**

A **retrospective study** is a study in which we initially identify two groups of individuals: (1) a group that has the disease under study (the cases) and (2) a group that does not have the disease under study (the controls). We then try to relate their *prior* health habits to their current disease status. ∎

What are the advantages of the two types of studies? A prospective study is usually more definitive because the patients' knowledge of their current health habits will be more precise than their (or related individuals') recall of their past health habits. Second, there is a greater chance of bias with a retrospective study because (1) it is much more difficult to obtain a representative sample of people who already have the disease in question, since, for example, some of the diseased individuals may have already died and we may be including only the mildest cases (or if it is a study of deceased cases, the most severe cases) and (2) the diseased individuals, if still alive, or their surrogates will tend to give biased answers about prior health habits if they *believe* there is a relationship between these prior health habits and the disease. For example, in Example 10.26 we may have difficulty in obtaining dietary histories from the relatives. However, a retrospective study is much less expensive to perform and can be completed in a much shorter period of time than a prospective study can. Thus, we may initially do an inexpensive retrospective study as a justification for the ultimate, definitive prospective study.

*Example 10.27*    ***Cardiovascular Disease, Nutrition*** Suppose we do a retrospective study on the deaths of all men aged 50–54 in a specific county over a 1-month period. We find that of 35 persons who died from CVD, 5 were on a high-salt diet before they died, whereas of 25 persons who died from other causes, 2 were on such a diet. These data, presented in Table 10.9, are in the form of a 2 × 2 contingency table, and thus the methods of Section 10.2.2 may be applicable. We find, however, that the expected values of this table are too small to validly use such methods. Indeed,

$$E_{11} = 7(25)/60 = 2.92$$

$$E_{21} = 7(35)/60 = 4.08$$

*Table 10.9*

*Data concerning the possible relationship between cause of death and high salt intake*

| | Type of diet | | |
|---|---|---|---|
| **Cause of death** | *High salt* | *Low salt* | *Total* |
| *Non-CVD* | 2 | 23 | 25 |
| *CVD* | 5 | 30 | 35 |
| *Total* | 7 | 53 | 60 |

and thus two of the four cells have expected values less than 5. How should we test for a relationship between cause of death and type of diet?    ■

We will introduce a method known as **Fisher's exact test,** which gives exact results for any 2 × 2 table but is only necessary for tables with small expected values, where the standard chi-square test as given in **(10.5)** is not applicable. For tables in which the use of the chi-square test is appropriate, the two tests give very similar results. Suppose the probability that a person was on a high-salt diet given that their cause of death was noncardiovascular (non-CVD) = $p_1$, and the probability that a person was on a high-salt diet given that their cause of death was cardiovascular (CVD) = $p_2$. We wish to test the hypothesis $H_0: p_1 = p_2 = p$ vs. $H_1: p_1 \neq p_2$. Table 10.10 gives the general layout of the data.

We will assume that the margins of this table are *fixed*; that is, the numbers of non-CVD deaths and CVD deaths are fixed at $a + b$ and $c + d$, respectively, whereas the numbers of persons on a high- and low-salt diet are fixed at $a + c$ and $b + d$, respectively. We can then show that the *exact* probability of observing the table with cells $a, b, c, d$ is given as follows:

---

**10.12** **Exact Probability of Observing a Table with Cells a, b, c, d**

$$Pr(a, b, c, d) = \frac{(a+b)!(c+d)!(a+c)!(b+d)!}{n!a!b!c!d!}$$

---

**Table 10.10**
General layout
of table for
Fisher's exact
test example

| Cause of death | Type of diet | | Total |
| --- | --- | --- | --- |
| | High salt | Low salt | |
| Non-CVD | $a$ | $b$ | $a+b$ |
| CVD | $c$ | $d$ | $c+d$ |
| Total | $a+c$ | $b+d$ | $n$ |

The formula in **(10.12)** is easy to remember, since the numerator is the product of factorials of each of the row and column margins, and the denominator is the product of the factorial of the grand total and the factorials of the individual cells.

**Example 10.28**    Suppose we have the $2 \times 2$ table as shown in Table 10.11. Compute the exact probability of obtaining this table assuming that the margins are fixed.

**Solution**    We have

$$Pr(2, 5, 3, 1) = \frac{7!4!5!6!}{11!2!5!3!1!} = \frac{(5040)(24)(120)(720)}{(39,916,800)(2)(120)(6)}$$

$$= \frac{1.0450944 \times 10^{10}}{5.7480192 \times 10^{10}} = 0.182$$

Note that in some cases we can cancel the factorials and simplify the computations. Indeed, we find that

$$Pr(2, 5, 3, 1) = \frac{7!4!5!6!}{11!2!5!3!1!} = \left(\frac{7!}{11!}\right) \times \left(\frac{4!}{2!}\right) \times \left(\frac{6!}{3!}\right)$$

$$= \frac{1}{11 \times 10 \times 9 \times 8} \times \frac{4 \times 3}{1} \times \frac{6 \times 5 \times 4}{1} = \frac{1440}{7920} = 0.182 \quad \blacksquare$$

Our basic strategy in testing the hypothesis will be to enumerate all possible tables with the same margins as in our observed table and compute the exact

**Table 10.11**
Hypothetical $2 \times 2$
contingency table
in Example 10.28

| | | |
| --- | --- | --- |
| 2 | 5 | 7 |
| 3 | 1 | 4 |
| 5 | 6 | 11 |

probability for each such table. A method for accomplishing this task is given as follows:

**10.13** **Enumeration of All Possible Tables with the Same Margins as the Observed Table**

*1.* Rearrange the rows and columns of our observed table so that the smaller row total is in the first row and the smaller column total is in the first column.

Suppose that after the rearrangement, the cells in our observed table are $a, b, c, d$, as depicted in Table 10.10.

*2.* We start with the table with 0 in the (1, 1) cell. The other cells in this table are then determined from the row and column margins. Indeed, to maintain the same row and column margins as our observed table, the (1, 2) element must be $a + b$, the (2, 1) cell must be $a + c$, and the (2, 2) element must be $(c + d) - (a + c) = d - a$.

*3.* We construct the next table by increasing the (1, 1) cell by 1 (i.e., from 0 to 1), decreasing the (1, 2) and (2, 1) cells by 1, and increasing the (2, 2) cell by 1.

*4.* We continue increasing and decreasing the cells by 1, as in step 3, until one of the cells is 0, at which point we have enumerated all possible tables with the given row and column margins. We will refer to each table in the sequence of tables by the (1, 1) element. Thus, the first table is the 0 table, the next table is the 1 table, and so on.

*Example 10.29*    **Cardiovascular Disease, Nutrition**  Enumerate all possible tables with the same row and column margins as the observed table in Table 10.9.

*Solution*    Our observed table has $a = 2, b = 23, c = 5, d = 30$. We do not need to rearrange rows or columns, since the first row total is smaller than the second row total, and the first column total is smaller than the second column total. We start with the 0 table, which has 0 in the (1, 1) cell, 25 in the (1, 2) cell, 7 in the (2, 1) cell, and $30 - 2$, or 28, in the (2, 2) cell. The 1 table then has 1 in the (1, 1) cell, $25 - 1 = 24$ in the (1, 2) cell, $7 - 1 = 6$ in the (2, 1) cell, and $28 + 1 = 29$ in the (2, 2) cell. We continue in this fashion until we reach the 7 table, which has 0 in the (2, 1) cell, at which point we have enumerated all possible tables with the given row and column margins. This collection of tables is shown in Table 10.12.

**Table 10.12**

*Enumeration of all possible tables with fixed margins for Example 10.29*

| 0 | 25 |
|---|----|
| 7 | 28 |

0.017

| 1 | 24 |
|---|----|
| 6 | 29 |

0.105

| 2 | 23 |
|---|----|
| 5 | 30 |

0.252

| 3 | 22 |
|---|----|
| 4 | 31 |

0.312

| 4 | 21 |
|---|----|
| 3 | 32 |

0.214

| 5 | 20 |
|---|----|
| 2 | 33 |

0.082

| 6 | 19 |
|---|----|
| 1 | 34 |

0.016

| 7 | 18 |
|---|----|
| 0 | 35 |

0.001

∎

We must now compute the exact probability of each of the tables we have enumerated. We could do this computation directly by evaluating the probability of each table individually, using the formula in **(10.12)**. However, a **recursion rule** is often easier for this purpose. The advantage of the recursion rule is that once all the tables are generated, we can calculate the probabilities of all tables *at once* without computing a single factorial. The recursion rule is given as follows:

| | |
|---|---|
| 10.14 | *Recursion Rule for Computing Exact Probabilities* |

*1*. We enumerate all possible tables with the same margins as our observed table, starting with the 0 table as presented in **(10.13)**. We will refer to the probability of the *a* table as $Pr(a)$. Suppose that the *a* table and $a + 1$ table are among the tables we have enumerated. We can show that:

*2*.
$$Pr(a + 1) = Pr(a) \times \frac{bc}{(a + 1)(d + 1)}$$

Notice that we can compute $bc/[(a + 1)(d + 1)]$ by starting at the lower left of the *a* table, multiplying by the terms along the dotted diagonal, and dividing by the terms along the dotted diagonal of the $a + 1$ table, as shown in Table 10.13. Note that the $(1, 2), (2, 1)$, and $(2, 2)$ cells of the $a + 1$ table must be $b - 1, c - 1$, and $d + 1$, provided that $b \geqslant 1, c \geqslant 1$, which we assume is true.

*3*. This procedure can be used to calculate the probabilities of all possible tables. Since we can express $Pr(1)$ in terms of $Pr(0)$, we can also express $Pr(2)$ in terms of $Pr(1)$, which can in turn be expressed in terms of $Pr(0)$, and so on. Thus, we can express the probability of each table as a multiple of $Pr(0)$, and since all the probabilities add up to 1, we can solve first for $Pr(0)$ and then for each of the other probabilities. In particular, suppose that the *k* table is the last table enumerated. If

$$Pr(1) = \lambda_1 Pr(0), Pr(2) = \lambda_2 Pr(0), \ldots, Pr(k) = \lambda_k Pr(0)$$

then

$$1 = Pr(0) + Pr(1) + \cdots + Pr(k)$$
$$= Pr(0) + \lambda_1 Pr(0) + \lambda_2 Pr(0) + \cdots + \lambda_k Pr(0)$$
$$= Pr(0)(1 + \lambda_1 + \lambda_2 + \cdots + \lambda_k)$$

Therefore,

$$Pr(0) = \frac{1}{1 + \lambda_1 + \lambda_2 + \cdots + \lambda_k}$$

$$Pr(1) = \frac{\lambda_1}{1 + \lambda_1 + \lambda_2 + \cdots + \lambda_k}$$

$$Pr(2) = \frac{\lambda_2}{1 + \lambda_1 + \lambda_2 + \cdots + \lambda_k}$$

$$\vdots$$

$$Pr(k) = \frac{\lambda_k}{1 + \lambda_1 + \lambda_2 + \cdots + \lambda_k}$$

**Table 10.13**

*Illustration of the recursion rule for computation of exact probabilities*

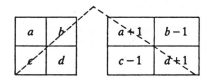

**Example 10.30**     ***Cardiovascular Disease, Nutrition*** Evaluate the exact probabilities of all tables enumerated in Table 10.12.

**Solution**     We refer to Table 10.12. Using the recursion rule, we have

$$Pr(0) = 1Pr(0)$$

$$Pr(1) = \frac{7 \times 25}{1 \times 29} Pr(0) = 6.034Pr(0)$$

$$Pr(2) = \frac{6 \times 24}{2 \times 30} Pr(1) = 2.40Pr(1) = 2.40 \times 6.034Pr(0) = 14.482Pr(0)$$

$$Pr(3) = \frac{5 \times 23}{3 \times 31} Pr(2) = 17.908Pr(0)$$

$$Pr(4) = \frac{4 \times 22}{4 \times 32} Pr(3) = 12.312Pr(0)$$

$$Pr(5) = \frac{3 \times 21}{5 \times 33} Pr(4) = 4.701Pr(0)$$

$$Pr(6) = \frac{2 \times 20}{6 \times 34} Pr(5) = 0.922Pr(0)$$

$$Pr(7) = \frac{1 \times 19}{7 \times 35} Pr(6) = 0.072Pr(0)$$

We also know that all these probabilities must add up to 1. Hence we have

$$Pr(0)(1 + 6.034 + 14.482 + 17.908 + 12.312 + 4.701 + 0.922 + 0.072) = 1$$

or

$$Pr(0)(57.431) = 1 \quad \text{or} \quad Pr(0) = 0.0174$$

We can now solve for all the other probabilities in terms of $Pr(0)$. These probabilities are listed under the corresponding tables in Table 10.12. It is advisable to check that these probabilities add up to 1. They do in this case, except for roundoff error.     ∎

The question now is what should we do with these probabilities to evaluate the significance of our results. The answer depends on whether we are using a one-sided or a two-sided alternative. In general, we can use the following procedure:

**10.15**    ### *Fisher's Exact Test: General Procedure and Computation of P-value*

If we wish to test the hypothesis $H_0: p_1 = p_2$ vs. $H_1: p_1 \neq p_2$, where the expected value of at least one cell is $< 5$ when the data are analyzed in the form of a $2 \times 2$ contingency table, then

**1.** Enumerate all possible tables with the same row and column margins as our table, as shown in **(10.13)**.

**2.** Compute the exact probability of each table enumerated in step 1, using either the direct method in **(10.12)** or the recursion rule in **(10.14)**.

**3.** Suppose that the observed table is the $a$ table and that the last table enumerated is the $k$ table.

**3a.** If we wish to test the hypothesis $H_0: p_1 = p_2$ vs. $H_1: p_1 \neq p_2$, then the $p$-value = $2 \times min[Pr(0) + Pr(1) + \cdots + Pr(a), Pr(a) + Pr(a+1) + \cdots + Pr(k)]$.

**3b.** If we wish to test the hypothesis $H_0: p_1 = p_2$ vs. $H_1: p_1 < p_2$, then the $p$-value = $Pr(0) + Pr(1) + \cdots + Pr(a)$.

**3c.** If we wish to test the hypothesis $H_0: p_1 = p_2$ vs. $H_1: p_1 > p_2$, then the $p$-value = $Pr(a) + Pr(a+1) + \cdots + Pr(k)$.

For each of these three alternative hypotheses, we can interpret the $p$-value as the probability of obtaining a table as extreme as or more extreme than our observed table.

---

*Example 10.31*    ### *Cardiovascular Disease, Nutrition*  Evaluate the statistical significance of the data in Example 10.27.

*Solution*    Suppose we have a two-sided alternative of the form $H_0: p_1 = p_2$ vs. $H_1: p_1 \neq p_2$. Our table is the 2 table in Table 10.12. Thus, we compute the smaller of the tail probabilities corresponding to the 2 table and double it. This strategy corresponds to our procedures for the various normal theory tests that we studied in Chapters 7 and 8. First we compute the left-hand tail area,

$$Pr(0) + Pr(1) + Pr(2) = 0.017 + 0.105 + 0.252 = 0.374$$

and the right-hand tail area,

$$Pr(2) + Pr(3) + \cdots + Pr(7) = 0.252 + 0.312 + 0.214 + 0.082 + 0.016 + 0.001 = 0.877$$

Then

$$p = 2 \times min(0.374, 0.877) = 2(0.374) = 0.748$$

If we use a one-sided alternative of the form $H_0: p_1 = p_2$ vs. $H_1: p_1 < p_2$, then the $p$-value equals

$$Pr(0) + Pr(1) + Pr(2) = 0.017 + 0.105 + 0.252 = 0.374$$

Thus, the two proportions in this example are *not* significantly different with either a one-sided or two-sided alternative, and we *cannot* say, on the basis of this limited amount of data, that there is a significant association between salt intake and cause of death.    ∎

# ■ *10.6 TWO-SAMPLE TEST FOR BINOMIAL PROPORTIONS FOR MATCHED-PAIR DATA (McNEMAR'S TEST)*

*Example 10.32*   *Cancer*  Suppose we want to compare two different treatments for a rare form of cancer. Since relatively few cases of this disease are seen, we want the two treatment groups to be as comparable as possible. To accomplish this goal, we set up a matched study such that a random member of each matched pair gets treatment A (chemotherapy), whereas the other member gets treatment B (surgery). The patients are assigned to pairs matched on age (within 5 years), sex, and clinical condition. The patients are followed for 5 years, with survival as the outcome variable. The data are displayed in a $2 \times 2$ table, as shown in Table 10.14. Notice the small difference in survival between the two treatment groups: the 5-year survival rate for treatment $A = 106/621 = 0.171$ and for treatment $B = 95/621 = 0.153$. Indeed, the Yates corrected chi-square statistic as given in **(10.5)** is 0.59 with 1 d.f., which is not significant. However, we must realize that *the use of this test is valid only if the two samples are independent.* We can see from the manner in which the samples were selected that they are *not* independent, since each pair of persons is similar in age, sex, and clinical condition. Thus, we *cannot* use the Yates corrected chi-square test. How can we compare the two treatments using a hypothesis test?

**Table 10.14**
*2 × 2 contingency table comparing treatments A and B for a rare form of cancer*

| | Outcome | | |
|---|---|---|---|
| Treatment | Survive for 5 years | Die within 5 years | Total |
| A | 106 | 515 | 621 |
| B | 95 | 526 | 621 |
| Total | 201 | 1041 | 1242 |

■

Suppose we construct a different kind of $2 \times 2$ table to illustrate these data. In Table 10.14 we selected the *person* as the basic unit and then had a sample size of 1242 persons. In Table 10.15 we use the *matched pair* as the basic unit and classify *pairs* according to whether or not each treatment worked for the members of that pair. Notice that this table has 621 units, rather than the 1242 in the previous table. Furthermore, there are 90 pairs in which both patients survived, 510 pairs in which both patients died, 16 pairs in which the treatment A patient survived and the

**Table 10.15**
*2 × 2 table with the matched pair as the sampling unit*

| Outcome of treatment A patient | Outcome of treatment B patient | | |
|---|---|---|---|
| | Survive | Die | Total |
| Survive | 90 | 16 | 106 |
| Die | 5 | 510 | 515 |
| Total | 95 | 526 | 621 |

treatment B patient died, and 5 pairs in which the treatment B patient survived and the treatment A patient died. We can illustrate the dependence of the two samples by noting that the probability that the treatment B member of the pair survived given that the treatment A member of the pair survived $= 90/106 = 0.849$, and the probability that the treatment B member of the pair survived given that the treatment A member of the pair died $= 5/515 = 0.010$. If the samples were independent, then these two probabilities should be about the same. Thus, we conclude that the samples are highly dependent and that we cannot use the chi-square test.

If we refer to Table 10.15, we see that for 600 pairs $(90 + 510)$ of persons, the outcomes of the two treatments are the same, whereas for 21 pairs $(16 + 5)$ of persons, the outcomes of the two treatments are different. We will give the following special names to each of these types of pairs:

**Definition 10.6**

A **concordant pair** is a matched pair in which the outcome is the same for each member of the pair. ∎

**Definition 10.7**

A **discordant pair** is a matched pair in which the outcomes are different for the members of the pair. ∎

**Example 10.33**    There are 600 concordant pairs and 21 discordant pairs for the data in Table 10.15. ∎

The concordant pairs give us no information about *differences between treatments*, and we will not use them in our assessment. Instead, we will focus on the discordant pairs. We will distinguish between two types of discordant pairs.

**Definition 10.8**

We define a **type A discordant pair** as a discordant pair in which the treatment A member of the pair has the event and the treatment B member of the pair does not. Similarly, a **type B discordant pair** is a discordant pair in which the treatment B member of the pair has the event and the treatment A member of the pair does not. ∎

**Example 10.34**    There are 16 type A discordant pairs and 5 type B discordant pairs from the data in Table 10.15. ∎

Let $p =$ probability that a discordant pair is of type A. If the treatments are equally effective, then we would expect about an equal number of type A and type B discordant pairs, and $p$ should $= \frac{1}{2}$. If treatment A is more effective than treatment B, then we would expect more type A than type B discordant pairs, and $p$ should be $> \frac{1}{2}$. Finally, if treatment B is more effective than treatment A, then we would expect more type B than type A discordant pairs, and $p$ should be $< \frac{1}{2}$.

Thus we wish to test the hypothesis $H_0: p = \frac{1}{2}$ vs. $H_1: p \neq \frac{1}{2}$.

## ☐ 10.6.1 Normal Theory Test

Suppose that of $n_D$ discordant pairs, $n_A$ are type A. Then under $H_0$, $E(n_A) = n_D/2$ and $Var(n_A) = n_D/4$, from the mean and variance of a binomial distribution, respectively. We will assume that the normal approximation to the binomial distribution holds, but we will use a continuity correction for a better approximation. This approximation will be valid if $npq = n_D/4 \geqslant 5$ or $n_D \geqslant 20$. We then can use the following test procedure, referred to as McNemar's test.

**10.16** | **McNemar's Test for Correlated Proportions—Normal Theory Test**

*1.* We form a 2 × 2 table of matched pairs, where the outcomes for the treatment A members of the matched pairs are listed along the rows and the outcomes for the treatment B members of the matched pairs are listed along the columns.

*2.* We count the total number of discordant pairs ($n_D$) and the number of type A discordant pairs ($n_A$).

*3.* We compute the test statistic

$$S = \left( \left| n_A - \frac{n_D}{2} \right| - \frac{1}{2} \right)^2 \Big/ \left( \frac{n_D}{4} \right)$$

*4.* For a two-sided level $\alpha$ test: If

$$S > \chi^2_{1,1-\alpha}$$

then we reject $H_0$; if

$$S \leqslant \chi^2_{1,1-\alpha}$$

then we accept $H_0$.

*5.* The exact p-value is given by $p = Pr(\chi^2_1 \geqslant S)$.

*6.* We will use this test only if $n_D \geqslant 20$.

The acceptance and rejection regions for this test are depicted in Figure 10.5. The computation of the p-value for McNemar's test is depicted in Figure 10.6.

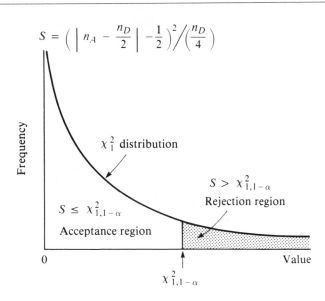

$$S = \left( \left| n_A - \frac{n_D}{2} \right| - \frac{1}{2} \right)^2 \Big/ \left( \frac{n_D}{4} \right)$$

$\chi^2_1$ distribution

$S > \chi^2_{1,1-\alpha}$
Rejection region

$S \leqslant \chi^2_{1,1-\alpha}$
Acceptance region

Frequency

0                                                          Value

$\chi^2_{1,1-\alpha}$

**Figure 10.5**
*Acceptance and rejection regions for McNemar's test— normal theory method*

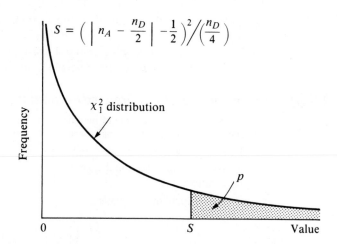

**Figure 10.6**
*Computation of
the p-value for
McNemar's test—
normal theory
method*

**Example 10.35**   *Cancer*  Assess the statistical significance of the data in Table 10.15.

**Solution**   We note that $n_D = 21$. Since $n_D(\frac{1}{2})(\frac{1}{2}) = 5.25 \geqslant 5$, we can use the normal approximation to the binomial distribution and the test in **(10.16)**. We have

$$S = \frac{(|16 - 10.5| - \frac{1}{2})^2}{(21/4)} = \frac{(5.5 - \frac{1}{2})^2}{5.25} = \frac{5^2}{5.25} = \frac{25}{5.25} = 4.76$$

From Table 6 in the appendix, we note that

$$\chi^2_{1,.95} = 3.84$$

$$\chi^2_{1,.975} = 5.02$$

Thus, $0.025 < p < 0.05$, and the results are statistically significant.     ∎

We conclude that *if the treatments give different results from each other*, then the treatment A member of the pair is significantly more likely to survive than the treatment B member of the pair. Thus, all other things being equal (such as side effects, cost, etc.), treatment A would be the treatment of choice.

## ☐ 10.6.2  Exact Test

If $n_D/4 < 5$, that is, if $n_D < 20$, then the normal approximation to the binomial distribution cannot be used, and a test based on exact binomial probabilities is required. The details of the test procedure are similar to the one-sample binomial test given in **(7.35)** and are summarized as follows:

**10.17**   *McNemar's Test for Correlated Proportions—Exact Test*

    *1*. We follow the procedure in step 1 in **(10.16)**.

    *2*. We follow the procedure in step 2 in **(10.16)**.

    **3.**

$$p = 2 \times \sum_{k=0}^{n_A} \binom{n_D}{k}\left(\frac{1}{2}\right)^{n_D} \qquad \text{if } n_A < n_D/2$$

$$p = 2 \times \sum_{k=n_A}^{n_D} \binom{n_D}{k}\left(\frac{1}{2}\right)^{n_D} \qquad \text{if } n_A \geqslant n_D/2$$

**4.** This test is valid for any number of discordant pairs ($n_D$) but is particularly useful for $n_D < 20$, when the normal theory test in **(10.16)** cannot be used.

The computation of the p-value for this test is depicted in Figure 10.7.

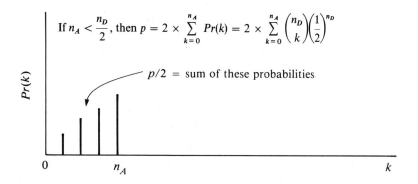

$$\text{If } n_A < \frac{n_D}{2}, \text{ then } p = 2 \times \sum_{k=0}^{n_A} Pr(k) = 2 \times \sum_{k=0}^{n_A} \binom{n_D}{k}\left(\frac{1}{2}\right)^{n_D}$$

$p/2 = $ sum of these probabilities

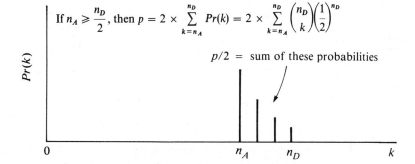

$$\text{If } n_A \geqslant \frac{n_D}{2}, \text{ then } p = 2 \times \sum_{k=n_A}^{n_D} Pr(k) = 2 \times \sum_{k=n_A}^{n_D} \binom{n_D}{k}\left(\frac{1}{2}\right)^{n_D}$$

$p/2 = $ sum of these probabilities

**Figure 10.7**
*Computation of the p-value for McNemar's test— exact method*

**Example 10.36**    **Hypertension** A recent phenomenon in the recording of blood pressure is the development of the automated blood pressure machine, where for a small fee a person can sit in a booth and have his or her blood pressure measured by a computer device. A study is conducted to compare the computer device with standard methods of measuring blood pressure. Twenty patients are recruited, and their hypertensive status is assessed by both the computer device and a trained observer. Hypertensive status is defined as either hypertensive ($+$), if either systolic $bp \geqslant 160$ or diastolic $bp \geqslant 95$, or normotensive ($-$) otherwise. The data are given in Table 10.16. Assess the statistical significance of these data.

**Solution**    We cannot use an ordinary Yates corrected chi-square test on these data, since each person is being used as his or her own control and we *do not have* two independent samples. We instead form a $2 \times 2$ table of matched pairs, as shown in Table 10.17. We note that 3 people are measured as hypertensive by both the computer device and the trained observer, 9 people are normotensive by both methods, 7 people are hypertensive by the computer device and normotensive by the trained observer, and 1 person is normotensive by the computer device and hypertensive by the trained observer. Therefore, we have 12 ($9 + 3$) concordant pairs and 8 ($7 + 1$) discordant pairs ($n_D$). Since $n_D < 20$, we must use the exact method. We see that $n_A = 7$, $n_D = 8$. Therefore, since $n_A \geqslant n_D/2 = 4$, it follows from **(10.17)** that

$$p = 2 \times \sum_{k=7}^{8} \binom{8}{k}\left(\frac{1}{2}\right)^{8}$$

**Table 10.16**

Hypertensive status of 20 patients as judged by a computer device and a trained observer

| Person | Computer device | Trained observer | Person | Computer device | Trained observer |
|---|---|---|---|---|---|
| | *Hypertensive status* | | | *Hypertensive status* | |
| 1 | − | − | 11 | + | − |
| 2 | − | − | 12 | + | − |
| 3 | + | − | 13 | − | − |
| 4 | + | + | 14 | + | − |
| 5 | − | − | 15 | − | + |
| 6 | + | − | 16 | + | − |
| 7 | − | − | 17 | + | − |
| 8 | + | + | 18 | − | − |
| 9 | + | + | 19 | − | − |
| 10 | − | − | 20 | − | − |

**Table 10.17**

Comparison of hypertensive status as judged by a computer device and a trained observer

| Computer device | Trained observer | |
|---|---|---|
| | + | − |
| + | 3 | 7 |
| − | 1 | 9 |

We can evaluate this expression using Table I in the appendix, where we refer to $n = 8$, $p = 0.5$ and note that $Pr(X \geqslant 7 | p = 0.5) = 0.0313 + 0.0039 = 0.0352$. Thus the two-tailed $p$-value = $2 \times 0.0352 = 0.070$.

Alternatively, we could use a computer program to perform the computations, as shown in Table 10.18. Note that the first and second columns have been interchanged so that the discordant pairs appear in the diagonal elements (and are easier to identify). In summary, the results are not statistically significant, and we cannot conclude that there is a significant

**Table 10.18**

Use of SPSS/PC McNemar Test program to evaluate the significance of the data in Table 10.17

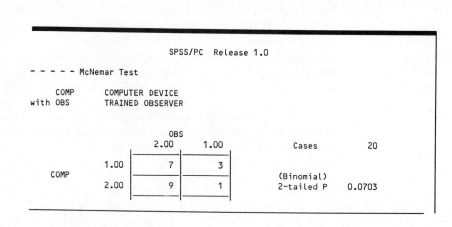

difference between the two methods, although we can detect a *trend* toward the computer device identifying more hypertensives than the trained observer. ∎

# ■ 10.7 *R×C CONTINGENCY TABLES*

## □ *10.7.1 Tests for Association for R × C Tables*

In the previous sections of this chapter, we studied methods of analyzing data in the form of a 2 × 2 contingency table, that is, where each of the variables under study has only two categories. Frequently, one or both variables under study have more than two categories.

**Definition 10.9**

We define an **R × C contingency table** as a table with $R$ rows and $C$ columns. It expresses the relationship between two variables, where the variable depicted in the rows has $R$ categories and the variable depicted in the columns has $C$ categories. ∎

**Table 10.19**

Data from the international study investigating the possible association between age at first birth and case/control status

| Case/control status | Age at first birth | | | | | |
|---|---|---|---|---|---|---|
| | < 20 | 20–24 | 25–29 | 30–34 | ≥ 35 | Total |
| Case | 320 | 1206 | 1011 | 463 | 220 | 3220 |
| Control | 1422 | 4432 | 2893 | 1092 | 406 | 10,245 |
| Total | 1742 | 5638 | 3904 | 1555 | 626 | 13,465 |
| % cases | 0.184 | 0.214 | 0.259 | 0.298 | 0.351 | 0.239 |

(Reprinted with permission of *WHO Bulletin* **43**: 209–221, 1970.)

**Example 10.37**

*Cancer* Suppose we wish to study further the relationship between age at first birth and development of breast cancer, as given in Example 10.4. In particular, we would like to know if the effect of age at first birth follows a consistent trend, that is, (1) more protection for women whose age at first birth is < 20 than for women whose age at first birth is 25–29 and (2) higher risk for women whose age at first birth is ≥ 35 than for women whose age at first birth is 30–34. We present the data in Table 10.19, where the case/control status is indicated along the rows and age at first birth is indicated along the columns. The data are arranged in the form of a 2 × 5 contingency table, since case/control status has two categories and age at first birth has five categories. We wish to test for a relationship between age at first birth and case/control status. How should we do this? ∎

Generalizing our experience from the 2 × 2 situation, we can form the expected table for an $R \times C$ table in the same way as for a 2 × 2 table.

**10.18** *Computation of the Expected Table for an R × C Contingency Table*

The expected number of units that fall in the $(i, j)$ cell = $E_{ij}$ = the product of the number of units in the $i$th row multiplied by the number of units in $j$th column, divided by the total number of units in the table.

*Example 10.38*    **Cancer** Compute the expected table for the data presented in Table 10.19.

**Solution**

$$\text{The expected value of the (1, 1) cell} = \frac{\text{first row total} \times \text{first column total}}{\text{grand total}} = \frac{3220(1742)}{13,465} = 416.6$$

$$\text{The expected value of the (1, 2) cell} = \frac{\text{first row total} \times \text{second column total}}{\text{grand total}} = \frac{(3220)(5638)}{13,465} = 1348.3$$

$$\vdots$$

$$\text{The expected value of the (2, 5) cell} = \frac{\text{second row total} \times \text{fifth column total}}{\text{grand total}} = \frac{(10,245)(626)}{13,465} = 476.3$$

All 10 expected values are given in Table 10.20.

**Table 10.20**

*Expected table for the international study data in Table 10.19*

| Case/control status | Age at first birth | | | | | |
|---|---|---|---|---|---|---|
| | < 20 | 20–24 | 25–29 | 30–34 | ≥ 35 | Total |
| Case | 416.6 | 1348.3 | 933.6 | 371.9 | 149.7 | 3220 |
| Control | 1325.4 | 4289.7 | 2970.4 | 1183.1 | 476.3 | 10,245 |
| Total | 1742 | 5638 | 3904 | 1555 | 626 | 13,465 |

■

The sum of the expected values across any row or column must equal the corresponding row or column total, as was the case for 2 × 2 tables. This fact provides a good check that the expected values are computed correctly. The expected values in Table 10.20 will fulfill this criterion except for roundoff error.

We again wish to compare the observed table with the expected table. The more similar these tables are, the more willing we will be to accept the null hypothesis that there is no relationship between the two variables. The more different the tables are, the more willing we will be to reject $H_0$. Again we will use the criterion $(O - E)^2/E$ to compare the observed and expected tables for a particular cell. Furthermore, we will sum $(O - E)^2/E$ over all the cells in the table to get an overall measure of how close the observed and expected tables are. We can show that under $H_0$, for an $R \times C$ contingency table, the sum of $(O - E)^2/E$ over the $RC$ cells in the table will approximately follow a chi-square distribution with $(R - 1) \times (C - 1)$ d.f. We will reject $H_0$ for large values of this sum and will accept $H_0$ for small values.

Generally speaking, the continuity correction is not used for contingency tables larger than 2 × 2, since it has been found empirically that it does not aid in the approximation of the test statistic by the chi-square distribution. As was the case for 2 × 2 tables, this test should not be used if the expected values of the cells are too small. Cochran has studied the validity of the approximation in this case and recommends its use under the following conditions [4]:

*1.* No more than $\frac{1}{5}$ of the cells have expected values $< 5$.

*2.* No cells have expected values $< 1$.

The test procedure can be summarized as follows:

**10.19** | *Chi-Square Test for an $R \times C$ Contingency Table*

Suppose we wish to test for the relationship between two discrete variables, where one variable has $R$ categories and the other has $C$ categories.

*1*. We analyze the data in the form of an $R \times C$ contingency table, where $O_{ij}$ represents the observed number of units in the $(i, j)$ cell.

*2*. We compute the expected table as shown in **(10.18)**, where $E_{ij}$ represents the expected number of units in the $(i, j)$ cell.

*3*. We compute the test statistic

$$T = (O_{11} - E_{11})^2/E_{11} + (O_{12} - E_{12})^2/E_{12} + \cdots + (O_{RC} - E_{RC})^2/E_{RC}$$

which under $H_0$ approximately follows a chi-square distribution with $(R - 1) \times (C - 1)$ d.f.

*4*. For a level $\alpha$ test, if

$$T > \chi^2_{(R-1) \times (C-1), 1-\alpha}$$

we reject $H_0$. If

$$T \leq \chi^2_{(R-1) \times (C-1), 1-\alpha}$$

we accept $H_0$.

*5*. The exact $p$-value is given by the area to the right of $T$ under a $\chi^2_{(R-1) \times (C-1)}$ distribution.

*6*. We will use this test only if the following two conditions are satisfied:
   **(a)** No more than $\frac{1}{5}$ of the cells should have expected values $<5$.
   **(b)** No cell should have expected value $<1$.

The acceptance and rejection regions for this test are depicted in Figure 10.8. The computation of the $p$-value for this test is illustrated in Figure 10.9.

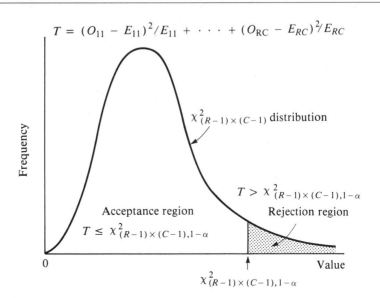

$$T = (O_{11} - E_{11})^2/E_{11} + \cdots + (O_{RC} - E_{RC})^2/E_{RC}$$

$\chi^2_{(R-1) \times (C-1)}$ distribution

$T > \chi^2_{(R-1) \times (C-1), 1-\alpha}$

Acceptance region

Rejection region

$T \leq \chi^2_{(R-1) \times (C-1), 1-\alpha}$

Frequency

0

Value

$\chi^2_{(R-1) \times (C-1), 1-\alpha}$

**Figure 10.8**
*Acceptance and rejection regions for the chi-square test for an $R \times C$ contingency table*

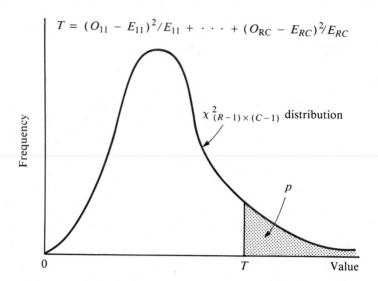

$$T = (O_{11} - E_{11})^2/E_{11} + \cdots + (O_{RC} - E_{RC})^2/E_{RC}$$

$\chi^2_{(R-1)\times(C-1)}$ distribution

$p$

Frequency

0                        $T$                  Value

**Figure 10.9**
Computation of
the p-value for the
chi-square test for
an R × C
contingency table

**Example 10.39**    *Cancer*  Assess the statistical significance of the data in Example 10.37.

**Solution**    From Table 10.20 we see that all expected values are $\geq 5$; so we can use the test procedure in **(10.18)**. We have from Tables 10.19 and 10.20 that

$$T = \frac{(320 - 416.6)^2}{416.6} + \frac{(1206 - 1348.3)^2}{1348.3} + \cdots + \frac{(406 - 476.3)^2}{476.3} = 130.33$$

Under $H_0$, $T$ follows a chi-square distribution with $(2 - 1) \times (5 - 1)$, or 4, d.f. Since

$$\chi^2_{4,.999} = 18.47 < 130.33 = T$$

it follows that

$$p < 1 - 0.999 = 0.001$$

Therefore, the results are very highly significant, and we can conclude that there is a relationship between age at first birth and the development of breast cancer.    ∎

### ☐ 10.7.2  Chi-Square Test for Trend in Binomial Proportions

Let us refer again to the international study data presented in Table 10.19. In Example 10.39 we used the test procedure in **(10.19)** to analyze these data. For the special case of a $2 \times k$ table, this test procedure enables us to test the hypothesis $H_0: p_1 = p_2 = \cdots = p_k$ vs. $H_1$: at least two of the $p_i$ are unequal, where $p_i$ = probability of success for the $i$th group = probability that an observation from the $i$th column falls in the first row. When we employed this test procedure in Example 10.39, we found a chi-square statistic of 130.33 with 4 d.f., which was highly significant ($p < 0.001$). As a result we were able to reject $H_0$ and conclude that the proportion of breast cancer cases in at least two of the five age at first birth groups were different. However, although this result shows us that some relationship exists between breast cancer and age at first birth, it does not tell us specifically about the nature of the relationship. In particular, from Table 10.19 we notice an increasing *trend* in the proportion of women with breast cancer in each succeeding column. We would like to employ a specific test for such trends. For this purpose we introduce a **score variable** $S_i$ to correspond to the $i$th group. The score variable can represent some particular numerical attribute of the group. In other instances, for simplicity 1 is assigned to the first group, 2 to the second group, ..., $k$ to the $k$th (last) group.

*Example 10.40*     *Cancer* Construct a score variable for the international study data in Table 10.19.

*Solution*     It is natural to use the average age at first birth within a group as the score variable for that group. This rule presents no problem for the second, third, and fourth groups, in which we estimate the average age as 22.5 [(20 + 25)/2], 27.5, and 32.5 years, respectively. However, we cannot perform a similar calculation for the first and fifth groups, since they are defined as <20 and ≥35, respectively. By symmetry, we could assign a score of 17.5 years to the first group and 37.5 years to the fifth group. However, since the scores are equally spaced, our purposes will be equally well served by assigning scores of 1, 2, 3, 4, and 5 to the five groups. We will adopt this scoring method for simplicity.     ■

We wish to relate the proportion of breast cancer cases in a group with the score variable for that group. In other words, we wish to test whether the proportion of breast cancer cases increases or decreases as age at first birth increases. For this purpose we introduce the following test procedure:

**10.20**     **Chi-Square Test for Trend in Binomial Proportions**

Suppose we have $k$ groups and wish to test if there is an increasing (or decreasing) trend in the proportion of "successes" $p_i$ (i.e., the proportion of units in the first row of the $i$th group) as $i$ increases.

*1.* We set up the data in the form of a $2 \times k$ contingency table, where success or failure is listed along the rows and the $k$ groups are listed along the columns.

*2.* We denote the number of successes in the $i$th group by $x_i$, the total number of units in the $i$th group by $n_i$, and the proportion of successes in the $i$th group by $\hat{p}_i = x_i/n_i$. We also denote the total number of successes over all groups by $x$, the total number of units over all groups by $N$, the overall proportion of successes by $\bar{p} = x/N$, and the overall proportion of failures by $\bar{q} = 1 - \bar{p}$.

*3.* We construct a score variable $S_i$ to correspond to the $i$th group. This variable will usually either be 1, 2, ..., $k$ for the $k$ groups or be defined to correspond to some other numerical attribute of the group.

*4.* To relate $p_i$ and $S_i$, we compute the test statistic $T_1 = A^2/B$, where

$$A = \sum_{i=1}^{k} n_i(\hat{p}_i - \bar{p})(S_i - \bar{S})$$

$$= \left( \sum_{i=1}^{k} x_i S_i \right) - x\bar{S}$$

$$= \left( \sum_{i=1}^{k} x_i S_i \right) - x\left( \sum_{i=1}^{k} n_i S_i \right)\bigg/ N$$

$$B = \bar{p}\bar{q}\left[ \left( \sum_{i=1}^{k} n_i S_i^2 \right) - \left( \sum_{i=1}^{k} n_i S_i \right)^2 \bigg/ N \right]$$

which under $H_0$ approximately follows a chi-square distribution with 1 d.f.

5. For a level $\alpha$ test, if

$$T_1 > \chi^2_{1,1-\alpha}$$

then we reject $H_0$. If

$$T_1 \leq \chi^2_{1,1-\alpha}$$

then we accept $H_0$.

6. The exact $p$-value is given by the area to the right of $T_1$ under an $\chi^2_1$ distribution.

7. The direction of the trend in proportions is indicated by the sign of $A$. If $A > 0$, then the proportions increase with increasing score; if $A < 0$, then the proportions decrease with increasing score.

8. We should use this test only if $N\bar{p}\bar{q} \geq 5.0$.

The acceptance and rejection regions for this test are depicted in Figure 10.10. The computation of the $p$-value is illustrated in Figure 10.11.

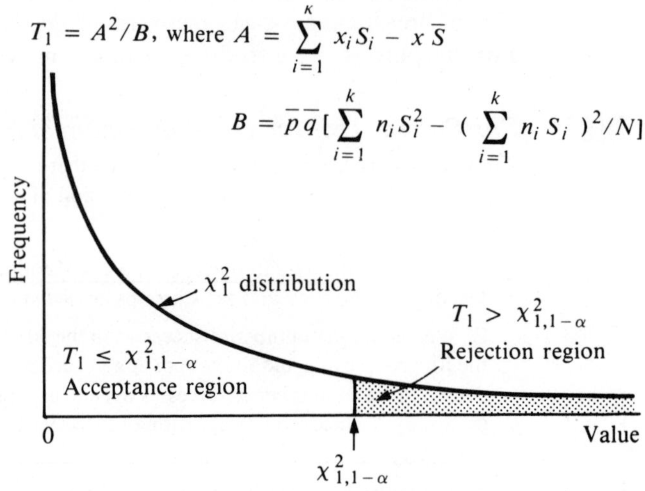

$T_1 = A^2/B$, where $A = \sum_{i=1}^{k} x_i S_i - x\bar{S}$
$B = \bar{p}\bar{q}[\sum_{i=1}^{k} n_i S_i^2 - (\sum_{i=1}^{k} n_i S_i)^2/N]$
Frequency
$\chi^2_1$ distribution
$T_1 > \chi^2_{1,1-\alpha}$
Rejection region
$T_1 \leq \chi^2_{1,1-\alpha}$
Acceptance region
0
Value
$\chi^2_{1,1-\alpha}$


*Figure 10.10* Acceptance and rejection regions for the chi-square test for trend in binomial proportions

$T_1 = A^2/B$, where $A = \sum_{i=1}^{k} x_i S_i - x\bar{S}$
$B = \bar{p}\bar{q}[\sum_{i=1}^{k} n_i S_i^2 - (\sum_{i=1}^{k} n_i S_i)^2/N]$
Frequency
$\chi^2_1$ distribution
$p$
0
$T_1$
Value


*Figure 10.11* Computation of the $p$-value for the chi-square test for trend in binomial proportions

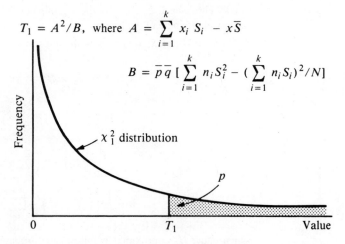

The test statistic in **(10.20)** is reasonable, since if $\hat{p}_i$ (or $\hat{p}_i - \bar{p}$) increases as $S_i$ increases, then $A > 0$, whereas if $\hat{p}_i$ decreases as $S_i$ increases, then $A < 0$. In either case $A^2$ and the test statistic $T_1$ will be large. On the other hand, if $\hat{p}_i$ shows no particular trend regarding $S_i$, then $A$ will be close to 0 and the test statistic $T_1$ will be small. Note that we can use this test even if some of the groups have small sample size, since the test is based on the overall trend in the proportions. This characteristic is in contrast to the overall chi-square test in **(10.19)**, which tests for heterogeneity among proportions and requires that the expected number of units in individual cells not be too small.

*Example 10.41*     *Cancer* Using the international study data in Table 10.19, assess whether or not there is an increasing trend in the proportion of breast cancer cases as age at first birth increases.

*Solution*     We note that $S_i = 1, 2, 3, 4, 5$ in the five groups, respectively. Furthermore, from Table 10.19 we see that $x_i = 320, 1206, 1011, 463, 220$, and $n_i = 1742, 5638, 3904, 1555, 626$ in the five respective groups, whereas $x = 3220$, $N = 13{,}465$, $\bar{p} = x/N = 0.239$, $\bar{q} = 1 - \bar{p} = 0.761$. From **(10.20)** it follows that

$A = (320)(1) + (1206)(2) + \cdots + (220)(5) - (3220)[1742(1) + 5638(2) + \cdots + 626(5)]/13{,}465$

$\quad = 8717 - (3220)(34{,}080)/13{,}465$

$\quad = 8717 - 8149.84$

$\quad = 567.16$

$B = (0.239)(0.761)\{1742(1^2) + 5638(2^2) + \cdots + 626(5^2)$

$\quad\quad -[1742(1) + (5638)(2) + \cdots + 626(5)]^2/13{,}465\}$

$\quad = (0.239)(0.761)[99{,}960 - (34{,}080)^2/13{,}465]$

$\quad = (0.239)(0.761)(99{,}960 - 86{,}256.70)$

$\quad = 2492.34$

Thus,

$$T_1 = A^2/B$$

$$= \frac{567.16^2}{2492.34}$$

$$= 129.06 \sim \chi_1^2 \text{ under } H_0$$

Since $\chi_{1,.999}^2 = 10.83 < 129.06 = T_1$, we can reject $H_0$ with $p < 0.001$ and conclude that there is a significant trend in the proportion of breast cancer cases among age at first birth groups. Since $A > 0$, it follows that as age at first birth increases, the proportion of breast cancer cases rises. ∎

Note that with a $2 \times k$ table, the chi-square test for trend in **(10.20)** is often more relevant to the hypotheses of interest than the chi-square test for heterogeneity in **(10.19)**, since the former procedure tests for specific trends in the proportions, whereas the latter tests for any differences in the proportions, where the proportions may follow any pattern. Other, more advanced methods for assessing $R \times C$ contingency tables are given in Maxwell's *Analyzing Qualitative Data* [5].

# ■ 10.8 MANTEL-HAENSZEL TEST

When looking at the relationship between a disease and an exposure variable, it is often important to control for the effect of some other variable that may be associated with either the disease or the exposure or both.

**Definition 10.10**

A **confounding variable** is a variable that may be associated with either disease or exposure or both. Such a variable must usually be controlled for before looking at the disease-exposure relationship.                                                                                     ■

**Example 10.42**    *Cancer* A recent study identified a group of 518 cancer cases ages 15–59 and a group of 518 age- and sex-matched controls by mail questionnaire [6]. The main purpose of the study was to look at the effect of passive smoking on cancer risk. In the study passive smoking was defined as exposure to the cigarette smoke of a spouse who smoked at least one cigarette per day for at least 6 months. One potential confounding variable was smoking by the test subjects themselves (i.e., personal smoking), since personal smoking is related to both cancer risk and spouse smoking. Therefore, it was important to control for personal smoking before looking at the relationship between passive smoking and cancer risk.                              ■

To analyze the data, a $2 \times 2$ table relating case-control status to passive smoking can be constructed for both nonsmokers and smokers. The data are given in Table 10.21 for nonsmokers and Table 10.22 for smokers.

**Table 10.21**
*Relationship of passive smoking to cancer risk among nonsmokers*

| Case-control status | Passive smoker | | |
| | Yes | No | Total |
|---|---|---|---|
| Case | 120 | 111 | 231 |
| Control | 80 | 155 | 235 |
| Total | 200 | 266 | 466 |

(Reprinted with permission of the *American Journal of Epidemiology* **121(1)**: 37–48, 1985.)

**Table 10.22**
*Relationship of passive smoking to cancer risk among smokers*

| Case-control status | Passive smoker | | |
| | Yes | No | Total |
|---|---|---|---|
| Case | 161 | 117 | 278 |
| Control | 130 | 124 | 254 |
| Total | 291 | 241 | 532 |

(Reprinted with permission of the *American Journal of Epidemiology* **121(1)**: 37–48, 1985.)

**Table 10.23**

Relationship of
disease to exposure
in the ith stratum

| Disease | Exposure | | Total |
|---|---|---|---|
| | Yes | No | |
| Yes | $a_i$ | $b_i$ | $a_i + b_i$ |
| No | $c_i$ | $d_i$ | $c_i + d_i$ |
| Total | $a_i + c_i$ | $b_i + d_i$ | $N_i$ |

We can assess the passive smoking effect separately for nonsmokers and smokers. Indeed, we notice from Table 10.21 that the odds ratio in favor of a case being exposed to cigarette smoke from a spouse who smokes vs. a control is $(120 \times 155)/(80 \times 111) = 2.1$ for nonsmokers, whereas the corresponding odds ratio for smokers is $(161 \times 124)/(130 \times 117) = 1.3$. Thus for both subgroups the trend is in the direction of more passive smoking among cases than controls. The key question is how to combine the results of the two tables to obtain an overall test of significance for the passive smoking effect.

In general, we will stratify our data into $k$ subgroups according to one or more confounding variables to make the units within a stratum as homogeneous as possible. The data for each stratum consist of a $2 \times 2$ contingency table relating exposure to disease, as shown in Table 10.23 for the $i$th stratum.

Our test procedure will be based on a comparison of the observed number of units in the $(1, 1)$ cell of each stratum (denoted by $O_i = a_i$) with the expected number of units in that cell (denoted by $E_i$). The test procedure is the same regardless of the order of the rows and columns; that is, which row (or column) is designated as the first row (or column) is arbitrary. Based on the margins, the expected number of units in the $(1, 1)$ cell of the $i$th stratum is given by

**10.21**

$$E_i = \frac{(a_i + b_i)(a_i + c_i)}{N_i}$$

We then sum the observed and expected numbers of units in the $(1, 1)$ cell over all strata, obtaining $O = \sum_{i=1}^{k} O_i$, $E = \sum_{i=1}^{k} E_i$, and base our test on $O - E$. It can be shown that the variance of $(O_i - E_i)$ is given by

**10.22**

$$V_i = \frac{(a_i + b_i)(c_i + d_i)(a_i + c_i)(b_i + d_i)}{N_i^2(N_i - 1)}$$

Furthermore, the variance of $O - E = V = \sum_{i=1}^{k} V_i$. Our test statistic is given by $T = (|O - E| - 0.5)^2/V$, which should follow a chi-square distribution with 1 d.f. under the null hypothesis of no association between disease and exposure. We reject $H_0$ if $T$ is large. This procedure is known as the Mantel-Haenszel test and is summarized as follows:

**10.23** *Mantel-Haenszel Test*

To assess the association between a dichotomous disease and a dichotomous exposure variable after controlling for one or more confounding variables, we use the following procedure:

1. We form $k$ strata, based on the level of the confounding variable(s), and construct a $2 \times 2$ table relating disease and exposure within each stratum, as shown in Table 10.23.

2. We compute the total observed number of units ($O$) in the (1, 1) cell over all strata, where

$$O = \sum_{i=1}^{k} O_i = \sum_{i=1}^{k} a_i$$

3. We compute the total expected number of units ($E$) in the (1, 1) cell over all strata, where

$$E = \sum_{i=1}^{k} E_i = \sum_{i=1}^{k} \frac{(a_i + b_i)(a_i + c_i)}{N_i}$$

4. We compute the variance ($V$) of the difference $O - E$, where

$$V = \sum_{i=1}^{k} V_i = \sum_{i=1}^{k} \frac{(a_i + b_i)(c_i + d_i)(a_i + c_i)(b_i + d_i)}{N_i^2(N_i - 1)}$$

5. Our test statistic is then given by

$$T_{MH} = \frac{(|O - E| - 0.5)^2}{V}$$

which under $H_0$ follows a chi-square distribution with 1 d.f. ($MH$ refers to Mantel-Haenszel).

6. For a test with significance level $\alpha$, if

$$T_{MH} > \chi^2_{1,1-\alpha}$$

then we reject $H_0$. If

$$T_{MH} \leqslant \chi^2_{1,1-\alpha}$$

then we accept $H_0$.

7. The exact $p$-value for this test is given by

$$p = Pr(\chi^2_1 > T_{MH})$$

8. We should use this test only if the variance $V \geqslant 5$.

9. Which row or column is designated as first is arbitrary. The test statistic $T_{MH}$ and the assessment of significance are the same regardless of the order of the rows and columns.

The acceptance and rejection regions for the Mantel-Haenszel test are depicted in Figure 10.12. The computation of the $p$-value for the Mantel-Haenszel test is illustrated in Figure 10.13.

---

**Example 10.43**  ***Cancer*** Assess the relationship between passive smoking and cancer risk using the data stratified by personal smoking status given in Tables 10.21 and 10.22.

**Solution**  We will denote the nonsmokers as stratum 1 and the smokers as stratum 2. We note that

$O_1$ = observed number of nonsmoking cases who are passive smokers = 120

$O_2$ = observed number of smoking cases who are passive smokers = 161

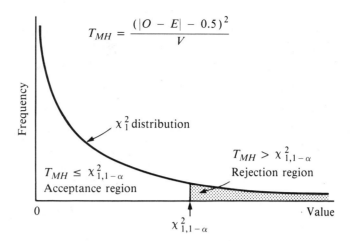

**Figure 10.12**
Acceptance and
rejection regions for
the Mantel-
Haenszel test

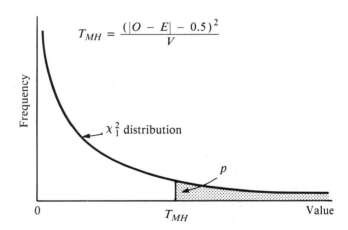

**Figure 10.13**
Computation of
the p-value for the
Mantel-Haenszel
test

Furthermore,

$$E_1 = \frac{231 \times 200}{466} = 99.1$$

$$E_2 = \frac{278 \times 291}{532} = 152.1$$

Thus, the total observed and expected numbers of cases who are passive smokers are, respectively,

$$O = O_1 + O_2 = 120 + 161 = 281$$

$$E = E_1 + E_2 = 99.1 + 152.1 = 251.2$$

Therefore, we have more cases who are passive smokers than we would expect based on their personal smoking habits. We now must compute the variance to assess if this difference is statistically significant. We have

$$V_1 = \frac{231 \times 235 \times 200 \times 266}{466^2 \times 465} = 28.60$$

$$V_2 = \frac{278 \times 254 \times 291 \times 241}{532^2 \times 531} = 32.95$$

Therefore,

$$V = V_1 + V_2 = 28.60 + 32.95 = 61.55$$

Thus, our test statistic $T_{MH}$ is given by

$$T_{MH} = \frac{(|281 - 251.2| - 0.5)^2}{61.55}$$

$$= \frac{858.49}{61.55}$$

$$= 13.95 \sim \chi_1^2 \text{ under } H_0$$

Since $\chi_{1,.999}^2 = 10.83 < 13.95 = T_{MH}$, it follows that $p < 0.001$. Thus, there is a highly significant association between case-control status and passive smoking exposure, *even after controlling for personal cigarette smoking habit.* ∎

## ☐ 10.8.1 Estimation of the Odds Ratio for Stratified Data

The Mantel-Haenszel test tells us about the statistical significance of the relationship between disease and exposure. However, it does not give us a measure of the strength of the association. Ideally, we would like a measure similar to the odds ratio presented for a single $2 \times 2$ contingency table in Definition 10.3. If we assume that the true odds ratio is the same for each stratum, then an estimate of the common odds ratio is provided by the Mantel-Haenszel estimator as follows:

**10.24**    **Mantel-Haenszel Estimator of the Common Odds Ratio for Stratified Data**

If we have a collection of $k$ $2 \times 2$ contingency tables, where the $i$th table corresponding to the $i$th stratum is denoted as in Table 10.23, then the Mantel-Haenszel estimator of the common odds ratio is given by

$$\widehat{OR}_{MH} = \frac{\sum_{i=1}^{k} (a_i d_i / N_i)}{\sum_{i=1}^{k} (b_i c_i / N_i)}$$

*Example 10.44*    **Cancer** Estimate the odds ratio in favor of passive smoking for cancer cases vs. controls after controlling for personal smoking habit.

**Solution**

From **(10.24)**, Table 10.21, and Table 10.22, we have

$$\widehat{OR}_{MH} = \frac{(120 \times 155/466) + (161 \times 124/532)}{(80 \times 111/466) + (130 \times 117/532)}$$

$$= \frac{77.44}{47.65}$$

$$= 1.63$$

Thus, the odds in favor of passive smoking for a breast cancer case is 1.6 times as large as that for a control. ■

We are also interested in estimating confidence limits for the odds ratio in **(10.24)**. We can use a test-based method similar to that presented for a single $2 \times 2$ contingency table in **(10.8)**. This method is given as follows:

**10.25** | *Interval Estimates for the Common Odds Ratio from a Collection of k 2 × 2 Contingency Tables (Test-Based Method)*

A two-sided $100\% \times (1 - \alpha)$ confidence interval for the common odds ratio from a collection of $k$ $2 \times 2$ contingency tables is given by

$$\left(\widehat{OR}_{MH}^{1 - \sqrt{\chi_{1,1-\alpha}^2/T_{MH}}}, \widehat{OR}_{MH}^{1 + \sqrt{\chi_{1,1-\alpha}^2/T_{MH}}}\right) \qquad \text{if } \widehat{OR}_{MH} \geq 1$$

$$\left(\widehat{OR}_{MH}^{1 + \sqrt{\chi_{1,1-\alpha}^2/T_{MH}}}, \widehat{OR}_{MH}^{1 - \sqrt{\chi_{1,1-\alpha}^2/T_{MH}}}\right) \qquad \text{if } \widehat{OR}_{MH} < 1$$

where $\widehat{OR}_{MH}$ is the Mantel-Haenszel estimator of the common odds ratio given in **(10.24)**, and $T_{MH}$ is the Mantel-Haenszel test statistic given in **(10.23)**. This method should be used only if $0.2 \leq \widehat{OR}_{MH} \leq 5.0$.

**Example 10.45**

*Cancer* Estimate 95% confidence limits for the common odds ratio using the data in Tables 10.21 and 10.22.

**Solution**

We note from Example 10.44 that our point estimate of the odds ratio $= \widehat{OR}_{MH} = 1.63$. Furthermore, from Example 10.43 the Mantel-Haenszel test statistic is 13.95. Finally, since we want a 95% confidence interval, it follows that $\chi_{1,1-\alpha}^2 = \chi_{1,.95}^2 = 3.84$. Therefore, using **(10.25)**, we have the following 95% confidence interval for $OR$:

$$(1.63^{1 - \sqrt{3.84/13.95}}, 1.63^{1 + \sqrt{3.84/13.95}})$$

$$= (1.63^{1 - 0.52}, 1.63^{1 + 0.52})$$

$$= (1.63^{0.48}, 1.63^{1.52})$$

$$= (1.26, 2.10)$$

Notice that the 95% confidence interval for $OR$ does not include 1, which agrees with the level of significance of the test statistic ($T_{MH} = 13.95, p < 0.001$). This relationship is one advantage of the test-based method: if the Mantel-Haenszel test statistic is significant at the 5% level, then the test-based 95% confidence interval for $OR$ will always exclude 1. If the Mantel-Haenszel test statistic is not significant at the 5% level, then the 95% confidence interval for

*OR* will always include 1. This relationship was also true for the test-based method for a single 2 × 2 contingency table in **(10.8)**.                                                                                      ■

As was the case for a single 2 × 2 contingency table, the test-based method should be used only if the estimated odds ratio is not too different from 1, that is, if $0.2 \leqslant \widehat{OR}_{MH} \leqslant 5.0$. If $\widehat{OR}_{MH}$ is outside this range, then more sophisticated methods should be used (see [2]).

Finally, one assumption made in the estimation of a common odds ratio in **(10.24)** is that the strength of association is the same in each stratum. If the underlying odds ratio is different in the various strata, then it makes little sense to estimate a common odds ratio. A method for testing for the homogeneity of the odds ratio over multiple strata is given in Fleiss [7].

# ■ *10.9  CHI-SQUARE GOODNESS-OF-FIT TEST*

In our previous work on estimation and hypothesis testing, we usually assumed that our data came from a specific underlying probability model and then proceeded to either estimate the parameters of the model or test hypotheses concerning different possible values of the parameters. In this section we present a general method of testing for the *goodness of fit of a probability model.* Consider the following problem:

*Example 10.46*    *Hypertension*  Suppose we collected diastolic blood pressure measurements at home in a community-wide screening program of 14,736 adults ages 30–69 in East Boston, Massachusetts, as part of a nationwide study to detect and treat hypertensive persons [8]. The persons in the study were each screened in the home with two measurements taken at one visit. A frequency distribution of the mean blood pressure is given in Table 10.24 in 10-mm intervals.

We would like to assume that these measurements came from an underlying normal distribution, since we then could apply standard methods of statistical inference on these data as presented in this text. How can we test if this assumption is valid?                                       ■

We can test this assumption by first computing what the expected frequencies would be in each group if the data did come from an underlying normal distribution and then comparing these expected frequencies to the corresponding observed frequencies.

*Example 10.47*    *Hypertension*  Compute the expected frequencies for the data in Table 10.24 assuming an underlying normal distribution.

**Table 10.24**
*Frequency distribution of mean diastolic blood pressure for adults 30–69 years old in a community-wide screening program in East Boston, Massachusetts*

| Group | Observed frequency | Expected frequency | Group | Observed frequency | Expected frequency |
|---|---|---|---|---|---|
| < 50 | 57 | 77 | ≥ 80, < 90 | 4604 | 4511 |
| ≥ 50, < 60 | 330 | 553 | ≥ 90, < 100 | 2119 | 2417 |
| ≥ 60, < 70 | 2132 | 2122 | ≥ 100, < 110 | 659 | 684 |
| ≥ 70, < 80 | 4584 | 4265 | ≥ 110, < 120 | 251 | 107 |
|  |  |  | Total | 14,736 | 14,736 |

**Solution**

We will assume that the mean and standard deviation of this hypothetical normal distribution are given by the sample mean and standard deviation, respectively ($\bar{x} = 80.68$, $s = 12.00$). The expected frequency within a group interval from $a$ to $b$ would then be given by

$$14{,}736\{\Phi[(b - \mu)/\sigma] - \Phi[(a - \mu)/\sigma]\}$$

Thus, the expected frequency within the ($\geqslant 50$, $< 60$) group would be

$$14{,}736 \times \{\Phi[(60 - 80.68)/12] - \Phi[(50 - 80.68)/12]\}$$

$$= 14{,}736 \times [\Phi(-1.72) - \Phi(-2.56)]$$

$$= 14{,}736 \times (0.0427 - 0.0052) = 14{,}736(0.0375) = 552.6$$

The expected frequencies for all the groups are given in Table 10.24. ∎

We will use the same measure of agreement between the observed and expected frequencies in a group as we did in our work on contingency tables, namely, $(O - E)^2/E$. Furthermore, we can summarize the agreement between observed and expected frequencies over the whole table by summing $(O - E)^2/E$ over all the groups. We can show that if we have the correct underlying model, then this sum will approximately follow a chi-square distribution with $g - 1 - p$ d.f., where $g$ = the number of groups and $p$ = the number of parameters estimated from the data to compute the expected frequencies. This approximation will again be valid only if the expected values in the groups are not too small. In particular, we require that no expected value be less than 1 and that no more than $\frac{1}{5}$ of the expected values be less than 5. If we have too many groups with small expected frequencies, then we should combine some of them with other groups so that the preceding rule is not violated. The test procedure can be summarized as follows:

**10.26**    *Chi-Square Goodness-of-Fit Test*

If we wish to test for the goodness of fit of a probability model, then:

*1.* We divide our raw data into groups. The considerations for grouping data are similar to those given in Section 2.7. In particular, we require that the groups not be too small, so that step 7 is not violated.

*2.* We estimate the $p$ parameters of the probability model from our data using the methods of Chapter 6.

*3.* We use the estimates in step 2 to compute the probability $\hat{p}$ of obtaining a value within a particular group and the corresponding expected frequency within that group ($n\hat{p}$), where $n$ is the total number of data points.

*4.* If $O$ and $E$ are, respectively, the observed and expected number of units within a particular group, then we compute

$$S = (O_1 - E_1)^2/E_1 + (O_2 - E_2)^2/E_2 + \cdots + (O_g - E_g)^2/E_g$$

where $g$ = the number of groups.

*5.* For a test with significance level $\alpha$, if

$$S > \chi^2_{g - p - 1, 1 - \alpha}$$

then we reject $H_0$; if

$$S \leqslant \chi^2_{g-p-1,1-\alpha}$$

then we accept $H_0$.

6. The exact $p$-value for this test is given by

$$Pr(\chi^2_{g-p-1} > S)$$

7. We will use this test only if
 (i) No more than $\frac{1}{5}$ of the expected values are $<5$
 (ii) No expected values are $<1$

The acceptance and rejection regions for this test are depicted in Figure 10.14. The computation of the $p$-value for this test is illustrated in Figure 10.15.

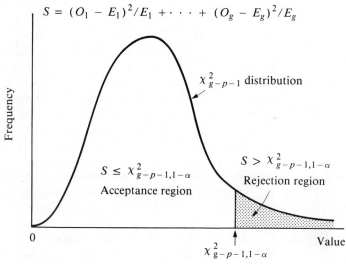

$$S = (O_1 - E_1)^2/E_1 + \cdots + (O_g - E_g)^2/E_g$$

$\chi^2_{g-p-1}$ distribution

$S \leq \chi^2_{g-p-1,1-\alpha}$
Acceptance region

$S > \chi^2_{g-p-1,1-\alpha}$
Rejection region

$\chi^2_{g-p-1,1-\alpha}$

**Figure 10.14**

*Acceptance and rejection regions for the chi-square goodness-of-fit test*

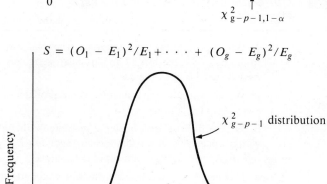

$$S = (O_1 - E_1)^2/E_1 + \cdots + (O_g - E_g)^2/E_g$$

$\chi^2_{g-p-1}$ distribution

$p$

**Figure 10.15**

*Computation of the p-value for the chi-square goodness-of-fit test*

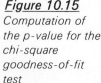
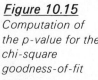

*Example 10.48*  **Hypertension** Test for the goodness-of-fit of the normal probability model using the data in Table 10.24.

*Solution*  We have estimated two parameters from the data ($\mu$, $\sigma^2$) and have eight groups. Therefore, $p = 2$, $g = 8$. Under $H_0$, $S$ follows a chi-square distribution with $8 - 2 - 1 = 5$ d.f.

$$S = (O_1 - E_1)^2/E_1 + \cdots + (O_8 - E_8)^2/E_8$$
$$= (57 - 77)^2/77 + \cdots + (251 - 107)^2/107$$
$$= 352.6 \sim \chi^2_5 \text{ under } H_0$$

Since $\chi^2_{5,.999} = 20.52 < 352.6 = S$, the $p$-value $< 1 - 0.999 = 0.001$ and the results are very highly significant.

Thus, we *do not* accept the adequacy of the normal model. The normal model appears to fit fairly well in the middle of the distribution (between 60 and 110 mm) but fails badly in the tails, predicting too many blood pressures below 60 mm and too few over 110 mm.  ∎

Note that the test procedure in **(10.26)** can be used to assess the goodness-of-fit of any probability model, not just the normal model. We would compute the expected frequencies from the probability distribution of the proposed model and then use the same goodness-of-fit test statistic as given in **(10.26)**.

# ■ *10.10 SUMMARY*

In this chapter we discussed the most widely used techniques for analyzing qualitative (or categorical) data. First we studied the problem of how to compare binomial proportions from two independent samples. For the large-sample case, we solved this problem in two different (but equivalent) ways: either the **two-sample test for binomial proportions** or the **chi-square test for 2 × 2 contingency tables**. The former method is similar to the *t* test methodology introduced in Chapter 8, whereas the contingency table approach can be easily generalized to more complex problems involving qualitative data. For the small-sample case, we need to use **Fisher's exact test** to compare binomial proportions in two independent samples. If we wish to compare binomial proportions in paired samples, such as when a person is used as his or her own control, then we should use **McNemar's test for correlated proportions**.

We then extended the 2 × 2 contingency table problem to the investigation of the relationship between two qualitative variables, in which one or both of the variables have more than two possible categories of response. We were able to develop a **chi-square test for $R \times C$ contingency tables**, which is a direct generalization of the 2 × 2 contingency table test. We also considered the question of how to compare two binomial proportions when confounding was present. Our approach was to partition the data into $k$ strata according to the values of one or more confounding variables. We then used the **Mantel-Haenszel test** to combine evidence over more than one stratum. Finally, we studied the problem of how to assess the goodness-of-fit of the probability models proposed in earlier chapters and used the **chi-square goodness-of-fit test** to address this problem. These strategies are illustrated in the shaded boxes of the flowchart in Figure 10.16.

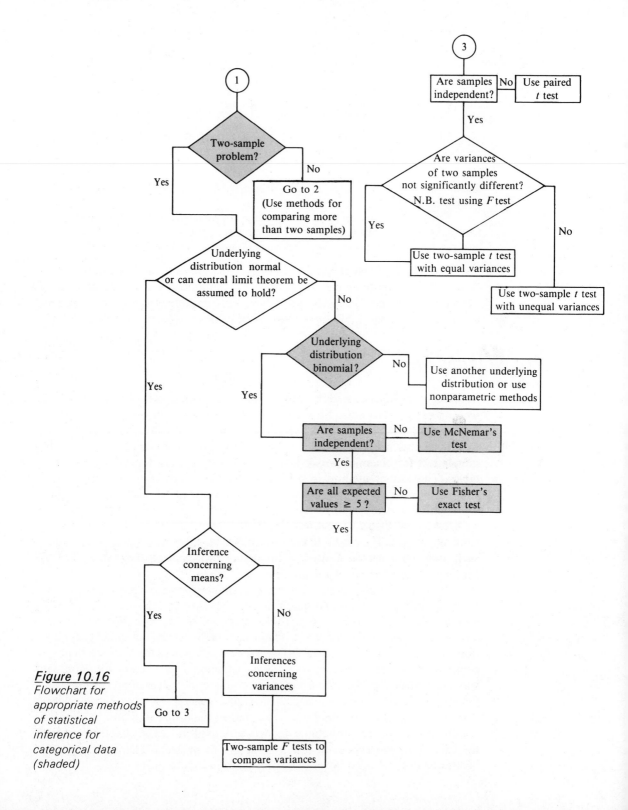

**Figure 10.16**
Flowchart for
appropriate methods
of statistical
inference for
categorical data
(shaded)

In this chapter we focused on how to assess the relationship between two qualitative variables. In the next two chapters, we will treat a similar problem, in which the variables under study are either all continuous or some are continuous and others are categorical.

# Problems

## Cardiovascular Disease

In a recent study of the effectiveness of streptokinase in the treatment of patients who have been hospitalized after myocardial infarction, 9 of 199 males receiving streptokinase and 13 of 97 males in the control group died within 12 months [9].

**10.1** Use the normal theory method to test for significant differences in 12-month mortality between the two groups.

**10.2** Construct the observed and expected contingency tables for these data.

**10.3** Perform the test in Problem 10.1 using the contingency table method.

**10.4** Compare your results in Problems 10.1 and 10.3.

## Gynecology

In a recent study of the relationship between contraceptive use and infertility, 89 out of 283 infertile women compared with 640 out of 3833 control women had used an IUD at some time in their lives [10].

**10.5** Use the normal theory method to test for significant differences in contraceptive use patterns between the two groups.

**10.6** Use the contingency table method to perform the test in Problem 10.5.

**10.7** Compare your results in Problems 10.5 and 10.6.

**10.8** Compute a 95% confidence interval for the difference in 12-month mortality rates between the streptokinase and control groups in Problem 10.1.

**10.9** Compute a 95% confidence interval for the difference in the proportion of women who have ever used IUD's between the case and control groups in Problem 10.5.

**10.10** Compute the odds ratio in favor of death within 12 months for streptokinase therapy vs. control therapy using the data in Problem 10.1.

**10.11** Provide a 95% confidence interval for the true odds ratio corresponding to your answer to Problem 10.10.

**10.12** What is the relationship between your answers to Problems 10.3 and 10.11?

**10.13** Compute the odds ratio in favor of ever using an IUD for infertile women vs. control women.

**10.14** Provide a 95% confidence interval for the true odds ratio corresponding to your answer to Problem 10.13.

**10.15** What is the relationship between your answers to Problems 10.6 and 10.14?

## Cardiovascular Disease

Suppose we plan a 5-year clinical trial comparing aspirin vs. placebo for the prevention of MI in men. We anticipate a 2.5% incidence rate of MI over 5 years among 40–64-year-old placebo males and a 2.0% rate over 5 years among comparably aged males taking aspirin.

**10.16** How many subjects do we need to enroll in each group to have an 80% chance of detecting a significant difference using a two-sided test with $\alpha = 0.05$?

**10.17** Answer Problem 10.16 if we wish to use a two-sided test with power = 0.9.

**10.18** Answer Problem 10.16 if we wish to use a one-sided test with power = 0.8.

**10.19** Suppose we actually enroll 5000 men in each treatment group. What would be the power of such a study if we were to use a two-sided test with $\alpha = 0.05$?

**10.20** Answer Problem 10.19 if we enroll 7000 men in each group.

## Cardiovascular Disease

In the streptokinase study in Problem 10.1, 2 of 15 females receiving streptokinase and 4 of 19 females in the control group died within 12 months.

**10.21** Why is Fisher's exact test the appropriate procedure to test for differences in 12-month mortality rates between these two groups?

*10.22* Write down all possible tables with the same row and column margins as given in the observed data.

*10.23* Calculate the probability of each of the tables enumerated in Problem 10.22.

*10.24* Evaluate whether or not there is a significant difference between the mortality rates for streptokinase and control group females using a two-sided test based on your results in Problem 10.23.
Refer to Table 2.11 (page 37).

*10.25* What significance test can be used to detect a relationship between receiving an antibiotic and receiving a bacterial culture, while in the hospital?

*10.26* Perform the test in Problem 10.25 and report a *p*-value.

*Gastroenterology*

Two drugs (A, B) are compared for the medical treatment of duodenal ulcer. For this purpose patients are carefully matched on age, sex, and clinical condition. The treatment results based on 200 matched pairs show that for 89 matched pairs both treatments are effective; for 90 matched pairs both treatments are ineffective; for 5 matched pairs drug A is effective, whereas drug B is ineffective; for 16 matched pairs drug B is effective, whereas drug A is ineffective.

*10.27* What test procedure can be used to assess the results?

*10.28* Perform the test in Problem 10.27 and report a *p*-value.

In the same study, if we focus on the 100 matched pairs consisting of male patients, then we get the following results: for 52 matched pairs both drugs are effective; for 35 matched pairs both drugs are ineffective; for 4 matched pairs drug A is effective, whereas drug B is ineffective; for 9 matched pairs drug B is effective, whereas drug A is ineffective.

*10.29* How many concordant pairs are among the male matched pairs?

*10.30* How many discordant pairs are among the male matched pairs?

*10.31* Perform a significance test to assess any differences in effectiveness between the drugs among males. Report a *p*-value.

*Gynecology*

Women were subdivided by duration of IUD use in the study presented in Problem 10.5. The data are given in Table 10.25.

**Table 10.25** *Relationship between duration of IUD use and infertility among IUD users*

| | Duration of IUD use (months) | | | |
|---|---|---|---|---|
| | < 3 | ≥ 3, < 18 | ≥ 18, ≤ 36 | > 36 |
| *Cases* | 10 | 23 | 20 | 36 |
| *Controls* | 53 | 200 | 168 | 219 |

(Reprinted with permission of the *New England Journal of Medicine* **312(15)**: 941–947, 1985.)

*10.32* Perform a test for heterogeneity of the proportions of cases in the four groups.

*10.33* Suppose we assign the score variable 1, 2, 3, 4 to the four duration groups. Perform a test for trend on these data; that is, does the proportion of cases increase or decrease as the duration of IUD use increases?

*10.34* Interpret your results in Problems 10.32 and 10.33.

Refer to the streptokinase data presented for males in Problem 10.1 and for females in Problem 10.21.

*10.35* Perform a significance test for association between treatment group and 12-month mortality, after stratifying the data by sex.

*10.36* Estimate the odds ratio in favor of 12-month mortality in the streptokinase group vs. the control group, after stratifying the data by sex.

*10.37* Provide a 95% confidence interval for the true odds ratio corresponding to your answer to Problem 10.36.

*10.38* Test for the goodness-of-fit of the normal model for the distribution of survival times of mice given in Table 6.11 (page 178).

*10.39* Test for the adequacy of the normal model for the distribution of duration of hospitalization given in Table 2.11 (page 37).

*10.40* Answer Problem 10.39 for the distribution of $\log_e$ (duration of hospitalization).

*Pulmonary Disease*

Suppose we wish to investigate the familial aggregation of respiratory disease on a disease-specific basis. We identify 100 families in which the head of household or spouse has asthma, which we refer to as type A families, and we identify 200 families in which neither the head of household nor the spouse has asthma, which we refer to as type B families. Suppose that in 15 of the type A families the first-born child has asthma, whereas in 3 other type A families the first-born child has some non-asthmatic respiratory disease. Furthermore, in 4 of the type B households the first-born child has asthma, whereas in 2 other type B households the first-born child has some nonasthmatic respiratory disease.

*10.41* Compare the prevalence rates of asthma in the two types of families. State all hypotheses being tested.

*10.42* Compare the prevalence rates of nonasthmatic respiratory disease in the two types of families. State all hypotheses being tested.

### Venereal Disease

Suppose we are performing an epidemiologic investigation of persons entering a VD clinic. We find that 160 of 200 patients who are diagnosed as having gonorrhea and 50 of 105 patients who are diagnosed as having nongonococcal urethritis (NGU) have had previous episodes of urethritis.

*10.43* Is there an association between the present diagnosis and prior episodes of urethritis?

### Cardiovascular Disease

A recent study investigated the relationship between cigarette smoking and subsequent mortality in men with a prior history of coronary disease [11]. It was found that 264 out of 1731 nonsmokers and 208 out of 1058 smokers had died in the 5-year period after the study began.

*10.44* Assuming that the age distributions of the two groups are comparable, compare the mortality rates in the two groups.

### Cancer

*10.45* A recent study was performed to investigate the relationship between the use of oral contraceptives and the development of endometrial cancer [12]. It was found that of 117 endometrial cancer patients, 6 had used the oral contraceptive Oracon at some time in their lives, whereas of 395 controls, 8 had used this agent. Test for an association between the use of Oracon and the incidence of endometrial cancer using a two-tailed test.

### Obstetrics

Suppose we have 500 pairs of pregnant women who participate in a prematurity study and are paired in such a way that the body weight of the 2 women in a pair are within 5 lb of each other. We then give one of the 2 women a placebo and the other drug A to see if drug A has an effect in preventing prematurity. Suppose that in 30 pairs

of women, *both* women in a pair have a premature child; in 420 pairs of women, *both* women have a normal child; in 35 pairs of women, the woman taking drug A has a normal child and the woman taking the placebo has a premature child; in 15 pairs of women, the woman taking drug A has a premature child and the woman taking the placebo has a normal child.

*10.46* Assess the statistical significance of these results.

### Ophthalmology

Retinitis pigmentosa is a disease that manifests itself via different genetic modes of inheritance. Cases have been documented with a dominant, recessive, and sex-linked mode of inheritance. It has been conjectured that the mode of inheritance is related to the ethnic origin of the individual. Cases of the disease have been surveyed in an English and a Swiss population with the following results: Out of 125 English cases, 46 had sex-linked disease, 25 had recessive disease, and 54 had dominant disease. Out of the 110 Swiss cases, 1 had sex-linked disease, 99 had recessive disease, and 10 had dominant disease.

*10.47* Do these data show a significant association between ethnic origin and genetic type?

### Cancer

Suppose we wish to compare the following two treatments for breast cancer: simple mastectomy (S) and radical mastectomy (R). We form matched pairs of women who are within the same decade of age and with the same clinical condition. They receive the two treatments, and we monitor their subsequent 5-year survival. The results are given in Table 10.26. We wish to test for significant differences between the treatments.

*10.48* What test should be used to analyze these data? State the hypothesis being tested.

*10.49* Conduct the test mentioned in Problem 10.48.

### Venereal Disease

Suppose we are interested in comparing the effectiveness of two different antibiotics, A and B, in treating gonorrhea. We match each person receiving antibiotic A with an equivalent person (age within 5 years, same sex), to whom we give antibiotic B. We ask these persons to return to the clinic within 1 week to see if the gonorrhea has been eliminated. Suppose the results are as follows:

(a) For 40 pairs of people, both antibiotics are successful.

(b) For 20 pairs of people, antibiotic A is effective whereas antibiotic B is not.

(c) For 16 pairs of people, antibiotic B is effective whereas antibiotic A is not.

**Table 10.26** Comparison of simple and radical mastectomy in treating breast cancer

| Pair | Treatment S woman | Treatment R woman |
|------|-------------------|-------------------|
| 1 | L* | L |
| 2 | L | D |
| 3 | L | L |
| 4 | L | L |
| 5 | L | L |
| 6 | D† | L |
| 7 | L | L |
| 8 | L | D |
| 9 | L | D |
| 10 | L | L |
| 11 | D | D |
| 12 | L | D |
| 13 | L | L |
| 14 | L | L |
| 15 | L | D |
| 16 | L | L |
| 17 | L | D |
| 18 | L | D |
| 19 | L | L |
| 20 | L | D |

*L = lived at least 5 years
†D = died within 5 years

(d) For 3 pairs of people, neither antibiotic is effective.

**10.50** Test for the relative effectiveness of the two antibiotics.

We compile the annual incidence in 1973 of a rare disease in two communities, A and B, and find that of 100,000 persons in community A, 5 have the disease, whereas of 200,000 persons in community B, only 1 has the disease.

**10.51** Test whether the underlying incidence rates are significantly different.

## Pulmonary Disease

One important aspect of medical diagnosis is its reproducibility. Suppose that two different doctors examine 100 patients for dyspnea in a respiratory disease clinic and that 15 patients are diagnosed as having dyspnea by doctor A, 10 patients are diagnosed as having dyspnea by doctor B, and 7 patients are diagnosed as having dyspnea by *both* doctor A and doctor B.

**10.52** Test whether or not the diagnoses of the two doctors are comparable.

## Cardiovascular Disease

Much controversy has arisen recently on the possible association of myocardial infarction (MI) and coffee drinking. Suppose we obtain the information given in Table 10.27 on coffee drinking and prior MI status from 200 60–64-year-old males in the general population.

**Table 10.27** Coffee drinking and prior MI status

| Coffee drinking (cups/day) | MI in last 5 years | Number of people |
|----------------------------|--------------------|------------------|
| 0 | Yes | 3 |
| 0 | No | 57 |
| 1 | Yes | 7 |
| 1 | No | 43 |
| 2 | Yes | 8 |
| 2 | No | 42 |
| 3 or more | Yes | 12 |
| 3 or more | No | 28 |
| | Total yes | 30 |
| | Total no | 170 |

**10.53** Test for the association between history of MI and coffee drinking status, which is categorized as follows: 0 cups, 1 or more cups.

**10.54** Suppose we categorize coffee drinking as follows: 0 cups, 1 cup, 2 cups, 3 or more cups. Perform a test to investigate whether or not there is a consistent association between these two variables using this categorization.

## Infectious Disease

Suppose we have a computerized data bank consisting of all charts of patients at nine hospitals in Cleveland, Ohio. One concern of the group conducting the study is the possibility that the attending physician under- or overreports various diagnoses that seem consistent with a patient's chart. An investigator notes that 50 out of the 10,000 people in the data bank are reported as having a particular viral infection by their attending physician. A computer using an automated method of diagnosis claims that 68 out of the 10,000 people have the infection, 48 of them from the attending physician's 50 positives and 20 from the attending physician's 9950 negatives.

**10.55** Test the hypothesis that the computer's and the attending physician's diagnoses are comparable.

## Obstetrics

*10.56* Test for the adequacy of the goodness-of-fit of the normal distribution when applied to the distribution of birthweights given in Figure 2.8 (page 31). The sample mean and standard deviation for these data are 111.26 oz and 20.95 oz, respectively.

## Cardiovascular Disease

An investigator wishes to study the effect of cigarette smoking on the development of myocardial infarction (MI) in women. In particular, there is some question in the literature as to the relationship of the timing of cigarette smoking to the development of disease. One school of thought says that current smokers are at much higher risk than ex-smokers. Another school of thought says that a considerable latent period of nonsmoking is needed before the risk of ex-smokers becomes less than that of current smokers. To test this hypothesis, 2000 disease-free currently smoking women and 1000 disease-free ex-smoking women, aged 50–59, are identified in 1976, and the incidence of MI between 1976 and 1978 is noted at follow-up visits 2 years later. Investigators find that 40 currently smoking women and 10 ex-smoking women have developed the disease.

*10.57* Is a one-sample or two-sample test needed here?

*10.58* Is a one-sided or two-sided test needed here?

*10.59* Which of the following test procedures should be used to test this hypothesis? (More than one may be necessary.)

    (a) $\chi^2$ test for $2 \times 2$ contingency tables

    (b) Fisher's exact test

    (c) McNemar's test

    (d) One-sample binomial test

    (e) One-sample $t$ test

    (f) Two-sample $t$ test with equal variances

*10.60* Carry out the test procedure(s) mentioned in Problem 10.59 and report a $p$-value.

## Cardiovascular Disease

A hypothesis has been suggested that a principal benefit of physical activity is to prevent sudden death from heart attack. The following study was designed to test this hypothesis: 100 men who died from a first heart attack and 100 men who survived a first heart attack in the age group 50–59 were identified and their wives were each given a detailed questionnaire concerning their husband's physical activity in the year preceding their heart attacks. The men were then classified as active or inactive. Suppose that 30 of the 100 who survived and 10 of the 100

who died were physically active. If we wish to test the hypothesis, then:

*10.61* Is a one-sample or two-sample test needed here?

*10.62* Which one of the following test procedures should be used to test the hypothesis?

    (a) Paired $t$ test

    (b) Two-sample $t$ test with independent samples

    (c) $\chi^2$ test for $2 \times 2$ contingency tables

    (d) Fisher's exact test

    (e) McNemar's test

*10.63* Carry out the test procedure(s) in Problem 10.62 and report a $p$-value.

*10.64* Compute the odds ratio in favor of prior physical activity for MI survivors vs. MI deceased.

*10.65* Compute a 95% confidence interval for the odds ratio referred to in Problem 10.64.

## Cardiovascular Disease

A longitudinal study in apparently normal men is organized to relate *changes* in cardiovascular risk parameters to subsequent mortality. The hypothesis being tested is that men whose cholesterol level rises have a different subsequent mortality than those whose cholesterol level drops. In particular, two groups of 50–59-year-old men with initially normal cholesterol levels are identified: (1) group A = 25 men whose cholesterol level rises by 50 mg% over a 5-year period and (2) group B = 25 men whose cholesterol level drops by 50 mg% over a 5-year period. The groups are then followed for mortality over the next 5 years. The results are given in Table 10.28.

*10.66* Is a one-sample or two-sample test needed here?

*10.67* Is a one-sided or two-sided test needed here?

*10.68* Which of the following test procedures should we use? (More than one may be necessary.)

    (a) Paired $t$ test

    (b) Two-sample $t$ test with equal variances

    (c) $\chi^2$ test for $2 \times 2$ tables

    (d) Fisher's exact test

    (e) McNemar's test

    (f) One-sample binomial test

*10.69* Carry out the test procedure in Problem 10.68 and report a $p$-value.

## Psychiatry

An observational study is set up to assess the effects of lithium in treating manic-depressive patients. New

**Table 10.28** *Association between cardiovascular mortality and cholesterol change (+ = dead within the next 5 years; − = alive after 5 years)*

| Number of pairs | Mortality outcome, group A | Mortality outcome, group B |
|:---:|:---:|:---:|
| 1 | − | − |
| 2 | + | − |
| 3 | − | − |
| 4 | − | + |
| 5 | − | − |
| 6 | − | − |
| 7 | − | − |
| 8 | + | − |
| 9 | − | − |
| 10 | − | − |
| 11 | + | − |
| 12 | − | − |
| 13 | − | − |
| 14 | − | − |
| 15 | − | − |
| 16 | − | − |
| 17 | + | − |
| 18 | − | − |
| 19 | − | − |
| 20 | − | − |
| 21 | + | − |
| 22 | − | − |
| 23 | − | − |
| 24 | − | − |
| 25 | − | − |

patients in an out-patient service are matched according to age, sex, and clinical condition, with one patient receiving lithium and the other a placebo. Suppose the outcome variable is whether or not the patient has any manic-depressive episodes in the next 3 months. The results are as follows: In 20 cases both the lithium and placebo members of the pair have manic-depressive episodes; in 10 cases only the placebo member has an episode (the lithium member does not); in 2 cases only the lithium member has an episode (the placebo member does not); in 36 cases neither member has an episode.

**10.70** State an appropriate hypothesis to test whether lithium has any effect in treating manic-depressive patients.

**10.71** Test the hypothesis mentioned in Problem 10.70.

*Cancer*

Several studies have investigated the possible association between breast cancer and the use of oral contraceptives. Suppose a cohort of 5000 women in the age group 31–40 with no previous history of breast cancer is established in 1970. Of these women, 3000 have used oral contraceptives at some point in their lives (ever users) and 2000 have never used oral contraceptives. This cohort is examined every 2 years until 1980 for the presence of breast cancer. During these 10 years, 1 of the ever users has developed the disease, whereas 4 of the never users have developed the disease. Let us assume that there are no dropouts from the study over the 10-year period.

**10.72** Test for the association between the use of oral contraceptives and breast cancer.

**10.73** Compute an odds ratio for breast cancer incidence among oral contraceptive users vs. nonusers.

**10.74** One possible problem with the study design is that some of the women who report that they are never users up to 1970 will become ever users by 1980. How might this change affect the results in Problem 10.72?

*Cancer*

The following data are survival rates for cancer of the pancreas for the years 1955–1964, published in the volume *End Results in Cancer* by the U.S. Department of Health, Education and Welfare [13]: there were 256 reported cases of disease in the under-45 age group, of whom 8% survived for at least 3 years; 710 reported cases of disease in the 45–54 age group, of whom 2% survived for at least 3 years; 1348 reported cases of disease in the 55–64 age group, of whom 2% survived for at least 3 years; 1768 cases of disease in the 65–74 age group, of whom 1% survived for at least 3 years; 1292 cases of disease in the 75+ age group, of whom 1% survived for at least 3 years.

**10.75** What significance test can be used to test if there is an age trend in the 3-year survival rates?

**10.76** Perform the test in Problem 10.75 and report a *p*-value.

*Cardiovascular Disease*

In some studies heart disease has been associated with being overweight. Suppose we examine this association in a large-scale epidemiological study and find that of 2000 men in the age group 55–59, 200 have myocardial infarctions in the next 5 years. Suppose we group the men by body weight as given in Table 10.29.

**10.77** Comment in detail on these data.

*Table 10.29* Association between body weight and myocardial infarctions

| Body weight (lb) | Number of myocardial infarctions | Total number of men |
|---|---|---|
| 120–139 | 10 | 300 |
| 140–159 | 20 | 700 |
| 160–179 | 50 | 600 |
| 180–199 | 95 | 300 |
| 200 + | 25 | 100 |
| Total | 200 | 2000 |

### Venereal Disease

Suppose we conduct a study to examine the relative efficacy of penicillin and spectinomycin in the treatment of gonorrhea. We look at 3 treatments: (1) penicillin, (2) spectinomycin, low dose, and (3) spectinomycin, high dose. We record three possible responses: (1) positive smear, (2) negative smear, positive culture, (3) negative smear, negative culture. We obtain the following data.

*Table 10.30* Efficacy of different treatments for gonorrhea

| Treatment | Response | | | |
|---|---|---|---|---|
| | + Smear | − Smear + Culture | − Smear − Culture | Total |
| Penicillin | 40 | 30 | 130 | 200 |
| Spectinomycin (low dose) | 10 | 20 | 70 | 100 |
| Spectinomycin (high dose) | 15 | 40 | 45 | 100 |
| Total | 65 | 90 | 245 | 400 |

*10.78* Is there any relationship between type of treatment and response? What form does the relationship take?

*10.79* Suppose we regard either a positive smear or a positive culture as a positive response and distinguish that from the negative smear, negative culture response. Is there an association between the type of treatment and this measure of response?

### Cerebrovascular Disease

Atrial fibrillation (AF) is widely recognized to predispose patients to embolic stroke. Although oral anticoagulant therapy has been suggested to decrease the number of embolic events, its benefits have not been proven. A study is proposed in which patients with AF are randomly divided into two groups: one receives the anticoagulant

Warfarin, the other a placebo. The groups are then followed for the incidence of embolic stroke.

*10.80* Suppose we anticipate that 5% of treated patients and 22% of control patients will experience an embolic stroke over 3 years. If 100 patients are to be randomized to each group, then how much power would such a study have of detecting a significant difference if a two-sided test is used with $\alpha = 0.05$?

*10.81* How large should such a study be to have an 80% chance of finding a significant difference given the same assumptions as in Problem 10.80?

*10.82* Answer Problem 10.81 for a power of 90% rather than 80%.

### Diabetes

Improvement in control of blood glucose levels is an important motivation for the use of insulin pumps for diabetic patients. However, certain side effects have been reported with pump therapy. Table 10.31 provides data on the occurrence of diabetic ketoacidosis (DKA) in patients before and after the onset of pump therapy [14].

*Table 10.31* Occurrence of DKA in patients before and after the onset of insulin pump therapy

| After pump therapy | Before pump therapy | |
|---|---|---|
| | No DKA | DKA |
| No DKA | 128 | 7 |
| DKA | 19 | 7 |

(Reprinted with permission of *JAMA* **252(23)**: 3265–3269, 1984.)

*10.83* What is the appropriate procedure to test if the

rate of DKA is different before and after the onset of pump therapy?

*10.84* Perform the significance test in Problem 10.83 and report a *p*-value.

### Pulmonary Disease

Each year approximately 4% of current smokers attempt to quit smoking, and about 50% of those who try to quit are successful; that is, they are able to abstain from smoking for at least 1 year from the date they quit. Investigators have attempted to identify risk factors that might influence these two probabilities. One such variable is the number of cigarettes currently smoked per day. In particular, the investigators found that among 75 current smokers who smoked $\leq 1$ pack/day, 5 attempted to quit, whereas among 50 current smokers who smoked more than 1 pack/day, 1 attempted to quit.

*10.85* Assess the statistical significance of these results and report a *p*-value.

Similarly, a different study reported that out of 311 persons who had attempted to quit smoking, 16 out of 33 with less than a high school education were successful quitters; 47 out of 76 who had finished high school but had not gone to college were successful quitters; 69 out of 125 who attended college but did not finish 4 years of college were successful quitters; and 52 out of 77 who had completed college were successful quitters.

*10.86* Do these data show an association between the number of years of education and the rate of successful quitting?

### Renal Disease

A study group of 586 working women 30–49 years old who took phenacetin-containing analgesics and a control group of 559 comparably aged women without such intake were identified in 1968 and followed-up for mortality and morbidity outcomes. One hypothesis to be tested was that phenacetin intake may influence renal (kidney) function and hence have an effect on specific indices of renal morbidity and mortality. The mortality data of these women were traced from 1968 to 1979. Ten of the women in the study group and two of the women in the control group died, where at least one of the causes of death was deemed to be renal [15].

*10.87* If we wish to test for differences in renal mortality between the two groups in either direction, what statistical test should we use?

*10.88* Implement the test in Problem 10.87 and report a *p*-value.

*10.89* Provide a 95% confidence interval for the dif-

ference in renal mortality rates between the two groups.

From the study group a subgroup of 309 women with a very high intake of phenacetin at baseline was identified, and 8 of them died during 1968–1979.

*10.90* What statistical test should be used to compare the renal mortality experience of the high-intake group with that of the control group?

*10.91* Implement the test in Problem 10.90 and report a *p*-value.

### Infectious Disease, Hepatic Disease

Read the article, "Foodborne Hepatitis A Infection: A Report of Two Urban Restaurant-Associated Outbreaks" by Denes, *et al.*, in *The American Journal of Epidemiology*, volume **105**, no. **2** (1977), pages 156–162, and answer the following questions based on it.

*10.92* The authors analyzed the results of Table 1 using a chi-square statistic. Is this method of analysis reasonable for this table? If not, suggest an alternative method.

*10.93* Analyze the results in Table 1 using the method suggested in Problem 10.92. Do your results agree with the authors'?

*10.94* Student's *t* test with 40 d.f. was used to analyze the results in Table 2. Is this method of analysis reasonable for this table? If not, suggest an alternative method.

*10.95* The authors claim that there is a significant difference ($p = 0.01$) between the rate of consumption of salad among those who did and did not feel well. Check this result using the method of analysis suggested in Problem 10.94.

### Cancer

Read "Smoking and Carcinoma of the Lung" by R. Doll and A. B. Hill, published in the *British Medical Journal*, Sept. 30, 1950, pp. 739–748. Refer to Table IV in this paper and answer the following questions based on it.

*10.96* Test for the association between cigarette smoking and disease status among males only.

*10.97* Compute the odds ratio in favor of cigarette smoking for male lung cancer cases vs. controls.

*10.98* Compute a 95% confidence interval for the odds ratio computed in Problem 10.97.

*10.99* Test for the association between cigarette smoking and disease status among females.

*10.100* Answer Problem 10.97 for females.

*10.101* Answer Problem 10.98 for females.

The persons in the study were also classified in Table V according to the number of cigarettes per day smoked regularly just prior to the onset of their present illness.

**10.102** Is there a consistent trend between the number of cigarettes smoked and disease status among males? Perform the appropriate significance test.

**10.103** Answer Problem 10.102 for females.

### Cancer

Suppose we perform a clinical trial to assess the effect of a new treatment for cancer of the esophagus. We do not attempt to match the patients in any way because the number of cases is too small. We find that of 100 patients who were given the standard treatment, 6 lived for a 3-year period and 5 lived for a 5-year period. Correspondingly, of 47 patients who were given the new treatment, 10 survived for a 3-year period, whereas 2 survived for a 5-year period.

**10.104** Is there any evidence that the new treatment is helpful for the 3-year prognosis of the patient?

**10.105** Is there any evidence that the new treatment is helpful for the 5-year prognosis?

**10.106** Suppose a person has survived for 3 years. Is there any evidence for a treatment effect on the prognosis for the next 2 years?

### Infectious Disease

The presence of bacteria in the urine (bacteriuria) has been associated with kidney disease. Conflicting results have been reported from several studies concerning the possible role of oral contraceptives (OC's) in bacteriuria. The following data were collected in a population-based group of nonpregnant premenopausal women below the age of 50 [16]. The data are presented on an age-specific basis in Table 10.32.

_Table 10.32_ Rates of bacteriuria in oral contraceptive users and nonusers

| | % with bacteriuria | | | |
|---|---|---|---|---|
| | OC users | | Non-OC users | |
| Age group | % | n | % | n |
| _16–19_ | 1.2 | 84 | 3.2 | 281 |
| _20–29_ | 5.6 | 284 | 4.0 | 552 |
| _30–39_ | 6.3 | 96 | 5.5 | 623 |
| _40–49_ | 22.2 | 18 | 2.7 | 482 |

(Reprinted with permission of the _New England Journal of Medicine_ **299**: 536–537, 1978.)

**10.107** Why is controlling for age important in looking at the relationship between bacteriuria and OC use?

**10.108** Perform a significance test to examine the association between OC use and bacteriuria after controlling for age.

**10.109** Estimate the odds ratio in favor of bacteriuria for OC users vs. non-OC users after controlling for age.

**10.110** Provide a 95% confidence interval for the odds ratio in Problem 10.109.

**10.111** How do your answers to Problems 10.108 and 10.110 relate to each other?

**10.112** Suppose we did not control for age in the preceding analyses. Calculate the crude (unadjusted for age) odds ratio in favor of bacteriuria for OC users vs. non-OC users.

**10.113** How do your answers to Problems 10.112 and 10.109 relate to each other? Try to explain any differences found.

### Diabetes, Ophthalmology

Diabetic retinopathy is an ocular condition that can result in significant visual loss and hence is of major concern to diabetic patients. A recent hypothesis is that use of aldose reductase inhibitors may lead to a major breakthrough in the prevention of diabetic retinopathy. To test this hypothesis, a treatment trial is planned for juvenile-onset, insulin-dependent diabetics, comparing the aldose reductase inhibitor Sorbinil with placebo. Suppose that, based on previous population estimates, 26% of patients on placebo are expected to show signs of diabetic retinopathy over a 30-month period.

**10.114** If the true rate of disease in the Sorbinil group is 50% of that in the placebo group, then how much power would a study based on 100 randomized patients in each group have if we use a two-sided test with $\alpha = 0.05$?

**10.115** Answer Problem 10.114 if the true rate of disease in the Sorbinil group is assumed to be 30%, rather than 50%, less than that of placebo.

**10.116** How large a sample is needed in each group to achieve 80% power under the assumptions stated in Problem 10.114?

**10.117** How large a sample is needed in each group to achieve 80% power under the assumptions stated in Problem 10.115?

### Infectious Disease, Cardiology

Kawasaki's syndrome is an acute illness of unknown cause that occurs predominantly in children under the age of 5. It is characterized by persistent high fever and other clinical signs and can result in death and/or coronary artery aneurysms. The standard therapy for this condition is currently aspirin to prevent blood clotting. Recently, a Japanese group began experimentally treating children with intravenous gamma globulin in addition to aspirin to prevent cardiac symptoms in these patients [17].

A clinical trial is planned in the United States to compare the combined therapy of gamma globulin and aspirin vs. aspirin therapy alone. Suppose the rate of coronary artery aneurysms is 15% in the aspirin-treated group, based on previous experience, and the investigators intend to use a two-sided significance test with $\alpha = 0.05$.

**10.118** If the rate of coronary aneurysms in the combined therapy group is 5%, then how much statistical power will such a study have if 125 patients are to be recruited in each treatment group?

**10.119** Answer Problem 10.118 if 150 patients are recruited in each group.

**10.120** How many patients would have to be recruited in each group to have a 95% chance of finding a significant difference?

### Cancer

One interesting hypothesis is that oral contraceptives (OC's) may influence the risk of breast cancer. To test this hypothesis, the following data were collected in the Nurses Health Study, an ongoing longitudinal study of nurses, ages 30–55, who were first ascertained in 1976 and were followed every 2 years thereafter [18]. The data show the relationship between OC use status in 1976 and the incidence of breast cancer from 1976 to 1980. Since both breast cancer incidence and OC use are related to age, the data are presented by age group in Table 10.33.

**10.121** Calculate the crude odds ratio in favor of breast cancer for ever OC users vs. never OC users by pooling data from all age groups together, and perform a significance test to assess the results.

**10.122** Perform a significance test for the association between ever OC use and breast cancer after controlling for age.

**10.123** Calculate the odds ratio in favor of breast cancer for ever OC users vs. never OC users after controlling for age.

**10.124** Provide 95% confidence limits for the age-adjusted odds ratio in Problem 10.123.

**10.125** Compare your answers to Problems 10.121 and 10.123. Why should the results be different?

**Table 10.33** *Age-specific incidence of breast cancer between 1976 and 1980 compared with oral contraceptive status in 1976*

| Age group | OC use, 1976 | Number of breast cancer cases | Number of women |
|---|---|---|---|
| 30–34 | Ever | 21 | 15,428 |
|  | Never | 12 | 4586 |
| 35–39 | Ever | 50 | 13,061 |
|  | Never | 23 | 7716 |
| 40–44 | Ever | 53 | 10,326 |
|  | Never | 64 | 11,866 |
| 45–49 | Ever | 56 | 6509 |
|  | Never | 107 | 14,651 |
| 50–55 | Ever | 34 | 3959 |
|  | Never | 150 | 18,228 |

### Emergency Medicine

Mannitol and Decadron are drugs that are often administered to patients with severe head injury when they are admitted to the emergency room of a hospital. One hypothesis is that this type of treatment would be more beneficial if administered by paramedics to patients in the field before they are transported to the hospital. To plan such a study, a pilot study is performed, whereby 4 of 10 patients with field treatment and 6 of 10 patients with no field treatment die before discharge from the hospital.

**10.126** If a clinical trial is planned based on a two-tailed test with $\alpha = 0.05$, assuming that the pilot study results are valid, how much power would such a study have if 20 patients are randomized to each of the two groups?

**10.127** How many patients are needed in each group to achieve an 80% power with the preceding study design if the differences found in the pilot study are assumed to be valid?

**10.128** If the true mortality rate in the field-treated group were actually 0.50 rather than 0.40, how would these new data affect the power estimate in Problem 10.126 and the sample size estimate in Problem 10.127? (Only provide a qualitative answer.)

### Pulmonary Disease

Read the paper "Influence of Passive Smoking and Parental Phlegm on Pneumonia and Bronchitis in Early Childhood" by J. R. T. Colley, W. W. Holland, and R. T. Corkhill, published in *The Lancet* (Nov. 2, 1974) pages

1031–1034, and answer the following questions based on it.

**10.129** Perform a statistical test comparing the incidence rates of pneumonia and bronchitis for children in their first year of life in families in which both parents are nonsmokers vs. families in which both parents are smokers.

**10.130** Compute an odds ratio to compare the incidence rates of pneumonia and bronchitis in families in which both parents are smokers with families in which both parents are nonsmokers.

**10.131** Compute a 95% confidence interval corresponding to the odds ratio computed in Problem 10.130.

**10.132** Compare the incidence rates of pneumonia and bronchitis for children in their first year of life in families in which both parents are nonsmokers vs. families in which one parent is a smoker.

**10.133** Answer Problem 10.130, comparing families in which one parent is a smoker with families in which both parents are nonsmokers.

**10.134** Compute a 95% confidence interval corresponding to the odds ratio computed in Problem 10.133.

**10.135** Is there a significant trend in the percentage of children with pneumonia and bronchitis in the first year of life according to the number of smoking parents? Report a *p*-value.

**10.136** Compare the incidence rates of pneumonia and bronchitis for children in their third year of life in families in which both parents are nonsmokers as compared with the rates for families in which both parents are smokers.

**10.137** Suppose we wish to compare the incidence rates of disease for children in their first and second years of life in families in which both parents are nonsmokers. Rates of 7.8% and 8.1% based on samples of size 372 and 358, respectively, are presented in Table II. Would it be reasonable to use a chi-square test to compare these rates?

**10.138** Perform a statistical test comparing the incidence rates of pneumonia and bronchitis for children in the first year of life when stratified by number of cigarettes per day. (Use the groupings in Table IV in the appendix.) Restrict your analysis to families in which one or both parents are current smokers and have normal respiratory function.

**10.139** Is there a consistent trend in the incidence rates referred to in Problem 10.138 as the number of cigarettes smoked increases?

**10.140** Does the number of siblings in the family affect the incidence rate of pneumonia and bronchitis for children in the first year of life in families in which one or both parents have respiratory disease and both parents are nonsmokers? (Specifically, in Table VI compare children with 0 siblings to children with 1 or more siblings.)

# References

[1] MacMahon, B., Cole, P., Lin, T. M., Lowe, C. R., Mirra, A. P., Ravnihar, B., Salber, E. J., Valaoras, V. G., and Yuasa, S. (1970) "Age at First Birth and Breast Cancer Risk," *Bulletin of the World Health Organization* **43**: 209–221.

[2] Kleinbaum, D. G., Kupper, L. L., and Morgenstern, H. (1982) *Epidemiologic Research: Principles and Quantitative Methods* (Belmont, California: Wadsworth, Inc.).

[3] Doll, R., Muir, C., and Waterhouse, J., eds. (1970) *Cancer in Five Continents*, Vol. II (Berlin: Springer-Verlag).

[4] Cochran, W. G. (1954) "Some Methods for Strengthening the Common $\chi^2$ Test," *Biometrics* **10**: 417–451.

[5] Maxwell, A. W. (1961) *Analyzing Qualitative Data* (London: Methuen, Inc.).

[6] Sandler, D. P., Everson, R. B., and Wilcox, A. J. (1985) "Passive Smoking in Adulthood and Cancer Risk," *American Journal of Epidemiology* **121(1)**: 37–48.

[7] Fleiss, J. (1981) *Statistical Methods for Rates and Proportions* (New York: John Wiley).

[8] Hypertension Detection and Follow-up Program Cooperative Group. (1977) "Blood

Pressure Studies in 14 Communities—A Two-Stage Screen for Hypertension," *Journal of the American Medical Association* **237(22)**: 2385–2391.

[9] Kennedy, J. W., Ritchie, J. L., Davis, K. B., Stadius, M. L., Maynard, C., and Fritz, J. K. (1985) "The Western Washington Randomized Trial of Intracoronary Streptokinase in Acute Myocardial Infarction: A 12-Month Follow-up Report," *New England Journal of Medicine* **312(17)**: 1073–1078.

[10] Cramer, D. W., Schiff, I., Schoenbaum, S. C., Gibson, M., Belisle, J., Albrecht, B., Stillman, R. J., Berger, M. J., Wilson, E., Stadel, B. V., and Seibel, M. (1985) "Tubal Infertility and the Intrauterine Device," *New England Journal of Medicine* **312(15)**: 941–947.

[11] The Coronary Drug Project Research Group. (1979) "Cigarette Smoking as a Risk Factor in Men with a History of Myocardial Infarction," *Journal of Chronic Diseases* **32(6)**: 415–425.

[12] Weiss, N. S. and Sayetz, T. A. (1980) "Incidence of Endometrial Cancer in Relation to the Use of Oral Contraceptives," *New England Journal of Medicine* **302(10)**: 551–554.

[13] *End Results in Cancer. Report No. 4* (1972) U.S. Department of Health, Education, and Welfare, Bethesda, Maryland: 84.

[14] Mecklenburg, R. S., Benson, E. A., Benson, J. W., Fredlung, P. N., Guinn, T., Metz, R. J., Nielsen, R. L., and Sannar, C. A. (1984) "Acute Complications Associated with Insulin Pump Therapy: Report of Experience with 161 Patients," *JAMA* **252(23)**: 3265–3269.

[15] Dubach, U. C., Rosner, B., and Pfister, E. (1983) "Epidemiological Study of Abuse of Analgesics Containing Phenacetin: 1968–1979. Renal Morbidity and Mortality," *New England Journal of Medicine* **308**: 357–362.

[16] Evans, D. A., Hennekens, C. H., Miao, L., Laughlin, L. W., Chapman, W. G., Rosner, B., Taylor, J. O., and Kass, E. H. (1978) "Oral Contraceptives and Bacteriuria in a Community-Based Study," *New England Journal of Medicine* **299**: 536–537.

[17] Furusko, K., Sato, K., Socda, T., et al. (1983) "High Dose Intravenous Gamma Globulin for Kawasaki's Syndrome," *Lancet, letter*, December 10: 1359.

[18] Barton, J., Bain, C., Hennekens, C. H., Rosner, B., Belanger, C., Roth, A., and Speizer, F. E. (1980) "Characteristics of Respondents and Non-respondents to a Mail Questionnaire," *American Journal of Public Health* **70**: 823–825.

# 11 Regression and Correlation Methods

## ■ 11.1 INTRODUCTION

In the previous chapters we were concerned with methods of estimation and hypothesis testing whereby we were interested in only one variable. Frequently, we wish to look at the relationship between two or more variables in a particular sample.

*Example 11.1*    **Obstetrics**  Obstetricians sometimes order tests for estriol levels from 24-hour urine specimens taken from pregnant women who are near term, since the level of estriol has been found to be related to the birthweight of the infant. The test can provide indirect evidence of an abnormally small fetus. We can quantify the relationship between estriol level and birthweight by fitting a *regression line* that relates the two variables.    ■

*Example 11.2*    **Hypertension**  Much discussion has taken place in recent years on the *familial aggregation of blood pressure*. In general, children whose parents have high blood pressure tend to have higher blood pressure than their peers. One way of expressing this relationship is to compute a *correlation coefficient* relating the blood pressure of parents and children over a large collection of families.    ■

In this chapter we will study methods of regression and correlation analysis in which we relate *two* different variables in the same sample. We will also briefly discuss the extension of these methods to the case of multiple regression analysis whereby we look at the relationship between more than two variables at a time.

## ■ 11.2 GENERAL CONCEPTS

*Example 11.3*    **Obstetrics**  Greene and Touchstone conducted a study to relate birthweight to the estriol level of pregnant women [1]. Figure 11.1 is a plot of the data from the study, and the actual data points are listed in Table 11.1. As we can see from the figure, there appears to be a linear rela-

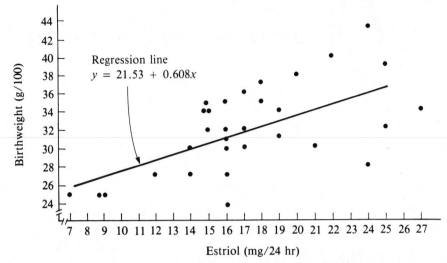

**Figure 11.1**
*Data from
Greene–Touchstone
study relating
birthweight and
estriol level in
pregnant women
near term.*

(Reprinted with permission of the *American Journal of Obstetrics and Gynecology* **85(1)**: 1–9, 1963.)

**Table 11.1**
*Sample data from
the Greene–
Touchstone study
relating birthweight
and estriol level in
pregnant women
near term*

| $i$ | Estriol (mg/24 hr) $x_i$ | Birthweight (g/100) $y_i$ | $i$ | Estriol (mg/24 hr) $x_i$ | Birthweight (g/100) $y_i$ |
|---|---|---|---|---|---|
| 1  | 7  | 25 | 17 | 17 | 32 |
| 2  | 9  | 25 | 18 | 25 | 32 |
| 3  | 9  | 25 | 19 | 27 | 34 |
| 4  | 12 | 27 | 20 | 15 | 34 |
| 5  | 14 | 27 | 21 | 15 | 34 |
| 6  | 16 | 27 | 22 | 15 | 35 |
| 7  | 16 | 24 | 23 | 16 | 35 |
| 8  | 14 | 30 | 24 | 19 | 34 |
| 9  | 16 | 30 | 25 | 18 | 35 |
| 10 | 16 | 31 | 26 | 17 | 36 |
| 11 | 17 | 30 | 27 | 18 | 37 |
| 12 | 19 | 31 | 28 | 20 | 38 |
| 13 | 21 | 30 | 29 | 22 | 40 |
| 14 | 24 | 28 | 30 | 25 | 39 |
| 15 | 15 | 32 | 31 | 24 | 43 |
| 16 | 16 | 32 | | | |

(Reprinted with permission of the *American Journal of Obstetrics and Gynecology* **85(1)**: 1–9, 1963.)

tionship between estriol level and birthweight, although this relationship is not consistent and considerable scatter exists throughout the plot. How can we quantify this relationship?  ∎

If we let $x$ = estriol level and $y$ = birthweight, then we may postulate a relationship between $y$ and $x$ that is of the following form:

**11.1**
$$E(y|x) = \alpha + \beta x$$

That is, for a given estriol level $x$, the expected birthweight $E(y|x)$ is $\alpha + \beta x$.

**Definition 11.1**

The line $y = \alpha + \beta x$ is defined as the **regression line**, where $\alpha$ is the intercept and $\beta$ is the slope of the line. ■

We do not expect that the relationship $y = \alpha + \beta x$ will hold exactly for every woman. Thus, we introduce an error term $e$ into our model, which respresents the variance of birthweight among all babies of women with a given estriol level $x$. We will assume that $e$ follows a normal distribution with mean 0 and variance $\sigma^2$. The full linear regression model then takes the following form:

**11.2**
$$y = \alpha + \beta x + e$$

where $e$ is normally distributed with mean 0 and variance $\sigma^2$.

**Definition 11.2**

For any linear regression equation of the form $y = \alpha + \beta x + e$, we will refer to $y$ as the **dependent variable** and $x$ as the **independent variable**, since we are trying to predict $y$ from $x$. ■

*Example 11.4*   ***Obstetrics*** Birthweight is the dependent variable and estriol is the independent variable for the problem posed in Example 11.3, since we are trying to use estriol levels to predict birthweight. ■

One interpretation of the regression line is that for a woman with estriol level $x$, the corresponding birthweight will be normally distributed with mean $\alpha + \beta x$ and variance $\sigma^2$. If $\sigma^2$ were 0, then every point would fall exactly on the regression line, whereas the larger $\sigma^2$ is, the more scatter occurs about the regression line. This effect is illustrated in Figure 11.2. How can we interpret $\beta$? If $\beta$ is greater than 0, then as $x$ increases, the expected value of $y = \alpha + \beta x$ will increase.

*Example 11.5*   ***Obstetrics*** This situation appears to be the case in Figure 11.3(a) for birthweight ($y$) and estriol ($x$), since as estriol increases, birthweight correspondingly increases. ■

If $\beta$ is less than 0, then as $x$ increases, the expected value of $y$ will decrease.

*Example 11.6*   ***Pediatrics*** This situation might occur in a plot of pulse rate ($y$) vs. age ($x$), as illustrated in Figure 11.3(b), since infants are born with rapid pulse rates that gradually decline with age. ■

If $\beta$ is equal to 0, then there is no relationship between $x$ and $y$.

*Example 11.7*   This situation might occur if we related birthweight to birthday, as shown in Figure 11.3(c), since there is no relationship between birthweight and birthday. ■

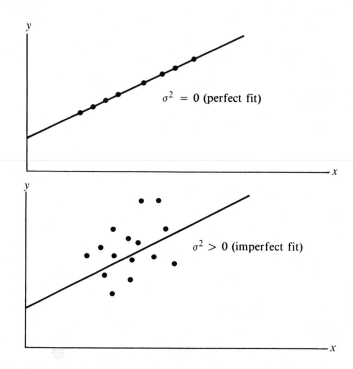

**Figure 11.2**
The effect of $\sigma^2$ on
the goodness-of-fit
of a regression line

# ■ 11.3 FITTING REGRESSION LINES—THE PRINCIPLE OF LEAST SQUARES

The question remains as to how to fit a regression line (or, equivalently, to obtain estimates of $\alpha$ and $\beta$, which we denote by $a$ and $b$, respectively) when given data that appear in the form of Figure 11.1. We could eyeball the data and draw a line that is not too distant from any of the points, but this approach is difficult in practice and can be quite imprecise with either a large number of points or a lot of scatter. A better method is to set up a specific criterion that defines the closeness of a line to a set of points and to find the line closest to the sample data according to this criterion.

Consider the data in Figure 11.4 and the proposed regression line $y = a + bx$. We could measure the distance $d_i$ of a typical sample point $(x_i, y_i)$ from the line along a direction parallel to the $y$-axis. If we let $(x_i, \hat{y}_i) = (x_i, a + bx_i)$ be the point on the regression line at $x_i$, then this distance is given by $d_i = y_i - \hat{y}_i = y_i - a - bx_i$. A good fitting line would make these distances as small as possible. Since the $d_i$ cannot all be 0, we can use the criterion $S_1 = $ sum of the absolute deviations of the sample points from the line $= \sum_{i=1}^{n} |d_i|$ and find the line that minimizes $S_1$. This strategy has proven to be analytically difficult. Instead, for both theoretical reasons and ease of derivation, the following **least squares criterion** is commonly used:

$S = $ sum of the squared distances of the points from the line

$$= \sum_{i=1}^{n} d_i^2 = \sum_{i=1}^{n} (y_i - a - bx_i)^2$$

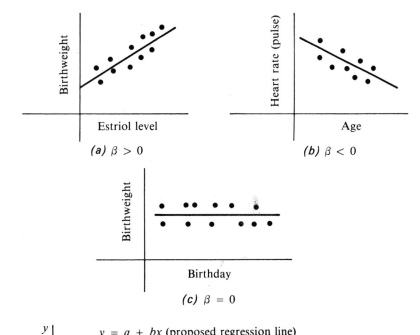

**Figure 11.3**
*The interpretation of the regression line for different values of β*

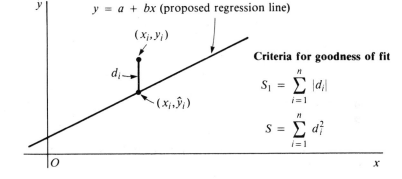

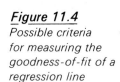

**Figure 11.4**
*Possible criteria for measuring the goodness-of-fit of a regression line*

Criteria for goodness of fit

$$S_1 = \sum_{i=1}^{n} |d_i|$$

$$S = \sum_{i=1}^{n} d_i^2$$

---

**Definition 11.3**

The **least squares line**, or **regression line**, is defined as the line $y = a + bx$ that minimizes the sum of squared distances of the sample points from the line given by

$$S = \sum_{i=1}^{n} d_i^2$$

This method of deriving the regression line is known as the **principle of least squares**. ∎

We now introduce the following notation, which we will need to define the slope and intercept of a regression line.

---

**Definition 11.4**

We define the **raw sum of squares for $x$** by

$$\sum_{i=1}^{n} x_i^2$$

We also define the **corrected sum of squares for x** by

$$\sum_{i=1}^{n} x_i^2 - \left(\sum_{i=1}^{n} x_i\right)^2 \Big/ n$$

which we denote by $L_{xx}$. Similarly, we define the **raw sum of squares for y** by

$$\sum_{i=1}^{n} y_i^2$$

We also define the **corrected sum of squares for y** by

$$\sum_{i=1}^{n} y_i^2 - \left(\sum_{i=1}^{n} y_i\right)^2 \Big/ n$$

which is denoted by $L_{yy}$.  ∎

Notice that $L_{xx}$ and $L_{yy}$ are simply the numerators of the expressions for the sample variances of $x$(i.e., $s_x^2$) and $y$(i.e., $s_y^2$), respectively, since

$$s_x^2 = \sum_{i=1}^{n} (x_i - \bar{x})^2/(n-1) \quad \text{and} \quad s_y^2 = \sum_{i=1}^{n} (y_i - \bar{y})^2/(n-1)$$

### Definition 11.5

We define the **raw sum of cross products** by

$$\sum_{i=1}^{n} x_i y_i$$

We also define the **corrected sum of cross products** by

$$\sum_{i=1}^{n} x_i y_i - \left(\sum_{i=1}^{n} x_i\right)\left(\sum_{i=1}^{n} y_i\right) \Big/ n$$

which we denote by $L_{xy}$.  ∎

We can show that the coefficients of the line that satisfy the least-squares criterion in Definition 11.3 are given as follows:

### 11.3  Estimation of the Least-Squares Line

The coefficients of the *least-squares line* $y = a + bx$ are given by

$$b = L_{xy}/L_{xx} \quad \text{and} \quad a = \bar{y} - b\bar{x} = \left(\sum_{i=1}^{n} y_i - b\sum_{i=1}^{n} x_i\right) \Big/ n$$

*Example 11.8*    **Obstetrics**  Derive the regression line for the data given in Table 11.1.

*Solution*    We first must obtain

$$\sum_{i=1}^{31} x_i \quad \sum_{i=1}^{31} x_i^2 \quad \sum_{i=1}^{31} y_i \quad \sum_{i=1}^{31} x_i y_i$$

so as to compute the corrected sums of squares ($L_{xx}$) and cross products ($L_{xy}$). These quantities are given as follows:

$$\sum_{i=1}^{31} x_i = 534 \qquad \sum_{i=1}^{31} x_i^2 = 9876 \qquad \sum_{i=1}^{31} y_i = 992 \qquad \sum_{i=1}^{31} x_i y_i = 17{,}500$$

We then compute $L_{xy}$ and $L_{xx}$ as follows:

$$L_{xy} = \sum_{i=1}^{31} x_i y_i - \left(\sum_{i=1}^{31} x_i\right)\left(\sum_{i=1}^{31} y_i\right)\Big/ 31 = 17{,}500 - (534)(992)/31 = 412$$

$$L_{xx} = \sum_{i=1}^{31} x_i^2 - \left(\sum_{i=1}^{31} x_i\right)^2\Big/ 31 = 9876 - (534)^2/31 = 677.42$$

Finally, we compute the slope of the regression line as follows:

$$b = L_{xy}/L_{xx} = 412/677.42 = 0.608$$

We also can compute the intercept of the regression line. For this purpose we need $\sum_{i=1}^{31} y_i = 992$. We then note from **(11.3)** that

$$a = \left(\sum_{i=1}^{31} y_i - 0.608 \sum_{i=1}^{31} x_i\right)\Big/ 31 = [992 - 0.608(534)]/31 = 21.53$$

Thus the regression line is given by $y = 21.53 + 0.608x$. This regression line is depicted in Figure 11.1. ∎

How can we use the regression line? One of its uses is to *predict* values of $y$ for given values of $x$.

| Definition 11.6 |
| --- |

We will denote the **predicted, or expected, value of y** for a given value of $x$, as obtained from the regression line, by $\hat{y} = a + bx$. Thus the point $(x, a + bx)$ is always on the regression line. ∎

*Example 11.9*    **Obstetrics** What is the expected birthweight if a pregnant woman has an estriol level of 15 mg/24 hr?

*Solution*    If the estriol level were 15 mg/24 hr, then the best prediction of birthweight would be

$$\hat{y} = 21.53 + 0.608(15) = 30.65 \times 100\,\text{g} = 3065\,\text{g} \qquad ∎$$

One possible use of estriol levels is to identify women who are carrying a low-birthweight fetus. If we can identify such women, then we might want to use drugs to prolong the pregnancy until the fetus grows larger, since low-birthweight infants are at greater risk than normal infants for (a) infant mortality in the first year of life and (b) poor growth and development in childhood.

*Example 11.10*    **Obstetrics** Let us define low birthweight as $\leqslant 2500$ g. For what estriol level would the expected birthweight be 2500 g?

*Solution*    We note that the expected birthweight

$$\hat{y} = 21.53 + 0.608x$$

If $\hat{y} = 2500/100 = 25$, then we can solve for $x$ from the equation

$$25 = 21.53 + 0.608x \quad \text{or} \quad x = (25 - 21.53)/0.608 = 3.47/0.608 = 5.71$$

Thus if a woman has an estriol level of 5.71 mg/24 hr, then the expected birthweight would be 2500 g. Furthermore, all women with estriol levels of $\leq 5.71$ mg/24 hr would be expected to have low-birthweight infants. This level could serve as a critical value for identifying high-risk women and attempting to prolong their pregnancies.   ∎

How can we interpret the slope of the regression line? The slope of the regression line tells us the amount that $y$ increases per unit increase in $x$.

**Example 11.11**   **Obstetrics**  Interpret the slope of the regression line for the birthweight-estriol data in Example 11.1.

**Solution**   The slope of 0.608 tells us that the expected birthweight increases by about $0.6 \times 100$ g per 1 mg/24 hr, or 60 g per 1 mg/24 hr, increase in estriol.   ∎

# ■ *11.4  TESTING THE GOODNESS-OF-FIT OF REGRESSION LINES (F TEST)*

In Section 11.3 we discussed the fitting of regression lines using the method of least squares. Since we can utilize this method with any set of points, we want to establish criteria for goodness-of-fit to distinguish regression lines that fit the data well from those that do not. Consider the typical situation depicted in Figure 11.5. We have drawn a hypothetical regression line and a representative sample point. First, we notice that the point $(\bar{x}, \bar{y})$ falls on the regression line. This feature is common to all regression lines, since we can represent a regression line as

$$y = a + bx = \bar{y} - b\bar{x} + bx = \bar{y} + b(x - \bar{x})$$

or, equivalently,

**11.4**

$$y - \bar{y} = b(x - \bar{x})$$

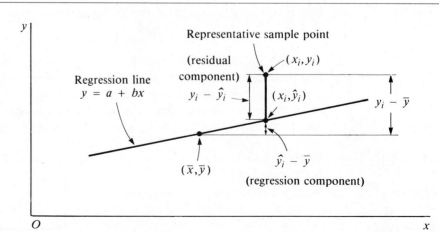

**Figure 11.5**
*Goodness-of-fit of a regression line*

If we substitute $\bar{x}$ for $x$ and $\bar{y}$ for $y$ in **(11.4)**, then we obtain 0 on both sides of the equation, which shows that *the point $(\bar{x}, \bar{y})$ must always fall on the regression line.* If we select a typical sample point $(x_i, y_i)$ and draw a line through this point parallel to the $y$-axis, then we obtain the representation in Figure 11.5.

**Definition 11.7**

For any sample point $(x_i, y_i)$, we define the **residual**, or **residual component**, of that point about the regression line by $y_i - \hat{y}_i$. ■

**Definition 11.8**

For any sample point $(x_i, y_i)$ we define the **regression component** of that point about the regression line by $\hat{y}_i - \bar{y}_i$. ■

We see in Figure 11.5 that the deviation $y_i - \bar{y}$ can be separated into residual $(y_i - \hat{y}_i)$ and regression $(\hat{y}_i - \bar{y})$ components. Note that if the point $(x_i, y_i)$ fell exactly on the regression line, then $y_i = \hat{y}_i$ and the residual component $y_i - \hat{y}_i$ would be 0 and $y_i - \bar{y} = \hat{y}_i - \bar{y}$. Generally speaking, a good fitting regression line will have regression components large in absolute value relative to the residual components, whereas the opposite is true for poor fitting regression lines. Some typical situations are depicted in Figure 11.6.

The best fitting regression line is depicted in (a), with large regression components and small residual components. The worst fitting regression line is depicted in (d), which has small regression components and large residual components. Intermediate situations for goodness-of-fit are depicted in (b) and (c).

How can we quantify what we see in Figure 11.6? One strategy is to square the deviations about the mean $y_i - \bar{y}$, sum them up over all points, and decompose this sum of squares into *regression* and *residual* components.

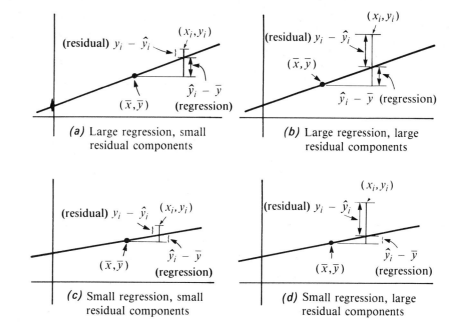

**Figure 11.6**
*Regression lines with varying goodness-of-fit relationships*

(a) Large regression, small residual components

(b) Large regression, large residual components

(c) Small regression, small residual components

(d) Small regression, large residual components

**Definition 11.9**

We define the **total sum of squares,** or Total SS, as the sum of squares of the deviations of the individual sample points from the sample mean:

$$\sum_{i=1}^{n} (y_i - \bar{y})^2$$ ∎

**Definition 11.10**

We define the **regression sum of squares,** or Reg SS, as the sum of squares of the regression components:

$$\sum_{i=1}^{n} (\hat{y}_i - \bar{y})^2$$ ∎

**Definition 11.11**

We define the **residual sum of squares,** or Res SS, as the sum of squares of the residual components:

$$\sum_{i=1}^{n} (y_i - \hat{y}_i)^2$$ ∎

It can be shown that the following relationship is true.

**11.5** _Decomposition of the Total Sum of Squares into Regression and Residual Components_

$$\sum_{i=1}^{n} (y_i - \bar{y})^2 = \sum_{i=1}^{n} (\hat{y}_i - \bar{y})^2 + \sum_{i=1}^{n} (y_i - \hat{y}_i)^2$$

or

$$\text{Total SS} = \text{Reg SS} + \text{Res SS}$$

The criterion for goodness-of-fit that we will use is the ratio of the regression sum of squares to the residual sum of squares. A large ratio indicates a good fit, whereas a small ratio indicates a poor fit. In hypothesis-testing terms we wish to test the hypothesis $H_0 : \beta = 0$ vs. $H_1 : \beta \neq 0$, where $\beta$ is the underlying slope of the regression line in **(11.2)**.

We will introduce the following terms for ease of notation in describing our hypothesis test:

**Definition 11.12**

We define the **regression mean square,** or Reg MS, as the Reg SS divided by the number of predictor variables ($k$) in our model. Thus Reg MS = Reg SS/$k$. For simple linear regression, which we have been discussing, $k = 1$ and thus Reg MS = Reg SS. For multiple regression in Section 11.8, $k$ will be $>1$. We will refer to $k$ as the degrees of freedom for the regression sum of squares, or Reg $df$. ∎

**Definition 11.13**

We define the **residual mean square**, or Res MS, as the ratio of the Res SS divided by $(n - k - 1)$, or Res MS = Res SS/$(n - k - 1)$. For simple linear regression, $k = 1$ and Res MS = Res SS/$(n - 2)$. We will refer to $n - k - 1$ as the degrees of freedom for the residual sum of squares, or Res *df*. Res MS is also sometimes denoted by $s_{y \cdot x}^2$ in the literature. ∎

We can show that under $H_0$, $\lambda$ = Reg MS/Res MS follows an $F$ distribution with 1 and $n - 2$ *df*, respectively. We wish to reject $H_0$ for large values of $\lambda$. Thus for a level $\alpha$ test, we will reject $H_0$ if $\lambda > F_{1,n-2,1-\alpha}$ and accept $H_0$ otherwise.

We can show that the expressions for the regression and residual sums of squares in **(11.5)** simplify for computational purposes as follows:

**11.6** **Short Computational Form for Regression and Residual SS**

Regression SS = $bL_{xy} = b^2 L_{xx} = L_{xy}^2/L_{xx}$

Residual SS = Total SS − Regression SS = $L_{yy} - L_{xy}^2/L_{xx}$

Thus we can summarize the test procedure as follows:

**11.7** **F Test for Simple Linear Regression**

If we wish to test $H_0: \beta = 0$ vs. $H_1: \beta \neq 0$, then:

*1.* We compute the test statistic

$$\lambda = \text{Reg MS/Res MS} = (L_{xy}^2/L_{xx})/[(L_{yy} - L_{xy}^2/L_{xx})/(n - 2)]$$

that follows an $F_{1,n-2}$ distribution under $H_0$.

*2.* For a two-sided test with significance level $\alpha$, if

$$\lambda > F_{1,n-2,1-\alpha}$$

then we reject $H_0$; if

$$\lambda \leq F_{1,n-2,1-\alpha}$$

then we accept $H_0$.

*3.* The exact *p*-value is given by $Pr(F_{1,n-2} > \lambda)$.

The acceptance and rejection regions for the regression $F$ test are illustrated in Figure 11.7. The computation of the exact *p*-value for the regression $F$ test is depicted in Figure 11.8. These results are typically summarized in an analysis of variance (ANOVA) table, as shown in Table 11.2.

**Table 11.2**

*ANOVA table for displaying regression results*

| | SS | df | MS | F Statistic | p-value |
|---|---|---|---|---|---|
| Regression | (a)* | 1 | (a)/1 | $\lambda = [(a)/1]/[(b)/(n - 2)]$ | $Pr(F_{1,n-2} > \lambda)$ |
| Residual | (b)† | $n - 2$ | (b)/(n − 2) | | |
| Total | (a) + (b) | | | | |

*(a) = Regression SS        †(b) = Residual SS

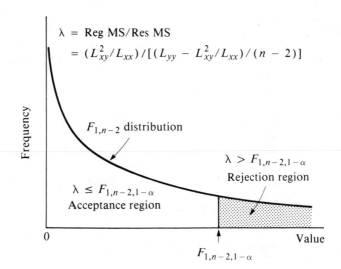

**_Figure 11.7_**
_Acceptance and
rejection regions for
the simple linear
regression F test_

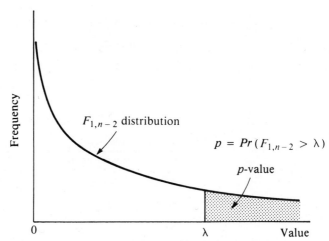

**_Figure 11.8_**
_Computation of the
p-value for the
simple linear
regression F test_

**_Example 11.12_**    **_Obstetrics_** Test for the significance of the regression line derived for the birthweight-estriol data in Example 11.8.

**_Solution_**    We have from Example 11.8 that

$$L_{xy} = 412, L_{xx} = 677.42$$

Furthermore,

$$\sum_{i=1}^{31} y_i^2 = 32{,}418 \qquad L_{yy} = \sum_{i=1}^{31} y_i^2 - \left(\sum_{i=1}^{31} y_i\right)^2 \Big/ 31 = 32{,}418 - (992)^2/31 = 674$$

Therefore,

$$\text{Reg SS} = L_{xy}^2/L_{xx} = \text{Reg MS} = (412)^2/677.42 = 250.57$$

$$\text{Total SS} = L_{yy} = 674$$

$$\text{Res SS} = \text{Total SS} - \text{Reg SS} = 674 - 250.57 = 423.43$$

$$\text{Res MS} = \text{Res SS}/(31 - 2) = \text{Res SS}/29 = 423.43/29 = 14.60$$

$$\lambda = \text{Reg MS}/\text{Res MS} = 250.57/14.60 = 17.16 \sim F_{1,29} \text{ under } H_0$$

From Table 8 in the appendix, we have

$$F_{1,29,.999} < F_{1,20,.999} = 14.82 < 17.16 = \lambda$$

Therefore,

$$p < 0.001$$

and we reject $H_0$ and accept the alternative hypothesis, namely, that the slope of the regression line is significantly different from 0, implying a *significant linear relationship* between birthweight and estriol level. These results are summarized in the ANOVA table (Table 11.3) using the SPSS/PC REGRESSION program.

**Table 11.3**

*ANOVA results for the birthweight-estriol data in Example 11.12*

| Analysis of Variance | | | |
|---|---|---|---|
| | DF | Sum of Squares | Mean Square |
| Regression | 1 | 250.57448 | 250.57448 |
| Residual | 29 | 423.42552 | 14.60088 |
| F = | 17.16160 | Signif F = 0.0003 | |

A summary measure of goodness-of-fit that is frequently referred to in the literature is $R^2$.

**Definition 11.14**

We define $R^2$ as Reg SS/Total SS.

$R^2$ can be thought of as the proportion of the variance of $y$ that can be explained by the variable $x$. If $R^2 = 1$, then all the variation in $y$ can be explained by the variation in $x$, and all the data points fall on the regression line. In other words, once we know $x$, we can predict $y$ exactly, with no error or variability in our prediction. If $R^2 = 0$, then $x$ gives us no information about $y$, and the variance of $y$ is the same with or without knowing $x$. If $R^2$ is between 0 and 1, then for a given value of $x$, the variance of $y$ is lower than it would be if $x$ were unknown but is still greater than 0. In particular, we can show that the best estimate of the variance of $y$ given $x$ [or $\sigma^2$ in the regression model in **(11.2)**] is given by Res MS (or $s_{y \cdot x}^2$). For large $n$, $s_{y \cdot x}^2 \approx s_y^2(1 - R^2)$. Thus $R^2$ represents the proportion of the variance of $y$ that is explained by $x$.

**Example 11.13**

**Solution**

**Obstetrics** Compute and interpret $R^2$ and $s_{y \cdot x}^2$ for the birthweight-estriol data.

From Table 11.3, the $R^2$ for the birthweight-estriol regression line is given by $250.57/674 = 0.372$. Thus about 37% of the variance of birthweight can be explained by estriol level. Furthermore, $s_{y \cdot x}^2 = 14.60$, as compared with

$$s_y^2 = \sum_{i=1}^{n} (y_i - \bar{y})^2/(n - 1) = 674/30 = 22.47$$

Thus, for the subgroup of women with a specific estriol level, such as 10 mg/24 hr, the variance of birthweight is 14.60, whereas for *all* women with any estriol level, the variance of birthweight is 22.47. Note that

$$s_{y \cdot x}^2/s_y^2 = 14.60/22.47 = 0.650 \approx 1 - R^2 = 1 - 0.372 = 0.628 \qquad \blacksquare$$

*Example 11.14*    **Pulmonary Function** Forced expiratory volume (FEV) is a standard measure of pulmonary function. To identify people with abnormal pulmonary function, we must be able to establish standards of FEV for normal people. One problem here is that FEV is related to both age and height. Let us focus on boys who are ages 10–15 and postulate a regression model of the form FEV = $\alpha + \beta$(height) + $e$. Data were collected on FEV and height for 655 boys in this age group residing in Tecumseh, Michigan [2]. The mean FEV in liters is presented for each of the twelve 4-cm height groups in Table 11.4. Find the best fitting regression line and test it for statistical significance. What proportion of the variance of FEV can be explained by height?

*Solution*    We fit a linear regression line to the points in Table 11.4. We have

$$\sum_{i=1}^{12} x_i = 1872 \qquad \sum_{i=1}^{12} x_i^2 = 294{,}320 \qquad \sum_{i=1}^{12} y_i = 32.3$$

$$\sum_{i=1}^{12} y_i^2 = 93.11 \qquad \sum_{i=1}^{12} x_i y_i = 5156.20$$

**Table 11.4**
*Mean FEV and height for boys ages 10–15 in Tecumseh, Michigan*

| Height (cm) | Mean FEV (liters) | Height (cm) | Mean FEV (liters) |
|---|---|---|---|
| 134* | 1.7 | 158 | 2.7 |
| 138 | 1.9 | 162 | 3.0 |
| 142 | 2.0 | 166 | 3.1 |
| 146 | 2.1 | 170 | 3.4 |
| 150 | 2.2 | 174 | 3.8 |
| 154 | 2.5 | 178 | 3.9 |

*The middle value of each 4-cm height group is given here.

(Reprinted with permission of the *American Review of Respiratory Disease* **108**: 258–272, 1973.)

Therefore,

$$L_{xy} = 5156.20 - \frac{(1872)(32.3)}{12} = 117.4$$

$$L_{xx} = 294{,}320 - \frac{(1872)^2}{12} = 2288$$

$$b = L_{xy}/L_{xx} = 0.051$$

$$a = \left(\sum_{i=1}^{12} y_i - b \sum_{i=1}^{12} x_i\right)\bigg/12 = [32.3 - 0.051(1872)]/12 = -5.264$$

Thus, the fitted regression line is

$$\text{FEV} = -5.264 + 0.051 \times \text{height}.$$

We test for statistical significance by computing the $F$ statistic in **(11.7)** as follows:

$$\text{Reg SS} = L_{xy}^2/L_{xx} = (117.4)^2/2288 = 6.024 = \text{Reg MS}$$

$$\text{Total SS} = L_{yy} = 93.11 - (32.3)^2/12 = 6.169$$

$$\text{Res SS} = 6.169 - 6.024 = 0.145$$

$$\text{Res MS} = \text{Res SS}/(n-2) = 0.145/10 = 0.0145$$

$$\lambda = \text{Reg MS/Res MS} = 415.4 \sim F_{1,10} \text{ under } H_0$$

Clearly, the fitted line is statistically significant because from Table 8 $F_{1,10,.999} = 21.04$, so that $p < 0.001$. These results can be displayed in an ANOVA table (Table 11.5).

Finally, the proportion of the variance of FEV that is explained by height is given by $R^2 = 6.024/6.169 = 0.976$. Thus, differences in height explain almost all the variability in FEV among boys in this age group. A scatter plot of the raw data and the fitted regression line is given in Figure 11.9. ∎

**Table 11.5**
*ANOVA table for the FEV-height regression results in Example 11.14*

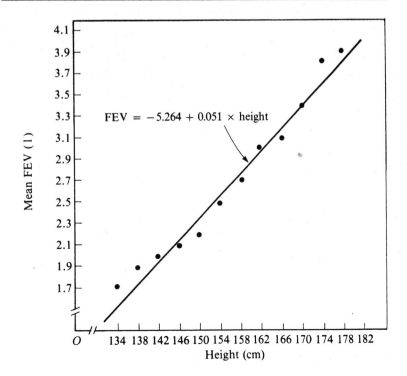

*Analysis of variance*

| | DF | Sum of Squares | Mean Square |
|---|---|---|---|
| Regression | 1 | 6.02393 | 6.02393 |
| Residual | 10 | 0.14523 | 0.01452 |

F = 414.77690     Signif F = 0.0000

**Figure 11.9**
*Scatter plot and estimated regression line of mean FEV by height in boys ages 10–15 in Tecumseh, Michigan*

The scatter plot is useful for looking at the goodness-of-fit of the regression line to the observed data. In particular, we can look for patterns in the residuals, that is, patterns in deviations of the observed data points from the fitted regression line. These patterns can give clues to an underlying curvilinear relationship between FEV and height, which would be missed by fitting a simple linear model. Also, the residuals can alert us to the presence of outlying values, which might exert undue influence on the fitting of the regression line. If we refer to Figure 11.9, we do not notice any particular pattern in the residuals nor are any outlying values evident. Thus we can conclude that the linear model seems to fit adequately in this age range. However, this fit might not be adequate if we had studied younger children, whose growth characteristics for FEV and height may be different.

# ■ 11.5  TESTING THE GOODNESS-OF-FIT OF REGRESSION LINES (t TEST)

In this section we present an alternative method for testing the hypothesis $H_0$: $\beta = 0$ vs. $H_1: \beta \neq 0$. This method is based on the $t$ test and is equivalent to the $F$ test presented in Section 11.4. The procedure is widely used and also provides interval estimates for $\beta$.

We will base our hypothesis test here on the sample regression coefficient $b$ or, more specifically, on $b/se(b)$, and we will reject $H_0$ if $|b|/se(b) > c$ for some constant $c$ and will accept $H_0$ otherwise.

We can show that the sample regression coefficient $b$ is an **unbiased estimator** of the population regression coefficient $\beta$ and, in particular, that under $H_0$, $E(b) = 0$. Furthermore, we can show that the variance of $b$ is given by

$$\sigma^2 \bigg/ \sum_{i=1}^{n} (x_i - \bar{x})^2 = \sigma^2/L_{xx}$$

In general, we do not know $\sigma^2$. However, we can show that the best estimate of $\sigma^2$ is given by $s_{y \cdot x}^2$. Hence

$$se(b) \approx s_{y \cdot x}/(L_{xx})^{1/2}$$

Finally, we can show that under $H_0$, $\gamma = b/se(b)$ follows a $t$ distribution with $n - 2\,df$. Therefore, we have the following test procedure for a two-sided test with significance level $\alpha$.

**11.8**    *t Test for Simple Linear Regression*

If we wish to test the hypothesis $H_0: \beta = 0$ vs. $H_1: \beta \neq 0$, then:

*1.* We compute the test statistic

$$\gamma = b/(s_{y \cdot x}^2/L_{xx})^{1/2}$$

*2.* For a two-sided test with significance level $\alpha$, if

$$\gamma > t_{n-2, 1-\alpha/2}$$

or

$$\gamma < t_{n-2,\alpha/2} = -t_{n-2,1-\alpha/2}$$

then we reject $H_0$; if

$$-t_{n-2,1-\alpha/2} \leq \gamma \leq t_{n-2,1-\alpha/2}$$

then we accept $H_0$.

**3.** The exact *p*-value is given by

$$p = 2 \times (\text{area to the left of } \gamma \text{ under a } t_{n-2} \text{ distribution}) \qquad \text{if } \gamma < 0$$

$$p = 2 \times (\text{area to the right of } \gamma \text{ under a } t_{n-2} \text{ distribution}) \qquad \text{if } \gamma \geq 0$$

The acceptance and rejection regions for this test are depicted in Figure 11.10. The computation of the exact *p*-value is illustrated in Figure 11.11.

We can show that the *t* test in this section and the *F* test in Section 11.4 are equivalent in that they always provide the same *p*-values. Which test is used is a matter of personal preference; both appear in the literature.

*Example 11.15*　**Obstetrics** Assess the statistical significance for the birthweight-estriol data using the *t* test in **(11.8)**.

*Solution*　We have from Example 11.8 that $b = L_{xy}/L_{xx} = 0.608$. Furthermore, from Table 11.3 and Example 11.12, we have

$$se(b) = (s_{y \cdot x}^2/L_{xx})^{1/2} = (14.60/677.42)^{1/2} = 0.147$$

Thus,

$$\gamma = b/se(b) = 0.608/0.147 = 4.14 \sim t_{29} \text{ under } H_0$$

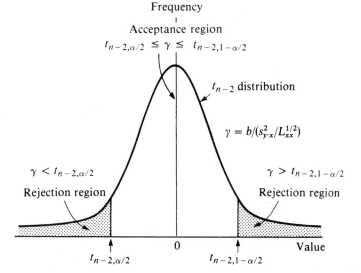

*Figure 11.10*
*Acceptance and rejection regions for the t test for simple linear regression*

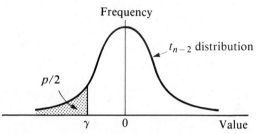

(a) If $\gamma < 0$, then $p = 2 \times$ (area to the left of $\gamma$ under a $t_{n-2}$ distribution).

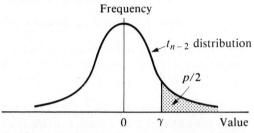

**Figure 11.11**
*Computation of the exact p-value for the t test for simple linear regression*

(b) If $\gamma \geq 0$, then $p = 2 \times$ (area to the right of $\gamma$ under a $t_{n-2}$ distribution).

Since

$$t_{29,.9995} = 3.659 < 4.14 = \gamma$$

we have

$$p < 2 \times (1 - 0.9995) = 0.001$$

This information is summarized in Table 11.6. Note that the *p*-values based on the *F* test in Table 11.3 and the *t* test in Table 11.6 are exactly the same ($p = 0.0003$).  ■

**Table 11.6**
*t test approach for the birthweight-estriol example*

```
* * * *   M U L T I P L E   R E G R E S S I O N   * * * *

Equation Number 1    Dependent Variable..   BWT   BIRTHWEIGHT

------------------ Variables in the Equation ------------------

Variable            B         SE B       Beta       T   Sig T

ESTRIOL          0.60819    0.14681    0.60973    4.143 0.0003
(Constant)      21.52343    2.62042               8.214 0.0000
```

# ■ 11.6 INTERVAL ESTIMATION FOR PARAMETERS OF A REGRESSION LINE

We often want to compute standard errors and interval estimates for the parameters of a regression line to obtain some idea of the precision of the estimates.

Furthermore, if we wish to compare our regression line with previously published regression coefficients $\beta_0$ and $\alpha_0$, where these estimates are based on much larger samples than our own, then, based on our data, we can check whether $\beta_0$ and $\alpha_0$ fall within the 95% confidence interval for $\beta$ and $\alpha$, respectively, to decide whether the two sets of results are comparable.

We can show that the standard errors of the estimated regression parameters are given as follows:

---

**11.9**    *Standard Errors of Estimated Parameters in Simple Linear Regression*

$$se(b) = \sqrt{\frac{s_{y \cdot x}^2}{L_{xx}}}$$

$$se(a) = \sqrt{s_{y \cdot x}^2 \left( \frac{1}{n} + \frac{\bar{x}^2}{L_{xx}} \right)}$$

---

Furthermore, the two-sided $100\% \times (1 - \alpha)$ confidence intervals for $\beta$ and $\alpha$ are given by:

---

**11.10**    *Two-Sided 100% × (1 − α) Confidence Intervals for the Parameters of a Regression Line*

If $b$ and $a$ are, respectively, the estimated slope and intercept of a regression line as given in **(11.3)** and $se(b)$, $se(a)$ are the estimated standard errors as given in **(11.9)**, then the two-sided $100\% \times (1 - \alpha)$ confidence intervals for $\beta$ and $\alpha$ are given by

$$b \pm t_{n-2, 1-\alpha/2} se(b) \qquad \text{and} \qquad a \pm t_{n-2, 1-\alpha/2} se(a)$$

respectively.

---

*Example 11.16*    **Obstetrics** Provide standard errors and 95% confidence intervals for the regression parameters of the birthweight-estriol data in Table 11.1.

*Solution*    The standard error of $b$ is given by

$$\sqrt{14.60/677.42} = 0.147$$

Thus, a 95% confidence interval for $\beta$ is obtained from

$$0.608 \pm t_{29,.975}(0.147) = 0.008 \pm 2.045(0.147) = 0.608 \pm 0.301 = (0.307, 0.909)$$

We need to compute $\bar{x}$ to obtain the standard error of $a$. From Example 11.8, we have

$$\bar{x} = \frac{\sum\limits_{i=1}^{31} x_i}{31} = \frac{534}{31} = 17.23$$

Thus, the standard error of $a$ is given by

$$\sqrt{14.60 \left[ \frac{1}{31} + \frac{(17.23)^2}{677.42} \right]} = 2.62$$

It follows that a 95% confidence interval for $\alpha$ is provided by

$$21.53 \pm t_{29,.975}(2.62) = 21.53 \pm 2.045(2.62) = 21.53 \pm 5.36 = (16.17, 26.89)$$

These intervals are rather wide, which is not surprising due to our small sample size.

Suppose we find another data set in the literature based on 500 pregnancies, where the birthweight-estriol regression line is estimated as $y = 25.04 + 0.52x$. Since 0.52 is within our 95% confidence interval for the slope and 25.04 is within our 95% confidence interval for the intercept, we can say that our results are compatible with the earlier study.    ∎

# ■ *11.7 INTERVAL ESTIMATION FOR PREDICTIONS MADE FROM REGRESSION LINES*

One important use for regression lines is in making predictions. Frequently, we must assess the accuracy of these predictions.

*Example 11.17*    *Pulmonary Function* Suppose we wish to use the FEV-height regression line computed in Example 11.14 to develop normal ranges for 10–15-year-old boys of particular heights. In particular, suppose we have John H., who is 12 years old and 160 cm tall and whose FEV is 2.5 l. Can we consider his FEV abnormal for his age and height?    ∎

In general, if we consider all boys of height $x$, then we can best estimate FEV for such boys from the regression equation by $\hat{y} = a + bx$. How accurate is this estimate? The answer to this question depends on whether we wish to make a prediction *for one specific boy* or for the *mean value of all boys of a given height*. The first estimate would be useful to a pediatrician interested in assessing the lung function of a particular patient, whereas the second estimate would be useful to a researcher interested in relationships between pulmonary function and height over *large populations of boys*. We can show that the standard error ($se_1$) of the first type of estimate and the resulting confidence interval are given as follows:

**11.11**    **Standard Error and Confidence Interval of Predictions Made from Regression Lines for a New Sample Point**

Suppose we wish to make predictions from a regression line for a new sample point with independent variable $x$ that was not used in constructing the regression line. The observed value of $y$ will be normally distributed with mean $= \hat{y} = a + bx$ and standard error given by

$$se_1(\hat{y}) = \sqrt{s_{y \cdot x}^2 \left[ 1 + \frac{1}{n} + \frac{(x - \bar{x})^2}{L_{xx}} \right]}$$

Furthermore, a two-sided $100\% \times (1 - \alpha)$ confidence interval for $y$ is given by

$$\hat{y} \pm t_{n-2, 1-\alpha/2} se_1(\hat{y})$$

*Example 11.18*    *Pulmonary Function* Construct a 95% confidence interval for the FEV of John H. in Example 11.17.

*Solution*    John's observed FEV is 2.5 l. The regression equation relating FEV and height was computed in Example 11.14 and is given by $y = -5.264 + 0.051 \times \text{height}$. Thus, his expected FEV is

$$\hat{y} = -5.264 + 160 \times 0.051 = 2.901$$

We need to obtain $\bar{x}$ before computing the $se(\hat{y})$. From Example 11.14 we have

$$\bar{x} = \frac{\sum\limits_{i=1}^{12} x_i}{12} = \frac{1872}{12} = 156.0$$

Thus, $se_1(\hat{y})$ is given by

$$se_1(\hat{y}) = \sqrt{(0.0145)\left[1 + \frac{1}{12} + \frac{(160 - 156)^2}{2288}\right]} = \sqrt{(0.0145)(1.090)} = 0.126$$

Finally, a 95% confidence interval for the FEV of John H. is given by

$$2.90 \pm t_{10,.975}(0.126) = 2.90 \pm 2.228(0.126) = 2.90 \pm 0.28 = (2.62, 3.18)$$

How can we use this confidence interval? We can say that since the observed FEV (2.5 l) does not fall within the confidence interval, John's lung function is abnormally low for a boy of his age and height, and, if possible, further exploration is needed to find a reason for this abnormality. ∎

Notice that the magnitude of the standard error in **(11.11)** depends on how far the observed value of $x$ for the new sample point is from the mean value of $x$ for the data points used in computing the regression line ($\bar{x}$). The standard error is smaller when $x$ is close to $\bar{x}$ than when $x$ is far from $\bar{x}$. In general, making predictions from a regression line for values of $x$ that are very far from $\bar{x}$ is dangerous, since the predictions are likely to be very inaccurate.

*Example 11.19*    **Pulmonary Function** Suppose that Bill Y. has a height of 190 cm with an FEV of 3.5 l. Compare the standard error of his predicted value with that for John H. given in Example 11.18.

*Solution*    From **(11.11)** we have

$$se_1(\hat{y}) = \sqrt{(0.0145)\left[1 + \frac{1}{12} + \frac{(190 - 156)^2}{2288}\right]}$$

$$= \sqrt{(0.0145)(1.589)} = 0.152 > 0.126 = se_1 \text{ (John H.)}$$

This result is expected, since 190 cm is further than 160 cm from $\bar{x} = 156$ cm. ∎

Suppose we want to assess the mean value of FEV for a large number of boys of a particular height rather than for one particular boy. This parameter might be of interest to a researcher interested in growth curves of pulmonary function in children. How can we estimate this mean FEV and obtain its standard error? The procedure is given as follows:

**11.12**    *Standard Error and Confidence Interval Predictions Made from Regression Lines for the Expected Value of y for a Given x*

Our best estimate of the expected value of $y$ for a given $x$ is $\hat{y} = a + bx$. Its standard error, which we denote by $se_2(\hat{y})$, is given by

$$se_2(\hat{y}) = \sqrt{s_{y\cdot x}^2 \left[ \frac{1}{n} + \frac{(x - \bar{x})^2}{L_{xx}} \right]}$$

Furthermore, a two-sided $100\% \times (1 - \alpha)$ confidence interval for the expected value of $y$ is

$$\hat{y} \pm t_{n-2, 1-\alpha/2} se_2(\hat{y})$$

*Example 11.20*    **Pulmonary Function**    Compute the standard error and 95% confidence interval for the mean value of FEV over a large number of boys with height of 160 cm.

*Solution*    We refer to the results of Example 11.18 for the necessary raw data to perform the computations. Our best estimate of the mean value of FEV is the same as our estimate for one boy (John H.), which was 2.901 as computed in Example 11.18. However, the standard error is computed differently. From **(11.12)** we have

$$se_2(\hat{y}) = \sqrt{(0.0145) \left[ \frac{1}{12} + \frac{(160 - 156)^2}{2288} \right]} = \sqrt{(0.0145)(0.090)} = 0.036$$

Therefore, a 95% confidence interval for the mean value of FEV over a large number of boys with height 160 cm is given by

$$2.90 \pm t_{10, .975}(0.036) = 2.90 \pm 2.228(0.036)$$

$$= 2.90 \pm 0.08 = (2.82, 2.98)$$

Notice that this standard error $[se_2(\hat{y}) = 0.036]$ is much smaller than the corresponding standard error $[se_1(y) = 0.126]$ computed in Example 11.18 for the FEV of one particular boy. Similarly, the 95% confidence interval is much narrower here (2.82, 2.98) than the corresponding confidence interval in Example 11.18 (2.62, 3.18). This disparity reflects the intuitive idea that we much much more precision in estimating the mean value of $y$ for a large number of boys with the same height $x$ than in estimating $y$ for one particular boy with height $x$. ∎

We note again that the standard error for the estimated expected value of $y$ for a given value of $x$ is not the same for all values of $x$, but gets larger the further $x$ is from the mean value of $x$ ($\bar{x}$) used to estimate the regression line.

*Example 11.21*    **Pulmonary Function** Compare the standard error of the expected FEV for boys of height 190 cm with that for boys of 160 cm.

*Solution*    From **(11.12)** we have

$$se_2(\hat{y}) = \sqrt{(0.0145) \left[ \frac{1}{12} + \frac{(190 - 156)^2}{2288} \right]} = \sqrt{(0.0145)(0.589)}$$

$$= 0.092 > 0.036 = se_2(\hat{y}) \text{ for } x = 160 \text{ cm}$$

This result is expected, since 190 cm is further than 160 cm from $\bar{x} = 156$ cm. ∎

# ■ 11.8 MULTIPLE REGRESSION

In Sections 11.2 through 11.7 we discussed problems in linear regression analysis in which we had one independent variable ($x$), one dependent variable ($y$), and a linear relationship between $x$ and $y$. In practice we often have more than one independent variable and would like to look at the relationship between each of the independent variables ($x_1, \ldots, x_k$) and the dependent variable ($y$) after taking into account the remaining independent variables. This type of problem forms the subject matter of **multiple regression analysis.**

**Example 11.22**    *Hypertension, Pediatrics* A topic of current interest in hypertension research is how the relationship between blood pressure levels of newborns and blood pressure levels of infants relates to the etiology of hypertension. One problem that arises is that the blood pressure of a newborn is affected by several extraneous factors that make this relationship difficult to study. In particular, newborn blood pressures are affected by (1) birthweight and (2) the day of life on which blood pressure is measured. We would like to be able to adjust the observed blood pressure for these two factors before looking at the relationship. ■

## □ 11.8.1 Estimation of the Regression Equation

Suppose we postulate a relationship between systolic blood pressure ($y$), birthweight ($x_1$), and age in days ($x_2$) that is of the form

**11.13**
$$y = \alpha + \beta_1 x_1 + \beta_2 x_2 + e$$

where $e$ is an error term that is normally distributed with mean 0 and variance $\sigma^2$. We would like to estimate the parameters of this model and test various hypotheses concerning it. We will use the same principle of least squares that we introduced in Section 11.3 for simple linear regression to fit the parameters of this multiple regression model. In particular, we will estimate $\alpha$, $\beta_1$, $\beta_2$ by $a$, $b_1$, and $b_2$, where we choose $a$, $b_1$, and $b_2$ to minimize the sum of

$$[y - (a + b_1 x_1 + b_2 x_2)]^2$$

over all the data points. For multiple regression, computation of the least squares estimators of the regression parameters involves matrix inversion and thus is sufficiently complex to almost always require a computer.

**Example 11.23**    *Hypertension, Pediatrics* Suppose we have measured systolic blood pressure, birthweight (oz), and age (days) for 16 infants and are given the data in Table 11.7. Estimate the parameters of the multiple regression equation in **(11.13)**.

**Solution**    We use the SPSS/PC REGRESSION program to obtain the least-squares estimators. The results are given in Table 11.8.

According to the B column, the regression equation is given by

$$y = 53.45 + 0.126x_1 + 5.89x_2$$

■

**Table 11.7**
Sample data for infant blood pressure, age and birthweight for 16 infants

| i | Birthweight in oz ($x_1$) | Age in days ($x_2$) | Systolic blood pressure (y) (mm Hg) |
|---|---|---|---|
| 1 | 135 | 3 | 89 |
| 2 | 120 | 4 | 90 |
| 3 | 100 | 3 | 83 |
| 4 | 105 | 2 | 77 |
| 5 | 130 | 4 | 92 |
| 6 | 125 | 5 | 98 |
| 7 | 125 | 2 | 82 |
| 8 | 105 | 3 | 85 |
| 9 | 120 | 5 | 96 |
| 10 | 90 | 4 | 95 |
| 11 | 120 | 2 | 80 |
| 12 | 95 | 3 | 79 |
| 13 | 120 | 3 | 86 |
| 14 | 150 | 4 | 97 |
| 15 | 160 | 3 | 92 |
| 16 | 125 | 3 | 88 |

**Table 11.8**
Least-squares estimators of the regression parameters for the newborn blood pressure data in Table 11.7 using the SPSS/PC REGRESSION program

```
                        SPSS/PC   Release 1.0

        * * * *   M U L T I P L E   R E G R E S S I O N   * * * *

Equation Number 1     Dependent Variable..    SYSBP   SYSTOLIC BLOOD PRESSURE

------------------ Variables in the Equation -------------------

Variable            B          SE B        Beta        T   Sig T

BWT             0.12558     0.03434      0.35208     3.657 0.0029
AGE             5.88772     0.68021      0.83323     8.656 0.0000
(Constant)     53.45019     4.53189                 11.794 0.0000
```

The regression equation tells us that for an average newborn the expected blood pressure increases by 0.126 mm per ounce of birthweight and 5.89 mm per day of age.

**Example 11.24**    *Hypertension, Pediatrics* Calculate the expected systolic blood pressure of a baby with birthweight 8 lb (128 oz) measured at 3 days of life.

**Solution**    The expected systolic blood pressure is given by

$$53.45 + 0.126(128) + 5.89(3) = 87.2 \text{ mm}$$    ∎

We are often interested in ranking the independent variables according to their predictive relationship with the dependent variable $y$. It is difficult to rank the variables based on the ordinary regression coefficients, since the independent variables are often in different units. Specifically, from the multiple regression model in **(11.13)**, we see that $b$ estimates the increase in $y$ per unit increase in $x$. If we increase $x$ by 1 standard deviation unit (i.e., $s_x$) to $x + s_x$, then we would expect $y$ to increase by $b \times s_x$ raw units or $(b \times s_x)/s_y$ standard deviation units of $y$ ($s_y$).

The **standardized regression coefficient** ($b_s$) is given by $b \times (s_x/s_y)$. It represents the predicted increase in $y$ (expressed in standard deviation units of $y$) that would be expected per standard deviation increase in $x$.                                                                                                              ■

Thus the standardized regression coefficient is a useful measure for comparing the predictive value of several independent variables, since it tells us the predicted increase in standard deviation units of $y$ that would be expected per standard deviation increase in $x$. By expressing change in standard deviation units of $x$, we can control for differences in the units of measurement for different independent variables.

*Example 11.25*    Compute the standardized regression coefficients for birthweight and age in days using the data in Table 11.7.

*Solution*    From Table 11.7 we have $s_y = 6.69$, $s_{x_1} = 18.75$, $s_{x_2} = 0.946$. Therefore, referring to the regression coefficients (B) in Table 11.8, we have

$$b_s \text{ (birthweight)} = \frac{0.1256 \times 18.75}{6.69} = 0.352$$

$$b_s \text{ (age in days)} = \frac{5.888 \times 0.946}{6.69} = 0.833$$

These quantities are given under the BETA column in Table 11.8. Thus, the expected increase in systolic blood pressure is 0.352 standard deviation units of blood pressure per standard deviation increase in birthweight and 0.833 standard deviation units of blood pressure per standard deviation increase in age in days. Thus, age in days appears to be the more important variable after controlling for both variables simultaneously in the multiple regression model.

                                                                                                              ■

## ☐ 11.8.2 Hypothesis Testing

*Example 11.26*    *Hypertension, Pediatrics* We would like to test various hypotheses concerning the data in Table 11.7. First, we would like to test the overall hypothesis that birthweight and age in days when taken together are significant predictors of blood pressure. How can we do this?    ■

Specifically, we will test the hypothesis $H_0$: $\beta_1 = \beta_2 = 0$ vs. $H_1$: either $\beta_1 \neq 0$ or $\beta_2 \neq 0$. The test of significance is similar to the $F$ test in Section 11.4. The test procedure for a level $\alpha$ test is given as follows:

**11.14**  *F Test for Testing the Hypothesis $H_0$: $\beta_1 = \beta_2 = 0$ Vs.*
*$H_1$: Either $\beta_1 \neq 0$ or $\beta_2 \neq 0$ in Multiple Linear Regression*

*1.* We compute

$$\text{Reg SS} \quad \text{and} \quad \text{Res SS}$$

*2.* We compute

$$\text{Reg MS} = \frac{\text{Reg SS}}{2} \quad \text{and} \quad \text{Res MS} = \frac{\text{Res SS}}{n-3}$$

*3.* We compute the test statistic

$$\lambda = \text{Reg MS/Res MS}$$

which follows an $F_{2,n-3}$ distribution under $H_0$.

*4.* For a level $\alpha$ test, if

$$\lambda > F_{2,n-3,1-\alpha}$$

then we reject $H_0$; if

$$\lambda \leq F_{2,n-3,1-\alpha}$$

then we accept $H_0$.

*5.* The exact $p$-value is given by the area to the right of $\lambda$ under an $F_{2,n-3}$ distribution $=$
$Pr(F_{2,n-3} > \lambda)$.

The acceptance and rejection regions for this test procedure are depicted in Figure
11.12. The computation of the exact $p$-value is illustrated in Figure 11.13.

*Example 11.27*  **Hypertension, Pediatrics**  Test the hypothesis $H_0$: $\beta_1 = \beta_2 = 0$ vs. $H_1$: either $\beta_1 \neq 0$
or $\beta_2 \neq 0$ using the data in Table 11.7.

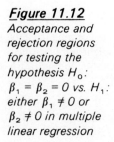

**Figure 11.12**
*Acceptance and
rejection regions
for testing the
hypothesis $H_0$:
$\beta_1 = \beta_2 = 0$ vs. $H_1$:
either $\beta_1 \neq 0$ or
$\beta_2 \neq 0$ in multiple
linear regression*

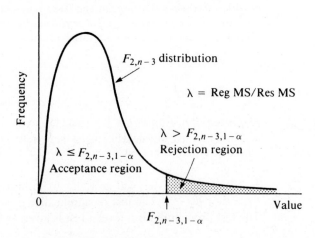

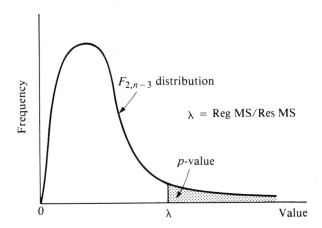

**Figure 11.13**
*Computation of the exact p-value for testing the hypothesis $H_0$: $\beta_1 = \beta_2$ vs. $H_1$: either $\beta_1 \neq 0$ or $\beta_2 \neq 0$ in multiple linear regression*

**Table 11.9**
*ANOVA table for newborn blood pressure data in Example 11.27*

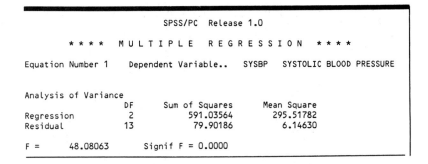

**Solution**

We refer to Table 11.9 and note that

$$\text{Regression SS} = 591.04$$

$$\text{Regression MS} = 591.04/2 = 295.52$$

$$\text{Residual SS} = 79.90$$

$$\text{Residual MS} = 79.90/13 = 6.146$$

$$\lambda = \text{Regression MS/Residual MS} = 48.08 \sim F_{2,13} \text{ under } H_0$$

Since

$$F_{2,13,.999} < F_{2,12,.999} = 12.97 < 48.08 = \lambda$$

we have that $p < 0.001$. Thus, we can conclude that the two variables when considered together are significant predictors of blood pressure. ∎

The significant $p$-value for this test could be attributed to either variable. We would like to perform significance tests to identify the independent contributions of each variable. How can we do this?

In particular, to assess the independent contribution of birthweight, we will assume that age in days is making a contribution under either hypothesis, and we will test the hypothesis $H_0: \beta_1 = 0, \beta_2 \neq 0$ vs. $H_1: \beta_1 \neq 0, \beta_2 \neq 0$. Similarly, to assess the independent contribution of age in days, we will assume that birthweight is making a contribution under either hypothesis and will test the hypothesis $H_0: \beta_2 = 0, \beta_1 \neq 0$ vs. $H_1: \beta_2 \neq 0, \beta_1 \neq 0$. Let us focus on assessing the independent contribution of birthweight. Our approach will be to compute the standard error of the regression coefficient for birthweight and base our test on $\gamma = b/se(b)$, which will follow a $t$ distribution with $n - 3$ d.f. under $H_0$. Specifically, we use the following test procedure for a level $\alpha$ test:

**11.15** *t Test for Testing the Hypothesis $H_0: \beta_1 = 0, \beta_2 \neq 0$ Vs. $H_1: \beta_1 \neq 0,$*
*$\beta_2 \neq 0$ in Multiple Linear Regression*

**1.** We compute

$$\gamma = b_1/se(b_1)$$

which should follow a $t$ distribution with $n - 3$ d.f. under $H_0$.

**2.** If

$$\gamma < t_{n-3,\alpha/2} \quad \text{or} \quad \gamma > t_{n-3,1-\alpha/2}$$

then we reject $H_0$; if

$$t_{n-3,\alpha/2} \leqslant \gamma \leqslant t_{n-3,1-\alpha/2}$$

then we accept $H_0$.

**3.** The exact $p$-value is given by

$$2 \times Pr(t_{n-3} > \gamma) \quad \text{if } \gamma \geqslant 0$$

$$2 \times Pr(t_{n-3} \leqslant \gamma) \quad \text{if } \gamma < 0$$

The acceptance and rejection regions for this test are depicted in Figure 11.14. The computation of the exact $p$-value is illustrated in Figure 11.15.

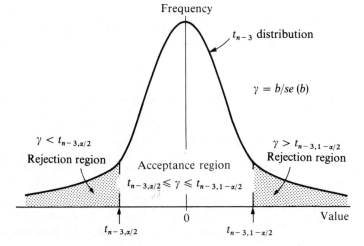

**Figure 11.14**

*Acceptance and rejection regions for the t test for multiple linear regression (two-variable case)*

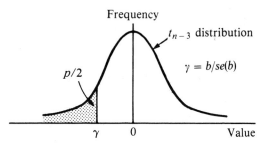

*(a) If $\gamma < 0$, then $p = 2 \times$ area to the left of $\gamma$ under a $t_{n-3}$ distribution.*

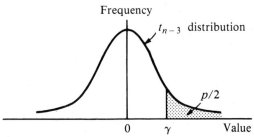

**Figure 11.15**
*Computation of the exact p-value for the t test for multiple linear regression (two-variable case)*

*(b) If $\gamma \geqslant 0$, then $p = 2 \times$ area to the right of $\gamma$ under a $t_{n-3}$ distribution.*

**Example 11.28**   **Hypertension, Pediatrics** Test for the independent contributions of birthweight and age in days in predicting systolic blood pressure in infants using the data in Table 11.8.

**Solution**   We have from Table 11.8 that

$$b_1 = 0.1256$$

$$se(b_1) = 0.0343$$

$$\gamma_1 = b_1/se(b_1) = 3.66$$

$$p = 2 \times Pr(t_{13} > 3.66) = 0.003$$

$$b_2 = 5.888$$

$$se(b_2) = 0.6802$$

$$\gamma_2 = b_2/se(b_2) = 8.66$$

$$p = 2 \times Pr(t_{13} > 8.66) < 0.001$$

Therefore, both birthweight and age in days have highly significant associations with systolic blood pressure even after controlling for the other variable.   ∎

It is possible that an independent variable $(x_1)$ will seem to have an important effect on a dependent variable $(y)$ when considered by itself, but will not be significant after adjusting for another independent variable $(x_2)$. This case usually occurs when $x_1$ and $x_2$ are strongly related to each other. Indeed, one of the advantages of multiple regression analysis is that it allows us to identify which few variables among a large set of independent variables have a significant relationship to the dependent variable *after adjusting for other important independent variables.*

**Example 11.29**    *Hypertension, Pediatrics* Suppose we consider the two independent variables $x_1 =$ birthweight, $x_2 =$ body length and try to use these variables to predict systolic blood pressure in newborns ($y$). Perhaps both $x_1$ and $x_2$, *when considered separately* in a simple linear regression model as given in **(11.2)**, have a significant relationship to blood pressure. However, since birthweight and body length are closely related to each other, after adjusting for birthweight, body length may not be significantly related to blood pressure based on the test procedure in **(11.15)**. One possible interpretation of this result is that the effect of body length on blood pressure can be explained by its strong relationship to birthweight. ∎

### ☐ 11.8.3 Extension to k Independent Variables

The methods of this section can be extended to the general case of $k$ independent variables. The general linear regression model is of the form

**11.16**

$$y = \alpha + \beta_1 x_1 + \beta_2 x_2 + \cdots + \beta_k x_k + e$$

The methods of estimation and hypothesis testing are similar to the procedures developed in this section. Specifically, to test the overall hypothesis $H_0$: $\beta_1 = \beta_2 = \cdots = \beta_k = 0$ vs. $H_1$: at least one of the $\beta_i \neq 0$, that is, at least some of the independent variables have an association with $y$, we proceed as follows:

**11.17**    *F Test for Testing the Hypothesis $H_0$: $\beta_1 = \beta_2 = \ldots = \beta_k = 0$ Vs. $H_1$: At Least One of the $\beta_i \neq 0$ in Multiple Linear Regression*

*1.* We fit the regression parameters using the method of least squares and compute Reg SS and Res SS.

*2.* We compute Reg MS = Reg SS/$k$, Res MS = Res SS/$(n - k - 1)$.

*3.* We compute the test statistic

$$\lambda = \text{Reg MS/Res MS}$$

which follows an $F_{k,n-k-1}$ distribution under $H_0$.

*4.* For a level $\alpha$ test, if

$$\lambda > F_{k,n-k-1,1-\alpha}$$

then we reject $H_0$; if

$$\lambda \leqslant F_{k,n-k-1,1-\alpha}$$

then we accept $H_0$.

*5.* The exact $p$-value is given by the area to the right of $\lambda$ under an $F_{k,n-k-1}$ distribution $= Pr(F_{k,n-k-1} > \lambda)$.

The acceptance and rejection regions for this test procedure are depicted in Figure 11.16. The computation of the exact $p$-value is illustrated in Figure 11.17.

This test will not identify which specific independent variables are associated with the dependent variable. We perform the following $t$ test to investigate the specific association of the $i$th independent variable with the dependent variable.

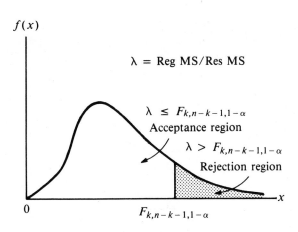

**Figure 11.16**
*Acceptance and rejection regions for testing the hypothesis $H_0$: $\beta_1 = \beta_2 = \ldots = \beta_k = 0$ vs. $H_1$: at least one of the $\beta_i \neq 0$ in multiple linear regression*

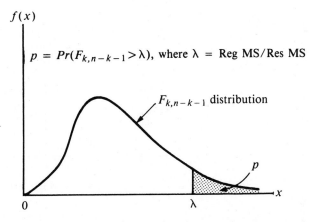

**Figure 11.17**
*Computation of the p-value for testing the hypothesis $H_0$: $\beta_1 = \beta_2 = \ldots = \beta_k = 0$ vs. $H_1$: at least $\beta_i \neq 0$ in multiple linear regression*

**11.18** ***t Test for Testing the Hypothesis $H_0$: $\beta_i = 0$, All Other $\beta_j \neq 0$ Vs. $H_1$: $\beta_i \neq 0$, All Other $\beta_j \neq 0$ in Multiple Linear Regression***

1. We compute

$$\gamma = b_i/se(b_i)$$

which should follow a $t$ distribution with $n - k - 1$ d.f. under $H_0$.

2. If

$$|\gamma| > t_{n-k-1,1-\alpha/2}$$

then we reject $H_0$; if

$$|\gamma| \leqslant t_{n-k-1,1-\alpha/2}$$

then we accept $H_0$.

3. The exact $p$-value is given by

$$2 \times Pr(t_{n-k-1} > \gamma) \qquad \text{if } \gamma \geqslant 0$$

$$2 \times Pr(t_{n-k-1} \leqslant \gamma) \qquad \text{if } \gamma < 0$$

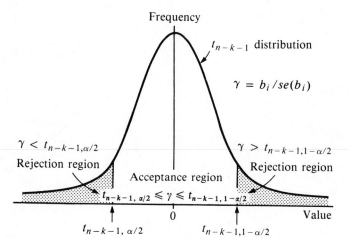

**Figure 11.18**
Acceptance and rejection regions for the t test for multiple linear regression (general case)

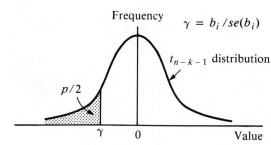

(a) If $\gamma < 0$, then $p = 2 \times$ (area to the left of $\gamma$ under a $t_{n-k-1}$ distribution).

**Figure 11.19**
Computation of the exact p-value for the t test for multiple linear regression (general case)

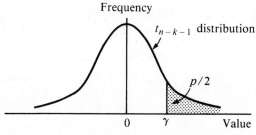

(b) If $\gamma \geq 0$, then $p = 2 \times$ (area to the right of $\gamma$ under a $t_{n-k-1}$ distribution).

The acceptance and rejection regions for this test are depicted in Figure 11.18. The computation of the exact p-value is illustrated in Figure 11.19.

**Example 11.30**    *Hypertension, Pediatrics* An example of the multiple regression methods in **(11.17)** and **(11.18)** is given in Table 11.10. The sample consists of 650 infants whose blood pressure was measured in the hospital shortly after birth. The dependent variable in this regression equation is MSYSHP = mean of three systolic blood pressure readings taken in the hospital. The

**Table 11.10**

*An example of multiple regression methods used to predict mean systolic blood pressure (MSYSHP) as a function of four other independent variables in a sample of 650 newborns*

|  | df | SS | MS | F | p |
|---|---|---|---|---|---|
| Regression | 4 | 10,580.44 | 2645.11 | 36.45 | <0.001 |
| Error | 645 | 46,806.44 | 72.57 |  |  |
| Total | 649 | 57,386.88 |  |  |  |

|  | b | se | t | p |
|---|---|---|---|---|
| INTERCEPT | 38.132 |  |  |  |
| ARMCIRHP | 2.758 | 0.386 | 7.15 | <0.001 |
| ARMLENHP | −0.796 | 0.385 | −2.07 | 0.039 |
| AGEHP | 3.252 | 0.356 | 9.13 | <0.001 |
| CONDHP | 2.236 | 0.677 | 3.30 | 0.001 |

independent variables are

ARMCIRHP = arm circumference (cm)

ARMLENHP = arm length (cm)

AGEHP = age (in days)

CONDHP = condition of infant at time of measurement (1 = awake, 0 = asleep)

Note that the overall $F$ statistic $= \lambda = 36.45 \sim F_{4,.645}$ and is statistically significant, with $p < 0.001$. This finding indicates that at least some of the variables are associated with systolic blood pressure. Furthermore, to test for the effects of specific variables, we perform $t$ tests as in **(11.18)**, which are given in the bottom of Table 11.10. For arm circumference we have $t = 7.15$, $p < 0.001$; for arm length we have $t = -2.07$, $p = 0.039$; for age we have $t = 9.13$, $p < 0.001$; for condition at the time of measurement, we have $t = 3.30$, $p = 0.001$. Thus, each of the variables is associated with systolic blood pressure even after controlling for the other three variables.

The final regression equation consists of

$$MSYSHP = 38.13 + 2.76 \times ARMCIRHP - 0.80 \times ARMLENHP$$

$$+ 3.25 \times AGEHP + 2.24 \times CONDHP \qquad \blacksquare$$

A more detailed treatment of multiple regression methods, including model selection strategies, is given in Draper and Smith [3] and Kleinbaum and Kupper [4].

# ■ 11.9 LIMITATIONS ON THE USE OF LINEAR REGRESSION

We made a number of assumptions in using the methods of simple and multiple linear regression in the previous sections of this chapter. What are some of these assumptions and what possible situations could we encounter that would make these assumptions not viable?

### Assumptions Made in Linear Regression Models

*1.* For any given value of $x$, the corresponding value of $y$ has an expected value $\alpha + \beta x$, which is a *linear function* of $x$.

*2.* For any given value of $x$, the corresponding value of $y$ is *normally distributed* about $\alpha + \beta x$ with the *same variance $\sigma^2$ for any $x$*.

*3.* For any two data points $(x_1, y_1)$, $(x_2, y_2)$, the error terms $e_1$, $e_2$ are *independent* of each other.

---

**Example 11.31**    **Pulmonary Disease** Cigarette smoking is one of the leading causes of pulmonary disease. One measure of cigarette consumption is the total number of *pack years* of cigarettes consumed in a lifetime. This measure is frequently estimated by multiplying the number of packs of cigarettes per day currently smoked (or last smoked, if the person is not a current smoker) by the number of years smoked. Thus, if a person smokes 2 packs per day for 20 years, then he or she has smoked 40 pack years. Suppose we wish to relate current level of FEV ($y$) to total number of pack years of cigarettes consumed ($x$) using a regression equation. How should we do this?  ∎

We could use a model of the form $y = \alpha + \beta x + e$ as in **(11.2)**. This model is not likely to work well because the distribution of the number of pack years is very skewed, and FEV is unlikely to be linearly related to this variable. Instead, we typically transform pack years to the scale of log(pack years $+ 1$) $= z$ and fit a regression model of the form

$$y = \alpha + \beta z + e$$

---

This transformation makes it much more likely that assumptions 1 and 2 in **(11.19)** will hold.

**Example 11.32**    **Hypertension, Pediatrics** A topic of current research interest is to look for risk factors in childhood for future cardiovascular disease. One such risk factor is blood pressure. One problem with quantifying blood pressure in children is that it is related to age. Another problem is that blood pressure tends to be more variable for older children than for younger children. Suppose we fit a linear regression model of the form $y = \alpha + \beta x + e$, where $y =$ systolic blood pressure and $x =$ age. A typical plot of blood pressure vs. age and the associated regression line is given in Figure 11.20.

The problem with this type of regression line is that there is more scatter about the regression line for older children than for younger children. This violates assumption 2 in **(11.19)**, which requires that the variance of blood pressure about the regression line for any given age be the same. One strategy that is frequently used to overcome this problem is to express blood pressure in the form of a $z$ score rather than in the form of raw blood pressure. For a child of age $x$ with blood pressure $y$, the $z$ score is defined as

$$z = \frac{(y - \bar{y})}{s}$$

where $\bar{y}$ and $s$ are the sample mean and standard deviation, respectively, of blood pressure for children of the same age group. Thus, if a 10-year-old child has a systolic blood pressure

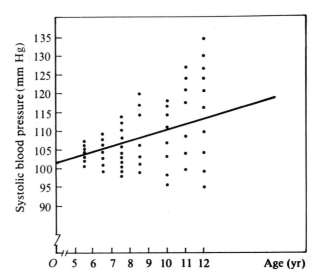

**Figure 11.20**
*Scatter plot and regression line of systolic blood pressure vs. age in children*

of 120 mm and the mean and standard deviation of systolic blood pressure for 10 year olds is 110 mm and 10 mm, respectively, then the z score = (120 − 110)/10 = 1.0. The advantage of the z score method is that regardless of age all blood pressure z scores are approximately normally distributed with mean 0 and variance 1. ∎

**Example 11.33** *Cerebrovascular Disease* Cerebral blood flow is sometimes measured to confirm or, in some cases, to predict the occurrence of stroke. Its advantage over an angiogram, which is the standard test used for this purpose, is that it is noninvasive and can be performed by placing several leads at various positions on the head so as to measure blood flow at different parts of the brain. Before this test can have wide clinical applicability, we must establish standards for blood flow in normal persons. For this purpose, we would like to fit a regression line predicting blood flow ($y$) as a linear function of age ($x$) in the form $y = \alpha + \beta x$, since blood flow is known to decline with age. Suppose we have made 10 measurements of blood flow at different parts of the brain on 50 persons of different ages. How should we use these data? ∎

Specifically, should we enter 500 points (50 persons × 10 measurements per person) and fit a simple linear regression model of the type in **(11.2)**? We probably should not, since this model would violate assumption 3 in **(11.19)**, namely that each sample point used to fit the regression line is independent of any other sample point. In particular, the 10 readings from one person are likely to be very similar to each other, and if the sample point corresponding to one of the readings is above the regression line, then most of the other readings for that person will be above the regression line as well. A simple method for dealing with this problem is to compute the average blood flow over all readings for a particular person and use one sample point for that person $(x, \bar{y})$ in fitting the regression line consisting of age and mean blood flow. This method would be used for each of the 50 people, and thus 50 sample points would be used to fit the regression line rather than 500. This method is valid although probably not the most efficient for handling this problem. (See Draper and Smith for a more advanced treatment of this subject [3].) The general issue here is that each sample point used in fitting a regression line should be independent of all other points, which is not likely to occur if several measurements are made for the same person, and each is considered as a separate data point in fitting a regression line.

# ■ *11.10 MULTIPLE LOGISTIC REGRESSION*

In the previous sections of this chapter we discussed methods for relating one or more independent variables to a normally distributed outcome variable. In many instances we are interested in performing similar analyses in which the outcome variable follows a binomial rather than a normal distribution.

*Example 11.34*    *Infectious Disease* Chlamydia trachomatis is a microorganism that has been established as an important cause of nongonococcal urethritis, pelvic inflammatory disease, and other infectious diseases. A study of risk factors for *Chlamydia trachomatis* was conducted in a population of 431 female college students [5]. Since multiple risk factors may be involved, we must simultaneously control for several risk factors in our analysis of variables associated with *Chlamydia trachomatis*. ■

We might consider a model of the form

**11.21**

$$p = \alpha + \beta_1 x_1 + \cdots + \beta_k x_k$$

However, since the right-hand side of **(11.21)** could be less than 0 or greater than 1 for certain values of $x_1, \ldots, x_k$, we could obtain predicted probabilities that are either less than 0 or greater than 1, which is impossible. Instead, we use the logit (logistic) transformation of $p$ as the dependent variable.

**Definition 11.16**

The logit transformation $\ell(p)$ is defined as

$$\ell(p) = \ln[p/(1 - p)]$$

Note that unlike $p$, the logit transformation can take on any value from $-\infty$ to $+\infty$. ■

*Example 11.35*    Compute logit(0.1), logit(0.95).

*Solution*    We have that

$$\ell(0.1) = \ln(0.1/0.9) = \ln(1/9) = -\ln(9) = -2.20$$

$$\ell(0.95) = \ln(0.95/0.05) = \ln(19) = 2.94$$

■

If we model $\ell(p)$ as a linear function of the independent variables $x_1, \ldots, x_k$, then we obtain the following multiple logistic regression model:

**11.22**    *Multiple Logistic Regression Model*

If $x_1, \ldots, x_k$ are a collection of independent variables and $y$ is a binomial outcome variable with probability of success = $p$, then the multiple logistic regression model is given by

$$\ell(p) = \ln\left(\frac{p}{1-p}\right) = \alpha + \beta_1 x_1 + \cdots + \beta_k x_k$$

or, equivalently, if we solve for $p$, then the model can be expressed in the form

$$p = \frac{e^{\alpha + \beta_1 x_1 + \cdots + \beta_k x_k}}{1 + e^{\alpha + \beta_1 x_1 + \cdots + \beta_k x_k}}$$

If we refer to the second form of the model, we see that $p$ must always lie between 0 and 1 regardless of the values of $x_1, \ldots, x_k$. Complex numerical algorithms are generally required to fit the parameters of the model in **(11.22)**. The best fitting model relating the prevalence of *Chlamydia trachomatis* to the risk factors (1) race and (2) the lifetime number of sexual partners is presented in Table 11.11.

**Table 11.11**
*Multiple logistic regression model relating prevalence of Chlamydia trachomatis to race and number of lifetime sexual partners*

| Risk factor | Regression coefficient $(\hat{\beta}_i)$ | Standard error $se(\hat{\beta}_i)$ | $\gamma$ $(\hat{\beta}_i/se(\hat{\beta}_i))$ |
|---|---|---|---|
| Constant | −1.637 | | |
| Black race | +2.242 | 0.529 | +4.24 |
| Lifetime number of sexual partners among users of nonbarrier* methods of contraception† | +0.102 | 0.040 | +2.55 |

*Barrier methods of contraception include diaphragm, diaphragm and foam, and condom; non-barrier methods include all other forms of contraception or no contraception.
†This variable is defined as 0 for users of barrier methods of contraception.
(Reprinted with permission of the *American Journal of Epidemiology* **121(1)**: 107–115, 1985.)

How can we interpret the results in Table 11.11? We would like to assess the significance of each of the independent variables after controlling for all other independent variables in the model. We can accomplish this task by first computing the test statistic $\gamma = \hat{\beta}_i/se(\hat{\beta}_i)$, which should follow a $N(0, 1)$ distribution under the null hypothesis that the $i$th independent variable has no association with the dependent variable after controlling for the other variables. We will reject $H_0$ for either large positive or large negative values of $\gamma$. This procedure is summarized as follows:

**11.23 Hypothesis Testing in Multiple Logistic Regression**

To test the hypothesis $H_0: \beta_i = 0$, all other $\beta_j \neq 0$, vs. $H_1:$ all $\beta_j \neq 0$ for the multiple logistic regression model given in **(11.22)**,

1. Compute the test statistic $\gamma = \hat{\beta}_i/se(\hat{\beta}_i) \sim N(0, 1)$ under $H_0$.
2. To conduct a two-sided test with significance level $\alpha$, if

$$\gamma > z_{1-\alpha/2} \quad \text{or} \quad \gamma < z_{\alpha/2}$$

then we reject $H_0$; if

$$z_{\alpha/2} \leqslant \gamma \leqslant z_{1-\alpha/2}$$

then we accept $H_0$.

3. The exact *p*-value is given by

$$2 \times [1 - \Phi(\gamma)] \qquad \text{if } \gamma \geqslant 0$$

$$2 \times \Phi(\gamma) \qquad \text{if } \gamma < 0$$

The acceptance and rejection regions for this test are depicted in Figure 11.21. The computation of the exact *p*-value is illustrated in Figure 11.22.

Distribution of $\gamma$ in **(11.23)** under $H_0 = N(0, 1)$ distribution

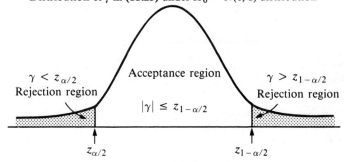

**Figure 11.21**

*Acceptance and rejection regions for the test of the hypothesis $H_0$: $\beta_i = 0$, all other $\beta_j \neq 0$, vs. $H_1$: all $\beta_j \neq 0$ in multiple logistic regression*

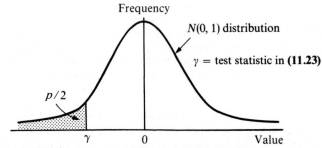

*(a) If $\gamma = \hat{\beta}_i / se(\hat{\beta}_i) < 0$, then $p = 2 \times$ (area to the left of $\gamma$ under a $N(0,1)$ distribution).*

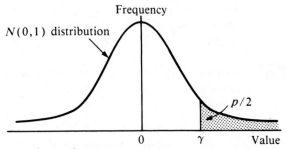

**Figure 11.22**

*Computation of the p-value for the test of the hypothesis $H_0$: $\beta_i = 0$, all other $\beta_j \neq 0$, vs. $H_1$: all $\beta_j \neq 0$ in multiple logistic regression*

*(b) If $\gamma = \hat{\beta}_i / se(\hat{\beta}_i) \geq 0$, then $p = 2 \times$ (area to the right of $\gamma$ under a $N(0,1)$ distribution).*

*Example 11.36*

**Infectious Disease** Assess the significance of the independent variables in the multiple logistic regression model presented in Table 11.11.

*Solution*

We first compute the test statistic $\gamma = \hat{\beta}_i / se(\hat{\beta}_i)$ for each of the independent variables, as shown in Table 11.11. For an $\alpha$ level of 0.05, we compare $|\gamma|$ with $z_{.975} = 1.96$ to assess statistical significance. Since both of the independent variables satisfy this criterion, they are both significant at the 5% level. The exact *p*-values are given by

$$p(\text{race}) = 2 \times [1 - \Phi(4.24)] < 0.001$$

$$p(\text{number of sexual partners}) = 2 \times [1 - \Phi(2.55)] = 0.011$$

Thus, both variables are significantly associated with *Chlamydia trachomatis*. Specifically, after controlling for the other variable in the model, there is an increased probability of infection for black women vs. white women and for women with greater previous sexual experience vs. women with lesser previous sexual experience. ∎

In addition to assessing statistical significance, we can also use an odds ratio to measure the strength of the association between each dichotomous independent variable and the dependent variable after controlling for the other variables in the model. This procedure is summarized as follows:

**11.24** | **Estimation of Odds Ratios in Multiple Logistic Regression for Dichotomous Independent Variables**

Suppose we have a dichotomous independent variable $(x_i)$, which is coded as 1 if present and 0 if absent. For the multiple logistic regression model in **(11.22)**, the odds ratio relating this independent variable to the dependent variable is estimated by

$$\widehat{OR} = e^{\hat{\beta}_i}$$

This relationship expresses the odds in favor of success if $x = 1$ divided by the odds in favor of success if $x = 0$ *after controlling for all other variables in the logistic regression model*. Furthermore, a two-sided $100\% \times (1 - \alpha)$ confidence interval for the true odds ratio is given by

$$\left[ e^{\hat{\beta}_i - z_{1-\alpha/2} se(\hat{\beta}_i)} \, , \, e^{\hat{\beta}_i + z_{1-\alpha/2} se(\hat{\beta}_i)} \right]$$

*Example 11.37*

**Infectious Disease** Estimate the odds in favor of infection with *chlamydia trachomatis* for black women compared with white women after controlling for previous sexual experience and provide a 95% confidence interval about this estimate.

*Solution*

From Table 11.11 we have
$$\widehat{OR} = e^{2.242} = 9.41$$

Thus, the odds in favor of infection for black women is 9 times as large as that for white women after controlling for previous sexual experience. Furthermore, since $z_{1-\alpha/2} = z_{.975} = 1.96$ and $se(\hat{\beta}_i) = 0.529$, a 95% confidence interval for *OR* is given by

$$\left[ e^{2.242 - 1.96(0.529)}, e^{2.242 + 1.96(0.529)} \right]$$

$$= (e^{1.205}, e^{3.279})$$

$$= (3.34, 26.55)$$

∎

We are also interested in expressing the strength of association between a continuous independent variable and the dependent variable in terms of an odds ratio after controlling for the other independent variables in the model.

---

**11.25**  ***Estimation of Odds Ratios in Multiple Logistic Regression for Nondichotomous Independent Variables***

Suppose we have a nondichotomous independent variable $(x_i)$. Consider two individuals who have values of $x + \Delta$ and $x$ for $x_i$, respectively, and have the same values for all other independent variables in the model. The odds ratio in favor of success for the first individual vs. the second individual is estimated by

$$\widehat{OR} = e^{\hat{\beta}_i \Delta}$$

Furthermore, a two-sided $100\% \times (1 - \alpha)$ confidence interval for $OR$ is given by

$$\left\{ e^{[\hat{\beta}_i - z_{1-\alpha/2} se(\hat{\beta}_i)]\Delta} \, , \, e^{[\hat{\beta}_i + z_{1-\alpha/2} se(\hat{\beta}_i)]\Delta} \right\}$$

---

Thus, $OR$ represents the odds in favor of success for an individual with level $x + \Delta$ for $x_i$ vs. an individual with level $x$ for $x_i$, after controlling for all other variables in the model.

*Example 11.38*    **Infectious Disease**  Based on the data in Table 11.11, what is the extra risk of infection for each additional sexual partner for women of a particular race who use nonbarrier methods of contraception? Provide a 95% confidence interval associated with this estimate.

*Solution*    We have that $\Delta = 1$. From Table 11.11, $\hat{\beta}_i = 0.102$, $se(\hat{\beta}_i) = 0.040$. Thus,

$$\widehat{OR} = e^{0.102 \times 1} = e^{0.102} = 1.11$$

Thus, the odds in favor of infection increases an estimated 11% for each additional sexual partner for women of a particular race who use nonbarrier methods of contraception. A 95% confidence interval for $OR$ is given by

$$\left\{ e^{[0.102 - 1.96(0.040)]}, e^{[0.102 + 1.96(0.040)]} \right\}$$

$$= (e^{0.0236}, e^{0.1804})$$

$$= (1.02, 1.20) \qquad ■$$

Finally, the 95% confidence intervals in **(11.24)** and **(11.25)** will contain 1 only if there is a nonsignificant association between $x_i$ and the dependent variable. Similarly, these intervals will not contain 1 only if there is a significant association between $x_i$ and the dependent variable. Thus, since both independent variables in Table 11.11 are statistically significant, the confidence intervals in Examples 11.37 and 11.38 both exclude 1.

# ■ *11.11 THE CORRELATION COEFFICIENT*

The primary focus of our work on linear regression analysis in Sections 11.2–11.9 of this chapter has been on methods of predicting one dependent variable ($y$) from one or more independent variables ($x_1, \ldots, x_k$). We referred to these methods as **simple linear regression** methods if we had only one independent variable and as **multiple linear regression** methods if we had more than one independent variable. Often we are interested not in predicting one variable from another but rather in merely investigating whether or not there is a relationship between two variables. We will see that the **correlation coefficient** is a useful tool for quantifying the relationship between variables and is better suited for this purpose than the regression coefficient.

*Example 11.39*    ***Cardiovascular Disease*** Serum cholesterol is an important risk factor in the etiology of cardiovascular disease. Much research has been devoted to understanding the environmental factors that cause elevated cholesterol levels. For this purpose cholesterol levels were measured on 100 genetically unrelated spouse pairs. We are not interested in predicting the cholesterol level of a husband from that of his wife, but rather we would like some quantitative measure of the relationship between their levels. What measure should we use?                   ■

**Definition 11.17**

We define the **sample (Pearson) correlation coefficient** ($r$) by

$$L_{xy}/\sqrt{L_{xx}L_{yy}}$$                   ■

We can easily show that the correlation is not affected by changes in location or scale in either variable and must lie between $-1$ and $+1$. We can interpret the correlation as follows:

**11.26**    *Interpretation of the Correlation Coefficient*

*1.* If the correlation is greater than 0, such as for birthweight and estriol, then the variables are said to be **positively correlated**. Two variables $(x, y)$ are positively correlated if as $x$ increases, $y$ tends to increase, whereas as $x$ decreases, $y$ tends to decrease.

*2.* If the correlation is less than 0, such as for pulse rate and age, then the variables are said to be **negatively correlated**. Two variables $(x, y)$ are negatively correlated if as $x$ increases, $y$ tends to decrease, whereas as $x$ decreases, $y$ tends to increase.

*3.* If the correlation is exactly 0, such as for birthweight and birthday, then the variables are said to be **uncorrelated**. Two variables $(x, y)$ are uncorrelated, if there is no relationship between $x$ and $y$.

Thus the correlation coefficient provides a *quantitative* measure of the dependence between two variables: the closer $|r|$ is to 1, the more closely related the variables are; if $|r| = 1$, then we can predict one variable exactly from the other. These definitions are illustrated in Figure 11.23.

*Example 11.40*    Suppose our two variables under study are temperature in F° ($y$) and temperature in C° ($x$). The correlation between these two variables must be 1, since one variable can be predicted exactly from the other ($y = \frac{9}{5}x + 32$).                   ■

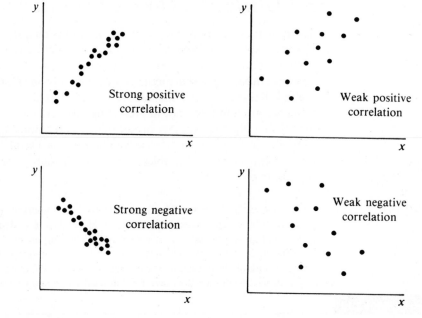

**Figure 11.23**
*Interpretation of various degrees of correlation*

**Example 11.41**    **Obstetrics** Compute the sample correlation coefficient for the birthweight-estriol data discussed in Examples 11.3, 11.8, and 11.12.

**Solution**    From Examples 11.8 and 11.12 we have

$$L_{xy} = 412 \qquad L_{xx} = 677.42 \qquad L_{yy} = 674$$

Therefore,

$$r = L_{xy}/\sqrt{L_{xx}L_{yy}} = 412/\sqrt{(677.42)(674)} = 412/675.71 = 0.61 \qquad \blacksquare$$

What is the relationship between the sample regression coefficient ($b$) and the sample correlation coefficient ($r$)? We can show after algebraic manipulation that

**11.27**

$$b = \frac{rs_y}{s_x}$$

How can we interpret **(11.27)**? We can interpret the regression coefficient ($b$) as a rescaled version of the correlation coefficient ($r$), where the scale factor is the ratio of the standard deviation of $y$ to that of $x$. Note that $r$ will be unchanged by a change in the units of $x$ or $y$ (or even by which variable we designate as $x$ and which we designate as $y$), whereas $b$ is in the units of $y/x$.

**Example 11.42**    **Pulmonary Function** Compute the correlation coefficient between FEV and height for the pulmonary function data in Example 11.14.

**Solution**    From Example 11.14 we have

$$L_{xy} = 117.4 \qquad L_{xx} = 2288 \qquad L_{yy} = 6.169$$

Therefore,

$$r = \frac{117.4}{\sqrt{(2288)(6.169)}} = \frac{117.4}{118.81} = 0.988$$

Thus, a very strong positive correlation exists between FEV and height. The sample regression coefficient $b$ was calculated as 0.051 in Example 11.14. Furthermore, we can compute the sample standard deviation of $x$ and $y$ as follows:

$$s_x = \sqrt{\frac{\sum_{i=1}^{n}(x_i - \bar{x})^2}{n-1}} = \sqrt{\frac{L_{xx}}{n-1}} = \sqrt{\frac{2288}{11}} = \sqrt{208} = 14.42$$

$$s_y = \sqrt{\frac{\sum_{i=1}^{n}(y_i - \bar{y})^2}{n-1}} = \sqrt{\frac{L_{yy}}{n-1}} = \sqrt{\frac{6.169}{11}} = \sqrt{0.561} = 0.749$$

and their ratio is thus given by

$$s_y/s_x = 0.749/14.42 = 0.052$$

Finally, we can express $b$ as a rescaled version of $r$ as

$$b = r(s_y/s_x) \quad \text{or} \quad 0.051 = (0.988)(0.052)$$

Notice that if we re-express height in inches rather than in centimeters (1 in. = 2.54 cm), then $s_x$ is divided by 2.54, and $b$ is multiplied by 2.54; that is,

$$b_{\text{in.}} = b_{\text{cm}} \times 2.54 = 0.051 \times 2.54 = 0.130$$

However, the correlation coefficient remains the same at 0.988. ∎

When should we use the regression coefficient and when the correlation coefficient? We should use the regression coefficient when we specifically wish to predict one variable from another. We should use the correlation coefficient when we simply wish to describe the relationship between two variables but do not wish to make predictions. In cases when it is not clear which of these two aims is primary, we can report both a regression and a correlation coefficient.

*Example 11.43*    ***Obstetrics, Pulmonary Disease, Cardiovascular Disease*** For the birthweight-estriol data in Example 11.3, the obstetrician is interested in using a regression equation to predict low birthweight from estriol levels. Thus the regression coefficient is more appropriate. Similarly, for the FEV-height data in Example 11.14, the pediatrician is interested in using a growth curve relating a child's pulmonary function to height, and again the regression coefficient is more appropriate. However, in collecting data on cholesterol levels in spouse pairs in Example 11.39, the geneticist is interested simply in describing if there is a relationship between cholesterol levels of spouse pairs and is not interested in prediction. Thus the correlation coefficient is more appropriate here. ∎

# ■ 11.12 HYPOTHESIS TESTING FOR CORRELATION COEFFICIENTS

In the previous section we defined the sample correlation coefficient. If we were able to sample every unit in our reference population, then we would find the sample correlation coefficient $(r)$ to be the same as the population correlation coefficient, which we denote by $\rho$.

**Definition 11.18**

We define the **population correlation coeffient** $(\rho)$ as the population analogue to the sample correlation coefficient; that is, if we were able to enumerate every member of the reference population, then the computed sample correlation $(r)$ would be the same as the population correlation $(\rho)$. For finite samples $r$ is used to estimate $\rho$.    ■

## □ 11.12.1 One-Sample t Test for a Correlation Coefficient

**Example 11.44**    *Cardiovascular Disease*  We would like to test hypotheses concerning $\rho$. In particular, suppose we measure serum cholesterol levels in spouse pairs and wish to determine if there is a correlation between levels in spouses. Specifically, suppose that $r = 0.25$ based on 100 spouse pairs. Is this evidence sufficient to warrant rejecting $H_0$?    ■

We wish to test the hypothesis $H_0: \rho = 0$ vs. $H_1: \rho \neq 0$. In this instance we would naturally base our hypothesis test on the sample correlation coefficient $r$ and reject $H_0$ if $|r|$ is sufficiently far from 0. If we assume that each of the random variables $x$ = serum cholesterol level for the husband and $y$ = serum cholesterol level for the wife are normally distributed, then we can show that the best procedure for testing the hypothesis is given as follows:

**11.28**    *One-Sample t Test for a Correlation Coefficient*

If we wish to test the hypothesis $H_0: \rho = 0$ vs. $H_1: \rho \neq 0$, then:

1. Compute the sample correlation coefficient $r$.

2. Compute the test statistic

$$T = r(n-2)^{1/2}/(1-r^2)^{1/2}$$

which under $H_0$ follows a $t$ distribution with $n-2$ *df*.

3. For a two-sided level $\alpha$ test, if

$$T > t_{n-2,1-\alpha/2} \quad \text{or} \quad T < -t_{n-2,1-\alpha/2}$$

then we reject $H_0$. If

$$-t_{n-2,1-\alpha/2} \leqslant T \leqslant t_{n-2,1-\alpha/2}$$

then we accept $H_0$.

4. The exact $p$-value is given by

$$p = 2 \times \text{(the area to the left of } T \text{ under a } t_{n-2} \text{ distribution)} \quad \text{if } T < 0$$

$$p = 2 \times \text{(area to the right of } T \text{ under a } t_{n-2} \text{ distribution)} \quad \text{if } T \geqslant 0$$

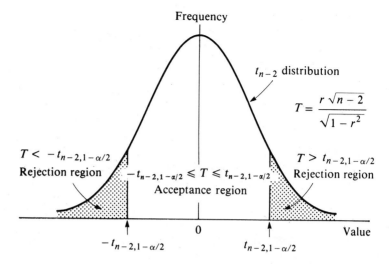

**Figure 11.24**

*Acceptance and rejection regions for the one-sample t test for a correlation coefficient*

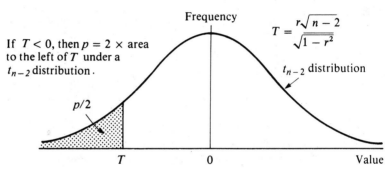

**Figure 11.25**

*Computation of the exact p-value for the one-sample t test for a correlation coefficient*

The acceptance and rejection regions for this test are depicted in Figure 11.24. The computation of the exact *p*-value is illustrated in Figure 11.25.

**Example 11.45**  Perform a test of significance for the data in Example 11.44.

**Solution**  We have $n = 100$, $r = 0.25$. Thus in this case,

$$T = (0.25)\sqrt{98}/\sqrt{1 - 0.25^2} = 2.475/0.968 = 2.56$$

From Table 5 in the appendix, we see that

$$t_{60,.99} = 2.39 \qquad t_{60,.995} = 2.66 \qquad t_{120,.99} = 2.358 \qquad t_{120,.995} = 2.617$$

Therefore, since $60 < 98 < 120$,

$$0.005 < p/2 < 0.01 \qquad \text{or} \qquad 0.01 < p < 0.02$$

and we reject $H_0$. We conclude that there is a significant aggregation of cholesterol among spouse pairs. This result is possibly due to common environmental factors such as diet. But it could also be due to the tendency for people of similar body build to marry each other, and their cholesterol levels may have been correlated at the time of marriage.  ∎

Interestingly, we can show that the test procedure for testing correlations in **(11.28)** is mathematically equivalent to the $F$ test in **(11.7)** and the $t$ test in **(11.8)** for testing regression coefficients, in that they always yield the same $p$-values. The question as to which test is more appropriate is best answered by whether a regression or a correlation coefficient is the parameter of primary interest.

## ☐ 11.12.2  One-Sample z Test for a Correlation Coefficient

In Section 11.12.1 we considered a test of the hypothesis $H_0: \rho = 0$ vs. $H_1: \rho \neq 0$. Sometimes we expect the correlation between two random variables to be some quantity $\rho_0$ other than 0 and wish to test the hypothesis $H_0: \rho = \rho_0$ vs. $H_1: \rho \neq \rho_0$.

*Example 11.46*   Suppose we measure the body weights of 100 fathers ($x$) and first-born sons ($y$) and find a sample correlation coefficient $r$ of 0.38. We might ask whether or not this sample correlation is compatible with an underlying correlation of 0.5 that might be expected on genetic grounds. How can we test this hypothesis?  ∎

In this case we wish to test the hypothesis $H_0: \rho = 0.5$ vs. $H_1: \rho \neq 0.5$. The problem with using the $t$ test formulation in **(11.28)** is that the sample correlation coefficient $r$ has a skewed distribution for nonzero $\rho$ that cannot be easily approximated by a normal distribution. Fisher considered this problem and proposed the following transformation to better approximate a normal distribution:

**11.29**   **Fisher's z Transformation of the Sample Correlation Coefficient r**

The $z$ transformation of $r$ given by

$$z = \frac{1}{2}\ln\left[\frac{(1 + r)}{(1 - r)}\right]$$

is approximately normally distributed under $H_0$ with mean

$$z_0 = \tfrac{1}{2}\ln[(1 + \rho_0)/(1 - \rho_0)]$$

and variance $1/(n - 3)$. The $z$ transformation is very close to $r$ for small values of $r$ but tends to deviate substantially from $r$ for larger values of $r$. A table of the $z$ transformation is given in Table 11 in the appendix.

*Example 11.47*    Compute the $z$ transformation of $r = 0.38$.

*Solution*    We can compute the $z$ transformation from **(11.29)** as follows:

$$z = \frac{1}{2} \ln \left[ \frac{(1 + 0.38)}{(1 - 0.38)} \right] = \frac{1}{2} \ln \left( \frac{1.38}{0.62} \right) = \frac{1}{2} \ln(2.226) = \frac{1}{2}(0.800) = 0.400$$

Alternatively, we could refer to Table 11 with $r = 0.38$ to obtain $z = 0.400$.      ∎

     We can use Fisher's $z$ transformation for our hypothesis test as follows: Under $H_0$, $z$ is normally distributed with mean $z_0$ and variance $1/(n - 3)$ or, equivalently,

$$\lambda = (z - z_0)\sqrt{n - 3} \sim N(0, 1)$$

We want to reject $H_0$ if $z$ is far from $z_0$. Thus, we use the following test procedure for a two-sided level $\alpha$ test:

**11.30**    **One-Sample z Test for a Correlation Coefficient**

If we wish to test the hypothesis $H_0: \rho = \rho_0$ vs. $H_1: \rho \neq \rho_0$, then:

*1.* We compute the sample correlation coefficient $r$ and the $z$ transformation of $r$.

*2.* We compute the test statistic

$$\lambda = (z - z_0)\sqrt{n - 3}$$

*3.* If

$$\lambda > z_{1 - \alpha/2} \quad \text{or} \quad \lambda < -z_{1 - \alpha/2}$$

we reject $H_0$. If

$$-z_{1 - \alpha/2} \leqslant \lambda \leqslant z_{1 - \alpha/2}$$

we accept $H_0$.

*4.* The exact $p$-value is given by

$$p = 2 \times \Phi(\lambda) \qquad \text{if } \lambda \leqslant 0$$
$$p = 2 \times [1 - \Phi(\lambda)] \qquad \text{if } \lambda > 0$$

The acceptance and rejection regions for this test are depicted in Figure 11.26. The computation of the exact $p$-value is illustrated in Figure 11.27.

*Example 11.48*    Perform a test of significance for the data in Example 11.46.

*Solution*    In this case $r = 0.38$, $n = 100$, $\rho_0 = 0.50$. From Table 11 we have

$$z_0 = \frac{1}{2} \ln \left[ \frac{(1 + 0.5)}{(1 - 0.5)} \right] = 0.549 \qquad z = \frac{1}{2} \ln \left[ \frac{(1 + 0.38)}{(1 - 0.38)} \right] = 0.400$$

Hence,

$$\lambda = (0.400 - 0.549)\sqrt{97} = (-0.149)(9.849) = -1.47 \sim N(0, 1)$$

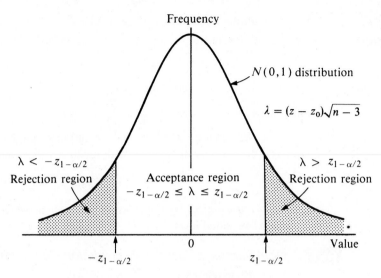

**Figure 11.26**
*Acceptance and rejection regions for the one-sample z test for a correlation coefficient*

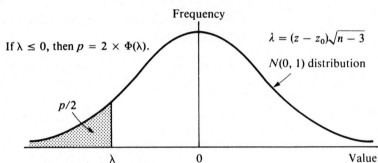

**Figure 11.27**
*Computation of the exact p-value for the one-sample z test for a correlation coefficient*

Thus, the *p*-value is given by

$$2 \times [1 - \Phi(1.47)] = 2 \times (1 - 0.9292) = 0.142$$

Therefore, we accept $H_0$ that our sample estimate of 0.38 is compatible with an underlying correlation of 0.50, which we would expect on purely genetic grounds. ∎

To sum up, we see that the *z* test in **(11.30)** is used to test hypotheses about nonzero null correlations, whereas the *t* test in **(11.28)** is used to test hypotheses about null correlations of zero. The $z$ test can also be used to test correlations of zero under the null hypothesis, but the $t$ test is slightly more powerful in this case and is preferred.

## ☐ *11.12.3 Two-Sample Tests for Correlations*

The use of Fisher's $z$ transformation can be extended to two-sample problems.

*Example 11.49*  **Hypertension** Suppose we have two groups of children. Children in one group live with their natural parents, whereas children in the other group live with adopted parents. One question that arises is whether or not the correlation between the blood pressure of mother and child is different in these two groups. A different correlation would suggest a genetic effect on blood pressure. Suppose we have 1000 mother-child pairs in the first group, with correlation 0.35, and 100 children in the second group, with correlation 0.06. How can we answer this question? ∎

We wish to test the hypothesis $H_0: \rho_1 = \rho_2$ vs. $H_1: \rho_1 \neq \rho_2$. It is reasonable to base our test on the difference between the $z$'s in the two samples. If this difference is large or small, then we will reject $H_0$; otherwise, we will accept $H_0$. This principle suggests the following test procedure for a two-sided level $\alpha$ test:

**11.31**  ### *Fisher's z Test for Comparing Two Correlation Coefficients*
If we wish to test the hypothesis $H_0: \rho_1 = \rho_2$ vs. $H_1: \rho_1 \neq \rho_2$, then:

*1.* We compute the sample correlation coefficients $(r_1, r_2)$ and Fisher's $z$ transformation $(z_1, z_2)$ for each of the two samples.

*2.* We compute the test statistic

$$\lambda = \frac{z_1 - z_2}{\sqrt{\dfrac{1}{n_1 - 3} + \dfrac{1}{n_2 - 3}}} \sim N(0, 1) \text{ under } H_0$$

*3.* If

$$\lambda > z_{1-\alpha/2} \qquad \text{or} \qquad \lambda < -z_{1-\alpha/2}$$

we reject $H_0$. If

$$-z_{1-\alpha/2} \leqslant \lambda \leqslant z_{1-\alpha/2}$$

we accept $H_0$.

*4.* The exact $p$-value is given by

$$p = 2\Phi(\lambda) \qquad \text{if } \lambda \leqslant 0;$$

$$p = 2 \times [1 - \Phi(\lambda)] \qquad \text{if } \lambda > 0.$$

The acceptance and rejection regions for this test are depicted in Figure 11.28. The computation of the exact $p$-value is illustrated in Figure 11.29.

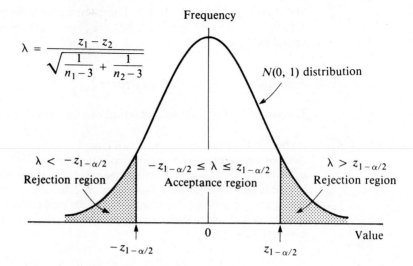

**Figure 11.28**
*Acceptance and rejection regions for Fisher's z test for comparing two correlation coefficients*

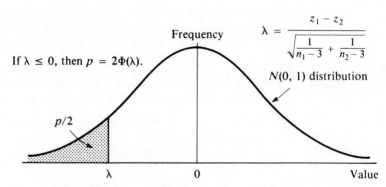

**Figure 11.29**
*Computation of the exact p-value for Fisher's z test for comparing two correlation coefficients*

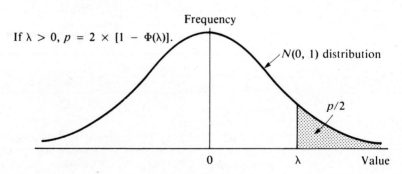

**Example 11.50**
**Solution**

Perform a significance test for the data in Example 11.49.

We have

$$r_1 = 0.35 \quad n_1 = 1000 \quad r_2 = 0.06 \quad n_2 = 100$$

Thus, from Table 11 we have

$$z_1 = 0.365 \quad z_2 = 0.060$$

and

$$\lambda = \frac{(0.365 - 0.060)}{\sqrt{\dfrac{1}{997} + \dfrac{1}{97}}} = 9.402(0.305) = 2.87 \sim N(0, 1) \text{ under } H_0$$

Hence the *p*-value is given by

$$2 \times [1 - \Phi(2.87)] = 0.004$$

Therefore, there is a significant difference between the mother-child correlations in the two groups, implying a significant genetic effect on blood pressure.    ∎

# ■ *11.13 RANK CORRELATION*

Sometimes we may want to look at the relationship between two variables, but one or both of these variables are either ordinal or have a distribution that is far from normal. The significance tests in Section 11.12 then will no longer be valid, and we need nonparametric analogues to these tests.

*Example 11.51*    **Obstetrics** The Apgar score was developed in 1952 as a measure of the physical condition of an infant at 1 and 5 minutes after birth [6]. The score is obtained by summing five components, each of which is rated as 0, 1, or 2 and represents different aspects of the condition of an infant at birth [7]. The method of scoring is indicated in Table 11.12. The score is routinely calculated for most newborn infants in U.S. hospitals. Suppose we are given the data in Table 11.13. We wish to relate the Apgar scores at 1 and 5 minutes and assess the significance of this relationship. How should we do this?    ∎

**Table 11.12**

*Method of Apgar scoring*

| Sign | Score 0 | Score 1 | Score 2 |
|------|---|---|---|
| Heart rate | Absent | Slow ($<100$) | $\geqslant 100$ |
| Respiratory effort | Absent | Weak cry; hypoventilation | Good; strong cry |
| Muscle tone | Limp | Some flexion of extremities | Well flexed |
| Reflex irritability | No response | Some motion | Cry |
| Color | Blue; pale | Body pink; extremities blue | Completely pink |

(Reprinted with permission of *JAMA* **168 (15)**: 1985–88, 1958.)

We do not wish to use the ordinary correlation coefficient developed in Section 11.11, since we can assess the significance of this measure only if we assume the distribution of each Apgar score to be normally distributed. Instead, we will use a nonparametric analogue to the correlation coefficient based on ranks.

**Table 11.13**
Apgar scores at 1
and 5 minutes for
24 newborns

| Infant | Apgar score, 1 min | Rank | Apgar score, 5 min | Rank | Rank difference $(d_i)$ |
|---|---|---|---|---|---|
| 1 | 10 | 23.5 | 10 | 19.5 | +4.0 |
| 2 | 3 | 1.5 | 6 | 2.0 | −0.5 |
| 3 | 8 | 10.0 | 9 | 8.5 | +1.5 |
| 4 | 9 | 18.5 | 10 | 19.5 | −1.0 |
| 5 | 8 | 10.0 | 9 | 8.5 | +1.5 |
| 6 | 9 | 18.5 | 10 | 19.5 | −1.0 |
| 7 | 8 | 10.0 | 9 | 8.5 | +1.5 |
| 8 | 8 | 10.0 | 9 | 8.5 | +1.5 |
| 9 | 8 | 10.0 | 9 | 8.5 | +1.5 |
| 10 | 8 | 10.0 | 9 | 8.5 | +1.5 |
| 11 | 7 | 4.5 | 9 | 8.5 | −4.0 |
| 12 | 8 | 10.0 | 9 | 8.5 | +1.5 |
| 13 | 6 | 3.0 | 9 | 8.5 | −5.5 |
| 14 | 8 | 10.0 | 10 | 19.5 | −9.5 |
| 15 | 9 | 18.5 | 10 | 19.5 | −1.0 |
| 16 | 9 | 18.5 | 10 | 19.5 | −1.0 |
| 17 | 9 | 18.5 | 10 | 19.5 | −1.0 |
| 18 | 9 | 18.5 | 9 | 8.5 | +10.0 |
| 19 | 8 | 10.0 | 10 | 19.5 | −9.5 |
| 20 | 9 | 18.5 | 9 | 8.5 | +10.0 |
| 21 | 3 | 1.5 | 3 | 1.0 | +0.5 |
| 22 | 9 | 18.5 | 9 | 8.5 | +10.0 |
| 23 | 7 | 4.5 | 10 | 19.5 | −15.0 |
| 24 | 10 | 23.5 | 10 | 19.5 | +4.0 |

---

**Definition 11.19**

We define the **Spearman rank correlation coefficient** $(r_s)$ as an ordinary correlation coefficient based on ranks.

Thus

$$r_s = \frac{L_{xy}}{\sqrt{L_{xx} \times L_{yy}}}$$

where the $L$'s are computed from the ranks rather than from the actual scores. However, a simpler method for the computation of $r_s$ is given as follows:

**11.32**  ***Method for Computing the Spearman Rank Correlation Coefficient***
If there are no ties,

$$r_s = 1 - \frac{6 \times \Sigma d_i^2}{n^3 - n}$$

If there are ties,

$$r_s = \frac{\frac{(n^3 - n)}{6} - \sum_{i=1}^{g_x} \frac{(t_i^3 - t_i)}{12} - \sum_{j=1}^{g_y} \frac{(t_j^3 - t_j)}{12} - \sum d_i^2}{2\sqrt{\left[\frac{(n^3 - n)}{12} - \sum_{i=1}^{g_x} \frac{(t_i^3 - t_i)}{12}\right]\left[\frac{(n^3 - n)}{12} - \sum_{j=1}^{g_y} \frac{(t_j^3 - t_j)}{12}\right]}}$$

where

$t_i$   refers to the $i$th group of tied observations for the first variable (of which there are $g_x$ tied groups in total)

$t_j$   refers to the $j$th group of tied observations for the second variable (of which there are $g_y$ tied groups in total)

$d_i$   equals the rank for the $i$th observation for the first variable minus the rank for the $i$th observation for the second variable

The rationale for this estimator is that if there were a perfect correlation between the two variables, then the ranks for each person on each variable would be the same. Thus, $d_i$ would equal 0 for each person, and in the absence of ties $r_s = 1$. The less perfect the correlation, the larger $\sum d_i^2$ would be and the smaller $r_s$ would be.

**Example 11.52**

**Obstetrics** Compute the Spearman rank correlation coefficient for the Apgar score data in Table 11.13.

**Solution**

We rank the collection of 24 Apgar 1-minute scores and 24 Apgar 5-minute scores in the usual way, assigning the average rank to tied values, as indicated in Table 11.14. The ranks and rank differences have been entered in Table 11.13. We now compute $\sum d_i^2$ as follows:

$$\sum d_i^2 = (4.0)^2 + (-0.5)^2 + \cdots + (4.0)^2 = 805.0$$

We then compute the correction terms for ties for the two scores. For Apgar 1-minute scores,

$$\frac{\sum (t_i^3 - t_i)}{12} = \frac{(2^3 - 2) + (2^3 - 2) + (9^3 - 9) + (8^3 - 8) + (2^3 - 2)}{12} = \frac{1242}{12} = 103.5$$

**Table 11.14**
Computation of average ranks for Apgar scores in Table 11.13

| Apgar score, 1 min | Frequency | Range of ranks | Mean rank | Apgar score, 5 min | Frequency | Range of ranks | Mean rank |
|---|---|---|---|---|---|---|---|
| 3 | 2 | 1–2 | 1.5 | 3 | 1 | 1 | 1.0 |
| 6 | 1 | 3 | 3.0 | 6 | 1 | 2 | 2.0 |
| 7 | 2 | 4–5 | 4.5 | 9 | 12 | 3–14 | 8.5 |
| 8 | 9 | 6–14 | 10.0 | 10 | 10 | 15–24 | 19.5 |
| 9 | 8 | 15–22 | 18.5 | | 24 | | |
| 10 | 2 | 23–24 | 23.5 | | | | |
| | 24 | | | | | | |

For Apgar 5-minute scores,

$$\frac{\sum (t_j^3 - t_j)}{12} = \frac{(12^3 - 12) + (10^3 - 10)}{12} = \frac{2706}{12} = 225.5$$

Thus, from **(11.32)** we have

$$r_s = \frac{\dfrac{(24^3 - 24)}{6} - 103.5 - 225.5 - 805.0}{2\sqrt{\left[\dfrac{(24^3 - 24)}{12} - 103.5\right] \times \left[\dfrac{(24^3 - 24)}{12} - 225.5\right]}}$$

$$= \frac{1166.0}{2\sqrt{(1046.5)(924.5)}} = \frac{1166.0}{1967.2} = 0.593 \qquad\blacksquare$$

We now would like to test the rank correlation for statistical significance. We can perform a similar test to that given in **(11.28)** as follows:

**11.33** **t Test for Spearman Rank Correlation**

*1.* We compute the test statistic

$$T_s = \frac{r_s\sqrt{n - 2}}{\sqrt{1 - r_s^2}}$$

which under the null hypothesis of no correlation follows a $t$ distribution with $n - 2$ degrees of freedom.

*2.* For a two-sided level $\alpha$ test, if

$$T_s > t_{n-2, 1-\alpha/2} \qquad \text{or} \qquad T_s < t_{n-2, \alpha/2}$$

then we reject $H_0$; otherwise, we accept $H_0$.

*3.* The exact $p$-value is given by

$$p = 2 \times \text{(the area to the left of } T_s \text{ under a } t_{n-2} \text{ distribution)} \qquad \text{if } T < 0$$
$$p = 2 \times \text{(the area to the right of } T_s \text{ under a } t_{n-2} \text{ distribution)} \qquad \text{if } T \geqslant 0$$

*4.* This test is valid only if $n \geqslant 10$.

The acceptance and rejection regions for this test are given in Figure 11.30. The computation of the exact $p$-value is illustrated in Figure 11.31.

*Example 11.53* **Obstetrics** Perform a significance test for the Spearman rank correlation coefficient based on the Apgar score data in Table 11.13.

*Solution* We note that $r_s = 0.593$ from Example 11.52. The test statistic is given by

$$T_s = \frac{r_s\sqrt{n - 2}}{\sqrt{1 - r_s^2}} = \frac{0.593\sqrt{22}}{\sqrt{1 - 0.593^2}} = \frac{2.781}{0.805} = 3.45$$

which follows a $t_{22}$ distribution under $H_0$. We note that

$$t_{22,.995} = 2.819 \qquad t_{22,.9995} = 3.792$$

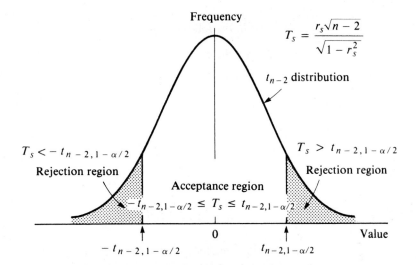

**Figure 11.30**
*Acceptance and rejection regions for the t test for a Spearman rank correlation coefficient*

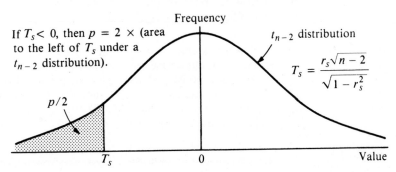

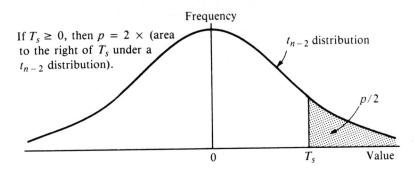

**Figure 11.31**
*Computation of the exact p-value for the t test for a Spearman rank correlation coefficient*

Thus, the two-tailed *p*-value is given by

$$2 \times (1 - 0.9995) < p < 2 \times (1 - 0.995) \quad \text{or} \quad 0.001 < p < 0.01$$

Thus, there is a significant rank correlation between the two scores.                    ∎

Note that the test procedure given in **(11.33)** is valid only for $n \geq 10$. If $n < 10$, then the *t* distribution is not a good approximation to the distribution of $T_s$, and we must use a table giving exact significance levels. For this purpose we present exact two-sided critical values for $r_s$ when $n \leqslant 9$ in Table 12. This table can be used in the following way:

1. Suppose the critical value in the table for significance level $\alpha$ is $c$.
2. We reject $H_0$ at level $\alpha$ if $r_s \geqslant c$ or $r_s \leqslant -c$ and accept $H_0$ otherwise.

**Example 11.54**    Suppose that $r_s = 0.750$ based on a sample of size 9. Assess the statistical significance of the results.

**Solution**    We see from Table 12 that the critical value for $\alpha = 0.05$, $n = 9$ is 0.683 and for $\alpha = 0.02$, $n = 9$ is 0.783. Since $0.683 < 0.750 < 0.783$, it follows that the two-tailed $p$-value is given by $0.02 \leqslant p < 0.05$. Similarly, the one-tailed $p$-value is given by $0.01 \leqslant p < 0.025$. ∎

# ■ *11.14 THE KAPPA STATISTIC*

In the previous sections we discussed the notion of correlation for continuous data and of rank correlation for ordinal data. We also want to have a measure of reproducibility for categorical data.

**Example 11.55**    *Nutrition*  A diet questionnaire was administered by mail to 537 female American nurses on two separate occasions several months apart. The questions asked included the quantities eaten of over 100 separate food items. The data obtained from the two surveys for beef consumption are presented in Table 11.15. Notice that the responses on the two surveys are the same only for $136 + 240 = 376$ out of 537 (70.0%) women. How can we quantify the reproducibility of response for these data? ∎

**Table 11.15**
*Beef consumption reported by 537 female American nurses at two different surveys*

|  | Survey 2 | | |
|---|---|---|---|
| *Survey 1* | *⩽ 1 serving/week* | *> 1 serving/week* | *Total* |
| *⩽ 1 serving/week* | 136 | 92 | 228 |
| *> 1 serving/week* | 69 | 240 | 309 |
| *Total* | 205 | 332 | 537 |

We could perform a chi-square test for association between the survey 1 and survey 2 responses. However, this test would not give us a quantitative measure of reproducibility between the responses at the two surveys. Instead, we will focus on the percentage of women with concordant responses in the two surveys. We noted in Example 11.55 that 70.0% of the women gave concordant responses. We would like to compare the observed concordance rate $(p_o)$ with the expected concordance rate $(p_e)$ if the responses of the women at the two surveys were statistically independent. The motivation behind this definition is that the questionnaire would be virtually worthless if the frequency of consumption reported at one survey had no relationship to the frequency of consumption reported at a second survey. Suppose there are $c$ response categories and the probability of response in the $i$th category is $a_i$ for the first survey and $b_i$ for the second survey. We can estimate these probabilities from the row and column margins of the contingency table. The expected concordance rate ($p_e$) if the survey responses are independent is given by $\sum (a_i b_i)$.

*Example 11.56*   **Nutrition** Compute the expected concordance rate using the beef consumption data in Table 11.15.

*Solution*   From Table 11.15 we have

$$a_1 = \frac{228}{537} = 0.425$$

$$a_2 = \frac{309}{537} = 0.575$$

$$b_1 = \frac{205}{537} = 0.382$$

$$b_2 = \frac{332}{537} = 0.618$$

Thus, we have

$$p_e = 0.425 \times 0.382 + 0.575 \times 0.618 = 0.518$$

Therefore, we would expect 51.8% concordance if the subjects were responding independently at the two surveys.                                                                              ∎

We could use $p_o - p_e$ as our measure of reproducibility. However, we prefer to use a measure that equals $+1.0$ in the case of perfect agreement and 0.0 if the responses on the two surveys are completely independent. Indeed, the maximum possible value for $p_o - p_e$ is $1 - p_e$, which is achieved when $p_o = 1$. Therefore, we use the Kappa statistic, which is defined as $(p_o - p_e)/(1 - p_e)$, as our measure of reproducibility:

**11.34**   **The Kappa Statistic**

*1.* If we have a categorical variable measured at two surveys, then we use the Kappa statistic ($\kappa$) to measure reproducibility between surveys, where

$$\kappa = \frac{p_o - p_e}{1 - p_e}$$

and

$p_o$ = observed probability of concordance between the two surveys

$p_e$ = expected probability of concordance between the two surveys

$= \sum (a_i b_i)$

where $a_i$, $b_i$ are the marginal probabilities for the $i$th category in the $c \times c$ contingency table relating the two surveys.

2. Furthermore,

$$se(\kappa) = \sqrt{\frac{1}{N(1 - p_e)^2} \times \left\{ p_e + p_e^2 - \sum_{i=1}^{c} [a_i b_i (a_i + b_i)] \right\}}$$

To test the hypothesis $H_0: \kappa = 0$ vs. $H_1: \kappa > 0$, we can use the test statistic

$$\lambda = \frac{\kappa}{se(\kappa)}$$

which follows a $N(0, 1)$ distribution under $H_0$.

3. We reject $H_0$ at level $\alpha$ if $\lambda > z_{1-\alpha}$ and accept $H_0$ otherwise.

4. The exact $p$-value is given by $p = 1 - \Phi(\lambda)$.

The acceptance and rejection regions for this test are depicted in Figure 11.32. The computation of the $p$-value is shown in Figure 11.33.

*Example 11.57*   **Nutrition** Compute the Kappa statistic and assess its statistical significance using the beef consumption data in Table 11.15.

*Solution*   From Examples 11.55 and 11.56 we have

$$p_o = 0.700$$

$$p_e = 0.518$$

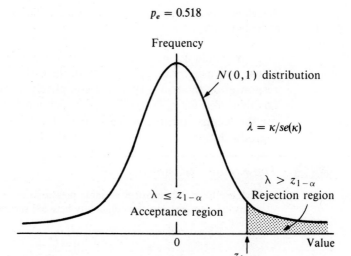

*Figure 11.32*
*Acceptance and rejection regions for the significance test for Kappa*

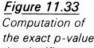
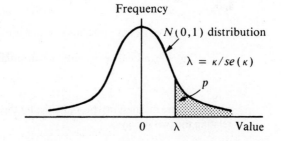

*Figure 11.33*
*Computation of the exact p-value for the significance test for Kappa*

Therefore, the Kappa statistic is given by

$$\kappa = \frac{0.700 - 0.518}{1 - 0.518}$$

$$= \frac{0.182}{0.482}$$

$$= 0.378$$

Furthermore, from **(11.34)** and the results of Example 11.56, the standard error of $\kappa$ is given by

$$se(\kappa) = \sqrt{\frac{1}{537(1 - 0.518)^2} \times \left\{0.518 + 0.518^2 - \sum [a_i b_i (a_i + b_i)]\right\}}$$

where

$$\sum [a_i b_i (a_i + b_i)] = 0.425 \times 0.382 \times (0.425 + 0.382) + 0.575 \times 0.618 \times (0.575 + 0.618)$$

$$= 0.555$$

Thus,

$$se(\kappa) = \sqrt{\frac{1}{537 \times 0.232} \times (0.518 + 0.268 - 0.555)}$$

$$= \sqrt{\frac{1}{124.6} \times 0.231}$$

$$= 0.0431$$

The test statistic is given by

$$\lambda = \frac{0.378}{0.0431}$$

$$= 8.8 \sim N(0, 1) \text{ under } H_0$$

The *p*-value is

$$p = 1 - \Phi(8.8) < 0.001$$

Thus, the Kappa statistic is highly significant, indicating significant reproducibility between the first and second surveys. ∎

Although the Kappa statistic was significant in Example 11.57, it still shows that the reproducibility was far from perfect. Indeed, Landis and Koch (1977) provide the following guidelines for the evaluation of Kappa [8]:

### 11.35    *Guidelines for the Evaluation of Kappa*

$\kappa > 0.75$ denotes *excellent* reproducibility.

$0.4 \leqslant \kappa \leqslant 0.75$ denotes *good* reproducibility.

$0 \leqslant \kappa < 0.4$ denotes *marginal* reproducibility.

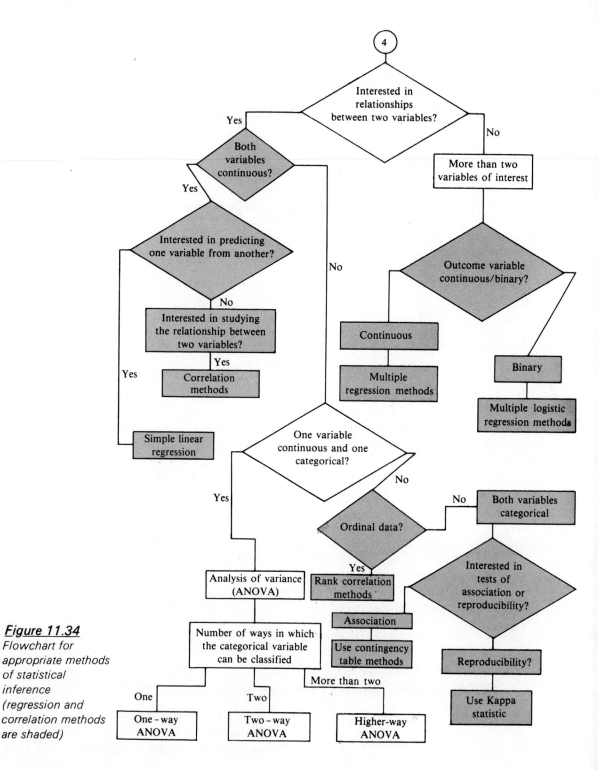

Figure 11.34
Flowchart for
appropriate methods
of statistical
inference (regression and
correlation methods
are shaded)

In general, reproducibility is not good for many items on dietary surveys, indicating the need for multiple dietary assessments to reduce variability. See Fleiss (1981) for further information about the Kappa statistic, including assessments of reproducibility for more than two surveys [9].

# ■ *11.15 SUMMARY*

In this chapter we studied methods of statistical inference that are appropriate for investigating the relationship between two or more variables. If we are studying only two variables, both of which are continuous, and we wish to predict one variable (the dependent variable) as a function of the other variable (the independent variable), then we can use **simple linear regression analysis.** If we simply wish to look at the association between the two variables without distinguishing between dependent and independent variables, then **Pearson correlation methods** are more appropriate. If our scale of measurement is ordinal rather than cardinal or our distributions are very far from being normal, then **rank correlation methods** are more appropriate than Pearson correlation methods for quantifying association. If both our variables of interest are categorical and we are interested in the association between the two variables, then we can invoke the contingency table methods of Chapter 10. If, on the other hand, we are almost certain that there will be some association between the two variables and we wish to quantify the degree of association, then we can use the **Kappa statistic.**

In many instances we are interested in more than two variables and we wish to predict the value of one variable (the dependent variable) as a function of several independent variables. If the dependent variable is normally distributed, then we can use **multiple regression methods**; similarly, if the dependent variable is binary, then we can employ **multiple logistic regression methods.** Multiple regression or multiple logistic regression methods can be very powerful, since the independent variables can be either continuous or categorical, or a combination of both. The preceding methods are summarized in the accompanying **flowchart**, on the preceding page and again in the back of the book.

In many situations we have a continuous outcome variable that we wish to relate to one or more categorical variables. In general, we can handle this situation with multiple regression methods. However, in many instances the formulation is easier if we use analysis of variance (ANOVA) methods, which we will discuss in detail in the next chapter.

# *P*roblems

**Cardiology**
The following data are given for 27 patients with acute dilated cardiomyopathy [10].

*11.1* Fit a regression line relating age ($x$) to LVEF ($y$).

*11.2* What is the expected LVEF for a 45-year-old patient with this condition?

*11.3* Test for the significance of the regression line in Problem 11.1 using the $F$ test.

**Table 11.16** *Data for patients with acute dilated cardiomyopathy*

| Patient number | Age x | Left ventricular ejection fraction (LVEF), y |
|:---:|:---:|:---:|
| 1 | 35 | 0.19 |
| 2 | 28 | 0.24 |
| 3 | 25 | 0.17 |
| 4 | 75 | 0.40 |
| 5 | 42 | 0.40 |
| 6 | 19 | 0.23 |
| 7 | 54 | 0.20 |
| 8 | 35 | 0.20 |
| 9 | 30 | 0.30 |
| 10 | 65 | 0.19 |
| 11 | 26 | 0.24 |
| 12 | 56 | 0.32 |
| 13 | 60 | 0.32 |
| 14 | 47 | 0.28 |
| 15 | 50 | 0.24 |
| 16 | 43 | 0.18 |
| 17 | 30 | 0.22 |
| 18 | 56 | 0.23 |
| 19 | 23 | 0.14 |
| 20 | 26 | 0.14 |
| 21 | 58 | 0.30 |
| 22 | 65 | 0.07 |
| 23 | 34 | 0.12 |
| 24 | 63 | 0.13 |
| 25 | 23 | 0.17 |
| 26 | 23 | 0.24 |
| 27 | 46 | 0.19 |

$\sum x_i = 1137$    $\sum x_i^2 = 54{,}749$    $\sum y_i = 6.05$
$\sum y_i^2 = 1.522$    $\sum x_i y_i = 262.93$

(Reprinted with permission of the *New England Journal of Medicine* 312(14): 885–890, 1985.)

**11.4** What is the $R^2$ for the regression line in Problem 11.1?

**11.5** What does $R^2$ mean in Problem 11.4?

**11.6** Test for the significance of the regression line in Problem 11.1 using the $t$ test.

**11.7** What are the standard errors of the slope and intercept for the regression line in Problem 11.1?

**11.8** Provide 95% confidence limits for the slope and intercept.

The following data are given for 9 patients with aplastic anemia [11].

**Table 11.17** *Hematologic data for patients with aplastic anemia*

| Patient number | % reticulytes | Lymphocytes (per mm³) |
|:---:|:---:|:---:|
| 1 | 3.6 | 1700 |
| 2 | 2.0 | 3078 |
| 3 | 0.3 | 1820 |
| 4 | 0.3 | 2706 |
| 5 | 0.2 | 2086 |
| 6 | 3.0 | 2299 |
| 7 | 0.0 | 676 |
| 8 | 1.0 | 2088 |
| 9 | 2.2 | 2013 |

(Reprinted with permission of the *New England Journal of Medicine* **312(16)**: 1015–1022, 1985.)

**11.9** Fit a regression line relating the percentage of reticulytes ($x$) to the number of lymphocytes ($y$).

**11.10** Test for the statistical significance of this regression line using the $F$ test.

**11.11** What is $R^2$ for the regression line in Problem 11.9?

**11.12** What does $R^2 s_{y\cdot x}^2$ mean in Problem 11.11?

**11.13** What is $s_{y\cdot x}^2$?

**11.14** Test for the statistical significance of the regression line using the $t$ test.

**11.15** What are the standard errors of the slope and intercept for the regression line in Problem 11.9?

*Endocrinology, Bone and Joint Disease*

A study was conducted to relate serum estrogens to bone metabolism.

**11.16** Suppose that a correlation of 0.52 is found between serum estradiol and the bone density of the lumbar region of the spine, as computed by CT scan among 23 postmenopausal women. Test for the statistical significance of these results and report a $p$-value.

**11.17** Similarly, a correlation of 0.34 is found between serum estradiol and the bone density of the distal radius of the nondominant arm among the same 23 post-menopausal women. Test for the statistical significance of these results and report a $p$-value.

**11.18** Finally, a correlation coefficient of 0.395 was computed between the two preceding measures of bone metabolism in Problems 11.16 and 11.17 based on the same group of women. Test for the statistical significance of these results and report a $p$-value.

**11.19** Suppose in a previous large study, other investigators found a correlation of 0.5 between the two measures of bone metabolism in Problems 11.16 and 11.17. Test for whether or not our sample results in Problem 11.18 are compatible with these previous results. Report a *p*-value.

**11.20** What is the *z* transformation of 0.34?

**11.21** What is the *z* transformation of 0.435?

## Pulmonary Function

Suppose the correlation coefficient between FEV for 100 sets of identical twins is 0.7, whereas the comparable correlation for 120 sets of fraternal twins is 0.38.

**11.22** What test procedure can we use to compare the two correlation coefficients?

**11.23** Perform the procedure in Problem 11.22 using the critical value method.

**11.24** What is the *p*-value of the test?

Suppose the correlation coefficient between weight is 0.78 for the 100 sets of identical twins and 0.50 for the 120 sets of fraternal twins.

**11.25** Test for whether or not the true correlation coefficients are different between these groups. Report a *p*-value.

## Psychiatry

Suppose as a reliability check the same psychiatric questionnaire is administered by two different observers to each of 30 psychiatric outpatients. An anxiety score is computed from each questionnaire. Since the investigators do not wish to assume normality for this score, the Spearman rank correlation coefficient is to be used as the index of reliability.

**11.26** If the estimated rank correlation coefficient is 0.4, then test whether or not the rank correlation is significantly *greater* than 0 using the critical value method.

**11.27** What is the *p*-value of the test?

Suppose the same procedure is employed for 8 psychiatric inpatients.

**11.28** If the estimated rank correlation is 0.7 for this group, then test whether or not the rank correlation is significantly *greater* than 0 for this subgroup. Report a *p*-value.

## Pathology

Two pathologists independently review biopsy specimens from 40 persons with self-reported malignant melanoma as ascertained by mail questionnaire. The results are given in Table 11.18.

**Table 11.18** *Pathology review for patients with self-reported malignant melanoma*

| Pathologist 1 diagnosis | Pathologist 2 diagnosis | | |
|---|---|---|---|
| | + | − | Total |
| + | 24 | 8 | 32 |
| − | 4 | 4 | 8 |
| Total | 28 | 12 | 40 |

**11.29** What index can we use to measure the reproducibility of the diagnoses made by the two pathologists?

**11.30** Compute the index in Problem 11.19.

**11.31** Test for whether or not the true index of reproducibility is significantly greater than 0 and report a *p*-value.

## Hypertension

Many hypertension studies involve more than one observer, and it is important to verify that the different observers are in fact comparable. A new observer and an experienced observer simultaneously take bp readings on 50 people $(x_i, y_i)$ $i = 1, \ldots, 50$, and the sample correlation coefficient is 0.75. Suppose the minimum acceptable population correlation is 0.9.

**11.32** Does the sample correlation fit in with this aim?

## Hospital Epidemiology

Refer to the data on hospital stays given in Table 2.11 (page 37).

**11.33** Find the best fitting linear relationship between duration of hospitalization and age.

**11.34** Test for the significance of this relationship. State any underlying assumptions you have used.

**11.35** What is $R^2$ for this regression?

## Hypertension

A frequently encountered phenomenon in Western society is the positive correlation of blood pressure and age. One finding of recent interest is the apparent absence of this correlation in many underdeveloped countries. Suppose that in a sample of 903 American males, the observed correlation is 0.402, whereas in a sample of 444 Polynesian males, the observed correlation is 0.053.

**11.36** Test for whether or not a significant difference exists between the two underlying correlations.

## Nutrition

In Table 10.3, data were presented relating reported

cholesterol intake for two different food frequency questionnaires. A test of association was performed on the data in Example 10.15. Suppose we wish to quantify the degree of reproducibility of reported cholesterol intake.

**11.37** What statistical index can we use to measure reproducibility in this case?

**11.38** Compute the index mentioned in Problem 11.37 and perform appropriate significance tests concerning this index.

**11.39** What information does this index provide that was not provided in the test for association in Example 10.15?

*Pathology*

**11.40** If we assume normality, then using the data in Table 2.10 (page 36), test if there is any relation between total heart weight and body weight within each of the two groups.

**11.41** Suppose we do not assume normality. Perform a nonparametric procedure to address the question posed in Problem 11.40.

**11.42** Which method of analysis do you feel is appropriate here?

*Hypertension*

Suppose that 20 married couples, each in the age group 25–34, have their systolic blood pressures taken with the data listed in Table 11.19.

**Table 11.19** *Systolic bp measurements from 20 married couples*

|    | Male | Female |    | Male | Female |
|----|------|--------|----|------|--------|
| 1  | 136  | 110    | 11 | 156  | 135    |
| 2  | 121  | 112    | 12 | 98   | 115    |
| 3  | 128  | 128    | 13 | 132  | 125    |
| 4  | 100  | 106    | 14 | 142  | 130    |
| 5  | 110  | 127    | 15 | 138  | 132    |
| 6  | 116  | 100    | 16 | 126  | 146    |
| 7  | 127  | 98     | 17 | 124  | 127    |
| 8  | 150  | 142    | 18 | 137  | 128    |
| 9  | 180  | 143    | 19 | 160  | 135    |
| 10 | 172  | 150    | 20 | 125  | 110    |

**11.43** Test the hypothesis that there is no correlation between the male and female scores.

**11.44** Suppose a study in the literature has found

$\rho = 0.1$ based on a sample of size 100. Do the data support this finding?

*Environmental Health*

Suppose we are interested in the relation between carbon monoxide concentrations and the density of cars in some geographical area. We measure the number of cars per hour to the nearest 500 cars per hour and the concentration of carbon monoxide (CO) in parts per million at a particular street corner and group the data by cars per hour. The data are given in Table 11.20.

**Table 11.20** *Carbon monoxide concentration and car density at a particular street corner*

| Cars/hour ($\times 10^3$) | CO concentrations | | | | Number of samples |
|---------------------------|------|------|------|------|-------------------|
| 1.0 | 9.0  | 6.8  | 7.7  |      | 3 |
| 1.5 | 9.6  | 6.8  | 11.3 |      | 3 |
| 2.0 | 12.3 | 11.8 |      |      | 2 |
| 3.0 | 20.7 | 19.2 | 21.6 | 20.6 | 4 |

**11.45** Is there an association between cars per hour and CO concentrations?

**11.46** What is the expected CO concentration if 2500 cars per hour are on the road?

**11.47** What is the standard error for the expected CO concentration over a large number of days when 2500 cars per hour are on the road?

*Hypertension*

It has been observed that blood pressure levels tend to be similar when measured in the same person over time. However, because of physiologic variations and measurement error, this similarity is far from being exact. Furthermore, an hypothesis has been proposed that older persons "track" better than younger persons in the sense that their blood pressure levels at two points in time tend to be more similar than those for younger persons. Suppose we measure systolic blood pressure at two points in time, 4 years apart, on a group of 300 50–54-year-old males and find a tracking correlation (i.e., a correlation between successive readings) of 0.6; whereas for a group of 200 30–34-year-old males, the estimated tracking correlation is 0.4.

**11.48** Is there a significant difference between the two underlying tracking correlations for these age groups?

*Obstetrics*

The data in Table 11.21 give the infant mortality rates

**Table 11.21** *U.S. infant mortality rates per 1000 live births, 1960–1979*

| x | y | x | y |
|------|------|------|------|
| 1960 | 26.0 | 1974 | 16.7 |
| 1965 | 24.7 | 1975 | 16.1 |
| 1970 | 20.0 | 1976 | 15.2 |
| 1971 | 19.1 | 1977 | 14.1 |
| 1972 | 18.5 | 1978 | 13.8 |
| 1973 | 17.7 | 1979 | 13.0 |

per 1000 live births in the United States for the period 1960–1979 [12].

Suppose we are given the following information:

$$\sum_{i=1}^{12} x_i = 23{,}670$$

$$\sum_{i=1}^{12} x_i^2 = 46{,}689{,}410$$

$$\sum_{i=1}^{12} y_i = 214.9$$

$$\sum_{i=1}^{12} y_i^2 = 4033.83$$

$$\sum_{i=1}^{12} x_i y_i = 423{,}643.3$$

**11.49** Fit a linear regression line relating infant mortality rate to chronological year using these data.

**11.50** Test for the significance of the linear relationship developed in Problem 11.49.

**11.51** If the present trends continue for the next 10 years, then what would be the expected mortality rate in 1989?

**11.52** Provide a standard error for the estimate in Problem 11.51.

**11.53** Can the linear relationship developed in Problem 11.49 be expected to continue indefinitely? Why or why not?

### Hypertension

The level of a catecholamine called kallikrein in the urine is a variable that has been associated in some studies with level of blood pressure in adults. Generally, persons with low levels of kallikrein tend to have high levels of blood pressure. A study was undertaken in a group of 18 infants to see if this relationship persisted. The following data were obtained:

**Table 11.22** *The relationship of Kallikrein to blood pressure*

| Observation | $\log_e^*$ (kallikrein), x | Systolic blood pressure z score,† y |
|:---:|:---:|:---:|
| 1 | 2.773 | 1.929 |
| 2 | 5.545 | −1.372 |
| 3 | 3.434 | −0.620 |
| 4 | 3.434 | 1.738 |
| 5 | 2.639 | 0.302 |
| 6 | 3.091 | 0.679 |
| 7 | 4.836 | 0.999 |
| 8 | 3.611 | 0.656 |
| 9 | 4.554 | 0.027 |
| 10 | 3.807 | −0.057 |
| 11 | 4.500 | 1.083 |
| 12 | 2.639 | −2.265 |
| 13 | 3.555 | 0.963 |
| 14 | 3.258 | −1.062 |
| 15 | 4.605 | 2.771 |
| 16 | 3.296 | −0.160 |
| 17 | 4.787 | −0.217 |
| 18 | 3.401 | −1.290 |

*The log transformation was used to better normalize the underlying distribution
†Instead of raw blood pressure a z score was used, which is defined as the raw blood pressure standardized for body weight and expressed in standard deviation units, with positive scores indicating high blood pressure and negative scores indicating low blood pressure.

Suppose that we are given the following statistics:

$$\sum_{i=1}^{18} x_i = 67.765 \qquad \sum_{i=1}^{18} x_i^2 = 267.217 \qquad \sum_{i=1}^{18} y_i = 4.104$$

$$\sum_{i=1}^{18} y_i^2 = 28.767 \qquad \sum_{i=1}^{18} x_i y_i = 17.249$$

**11.54** Assuming that a linear relationship exists between systolic blood pressure z score and $\log_e$ kallikrein, derive the best fitting linear relationship between these two variables.

**11.55** Is there a significant relationship between these

two variables based on your answer to Problem 11.54? Report a p-value.

11.56 In words, what does a p-value mean in the context of Problem 11.55?

## Nutrition

The assessment of the relationship between dietary intake and disease is one of the more prominent areas of current medical research. One of the problems is the difficulty in accurately assessing a person's diet, since the reported dietary intake varies over different surveys because of both (a) faulty memory of the actual diet and (b) true changes in diet over time. To assess reproducibility, a food frequency questionnaire with over 100 food items was administered to 537 American nurses at two different points in time 6 months apart. A number of food nutrients, such as total protein and fat, were calculated on the basis of the individual items, and correlations were calculated over the responses to the two questionnaires. Suppose the correlation coefficient for total protein intake as assessed at two points in time is 0.362. We wish to test for a significant relationship between reported total protein intake at two points in time.

11.57 Is a one-sided or two-sided test appropriate here?

11.58 Perform a significance test for this relationship and report a p-value.

An alternative method for assessing dietary intake is the 7-day diet record, in which a person writes down each food item eaten over a 1-week period, and the total nutrient intake is computed from these data. Suppose that two 7-day diet records 6 months apart are completed for a group of 50 nurses (different from the first group of 537 nurses), and it is found that the correlation between total protein intake is 0.45 using this method. We wish to test if the two methods are equally reproducible.

11.59 Is a one-sided or two-sided test needed here?

11.60 Perform a significance test for this hypothesis and report a p-value.

## Hypertension

The variability of blood pressure is important in planning screening programs for detecting persons with high blood pressure. There are two schools of thought concerning this variability; Some researchers feel that a subgroup of persons has extremely variable blood pressures, whereas most persons have relatively stable blood pressures; other researcher's feel that this variability is common to all people. A study was set up to answer this question. A group of 15 persons had their blood pressures measured on three separate visits in each of 2 years, and the between-visit variance of blood pressure was measured each year. The results for systolic blood pressure are given in Table 11.23.

**Table 11.23** Blood pressure variability measured at two points in time

| Person | Between-visit variance, year 1 | Between-visit variance, year 2 |
|---|---|---|
| 1 | 8.8 | 19.0 |
| 2 | 10.0 | 25.7 |
| 3 | 6.7 | 17.9 |
| 4 | 13.3 | 95.7 |
| 5 | 10.0 | 16.7 |
| 6 | 6.2 | 15.2 |
| 7 | 35.0 | 3.9 |
| 8 | 51.2 | 11.9 |
| 9 | 30.9 | 14.6 |
| 10 | 61.0 | 21.6 |
| 11 | 5.4 | 31.3 |
| 12 | 46.6 | 21.4 |
| 13 | 37.0 | 10.1 |
| 14 | 2.6 | 18.7 |
| 15 | 2.0 | 22.7 |

We wish to assess if there is any relationship between the year 1 and year 2 variances.

11.61 Why might a rank correlation be a useful method for expressing such a relationship?

11.62 Test for the significance of the rank correlation based on the previous data.

11.63 What are your conclusions based on these data?

## Pediatrics

It is often mentioned anecdotally that very young children have a higher metabolism that gives them more energy than older children and adults. We decide to test this hypothesis by measuring the pulse rates on a selected group of children. The children are randomly chosen from a community census so that two male children are selected from each 2-year age group starting with age 0 and ending with age 21 (i.e., 0–1/2–3/4–5/.../20–21). The data are given in Table 11.24.

We are given the following basic statistics:

$$n = 22 \qquad \sum_{i=1}^{22} y_i = 1725 \qquad \sum_{i=1}^{22} y_i^2 = 140{,}933,$$

$$\sum_{i=1}^{22} x_i = 233 \qquad \sum_{i=1}^{22} x_i^2 = 3345 \qquad \sum_{i=1}^{22} x_i y_i = 16{,}748$$

**11.64** Suppose we hypothesize that there is a linear regression model relating pulse rate and age. What are the assumptions for such a model?

**11.65** Fit the parameters for the model in Problem 11.64.

**11.66** Test the model fitted in Problem 11.65 for statistical significance.

**11.67** What is the predicted pulse for an average 12-year-old child?

**11.68** What is the standard error of the estimate in Problem 11.67?

**11.69** Suppose John Smith is 12 years old. What is his estimated pulse rate from the regression line?

**11.70** What is the standard error of the estimate in Problem 11.69?

**11.71** How does John compare with other children in his age group if his actual pulse rate is 75?

**11.72** What is the difference between the two predictions and standard errors in Problems 11.67, 11.68, 11.69, and 11.70?

*Hypertension*
Adults show a strong relationship between blood pressure and age. Data were collected from schoolchildren in Muscatine, Iowa, to see if this relationship continued to hold in the age group 5–18 [13]. The data in Table 11.25 were obtained from boys in this age group.

*Table 11.24* Pulse rate and age in children aged 0–21

| Age group | Age, $x_i$ | Pulse rate, $y_i$ |
|-----------|-----------|-------------------|
| 0–1 | 1 | 103 |
|     | 0 | 125 |
| 2–3 | 3 | 102 |
|     | 3 | 86 |
| 4–5 | 5 | 88 |
|     | 5 | 78 |
| 6–7 | 6 | 77 |
|     | 6 | 68 |
| 8–9 | 9 | 90 |
|     | 8 | 75 |
| 10–11 | 11 | 78 |
|       | 11 | 66 |
| 12–13 | 12 | 76 |
|       | 13 | 82 |
| 14–15 | 14 | 58 |
|       | 14 | 56 |
| 16–17 | 16 | 72 |
|       | 17 | 70 |
| 18–19 | 19 | 56 |
|       | 18 | 64 |
| 20–21 | 21 | 81 |
|       | 21 | 74 |

*Table 11.25* The relationship between blood pressure and age

| Age, x | Mean systolic blood pressure, y (mm Hg) |
|--------|------------------------------------------|
| 5 | 94.4 |
| 6 | 97.7 |
| 7 | 101.9 |
| 8 | 104.5 |
| 9 | 106.3 |
| 10 | 109.3 |
| 11 | 112.6 |
| 12 | 113.8 |
| 13 | 117.7 |
| 14 | 121.6 |
| 15 | 122.3 |
| 16 | 123.6 |
| 17 | 124.9 |
| 18 | 131.0 |

$$\sum x_i = 161 \qquad \sum x_i^2 = 2079$$
$$\sum y_i = 1581.6 \qquad \sum y_i^2 = 180{,}271$$
$$\sum x_i y_i = 18{,}787.3$$

**11.73** Fit a linear model relating blood pressure to age using the method of least squares.

**11.74** What are the standard errors of the regression parameters obtained in Problem 11.73?

**11.75** Test for the significance of the regression line in Problem 11.73 and report a *p*-value.

**11.76** What is the expected blood pressure for an

average 13-year-old boy as predicted from the regression line?

**11.77** What is the standard error of the estimate in Problem 11.76?

**11.78** What is the expected value and standard error for the change in blood pressure over the next 5 years for an average 13-year-old boy (i.e., from 13–18 years of age)?

### Hypertension, Genetics

Much research has been devoted to the etiology of hypertension. One general problem is to determine to what extent hypertension is a genetic phenomenon. We can examine this issue in 20 families by measuring the systolic bp of the mother, father, and the first-born child in the family. The data are given in Table 11.26.

**11.79** Test the assumption that the mother's bp and father's bp are uncorrelated. (We would expect a lack

of correlation, since the mother and father are genetically unrelated.)

**11.80** We would expect from genetic principles that the correlation between the mother's bp and the child's bp is 0.5. Can we test this expectation?

**11.81** Suppose we have found a nonzero correlation in Problem 11.80. Is there some explanation other than a genetic one for the existence of this correlation?

We would like to be able to predict the child's bp on the basis of the parents' bp.

**11.82** Find the best fitting linear relationship between the child's bp and the mother's bp.

**11.83** Test for the significance of this relationship.

**11.84** What would be the expected average child's bp if the mother's bp is 130?

**11.85** What would be the expected average child's bp if the mother's bp is 150?

**Table 11.26** *Familial blood pressure relationships*

| Family | Systolic bp Mother, y (mm Hg) | Systolic bp Father, x (mm Hg) | Systolic bp Child, t (mm Hg) | |
|--------|------|------|------|---|
| 1  | 130 | 140 | 90  | $\sum_{i=1}^{20} x_i = 2980$ |
| 2  | 125 | 120 | 85  | |
| 3  | 140 | 180 | 120 | |
| 4  | 110 | 150 | 100 | $\sum_{i=1}^{20} x_i^2 = 451{,}350$ |
| 5  | 145 | 175 | 105 | |
| 6  | 160 | 120 | 100 | |
| 7  | 120 | 145 | 110 | $\sum_{i=1}^{20} y_i = 2620$ |
| 8  | 180 | 160 | 140 | |
| 9  | 120 | 190 | 115 | |
| 10 | 130 | 135 | 105 | $\sum_{i=1}^{20} y_i^2 = 351{,}350$ |
| 11 | 125 | 150 | 100 | |
| 12 | 110 | 125 | 80  | |
| 13 | 90  | 140 | 70  | $\sum_{i=1}^{20} x_i y_i = 390{,}825$ |
| 14 | 120 | 170 | 115 | |
| 15 | 150 | 150 | 90  | |
| 16 | 145 | 155 | 90  | $\sum_{i=1}^{20} t_i = 2030$ |
| 17 | 130 | 160 | 115 | |
| 18 | 155 | 125 | 110 | $\sum_{i=1}^{20} t_i^2 = 210{,}850$ |
| 19 | 110 | 140 | 90  | |
| 20 | 125 | 150 | 100 | |
|    |     |     |     | $\sum_{i=1}^{20} x_i t_i = 305{,}700$ |
|    |     |     |     | $\sum_{i=1}^{20} y_i t_i = 269{,}550$ |

**Table 11.27** Two-variable regression models predicting child's blood pressure as a function of the parental blood pressures

```
* * * * MULTIPLE REGRESSION * * * *
Equation Number 1      Dependent Variable..    CBP      CHILD BP
Variable(s) Entered on Step Number
1..    FBP      FATHER BP
2..    MBP      MOTHER BP
Analysis of Variance
              DF       Sum of Squares      Mean Square
Regression     2        2870.08458         1435.04229
Residual      17        1934.91542          113.81855

* * * * MULTIPLE REGRESSION * * * *
Equation Number 1      Dependent Variable..    CBP      CHILD BP
Variable         B          SE B
FBP           0.41500      0.12482
MBP           0.42255      0.11852
(Constant)   −15.68925    23.65025
```

**11.86** What would be the expected average child's bp if the mother's bp is 170?

**11.87** Find the standard errors for the estimates in Problems 11.84, 11.85, and 11.86.

**11.88** Why are the three standard errors calculated in Problem 11.87 not the same?

The two-variable regression model with the father's bp and mother's bp as independent variables and the child's bp as the dependent variable is fitted in Table 11.27.

Suppose we wish to assess the independent effects of the mother's bp and father's bp.

**11.89** What hypotheses should we test for this assessment?

**11.90** Test the hypotheses proposed in Problem 11.89.

**11.91** What are the standardized regression coefficients in Table 11.27 and what do they mean?

_Cancer_

The following statistics are taken from an article by P. Burch relating cigarette smoking to lung cancer [14]. The article presents some data relating mortality from lung cancer to average cigarette consumption (lb/person) for females in England and Wales over a 40-year period. These data are given in Table 11.28.

**11.92** Compute the correlation between 5-year mortality and annual cigarette consumption when expressed in the $\log_{10}$ scale.

**11.93** Test this correlation for statistical significance and report a _p_-value.

**Table 11.28** Cigarette consumption and lung cancer mortality in England and Wales, 1930–1969

| Period | $\log_{10}$ mortality, y (over 5 years) | $\log_{10}$ annual cigarette consumption, x (lb/person) |
|---|---|---|
| 1930–1934 | −2.35 | −0.26 |
| 1935–1939 | −2.20 | −0.03 |
| 1940–1944 | −2.12 | 0.30 |
| 1945–1949 | −1.95 | 0.37 |
| 1950–1954 | −1.85 | 0.40 |
| 1955–1959 | −1.80 | 0.50 |
| 1960–1964 | −1.70 | 0.55 |
| 1965–1969 | −1.58 | 0.55 |

(Reprinted with permission of the _Journal of the Royal Statistical Society_, A. **141**: 437–477, 1978.)

$$\left( \sum_{i=1}^{8} x_i = 2.38 \quad \sum_{i=1}^{8} x_i^2 = 1.31 \quad \sum_{i=1}^{8} y_i = -15.55 \quad \sum_{i=1}^{8} y_i^2 = 30.71 \quad \sum_{i=1}^{8} x_i y_i = -4.12 \right)$$

**11.94** Fit a regression line relating 5-year mortality to annual cigarette consumption.

**11.95** If we wish to test the significance of this regression line, is it necessary to perform any additional tests other than those in Problem 11.93? If so, perform them.

**11.96** What is the expected mortality rate with an annual cigarette consumption of 1 lb/person?

**11.97** Why are the variables mortality rate and annual cigarette consumption expressed in the log scale?

### Cardiovascular Disease

Many studies have demonstrated that the level of HDL cholesterol (high-density lipoprotein cholesterol) is positively related to alcohol consumption. This relationship has intrigued researchers because the level of HDL cholesterol is inversely correlated with the incidence of heart disease.

One possible mechanism was explored by Kuller et al. in an analysis of participants in the MRFIT study relating the level of HDL cholesterol to the level of SGOT, a parameter commonly used to assess liver function [15]. The data in Table 11.29 were presented.

**Table 11.29** *The relationship of HDL cholesterol to SGOT in the MRFIT population*

| SGOT | Mean HDL cholesterol |
|------|----------------------|
| ≤9 | 40.0 |
| 10–12 | 41.2 |
| 13–14 | 42.3 |
| 15–16 | 42.8 |
| 17–18 | 43.8 |
| 19–20 | 43.6 |
| ≥21 | 46.5 |

(Reprinted with permission of the *American Journal of Epidemiology* **117(4)**: 406–418, 1983.)

**11.98** Fit a regression line predicting mean HDL cholesterol as a function of SGOT. For this purpose assume that all levels of SGOT $\leq 9$ and $\geq 21$ are 9.5 and 20.5, respectively, and that levels of SGOT within all other groups occur at the midpoint of the group. Assume also that group assignments are made after rounding; for example, 10–12 represents an actual range from 9.5 to 12.5. Using this convention, if $x = $ SGOT

and $y = $ mean HDL cholesterol, then

$$\sum_{i=1}^{7} x_i = 107 \qquad \sum_{i=1}^{7} x_i^2 = 1740.5 \qquad \sum_{i=1}^{7} y_i = 300.2$$

$$\sum_{i=1}^{7} y_i^2 = 12{,}900.2 \qquad \sum_{i=1}^{7} x_i y_i = 4637.6$$

**11.99** Test the line fitted in Problem 11.98 for statistical significance and report a *p*-value.

**11.100** What is our best estimate of the HDL cholesterol for an average person with SGOT level of 11, and what is the standard error of this estimate?

**11.101** Suppose that we have made a mistake in Problem 11.98 and that the SGOT groups were assigned by truncation rather than rounding (e.g., 10–12 would represent 10.0–12.99 rather than 9.5–12.5). It would follow that average levels of SGOT within each group would increase by 0.5 (assume this is also the case for

**Table 11.30** *Multiple regression of change in HDL cholesterol from the second screening visit to the 48-month follow-up visit (follow-up minus baseline) among participants receiving standard medical care (n = 5, 112)*

| Variable | Regression coefficient | Regression coefficient per standard error |
|----------|------------------------|-------------------------------------------|
| Age (years) | −0.0054 | −0.3 |
| Screen 2 HDL cholesterol (mg/dl) | −0.3109 | −29.3 |
| Screen 1 diastolic blood pressure (mm Hg) | −0.0322 | −1.7 |
| Screen 1 cigarettes/day | −0.0324 | −4.6 |
| Change in diastolic blood pressure (mm Hg) | 0.1233 | 9.1 |
| Change in thiocyanate* (mg/l) | 0.0106 | −4.4 |
| Change in body mass index (kg/m²) | −1.2702 | −18.0 |
| Change in drinks/week | 0.1053 | 9.5 |
| Change in SGOT (IU/l) | 0.1160 | 8.4 |

*A biochemical marker used to measure the actual number of cigarettes smoked recently.

the groups $\leqslant 9$ and $\geqslant 21$, respectively). What effect does the truncation assignment rule have on the estimates of the regression parameters in Problem 11.98? (No further calculation should be necessary.)

As part of the same study, a multiple regression analysis was performed relating the change in HDL cholesterol to baseline levels and changes in other risk factors. The results are presented in Table 11.30.

**11.102** Interpret the coefficients for change in SGOT and drinks/week in the multiple regression model.

### Cardiovascular Disease

Sudden death is an important, lethal cardiovascular end point. Most previous studies of risk factors for sudden death have focused on men. Looking at this issue for women is important as well. For this purpose data were used from the Framingham Heart Study [16]. Several potential risk factors, such as age, blood pressure, and cigarette smoking, are of interest and need to be controlled for simultaneously. Therefore, a multiple logistic regression model was fitted to these data, as shown in Table 11.31.

**11.103** Assess the statistical significance of the individual risk factors.

**11.104** What do these statistical tests mean in this instance?

**11.105** Compute the odds ratio relating the additional risk of sudden death per 100 centiliter decrease in vital capacity after adjustment for the other risk factors.

**11.106** Provide a 95% confidence interval for the estimate in Problem 11.105.

### Ophthalmology

A study was conducted using 225 lenses to assess the interobserver reproducibility of the classification of cataracts using the Cooperative Cataract Research Group classification system [17]. One aspect of the study involved the rating of cataracts by two different

*Table 11.31* Multiple logistic regression model relating 2-year incidence of sudden deaths in females without prior coronary heart disease (data taken from the Framingham Heart Study) to several risk factors

| Risk factor | Regression coefficient, $\hat{\beta}_i$ | se, $(\hat{\beta}_i)$ |
|---|---|---|
| Constant | −15.3 | |
| Systolic blood pressure (mm Hg) | 0.0019 | 0.0070 |
| Framingham relative weight (%) | −0.0060 | 0.0100 |
| Cholesterol (mg/100 ml) | 0.0056 | 0.0029 |
| Glucose (mg/100 ml) | 0.0066 | 0.0038 |
| Cigarette smoking (cigarettes/day) | 0.0069 | 0.0199 |
| Hematocrit (%) | 0.111 | 0.049 |
| Vital capacity (centiliters) | −0.0098 | 0.0036 |
| Age (years) | 0.0686 | 0.0225 |

(Reprinted with permission of the *American Journal of Epidemiology* **120(6)**: 888–899, 1984.)

observers as either immature, mature, or hypermature. The results are given in Table 11.32.

**11.107** Compute a measure of reproducibility between observers for this index.

**11.108** Assess the statistical significance of this measure.

### Obstetrics

Interest has increased in possible relationships between the health habits of the mother during pregnancy and

*Table 11.32* Reproducibility of the classification of cataracts

| Observer 1 | Observer 2 | | | |
|---|---|---|---|---|
| | Hypermature | Mature | Immature | Total |
| Hypermature | 8 | 2 | 0 | 10 |
| Mature | 1 | 8 | 3 | 12 |
| Immature | 0 | 1 | 202 | 203 |
| Total | 9 | 11 | 205 | 225 |

**Table 11.33** *Multiple logistic regression analysis relating the occurrence of major congenital malformations to several risk factors, using 12,424 women in the DIP study*

| Variable* | Regression coefficient | Standard error |
|---|---|---|
| Marijuana usage (any frequency) | 0.307 | 0.173 |
| Any previous miscarriage | 0.239 | 0.141 |
| White race | 0.191 | 0.161 |
| Alcohol use in pregnancy | 0.174 | 0.145 |
| Age 35+ | 0.178 | 0.186 |
| Any previous stillbirth | 0.049 | 0.328 |
| On welfare | 0.030 | 0.182 |
| Smoking 3+ cigarettes per day at delivery | −0.174 | 0.144 |
| Any previous induced abortion | −0.198 | 0.168 |
| Parity > 1† | −0.301 | 0.113 |

*All variables are coded as 1 if yes and 0 if no.
†Women with at least one previous pregnancy.
(Reprinted with permission of the *American Journal of Public Health* **73(10)**: 1161–1164, 1983.)

adverse delivery outcomes. An issue that is receiving attention is the effect of marijuana usage on the occurrence of congenital malformations. One potential problem is that many other maternal factors are associated with adverse pregnancy outcomes, including age, race, socioeconomic status (SES), smoking, and so forth. Since these factors may also be related to marijuana usage, they need to be simultaneously controlled for in the analysis. Therefore, data from the Delivery Interview Program (DIP) were utilized, and a multiple logistic regression was performed relating the occurrence of major congenital malformations to several maternal risk factors [18]. The results are given in Table 11.33.

**11.109** Perform a test to assess the significance of each of the risk factors after controlling for the other risk factors.

**11.110** Compute an odds ratio and an associated 95% confidence interval relating the presence or absence of each independent variable to the risk of malformations.

**11.111** How do you interpret the effect of marijuana usage on congenital malformations based on your findings in Problems 11.109 and 11.110?

# References

[1] Greene, J. and Touchstone, J. (1963) "Urinary Tract Estriol: An Index of Placental Function," *American Journal of Obstetrics and Gynecology* **85(1)**: 1–9.

[2] Higgins, M. and Keller, J. (1973) "Seven Measures of Ventilatory Lung Function," *American Review of Respiratory Disease* **108**: 258–272.

[3] Draper, N. and Smith, H. (1966) *Applied Regression Analysis* (New York: John Wiley).

[4] Kleinbaum, D. and Kupper, L. (1978) *Applied Regression Analysis and Other Multivariable Methods* (Boston: Duxbury Press).

[5] McCormack, W. M., Rosner, B., McComb, D. E., Evrard, J. R., and Zinner, S. H. (1985) "Infection with Chlamydia Trachomatis in Female College Students," *American Journal of Epidemiology* **121(1)**: 107–115.

[6] Apgar, V. (1953) "A Proposal for a New Method of Evaluation of the Newborn Infant," *Current Researches in Anesthesia and Analgesia* 260–267.

[7] Apgar, V. et al. (1958) "Evaluation of the Newborn Infant—Second Report," *Journal of American Medical Association* **168(15)**: 1985–1988.

[8] Landis, J. R. and Koch, G. G. (1977) "The Measurement of Observer Agreement for Categorical Data," *Biometrics* **33**: 159–174.

[9] Fleiss, J. L. (1981) *Statistical Methods for Rates and Proportions* (New York: John Wiley).

[10] Dec, G. W., Palacios, I. F., Fallon, J. T., Aretz, H. T., Mills, J., Lee, D. C. S., and Johnson,

R. A. (1985) "Active Myocarditis in the Spectrum of Acute Dilated Cardiomyopathies: Clinical Features, Histologic Correlates and Clinical Outcome," *New England Journal of Medicine* **312(14)**: 885–890.

[*11*] Torok-Storb, B., Doney, K., Sale, G., Thomas, E. D., and Storb, R. (1985) "Subsets of Patients with Aplastic Anemia Identified by Flow Microfluorometry," *New England Journal of Medicine* **312(16)**: 1015–1022.

[*12*] *Monthly Vital Statistics Report, Annual Summary* (1979). National Center for Health Statistics, Hyattsville, Maryland.

[*13*] Report of the Task Force on Blood Pressure Control in Children. (1977) *Pediatrics* **59** (5, part 2): 797–820.

[*14*] Burch, P. R. B. (1978) "Smoking and Lung Cancer: The Problem of Inferring Cause," *Journal of the Royal Statistical Society A* **141**: 437–477.

[*15*] Kuller, L. H., Hulley, S. B., Laporte, R. E., Neaton, J., and Dai, W. S. (1983) "Environmental Determinants, Liver Function, and High Density Lipoprotein Cholesterol Levels," *American Journal of Epidemiology* **117(4)**: 406–418.

[*16*] Schatzkin, A., Cupples, L. A., Heeren, T., Morelock, S., and Kannel, W. S. (1984) "Sudden Death in the Framingham Heart Study: Differences in Incidence and Risk Factors by Sex and Coronary Disease Status," *American Journal of Epidemiology* **120(6)**: 888–899.

[*17*] Chylack, L. T., Jr., White, O., and Tung, W. H. (1984) "Classification of Human Senile Cataractous Change by the American Cooperative Cataract Research Group (CCRG) Method: II. Staged Simplification of Cataract Classification," *Investigative Ophthalmology and Visual Science* **25**: 166–173.

[*18*] Linn, S., Schoenbaum, S. C., Monson, R. R., Rosner, B., Stubblefield, P. C., and Ryan, K. J. (1983) "The Association of Marijuana Use with Outcome of Pregnancy," *American Journal of Public Health* **73(10)**: 1161–1164.

# 12 Analysis of Variance

## ■ 12.1 INTRODUCTION

In Chapter 8 we were concerned with comparing the means of two normal distributions using the two-sample $t$ test for independent samples. Frequently, we are concerned with comparing the means of more than two distributions.

*Example 12.1*

**Pulmonary Disease** A topic of recent public health interest is whether or not *passive smoking* (i.e., exposure to cigarette smoke in the atmosphere among nonsmokers) has a measurable effect on pulmonary health. White and Froeb studied this question by measuring pulmonary function in several ways in the following six groups [1]:

1. **Nonsmokers (NS)** People who themselves did not smoke and were not exposed to cigarette smoke either at home or on the job.

2. **Passive Smokers (PS)** People who themselves did not smoke and were not exposed to cigarette smoke in the home, but were employed for 20 or more years in an enclosed working area that routinely contained tobacco smoke.

3. **Noninhaling Smokers (NI)** People who smoked pipes, cigars, or cigarettes, but who did not inhale.

4. **Light Smokers (LS)** People who smoked and inhaled 1–10 cigarettes per day for 20 or more years. (Note: There are 20 cigarettes in a pack.)

5. **Moderate Smokers (MS)** People who smoked and inhaled 11–39 cigarettes per day for 20 or more years.

6. **Heavy Smokers (HS)** People who smoked and inhaled 40 or more cigarettes per day for 20 or more years.

A principal measure used by the authors to assess pulmonary function was forced midexpiratory flow (FEF). The authors were interested in comparing FEF in the six groups.  ■

We shall see that the $t$ test methodology generalizes nicely in this case to a procedure referred to as the **one-way analysis of variance**.

In some instances the comparison groups can be classified in two different ways.

*Example 12.2*    **Cardiovascular Disease** Suppose we wish to look at the relationship between serum cholesterol level as measured in 1976 and oral contraceptive (OC) use as assessed at two different points in time (in 1973 and 1976). We can categorize women as OC users or non-OC users in 1976 and also as OC users or non-OC users in 1973. This classification might be useful if we wish to look at the effect of both current and past uses of OCs on serum cholesterol level.    ∎

In this type of example, when the groups can be classified in the form of a $2 \times 2$ contingency table, we shall see that the data can be analyzed by a technique known as the **two-way analysis of variance**.

# ∎ *12.2 ONE-WAY ANALYSIS OF VARIANCE—GENERAL MODEL*

*Example 12.3*    **Pulmonary Disease** Let us refer to Example 12.1. The authors were able to identify 200 males and 200 females in each of the six groups except for the NI group, which because of the small number of such people available, was limited to 50 males and 50 females. The mean and standard deviation of FEF for each of the six groups for males are presented in Table 12.1. How can we compare the means of these six groups?    ∎

Suppose that there are $k$ groups with $n_i$ observations in the $i$th group. Let us denote the $j$th observation in the $i$th group by $y_{ij}$. We will assume that the following model holds:

**12.1**
$$y_{ij} = \mu + \alpha_i + e_{ij}$$

where $\mu$ is a constant, $\alpha_i$ is a constant that is different for each group, and $e_{ij}$ is an error term, which is normally distributed with mean 0 and variance $\sigma^2$. The $\alpha_i$ are typically constrained in this model, so that the sum of the $\alpha_i$'s over all groups

**Table 12.1**
FEF data for smoking and nonsmoking males

| Group number, $i$ | Group name | Mean FEF ($l/s$) | sd FEF ($l/s$) | $n_i$ |
|---|---|---|---|---|
| 1 | NS | 3.78 | 0.79 | 200 |
| 2 | PS | 3.30 | 0.77 | 200 |
| 3 | NI | 3.32 | 0.86 | 50 |
| 4 | LS | 3.23 | 0.78 | 200 |
| 5 | MS | 2.73 | 0.81 | 200 |
| 6 | HS | 2.59 | 0.82 | 200 |

(Reprinted by permission of *The New England Journal of Medicine* **302 (13)**: 720–723, 1980.)

is 0. Thus, a typical observation from the $i$th group is normally distributed with mean $\mu + \alpha_i$ and variance $\sigma^2$.

---

**Definition 12.1**

We define the model given in **(12.1)** as a **one-way analysis of variance** or a **one-way ANOVA** model. This model will permit us to compare the means of an arbitrary number of groups, each of which follows a normal distribution. It will enable us to determine whether the variability in our data comes mostly from variability within groups or can truly be attributed to variability between groups.   ∎

We can interpret he parameters in **(12.1)** as follows:

**12.2**  *Interpretation of the Parameters of a One-Way Analysis of Variance Model*

> *1.* $\mu$ represents the underlying mean of all groups taken together.
>
> *2.* $\alpha_i$ represents the difference between the mean of the $i$th group and the overall mean.
>
> *3.* $e_{ij}$ represents random error about the mean $\mu + \alpha_i$ for an individual observation from the $i$th group.

---

# ■ *12.3 HYPOTHESIS TESTING IN ONE-WAY ANOVA*

Our null hypothesis ($H_0$) in this case is that the underlying mean FEF of each of the six groups is the same. This hypothesis is equivalent to stating that each $\alpha_i = 0$, since the $\alpha_i$ sum up to 0. Our alternative hypothesis ($H_1$) is that at least two of the group means are not the same. This hypothesis is equivalent to stating that at least one $\alpha_i \neq 0$. Thus, we wish to test the hypothesis $H_0$: all $\alpha_i = 0$ vs. $H_1$: at least one $\alpha_i \neq 0$.

## □ *12.3.1 F Test for Overall Comparison of Group Means*

Let us denote the mean FEF for the $i$th group by $\bar{y}_i$. Let us also denote the mean FEF over all groups by $\bar{\bar{y}}$. We can represent the deviation of an individual observation from the overall mean as

**12.3**
$$y_{ij} - \bar{\bar{y}} = (y_{ij} - \bar{y}_i) + (\bar{y}_i - \bar{\bar{y}})$$

---

The first term on the right-hand side $(y_{ij} - \bar{y}_i)$ represents the deviation of an individual observation from the group mean for that observation and is an indication of *within-group variability*. The second term on the right-hand side $(\bar{y}_i - \bar{\bar{y}})$ represents the deviation of a group mean from the overall mean and is an indication of *between-group variability*. These terms are depicted in Figure 12.1.

Generally speaking, if the between-group variability is large and the within-

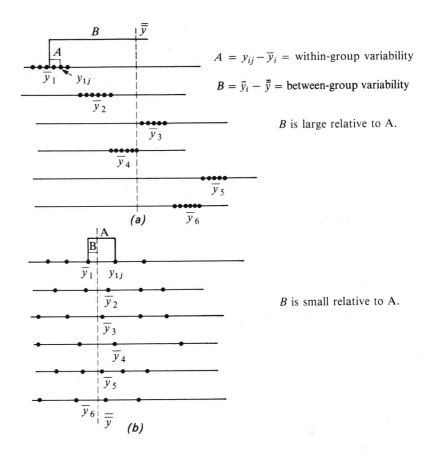

$A = y_{ij} - \bar{y}_i$ = within-group variability

$B = \bar{y}_i - \bar{\bar{y}}$ = between-group variability

$B$ is large relative to A.

$B$ is small relative to A.

**_Figure 12.1_**
_Comparison of
between-group and
within-group
variability_

group variability is small, as in Figure 12.1(a), then we will reject $H_0$ and declare that the underlying group means are significantly different. Conversely, if the between-group variability is small and the within-group variability is large, as in Figure 12.1(b), then we will accept $H_0$ that the underlying group means are the same.

If we square both sides of **(12.3)** and sum the squared deviations over all observations over all groups, then we obtain the relationship

**12.4**
$$\sum_{i=1}^{k} \sum_{j=1}^{n_i} (y_{ij} - \bar{\bar{y}})^2 = \sum_{i=1}^{k} \sum_{j=1}^{n_i} (y_{ij} - \bar{y}_i)^2 + \sum_{i=1}^{k} \sum_{j=1}^{n_i} (\bar{y}_i - \bar{\bar{y}})^2$$

**Definition 12.2**

We denote the term

$$\sum_{i=1}^{k} \sum_{j=1}^{n_i} (y_{ij} - \bar{\bar{y}})^2$$

as the **Total Sum of Squares (Total SS).** ∎

**Definition 12.3**

We denote the term

$$\sum_{i=1}^{k} \sum_{j=1}^{n_i} (y_{ij} - \bar{y}_i)^2$$

as the **Within Sum of Squares (Within SS)**.

**Definition 12.4**

We denote the term

$$\sum_{i=1}^{k} \sum_{j=1}^{n_i} (\bar{y}_i - \bar{\bar{y}})^2$$

as the **Between Sum of Squares (Between SS)**.

Thus, the relationship in **(12.4)** can be written as Total SS = Within SS + Between SS. The Within SS and Between SS play an analogous role to the Residual SS and Regression SS in linear regression analysis in Chapter 11.

It will be easier to use the short computational forms for the Within SS and Between SS in **(12.5)** for performing our hypothesis test.

**12.5** *Short Computational Forms for the Between SS and Within SS Based on Raw Data*

Let

$$y_{i.} = \sum_{j=1}^{k} y_{ij} = \text{sum of the observations in the } i\text{th group}$$

$$y_{..} = \sum_{i=1}^{k} \sum_{j=1}^{n_i} y_{ij} = \text{sum of the observations across all groups}$$

$$n = \sum_{i=1}^{k} n_i = \text{total number of observations over all groups}$$

The short computational forms are given as follows:

$$\text{Between SS} = \sum_{i=1}^{k} \frac{y_{i.}^2}{n_i} - \frac{y_{..}^2}{n}$$

$$\text{Total SS} = \sum_{i=1}^{k} \sum_{j=1}^{n_i} y_{ij}^2 - \frac{y_{..}^2}{n}$$

$$\text{Within SS} = \text{Total SS} - \text{Between SS}$$

This computational method is preferable if the raw data are available, since it minimizes roundoff error. This procedure is also used in most computer programs. Alternatively, if the raw data are not available, but rather the data are presented in terms of group means and variances, then we can use the following computational formula:

**12.6** **Short Computational Forms for the Between SS and Within SS Based on Grouped Data**

$$\text{Between SS} = \sum_{i=1}^{k} n_i \bar{y}_i^2 - \frac{\left( \sum_{i=1}^{k} n_i \bar{y}_i \right)^2}{n}$$

$$\text{Within SS} = \sum_{i=1}^{k} (n_i - 1) s_i^2$$

*Example 12.4*

**Pulmonary Disease** Compute the Within SS and Between SS for the FEF data in Table 12.1.

*Solution*

Since we are presented with grouped data, we use the computational form in **(12.6)**. We have

$$\text{Between SS} = [200(3.78)^2 + 200(3.30)^2 + \cdots + 200(2.59)^2$$

$$- \frac{[200(3.78) + 200(3.30) + \cdots + 200(2.59)]^2}{1050}$$

$$= 10{,}505.58 - (3292)^2/1050$$

$$= 10{,}505.58 - 10{,}321.20 = 184.38.$$

$$\text{Within SS} = 199(0.79)^2 + 199(0.77)^2 + 49(0.86)^2 + 199(0.78)^2$$

$$+ 199(0.81)^2 + 199(0.82)^2$$

$$= 124.20 + 117.99 + 36.24 + 121.07 + 130.56 + 133.81$$

$$= 663.87 \qquad\blacksquare$$

Finally, we have the following definitions

*Definition 12.5*

$$\textbf{Between Mean Square} = \textbf{Between MS} = \text{Between SS}/(k-1) \qquad\blacksquare$$

*Definition 12.6*

$$\textbf{Within Mean Square} = \textbf{Within MS} = \text{Within SS}/(n-k) \qquad\blacksquare$$

We will base our significance test on the ratio of the Between MS to the Within MS. If this ratio is large, then we will reject $H_0$; if it is small, we will accept $H_0$.

Thus, we will use the following test procedure for a level $\alpha$ test:

**12.7** **Overall F Test for One-Way ANOVA**

*1.* We compute the Between SS, Between MS, Within SS, and Within MS using either **(12.5)** or **(12.6)** and Definitions 12.5 and 12.6.

2. We compute the test statistic $\lambda = $ Between MS/Within MS, which follows an $F$ distribution with $k - 1$ and $n - k$ $df$ under $H_0$.

3. If

$$\lambda > F_{k-1,n-k,1-\alpha}$$

then we reject $H_0$. If

$$\lambda \leqslant F_{k-1,n-k,1-\alpha}$$

then we accept $H_0$.

4. The exact $p$-value is given by the area to the right of $\lambda$ under an $F_{k-1,n-k}$ distribution $= Pr(F_{k-1,n-k} > \lambda)$.

The acceptance and rejection regions for this test are depicted in Figure 12.2. The computation of the exact $p$-value is illustrated in Figure 12.3. The results from the analysis of variance are typically displayed in an ANOVA table, as in Table 12.2.

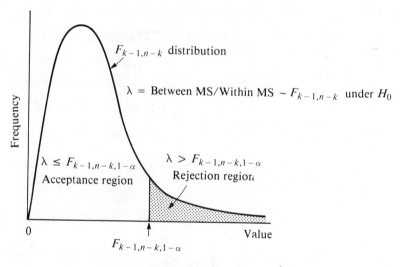

**Figure 12.2**
*Acceptance and rejection regions for the overall F test for one-way ANOVA*

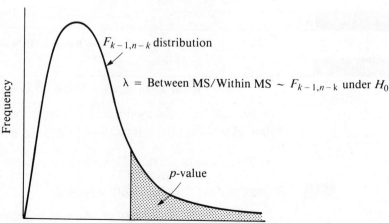

**Figure 12.3**
*Computation of the exact p-value for the overall F test for one-way ANOVA*

**Table 12.2**
*Display of one-way ANOVA results*

| Source of variation | SS | df | MS | F statistic | p-value |
|---|---|---|---|---|---|
| Between | $\displaystyle\sum_{i=1}^{k} \frac{y_{i.}^2}{n_i} - \frac{y_{..}^2}{n} = A$ | $k-1$ | $\dfrac{A}{k-1}$ | $\dfrac{A/(k-1)}{B/(n-k)} = \lambda$ | $Pr(F_{k-1,n-k} > \lambda)$ |
| Within | Total SS $-$ Between SS $= B$ | $n-k$ | $\dfrac{B}{n-k}$ | | |
| Total | $\displaystyle\sum_{i=1}^{k}\sum_{j=1}^{n_i} y_{ij}^2 - \frac{y_{..}^2}{n}$ | | | | |

**Example 12.5**

**Pulmonary Disease** Test if the mean FEF scores are significantly different in the six groups in Table 12.1.

**Solution**

We have from Example 12.4 that Between SS = 184.38 and Within SS = 663.87. Therefore, since there are 1050 observations combined over all groups, it follows that

$$\text{Between MS} = 184.38/5 = 36.876$$

$$\text{Within MS} = 663.87/(1050 - 6) = 663.87/1044 = 0.636$$

$$\lambda = \text{Between MS/Within MS} = 36.876/0.636 = 58.0 \sim F_{5,1044} \text{ under } H_0$$

We refer to Table 8 in the appendix and find that

$$F_{5,120,.999} = 4.42$$

Since

$$F_{5,1044,.999} < F_{5,120,.999} = 4.42 < 58.0 = \lambda$$

it follows that $p < 0.001$. Therefore, we can reject $H_0$ that all the means are equal and conclude that at least two of the means are not the same. These results are displayed in an ANOVA table (Table 12.3). ∎

**Table 12.3**
*ANOVA table for FEF data in Table 12.1*

| | SS | df | MS | F statistic | p-value |
|---|---|---|---|---|---|
| Between | 184.38 | 5 | 36.876 | 58.0 | $p < 0.001$ |
| Within | 663.87 | 1044 | 0.636 | | |
| Total | 848.25 | | | | |

# ■ 12.4 COMPARISONS OF SPECIFIC GROUPS IN ONE-WAY ANOVA

In the previous section we presented a test of the hypothesis $H_0$: all group means are equal vs. $H_1$: at least two group means are different. This test enables us to detect when at least two groups have different underlying means, but it does not allow us to state which of the groups have means that are different from each other. The usual practice is to perform the overall $F$ test just discussed. If we reject $H_0$, then we proceed to comparisons of specific groups, as discussed in this section.

## ☐ 12.4.1  t Test for Comparison of Pairs of Groups

Suppose we wish at this point to test if groups 1 and 2 have means that are significantly different from each other. From our underlying model in (12.1), we have that under either hypothesis

**12.8**

$\bar{y}_1$ is normally distributed with mean $\mu + \alpha_1$ and variance $\sigma^2/n_1$

and

$\bar{y}_2$ is normally distributed with mean $\mu + \alpha_2$ and variance $\sigma^2/n_2$

We shall use the difference of the sample means $(\bar{y}_1 - \bar{y}_2)$ as a test criterion. Thus, from (12.8) it follows that

**12.9**

$$\bar{y}_1 - \bar{y}_2 \sim N\left[\alpha_1 - \alpha_2, \sigma^2\left(\frac{1}{n_1} + \frac{1}{n_2}\right)\right]$$

However, under $H_0$, $\alpha_1 = \alpha_2$ and (12.9) reduces to

**12.10**

$$\bar{y}_1 - \bar{y}_2 \sim N\left[0, \sigma^2\left(\frac{1}{n_1} + \frac{1}{n_2}\right)\right]$$

If $\sigma^2$ were known, then we could divide by the standard error

**12.11**

$$\sigma\sqrt{\frac{1}{n_1} + \frac{1}{n_2}}$$

and obtain the test statistic

$$\delta^* = \frac{\bar{y}_1 - \bar{y}_2}{\sqrt{\sigma^2\left(\frac{1}{n_1} + \frac{1}{n_2}\right)}}$$

which would follow a $N(0, 1)$ distribution under $H_0$. Since $\sigma^2$ is in general unknown, we will substitute our best estimate of it, which we denote by $s^2$, and revise our test statistic accordingly.

How should we estimate $\sigma^2$? We recall that when we had to obtain a pooled estimate of the variance from two independent samples in Chapter 8, we used a weighted average of the sample variances from the individual samples, where the weights were the number of degrees of freedom in each sample. In particular, from **(8.9)** we used

$$s^2 = [(n_1 - 1)s_1^2 + (n_2 - 1)s_2^2]/(n_1 + n_2 - 2)$$

For the one-way ANOVA, we have $k$ sample variances and we use a similar approach to estimate $\sigma^2$ by computing a weighted average of $k$ individual sample variances, where the weights are the number of degrees of freedom in each of the $k$ samples. This formula is given as follows:

| **12.12** | **Pooled Estimate of the Variance for One-Way ANOVA** |
| --- | --- |

$$s^2 = \sum_{i=1}^{k} (n_i - 1)s_i^2 \Bigg/ \sum_{i=1}^{k} (n_i - 1) = \left[ \sum_{i=1}^{k} (n_i - 1)s_i^2 \right] \Bigg/ (n - k)$$

$$= \text{Within MS}$$

However, we note from **(12.6)**, **(12.12)**, and Definition 12.6 that this weighted average is the same as the Within MS. Thus, we use the Within MS to estimate $\sigma^2$. Note that $s^2$ had $(n_1 - 1) + (n_2 - 1) = n_1 + n_2 - 2 \; df$ in the two-sample case. Similarly, for the one-way ANOVA, $s^2$ has

$$(n_1 - 1) + (n_2 - 1) + \cdots + (n_k - 1) \, df = (n_1 + n_2 + \cdots + n_k) - k = n - k \, df$$

*Example 12.6*  **Pulmonary Disease** What is the best estimate of $\sigma^2$ for the FEF data in Table 12.1 and how many *df* does it have?

*Solution*  From Table 12.3 we see that our best estimate of the variance is the Within MS = 0.636, and it has $n - k \, df = 1044 \, df$. ∎

Hence, we will revise our test statistic in **(12.11)**, substituting $s^2$ for $\sigma^2$, with the new test statistic distributed as $t_{n-k}$ rather than $N(0, 1)$. The test procedure is given as follows:

| **12.13** | ***t* Test for the Comparison of Pairs of Groups in One-Way ANOVA** |
| --- | --- |

Suppose we wish to compare two specific groups, which we arbitrarily label as groups 1 and 2, among $k$ groups:

*1.* We compute the pooled estimate of the variance $s^2$ = Within MS from the one-way ANOVA.

*2.* We compute the test statistic

$$\delta = \frac{\bar{y}_1 - \bar{y}_2}{\sqrt{s^2\left(\dfrac{1}{n_1} + \dfrac{1}{n_2}\right)}}$$

which follows a $t_{n-k}$ distribution under $H_0$.

*3.* For a level $\alpha$ test, if

$$\delta > t_{n-k,1-\alpha/2} \qquad \text{or} \qquad \delta < t_{n-k,\alpha/2}$$

then we reject $H_0$; if

$$t_{n-k,\alpha/2} \leqslant \delta \leqslant t_{n-k,1-\alpha/2}$$

then we accept $H_0$.

*4.* The exact *p*-value is given by

$$p = 2 \times \text{the area to the left of } \delta \text{ under a } t_{n-k} \text{ distribution if } \delta < 0$$

$$= 2 \times Pr(t_{n-k} < \delta)$$

$$p = 2 \times \text{the area to the right of } \delta \text{ under a } t_{n-k} \text{ distribution if } \delta \geqslant 0$$

$$= 2 \times Pr(t_{n-k} > \delta).$$

The acceptance and rejection regions for this test are given in Figure 12.4. The computation of the exact *p*-value is illustrated in Figure 12.5.

---

**Example 12.7**    **Pulmonary Disease**  Compare each pair of groups for the FEF data in Table 12.1 and report any significant differences found.

**Solution**    We first plot the mean $\pm$ *se* of the FEF values for each of the six groups in Figure 12.6 to obtain some idea of the magnitude of the differences between groups. The standard error for an

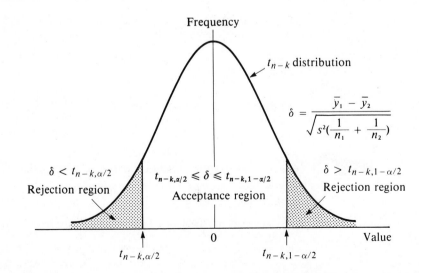

**Figure 12.4**
*Acceptance and rejection regions for the t test for the comparison of pairs of groups in one-way ANOVA*

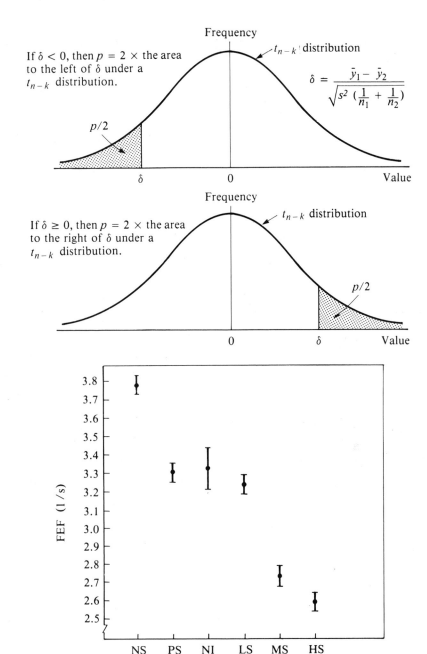

If $\delta < 0$, then $p = 2 \times$ the area to the left of $\delta$ under a $t_{n-k}$ distribution.

$$\delta = \frac{\bar{y}_1 - \bar{y}_2}{\sqrt{s^2 \left( \frac{1}{n_1} + \frac{1}{n_2} \right)}}$$

If $\delta \geq 0$, then $p = 2 \times$ the area to the right of $\delta$ under a $t_{n-k}$ distribution.

**Figure 12.5**

*Computation of the exact p-value for the t test for the comparison of pairs of groups in one-way ANOVA*

**Figure 12.6**

*Mean ± se for FEF for each of six smoking groups.*

(Reprinted by permission of the *New England Journal of Medicine* **302(13)**: 720–723, 1980.)

individual group mean is estimated by $s/\sqrt{n_i}$, where $s^2 =$ Within MS. Notice that the non-smokers have the best pulmonary function; the passive smokers, noninhaling smokers, and light smokers have about the same pulmonary function and are worse off than the non-smokers; and the moderate and heavy smokers have the poorest pulmonary function. Note also that the standard error bars are wider for the noninhaling smokers than for the other

**Table 12.4**

*t test results for comparisons of specific pairs of groups for FEF data in Table 12.1*

| Groups compared | Test statistic | p-value |
|---|---|---|
| NS, PS | $\delta = \dfrac{3.78 - 3.30}{\sqrt{0.636\left(\dfrac{1}{200} + \dfrac{1}{200}\right)}} = \dfrac{0.48}{0.08} = 6.00 \sim t_{1044}$ | $<0.001$ |
| NS, NI | $\delta = \dfrac{3.78 - 3.32}{\sqrt{0.636\left(\dfrac{1}{200} + \dfrac{1}{50}\right)}} = \dfrac{0.46}{0.126} = 3.65 \sim t_{1044}$ | $<0.001$ |
| NS, LS | $\delta = \dfrac{3.78 - 3.23}{\sqrt{0.636\left(\dfrac{1}{200} + \dfrac{1}{200}\right)}} = \dfrac{0.55}{0.08} = 6.88 \sim t_{1044}$ | $<0.001$ |
| NS, MS | $\delta = \dfrac{3.78 - 2.73}{0.080} = \dfrac{1.05}{0.08} = 13.13 \sim t_{1044}$ | $<0.001$ |
| NS, HS | $\delta = \dfrac{3.78 - 2.59}{0.080} = \dfrac{1.19}{0.08} = 14.88 \sim t_{1044}$ | $<0.001$ |
| PS, NI | $\delta = \dfrac{3.30 - 3.32}{0.126} = \dfrac{-0.02}{0.126} = -0.16 \sim t_{1044}$ | NS |
| PS, LS | $\delta = \dfrac{3.30 - 3.23}{0.080} = \dfrac{0.07}{0.08} = 0.88 \sim t_{1044}$ | NS |
| PS, MS | $\delta = \dfrac{3.30 - 2.73}{0.080} = \dfrac{0.57}{0.08} = 7.13 \sim t_{1044}$ | $<0.001$ |
| PS, HS | $\delta = \dfrac{3.30 - 2.59}{0.080} = \dfrac{0.71}{0.08} = 8.88 \sim t_{1044}$ | $<0.001$ |
| NI, LS | $\delta = \dfrac{3.32 - 3.23}{0.126} = \dfrac{0.09}{0.126} = 0.71 \sim t_{1044}$ | NS |
| NI, MS | $\delta = \dfrac{3.32 - 2.73}{0.126} = \dfrac{0.59}{0.126} = 4.68 \sim t_{1044}$ | $<0.001$ |
| NI, HS | $\delta = \dfrac{3.32 - 2.59}{0.126} = \dfrac{0.73}{0.126} = 5.79 \sim t_{1044}$ | $<0.001$ |
| LS, MS | $\delta = \dfrac{3.23 - 2.73}{0.08} = \dfrac{0.50}{0.08} = 6.25 \sim t_{1044}$ | $<0.001$ |
| LS, HS | $\delta = \dfrac{3.23 - 2.59}{0.08} = \dfrac{0.64}{0.08} = 8.00 \sim t_{1044}$ | $<0.001$ |
| MS, HS | $\delta = \dfrac{2.73 - 2.59}{0.08} = \dfrac{0.14}{0.08} = 1.75 \sim t_{1044}$ | NS |

groups, since this group has only 50 persons compared with 200 for all other groups. Let us see if the observed differences in the figure are statistically significant as assessed by the $t$ test procedure in **(12.13)**. The results are presented in Table 12.4.

We see that there are very highly significant differences (1) between the nonsmokers and all other groups, (2) between the passive smokers and the moderate and heavy smokers, (3) between the noninhalers and the moderate and heavy smokers, and (4) between the light smokers and the moderate and heavy smokers. There are no significant differences between the passive smokers, noninhalers, and light smokers and no significant differences between the moderate and heavy smokers, although there is a trend toward significance with the latter comparison. Thus, these results tend to confirm what we saw in the figure. They are very interesting because they show that the pulmonary function of passive smokers is significantly worse than that of nonsmokers and is essentially the same as that of noninhaling and light inhaling smokers ($\leqslant \frac{1}{2}$ pack cigarettes per day). In this case we have used the $N(0, 1)$ distribution to evaluate the $p$-values in Table 12.4, since the $t_{1044}$ and the $N(0, 1)$ distributions are essentially identical, and we have a table of $N(0, 1)$ percentiles in Table 3 in the appendix. ∎

A frequent error in performing the $t$ test in **(12.13)** when comparing groups 1 and 2 is to use only the sample variances from *these two groups* rather than from *all $k$ groups* to estimate $\sigma^2$. If we use the sample variances from only two groups, then we get different estimates of $\sigma^2$ for each pair of groups considered, which is not reasonable because *all* the groups have the same underlying variance $\sigma^2$. Furthermore, the estimate of $\sigma^2$ obtained by using all $k$ groups will be more accurate than that obtained from using any two groups, since the estimate of the variance will be based on more information. This is the principal advantage of performing the $t$ tests in the framework of a one-way ANOVA rather than by considering each pair of groups separately and performing $t$ tests for two independent samples as given in **(8.10)** for each pair of samples.

## ☐ 12.4.2  Linear Contrasts

In Section 12.4.1 we developed methods for comparing specific groups within the context of the analysis of variance. We frequently desire more general comparisons, such as the comparison of a collection of $\ell_1$ groups with another collection of $\ell_2$ groups.

*Example 12.8*    **Pulmonary Disease**  Suppose we wish to compare the pulmonary function of the group of smokers who inhale cigarettes with the group of nonsmokers. We could just combine the three groups of inhaling smokers in Table 12.1 to form one group of 600 inhaling smokers. However, these three groups were selected so as to be of the same size whereas in the general population the proportions of light, moderate, and heavy smokers is not likely to be the same. Suppose we know from large population surveys that 70% of inhaling smokers are moderate smokers, 20% are heavy smokers, and 10% are light smokers. How can we compare inhaling smokers as a group with nonsmokers? ∎

It is for this type of question that we shall study the estimation and testing of hypotheses for linear contrasts.

**Definition 12.7**

A **linear contrast** ($L$) is any linear combination of the individual group means such that the linear coefficients add up to 0. Specifically,

$$L = \sum_{i=1}^{k} \lambda_i \bar{y}_i$$

where

$$\sum_{i=1}^{k} \lambda_i = 0$$    ∎

Notice that the comparison of two means that we considered in the previous section is a special case of a linear contrast.

*Example 12.9*

**Pulmonary Disease** Suppose we wish to compare the pulmonary function of the nonsmokers and passive smokers. Represent this comparison as a linear contrast.

*Solution*

Since the nonsmokers are the first group and the passive smokers are the second group, we can represent this comparison by the linear contrast

$$L = \bar{y}_1 - \bar{y}_2$$

that is,

$$\lambda_1 = +1 \qquad \lambda_2 = -1$$    ∎

*Example 12.10*

**Pulmonary Disease** Suppose we wish to compare the pulmonary function of nonsmokers with that of the total group of inhaling smokers, assuming that 10% of inhaling smokers are light smokers, 70% are moderate smokers, and 20% are heavy smokers. Represent this comparison as a linear contrast.

*Solution*

We can represent this comparison by the linear contrast

$$\bar{y}_1 - 0.1\bar{y}_4 - 0.7\bar{y}_5 - 0.2\bar{y}_6$$

since the nonsmokers are group 1, the light smokers group 4, the moderate smokers group 5, and the heavy smokers group 6.    ∎

How can we test if a linear contrast is different from 0? In general, for any linear contrast,

$$L = \lambda_1 \bar{y}_1 + \lambda_2 \bar{y}_2 + \cdots + \lambda_k \bar{y}_k$$

We wish to test the hypothesis $H_0: \mu_L = 0$ vs. $H_1: \mu_L \neq 0$, where $\mu_L$ is the mean of the linear contrast $L$:

$$\lambda_1 \alpha_1 + \lambda_2 \alpha_2 + \cdots + \lambda_k \alpha_k$$

We can show that the following test procedure can be used, which is analogous to the *t* test for pairs of groups in **(12.13)**.

**12.14**    *t Test for Linear Contrasts in One-Way ANOVA*

Suppose we wish to test if the mean of a specific linear contrast $L$ is significantly different from 0.

*1.* We compute the pooled estimate of the variance $s^2 = $ Within MS from the one-way ANOVA.

*2.* We compute the linear contrast

$$L = \sum_{i=1}^{k} \lambda_i \bar{x}_i$$

3. We compute the test statistic

$$T = \frac{L}{\sqrt{s^2 \sum_{i=1}^{k} \frac{\lambda_i^2}{n_i}}}$$

4. If

$$T > t_{n-k, 1-\alpha/2} \quad \text{or} \quad T < t_{n-k, \alpha/2}$$

then we reject $H_0$. If

$$t_{n-k, \alpha/2} \leqslant T \leqslant t_{n-k, 1-\alpha/2}$$

then we accept $H_0$.

5. The exact $p$-value is given by

$p = 2 \times$ the area to the left of $T$ under a $t_{n-k}$ distribution if $T < 0 = 2 \times Pr(t_{n-k} < T)$

$p = 2 \times$ the area to the right of $T$ under a $t_{n-k}$ distribution if $T \geqslant 0 = 2 \times Pr(t_{n-k} > T)$

---

**Example 12.11**  **Pulmonary Disease** Test the hypothesis that the linear contrast defined in Example 12.10 is significantly different from 0.

**Solution**  We have $s^2 = 0.636$ from Table 12.3. Furthermore, the linear contrast $L$ is given by

$$L = \bar{y}_1 - 0.1\bar{y}_4 - 0.7\bar{y}_5 - 0.2\bar{y}_6 = 3.78 - 0.1(3.23) - 0.7(2.73) - 0.2(2.59) = 1.03$$

The standard error of this linear contrast is given by

$$se(L) = \sqrt{s^2 \sum_{i=1}^{k} \frac{\lambda_i^2}{n_i}}$$

$$= \sqrt{(0.636)\left[\frac{(1)^2}{200} + \frac{(-0.1)^2}{200} + \frac{(-0.7)^2}{200} + \frac{(-0.2)^2}{200}\right]} = 0.070$$

Thus,

$$T = L/se(L) = 1.03/0.070 = 14.71 \sim t_{1044} \text{ under } H_0$$

Clearly, this linear contrast is very highly significant ($p < 0.001$), and the inhaling smokers as a group have strikingly poorer pulmonary function than the nonsmokers. ∎

Another useful application of linear contrasts is when the different groups correspond to different dose levels of a particular quantity, and the coefficients of the contrast are chosen to reflect a particular dose-response relationship. This application is particularly useful if the sample sizes of the individual groups are small and a comparison of any pair of groups does not show a significant difference, but the overall trend is consistent in one direction.

**Example 12.12**  **Pulmonary Disease** Suppose we wish to study whether or not the amount of smoke inhaled is related to level of FEF among those smokers who inhale cigarettes. Perform a test of significance for this trend.

**Solution**

We focus on the light smokers, moderate smokers, and heavy smokers in this analysis. We know that the light smokers smoke from 1 to 10 cigarettes per day, and we will assume that they smoke an average of $(1 + 10)/2 = 5.5$ cigarettes per day. We know that the moderate smokers smoke from 11 to 39 cigarettes per day, and we will assume they smoke an average of $(11 + 39)/2 = 25$ cigarettes per day. The heavy smokers smoke at least 40 cigarettes per day. We will assume that they smoke exactly 40 cigarettes per day, which will underestimate the trend but is the best we can do with the information presented. We wish to test the contrast

$$L = 5.5\bar{y}_4 + 25\bar{y}_5 + 40\bar{y}_6$$

for statistical significance. The problem is that the coefficients of this contrast do not add up to 0; indeed, they add up to $5.5 + 25 + 40 = 70.5$. However, if we subtract $70.5/3 = 23.5$ from each coefficient, then they will add up to 0. Thus, we wish to test the contrast

$$L = (5.5 - 23.5)\bar{y}_4 + (25 - 23.5)\bar{y}_5 + (40 - 23.5)\bar{y}_6 = -18\bar{y}_4 + 1.5\bar{y}_5 + 16.5\bar{y}_6$$

for statistical significance. This contrast represents the increasing number of cigarettes per day smoked in the three groups. We have from **(12.14)** that

$$L = -18(3.23) + 1.5(2.73) + 16.5(2.59) = -58.14 + 4.10 + 42.74 = -11.30$$

$$se(L) = \sqrt{0.636\left[\frac{(-18)^2}{200} + \frac{(1.5)^2}{200} + \frac{(16.5)^2}{200}\right]} = \sqrt{0.636(2.99)} = \sqrt{1.902} = 1.38$$

Thus,

$$T = L/se(L) = -11.30/1.38 = -8.19 \sim t_{1044} \text{ under } H_0$$

Clearly, this trend is very highly significant ($p < 0.001$), and we can say that among smokers who inhale, the greater the number of cigarettes smoked per day, the worse the pulmonary function. ∎

### □ *12.4.3 Multiple Comparisons*

In many studies the comparisons of interest are specified before looking at the actual data, in which case the $t$ test procedure in **(12.13)** and the linear contrast procedure in **(12.14)** are appropriate. In other instances the comparisons of interest will only be specified after looking at the data. In this case a large number of potential comparisons are often possible. Specifically, if we have a large number of groups and we compare every pair of groups using the $t$ test procedure in **(12.13)**, then we are likely to find some significant differences just by chance.

*Example 12.13*

Suppose we have 10 groups. Thus, there are $\binom{10}{2} = 45$ possible pairs of groups to be compared. Using a 5% level of significance would imply that $0.05(45)$, or about two comparisons, are likely to be significant by chance alone. How can we protect ourselves against the detection of falsely significant differences resulting from making too many comparisons? ∎

Several procedures, referred to as **multiple comparisons procedures,** ensure that we do not declare too many falsely significant differences. The basic idea of these procedures is to ensure that the *overall probability of declaring any significant differences between all possible pairs of groups* is maintained at some fixed significance level (say $\alpha$). One such procedure that we will study here is called the **Newman–Keuls procedure,** which is in common use today. We will not discuss the several other multiple-comparison procedures for one-way ANOVA. (See Kleinbaum and Kupper for more details [2].)

To use this procedure, we need to learn how to use the studentized range statistic.

<hr>

**Definition 12.8**

Suppose we have a group of $c$ means, the largest of which is $\bar{y}_1$ with sample size $n_1$ and the smallest of which is $\bar{y}_2$ with sample size $n_2$. The $c$ means can be either all the means or a subset of the means identified in a one-way ANOVA problem. Let $s^2 =$ Within MS from the one-way ANOVA. The **studentized range statistic** $q$ for this group of means is defined by

$$q = \frac{\bar{y}_1 - \bar{y}_2}{\sqrt{\dfrac{s^2}{2}\left(\dfrac{1}{n_1} + \dfrac{1}{n_2}\right)}}$$

∎

The basic idea for using this statistic is that if $q$ is sufficiently small, then all of the means in the group are considered equal; otherwise, some of the means are considered significantly different. Table 13 gives the 5th and 1st percentiles of the studentized range statistic for varying values of $c =$ the number of means in the group and $d =$ the number of degrees of freedom for $s^2$. The appropriate critical value in the table is found in the $c$th column and the $d$th row of the table.

<hr>

**Definition 12.9**

We denote the *upper $\alpha$ percentile of the studentized range statistic* based on $c$ means, where the Within MS has $d$ degrees of freedom by $q_{c,d,1-\alpha}$.

∎

Thus, $q_{c,d,1-\alpha}$ is found in the entry at the $c$th column and $d$th row of the table for either $\alpha = 0.05$ or $\alpha = 0.01$.

*Example 12.14*    Find the upper 5% point of the studentized range statistic based on four means, where the Within MS is based on 10 *df.*

*Solution*    We refer to the 4th column and the 10th row in the $\alpha = 0.05$ table. We find that $q_{4,10,.95} = 4.33$.

∎

The basic strategy for declaring whether a group of $c$ means is significantly different or not is summarized as follows:

**12.15    *Use of the Studentized Range Statistic to Decide Whether a Group of Means Is Significantly Different***

If we have a group of $c$ means, the largest of which is $\bar{y}_1$ with sample size $n_1$ and the smallest of which is $\bar{y}_2$ with sample size $n_2$, and a Within MS $= s^2$ with $d$ degrees of freedom, then:

1. We compute

$$q = \frac{\bar{y}_1 - \bar{y}_2}{\sqrt{\dfrac{s^2}{2}\left(\dfrac{1}{n_1} + \dfrac{1}{n_2}\right)}}$$

2. For a level $\alpha$ test, if

$$q \leq q_{c,d,1-\alpha}$$

then we declare *all* the means in the group as *not significantly different*; if

$$q > q_{c,d,1-\alpha}$$

then we declare *some* of the means in the group as *significantly different*.

---

*Example 12.15*

Suppose we have a group of three means, the largest of which is 28.0 based on a sample of size 10 and the smallest of which is 15.0 based on a sample of size 5. Suppose also that the Within MS = 72 based on 20 df. Test if the means when considered as a group are significantly different at the 5% level.

*Solution*

We compute the studentized range statistic as follows:

$$q = \frac{28 - 15}{\sqrt{\dfrac{72}{2}\left(\dfrac{1}{10} + \dfrac{1}{5}\right)}} = \frac{13.0}{3.286} = 3.96$$

We find $q_{3,20,.95}$ from the 3 column and 20 row of the 5% table = 3.58. Since $q = 3.96 > 3.58$, we declare that some of the three means in this group are significantly different. ∎

Notice that from Table 13 the larger the number of means in the group, the more difficult it is to declare significant differences among means.

*Example 12.16*

Suppose our group in Example 12.15 consisted of five means rather than three means. Test if the means when considered as a group are significantly different.

*Solution*

We find $q_{5,20,.95}$ from the 5 column and 20 row of the table = 4.23. Since $q = 3.96 < 4.23$, we would declare that the group of five means is *not* significantly different. ∎

We still have the problem that if we decide from **(12.15)** that a *group* of means is significantly different, then we still do not know which means are actually different. We need a unified strategy for dealing with the problem of deciding which of $k$ means in a one-way ANOVA setting are significantly different. This strategy is given by the following Newman–Keuls multiple comparisons procedure:

### 12.16    *Newman–Keuls Multiple Comparisons Procedure*

*1.* Rank order the $k$ group means from smallest to largest and renumber the groups so that group 1 has the smallest mean, group 2 has the next smallest mean, . . . , and group $k$ has the largest mean.

*2.* For a level $\alpha$ test, compare the entire group of $k$ means using the studentized range procedure in **(12.15)** with significance level $\alpha$. If all means in the group are not significantly different, then stop; otherwise, go on to step 3.

*3.* Compare all possible subgroups of $(k-1)$ means using **(12.15)**. If *all* subgroups of $(k-1)$ means are not significantly different, then stop; otherwise, go on to step 4.

*4.* Compare all possible subgroups of $(k-2)$ means within the groups of $(k-1)$ means that were declared significantly different in step 3. If all such subgroups of $(k-2)$ means are not significantly different, then stop; otherwise, go on to step 5.

*5.* We continue this process until we are comparing subgroups of two means or until we have stopped at an earlier step. Notice that because of this procedure, any two means will be considered significantly different only if all subgroups of means that contain these two means are also declared significantly different at an earlier step of the procedure.

---

*Example 12.17*

**Pulmonary Disease** Perform a significance test at the 5% level for all pairs of means in the FEF data of Table 12.1 using the Newman–Keuls multiple comparisons procedure.

*Solution*

First, we renumber the groups from smallest to largest. Thus, we have the renumbered group means as shown in Table 12.5. Furthermore, the Within MS = 0.636 with 1044 *df* from Table 12.3. We will use the row marked $\infty$ *df* in Table 13 and $\alpha = 0.05$ for simplicity, since the actual percentiles for 1044 *df* will be close to these percentiles. (We could actually use harmonic interpolation, as we did for the $F$ distribution in **(8.14)**, to obtain the exact percentiles.) We first compare the entire group of six means. We have

$$q = \frac{3.78 - 2.59}{\sqrt{\dfrac{0.636}{2}\left(\dfrac{1}{200} + \dfrac{1}{200}\right)}} = \frac{1.19}{0.0564} = 21.1$$

We refer to $q_{6,\infty,.95} = 4.03$. Since $21.1 > 4.03$, we declare that some of the six means are significantly different. We next compare subgroups of five means. We start by comparing groups 1–5. We have

$$q = \frac{3.32 - 2.59}{\sqrt{\dfrac{0.636}{2}\left(\dfrac{1}{200} + \dfrac{1}{50}\right)}} = \frac{0.73}{0.0892} = 8.18$$

*Table 12.5*

Renumbered group means of FEF data for use with the Newman–Keuls procedure

| Group number | Group name | Mean $(\bar{y}_i)$ | Number in group $(n_i)$ |
|---|---|---|---|
| 1 | HS | 2.59 | 200 |
| 2 | MS | 2.73 | 200 |
| 3 | LS | 3.23 | 200 |
| 4 | PS | 3.30 | 200 |
| 5 | NI | 3.32 | 50 |
| 6 | NS | 3.78 | 200 |

(Reprinted with permission of *The New England Journal of Medicine* **302** (13): 720–723, 1980.)

We compare this value with $q_{5,\infty,.95} = 3.86$. Since $8.18 > 3.86$, we declare that some of these five means are significantly different. Similarly, we compare groups 2–6. We have

$$q = \frac{3.78 - 2.73}{0.0564} = 18.6 > q_{5,\infty,.95} = 3.86$$

Thus, some of the means in groups 2–6 are significantly different as well. We now focus on subgroups of four means. We will test groups 1–4, 2–5, and 3–6. We have the following test statistics:

$$\text{Groups 1–4: } q = \frac{3.30 - 2.59}{0.0564} = 12.6 > q_{4,\infty,.95} = 3.63$$

$$\text{Groups 2–5: } q = \frac{3.32 - 2.73}{0.0892} = 6.61 > 3.63$$

$$\text{Groups 3–6: } q = \frac{3.78 - 3.23}{0.0564} = 9.75 > 3.63$$

Thus each of these subgroups of means contains means that are significantly different.

We now focus on subgroups of three means. We will test groups 1–3, 2–4, 3–5, and 4–6. We have the following test statistics:

$$\text{Groups 1–3: } q = \frac{3.23 - 2.59}{0.0564} = 11.3 > q_{3,\infty,.95} = 3.31$$

$$\text{Groups 2–4: } q = \frac{3.30 - 2.73}{0.0564} = 10.1 > 3.31$$

$$\text{Groups 3–5: } q = \frac{3.32 - 3.23}{0.0892} = 1.01 < 3.31$$

$$\text{Groups 4–6: } q = \frac{3.78 - 3.30}{0.0564} = 8.51 > 3.31$$

Thus some means in groups 1–3, 2–4, and 4–6 are significantly different but none in groups 3–5. Finally, we look at subgroups of two means within the groups 1–3, 2–4, or 4–6 but *not* within the groups 3–5. Therefore, we will test groups 1–2, 2–3, and 5–6 but not 3–4 or 4–5, since these groups are contained in groups 3–5, which have already been declared not significantly different. We have the following test statistics:

$$\text{Groups 1–2: } q = \frac{2.73 - 2.59}{0.0564} = 2.48 < q_{2,\infty,.95} = 2.77$$

$$\text{Groups 2–3: } q = \frac{3.23 - 2.73}{0.0564} = 8.87 > 2.77$$

$$\text{Groups 5–6: } q = \frac{3.78 - 3.32}{0.0892} = 5.16 > 2.77$$

Thus groups 2–3 and 5–6 are significantly different, whereas groups 1–2 are not. Thus our conclusion is that there are three distinct groups of means, groups 1–2, 3–5, and 6. The means are not significantly different within groups but are significantly different between groups. The results of the multiple comparisons procedure are typically displayed as in Figure 12.7. A line

**Figure 12.7**

*Display of results of Newman– Keuls multiple comparisons procedure on FEF data in Table 12.1.*

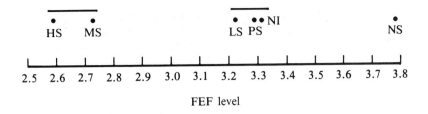

is drawn between the names or numbers of each pair of means that are *not* significantly different. This line enables us to visually summarize the results of many comparisons of pairs of means in one concise display. ∎

Note that the results of our *t* tests in Table 12.4 and our multiple comparisons procedures in Example 12.17 are the same. Namely, we have three distinct groups of persons: heavy and moderate smokers; light smokers, passive smokers, and noninhaling smokers; and nonsmokers. In general, the multiple comparison procedures are more strict than the ordinary *t* tests if we are comparing more than two means. That is, there are comparisons between pairs of groups for which the *t* test would declare a significant difference but the multiple comparisons procedure would not. This is the price we pay for trying to fix the $\alpha$ level of finding *any* significant difference among pairs of groups in using the multiple comparisons procedure rather than for *particular* pairs of groups in using the *t* test. If we are comparing only two means, then the *p*-values obtained from using the two procedures are identical.

We also note from Example 12.17 that the further apart two means are in the rank ordering of means, the larger our critical value for declaring significance. Thus if there are two means between our pair of means considered, then the critical value is 2.77, whereas if there are three means, then the critical value is 3.31, and so forth. This property illustrates another difference between the procedures, since for the *t* test in **(12.13)**, the same critical value is used $(t_{n-k, 1-\alpha/2})$ regardless of how many means are between the pair of means considered.

When should we use the more conservative multiple comparisons procedure in **(12.16)** rather than the *t* test procedure in **(12.13)** to identify specific differences between groups? This area is controversial. Some research workers routinely use multiple comparisons procedures for all one-way ANOVA problems; others never use them. My opinion is that multiple comparisons procedures should be used if there are many groups and not all comparisons between individual groups have been thought out in advance. On the other hand, if there are relatively few groups and only specific comparisons of interest are intended, which have been thought out in advance, then I prefer to use ordinary *t* tests rather than multiple comparison procedures.

# ∎ *12.5 BARTLETT'S TEST FOR HOMOGENEITY OF VARIANCE*

In our previous work on the analysis of variance, we *assumed in the underlying model in* **(12.1)** *that the population variances of the k groups are the same.* This assumption should be tested before using the analysis of variance, and in this section we present a test for the homogeneity of variance over $k$ groups.

We have already studied the $F$ test for the equality of two variances given in Section 8.4.3. The test presented here is a generalization of this test to the $k$ group situation. We wish to test the hypothesis $H_0: \sigma_1^2 = \sigma_2^2 = \cdots = \sigma_k^2$ vs. $H_1$: at least two of the $\sigma_i^2$ are unequal. Let $s_i^2 =$ sample variance of the $i$th group and let $s^2 =$ Within Mean Square from the one-way ANOVA table, which represents our best estimate of the common variance $\sigma^2$ under $H_0$. Our test will be based on deviations of the individual sample variances $s_i^2$ from $s^2$. Specifically, Bartlett devised a test based on the deviations of each of the $\log(s_i^2)$ from $\log(s^2)$. If these deviations are large, then we reject $H_0$; otherwise, we accept $H_0$. In particular, Bartlett has shown that the following test procedure can be used:

---

**12.17**    **Bartlett's Test for the Homogeneity of Variances**

If we wish to test the hypothesis $H_0: \sigma_1^2 = \sigma_2^2 = \cdots = \sigma_k^2$ vs. $H_1$: at least two of the $\sigma_i^2$ are unequal, then:

**1.** Compute the test statistic $\lambda^* = \lambda/c$, which follows a $\chi_{k-1}^2$ distribution under $H_0$, where

$$\lambda = 2.326 \sum_{i=1}^{k} (n_i - 1) \log_{10}\left(\frac{s^2}{s_i^2}\right) = \sum_{i=1}^{k} (n_i - 1) \ln\left(\frac{s^2}{s_i^2}\right)$$

$$c = 1 + \frac{1}{3(k-1)}\left[\left(\sum_{i=1}^{k} \frac{1}{n_i - 1}\right) - \frac{1}{n-k}\right]$$

$$s_i^2 = \text{sample variance of the } i\text{th group}$$

$$s^2 = \text{Within MS from the one-way ANOVA}$$

**2.** If

$$\lambda^* > \chi_{k-1,1-\alpha}^2$$

then we reject $H_0$; if

$$\lambda^* \leqslant \chi_{k-1,1-\alpha}^2$$

then we accept $H_0$.

**3.** The exact $p$-value is given by $p =$ the area to the right of $\lambda^*$ under a $\chi_{k-1}^2$ distribution $= Pr(\chi_{k-1}^2 > \lambda^*)$.

The acceptance and rejection regions for this test are depicted in Figure 12.8. The computation of the exact $p$-value is given in Figure 12.9.

---

**Example 12.18**    **Pulmonary Disease** Test for the homogeneity of variances for the FEF data in Table 12.1.

**Solution**    We have from Table 12.1 that

$$s_1 = 0.79, \quad s_2 = 0.77, \quad s_3 = 0.86, \quad s_4 = 0.78, \quad s_5 = 0.81, \quad s_6 = 0.82$$

$$n_1 = n_2 = n_4 = n_5 = n_6 = 200 \quad \text{and} \quad n_3 = 50$$

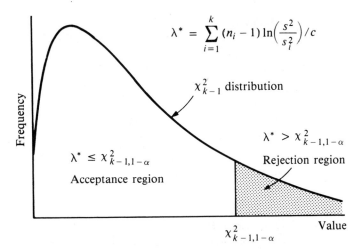

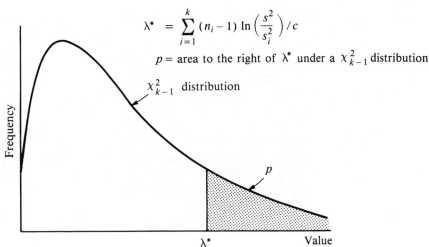

**Figure 12.8**
*Acceptance and rejection regions for Bartlett's test for the homogeneity of variances*

**Figure 12.9**
*Computation of the exact p-value for Bartlett's test for the homogeneity of variances*

Furthermore, from Table 12.3 we have

$$s^2 = 0.636 = (0.797)^2$$

Thus,

$$\lambda = 2.326 \left[ 199 \log_{10} \left( \frac{0.797}{0.79} \right)^2 + 199 \log_{10} \left( \frac{0.797}{0.77} \right)^2 + 49 \log_{10} \left( \frac{0.797}{0.86} \right)^2 \right.$$

$$\left. + 199 \log_{10} \left( \frac{0.797}{0.78} \right)^2 + 199 \log_{10} \left( \frac{0.797}{0.81} \right)^2 + 199 \log_{10} \left( \frac{0.797}{0.82} \right)^2 \right]$$

$$= 2.326[199(0.008) + 199(0.030) + 49(-0.066) + 199(0.019) + 199(-0.014)$$

$$+ 199(-0.025)]$$

$$= 2.326(1.592 + 5.970 - 3.234 + 3.781 - 2.786 - 4.975)$$

$$= 2.326(0.348) = 0.809$$

Furthermore,

$$c = 1 + \frac{1}{3(5)}\left[\frac{1}{199} + \frac{1}{199} + \frac{1}{49} + \frac{1}{199} + \frac{1}{199} + \frac{1}{199} - \frac{1}{1044}\right] = 1 + \frac{1}{15}(0.045)$$

$$= 1.003$$

Thus,

$$\lambda^* = 0.809/1.003 = 0.807 \sim \chi_5^2 \text{ under } H_0$$

From Table 6 we see that

$$\chi_{5,.95}^2 = 11.07 > 0.807 = \lambda^*$$

Thus, we accept $H_0$ that the variances are *not* significantly different. This result justifies our use of the one-way ANOVA procedure on these data.  ∎

    The question arises as to what can be done in comparing the means of $k$ groups if the variances *are* found to be significantly different using Bartlett's test. One possibility is to rescale the data using either a log or another transformation in an attempt to make the variances of the groups more homogeneous. Also such a transformation often has the effect of stabilizing the underlying distribution and making the data appear more bell shaped or at least more symmetric. If there is still a demonstrated heterogeneity of variances after transforming the data or if transforming the data does not seem advisable, then we can compare the groups in a pairwise fashion using $t$ tests with either equal or unequal variances, as given in Chapter 8, since there is no obvious advantage in considering the $k$ groups together. The general procedure for comparing the means of $k$ independent samples is summarized in Figure 12.10.

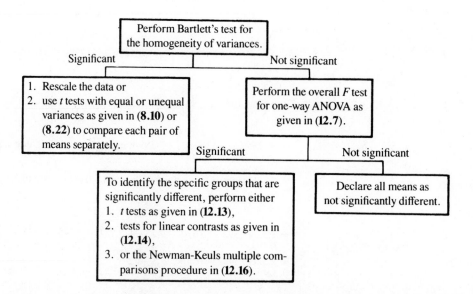

**Figure 12.10**

*General procedure for comparing the means of k independent normally distributed samples*

# ■ *12.6 THE KRUSKAL–WALLIS TEST*

In some instances we wish to compare means among more than two samples, but either our underlying distribution is far from being normal or we have ordinal data. In these cases we need to develop a nonparametric alternative to the one-way ANOVA described previously in this chapter.

*Example 12.19*    **Ophthalmology**   Arachidonic acid is well known to have an effect on ocular metabolism. In particular, topical application of arachidonic acid has caused lid closure, itching, and ocular discharge, among other effects. A study was conducted to compare the anti-inflammatory effects of four different drugs in Albino rabbits after administration of arachidonic acid [3]. For all groups the anti-inflammatory agent was administered to one eye and a saline solution was administered to the other eye. Ten minutes later arachidonic acid (sodium arachidonate) was delivered to both eyes. Both eyes were evaluated every 15 minutes thereafter for lid closure. At each assessment the lids of both eyes were examined and a lid closure score from 0–3 was determined, where $0$ = eye completely open, $3$ = eye completely closed, and $1, 2$ = intermediate states. The measure of effectiveness ($x$) is the change in lid closure scores (from baseline to follow-up) in the treated eye minus the change in lid closure scores in the saline eye. A high value for $x$ is indicative of an effective drug. The data, after 15 minutes of follow-up, are presented in Table 12.6. Since the scale of measurement was ordinal (0, 1, 2, 3), the use of a nonparametric technique to compare the four treatment groups is appropriate.   ■

We would like to generalize the Wilcoxon rank sum test to enable us to compare more than two samples. To accomplish this aim, we pool the observations in all treatment groups and assign ranks to each observation in the combined sample. We then compare the average ranks ($\bar{R}_i$) in the individual treatment groups. If the average ranks are close to each other, then we will accept $H_0$ that the treatments are equally effective. If the average ranks are far apart, then we will reject $H_0$ and conclude that at least some of the treatments are different. The test procedure for accomplishing this goal is known as the Kruskal–Wallis test.

**12.18**   *The Kruskal–Wallis Test*

To compare the means of $k$ samples ($k > 2$) using nonparametric methods, we:

    *1.* Pool the observations over all samples, thus constructing a combined sample of size $N = \sum n_i$.

    *2.* Assign ranks to the individual observations, using the average rank in the case of tied observations.

    *3.* Compute the rank sum $R_i$ for each of the $k$ samples.

    *4.* If there are no ties, compute the test statistic

$$H = H^* = \frac{12}{N(N+1)} \times \sum_{i=1}^{k} \frac{R_i^2}{n_i} - 3(N+1)$$

If there are ties, compute the test statistic

$$H = \frac{H^*}{1 - \dfrac{\sum_{j=1}^{g}(t_j^3 - t_j)}{N^3 - N}}$$

where $t_j$ refers to the $j$th cluster of tied observations.

**Table 12.6**

*Ocular anti-inflammatory effects of four drugs on lid closure after administration of arachidonic acid*

| Rabbit number | Indomethicin Score* | Indomethicin Rank | Aspirin Score | Aspirin Rank | Piroxicam Score | Piroxicam Rank | BW755C Score | BW755C Rank |
|---|---|---|---|---|---|---|---|---|
| 1 | +2 | 13.5 | +1 | 9.0 | +3 | 20.0 | +1 | 9.0 |
| 2 | +3 | 20.0 | +3 | 20.0 | +1 | 9.0 | 0 | 4.0 |
| 3 | +3 | 20.0 | +1 | 9.0 | +2 | 13.5 | 0 | 4.0 |
| 4 | +3 | 20.0 | +2 | 13.5 | +1 | 9.0 | 0 | 4.0 |
| 5 | +3 | 20.0 | +2 | 13.5 | +3 | 20.0 | 0 | 4.0 |
| 6 | 0 | 4.0 | +3 | 20.0 | +3 | 20.0 | −1 | 1.0 |

*(Lid closure score at baseline − lid closure score at 15 minutes)$_{treated\ eye}$ − (lid closure score at baseline − lid closure score at 15 minutes)$_{saline\ eye}$

**5.** For a level $\alpha$ test, if

$$H > \chi^2_{k-1, 1-\alpha}$$

then we reject $H_0$; if

$$H \leq \chi^2_{k-1, 1-\alpha}$$

then we accept $H_0$.

**6.** To assess statistical significance, the *p*-value is given by

$$p = Pr(\chi^2_{k-1} > H)$$

**7.** This test procedure should be used only if minimum $n_i \geq 5$ (i.e., if the smallest sample size for an individual group is at least 5).

The acceptance and rejection regions for this test are depicted in Figure 12.11. The computation of the exact *p*-value is given in Figure 12.12.

**Example 12.20**    **Ophthalmology**  Apply the Kruskal–Wallis test procedure to the ocular data in Table 12.6 and assess the statistical significance of the results.

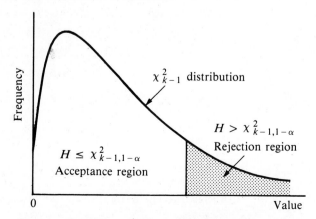

**Figure 12.11**

*Acceptance and rejection regions for the Kruskal–Wallis test*

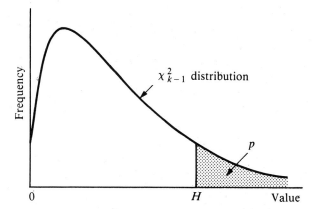

**Figure 12.12**
*Computation of the exact p-value for the Kruskal–Wallis test*

**Solution**

We first must pool the samples together and assign ranks to the individual observations. This procedure is performed in Table 12.7, with ranks given in Table 12.6.

**Table 12.7**
*Assignment of ranks to the individual observations in Table 12.6*

| Lid closure score | Frequency | Range of ranks | Average rank |
|---|---|---|---|
| −1 | 1 | 1 | 1.0 |
| 0 | 5 | 2–6 | 4.0 |
| +1 | 5 | 7–11 | 9.0 |
| +2 | 4 | 12–15 | 13.5 |
| +3 | 9 | 16–24 | 20.0 |

We then compute the rank sum in the four treatment groups:

$$R_1 = 13.5 + 20.0 + \cdots + 4.0 = 97.5$$

$$R_2 = 9.0 + 20.0 + \cdots + 20.0 = 85.0$$

$$R_3 = 20.0 + 9.0 + \cdots + 20.0 = 91.5$$

$$R_4 = 9.0 + 4.0 + \cdots + 1.0 = 26.0$$

Since there are ties, we now compute the Kruskal–Wallis test statistic $H$ as follows:

$$H = \frac{\dfrac{12}{24 \times 25} \times \left[ \dfrac{97.5^2}{6} + \dfrac{85.0^2}{6} + \dfrac{91.5^2}{6} + \dfrac{26.0^2}{6} \right] - 3(25)}{1 - \dfrac{(1^3 - 1) + (5^3 - 5) + (5^3 - 5) + (4^3 - 4) + (9^3 - 9)}{(24^3 - 24)}}$$

$$= \frac{0.020 \times 4296.583 - 75}{1 - \dfrac{1020}{13{,}800}}$$

$$= \frac{10.932}{0.926}$$

$$= 11.806$$

To assess statistical significance, we compare $H$ with a chi-square distribution with $k - 1 = 4 - 1 = 3\ df$. We note from Table 5 that $\chi^2_{3,.99} = 11.34$, $\chi^2_{3,.995} = 12.84$. Since $11.34 < H < 12.84$, it follows that $0.005 < p < 0.01$. Thus, there is a significant difference in the anti-inflammatory potency of the four drugs.  ∎

Note that although the sample sizes in the individual treatment groups were the same in Table 12.6, we can, in fact, use the Kruskal–Wallis test procedure for samples of unequal size. Also, if there are no ties, we can show that the Kruskal–Wallis test statistic $H$ in **(12.18)** can be written in the form

**12.19**

$$H = \frac{12}{N(N+1)} \sum_{i=1}^{k} n_i (\bar{R}_i - \bar{\bar{R}})^2$$

where $\bar{R}_i$ = average rank in the $i$th sample and $\bar{\bar{R}}$ = average rank over all samples combined. Thus, if the average rank is about the same in all samples, then $|\bar{R}_i - \bar{\bar{R}}|$ will tend to be small and we will accept $H_0$. On the contrary, if the average rank is very different across samples, then $|\bar{R}_i - \bar{\bar{R}}|$ will tend to be large and we will reject $H_0$.

The test procedure in **(12.18)** is only applicable if minimum $n_i \geq 5$. If one of our sample sizes is smaller than 5, then either the sample should be combined with another sample or special small-sample tables should be utilized. Table 14 provides critical values for selected sample sizes for the case of three samples (i.e., $k = 3$). The procedure for using this table is as follows:

*1.* Reorder the samples so that $n_1 \leq n_2 \leq n_3$, that is, so that the first sample has the smallest sample size, whereas the third sample has the largest sample size.

*2.* For a level $\alpha$ test, refer to the $\alpha$ column and the row corresponding to the sample sizes $n_1, n_2, n_3$ to find the critical value $c$.

*3.* If $H \geq c$, then we reject $H_0$ at level $\alpha$ (i.e., $p < \alpha$); if $H < c$, then we accept $H_0$ at level $\alpha$ (i.e., $p \geq \alpha$).

*Example 12.21*  Suppose we have three samples of sizes 2, 4, and 5 and $H = 6.141$. Assess the statistical significance of the results.

*Solution*  We refer to the $n_1 = 2, n_2 = 4, n_3 = 5$ row. The critical values for $\alpha = 0.05$ and $\alpha = 0.02$ are 5.273 and 6.541, respectively. Since $H \geq 5.273$, it follows that the results are statistically significant ($p < 0.05$). Since $H < 6.541$, it follows that $p \geq 0.02$. Thus, $0.02 \leq p < 0.05$.  ∎

## □ 12.6.1 Comparison of Specific Groups Under the Kruskal–Wallis Test

In Example 12.20 we determined that the treatments were not all equally effective. To determine which pairs of treatment groups are different, we can use the following procedure:

**12.20**  *Comparison of Specific Groups Under the Kruskal–Wallis Test (Dunn Procedure)*

To compare the $i_1$th and $i_2$th treatment groups under the Kruskal–Wallis test, we:

*1*. Compute

$$\lambda = \frac{\bar{R}_{i_1} - \bar{R}_{i_2}}{\sqrt{\dfrac{N(N+1)}{12} \times \left(\dfrac{1}{n_{i_1}} + \dfrac{1}{n_{i_2}}\right)}}$$

*2*. For a two-sided level $\alpha$ test, if

$$|\lambda| > z_{1-\alpha*}$$

then we reject $H_0$; if

$$|\lambda| \leq z_{1-\alpha*}$$

then we accept $H_0$, where

$$\alpha* = \frac{\alpha}{k(k-1)}$$

The acceptance and rejection regions for this test are depicted in Figure 12.13.

$N(0, 1)$ distribution $+$ distribution of $\lambda$ in **(12.20)** under $H_0$

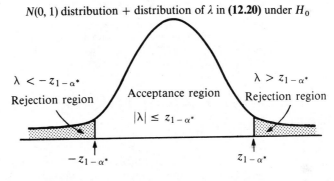

**Figure 12.13**
*Acceptance and rejection regions for the Dunn procedure*

*Example 12.22*    **Ophthalmology** Determine which specific groups are different using the ocular data in Table 12.6.

*Solution*    From Example 12.20 we have

$$\bar{R}_1 = \frac{97.5}{6} = 16.25$$

$$\bar{R}_2 = \frac{85.0}{6} = 14.17$$

$$\bar{R}_3 = \frac{91.5}{6} = 15.25$$

$$\bar{R}_4 = \frac{26.0}{6} = 4.33$$

Therefore, we have the following test statistics to compare each pair of groups:

$$\text{Groups 1 and 2: } \lambda_{12} = \frac{16.25 - 14.17}{\sqrt{\dfrac{24 \times 25}{12} \times \left(\dfrac{1}{6} + \dfrac{1}{6}\right)}} = \frac{2.08}{4.082} = 0.51$$

$$\text{Groups 1 and 3: } \lambda_{13} = \frac{16.25 - 15.25}{4.082} = \frac{1.0}{4.082} = 0.24$$

$$\text{Groups 1 and 4: } \lambda_{14} = \frac{16.25 - 4.33}{4.082} = \frac{11.92}{4.082} = 2.92$$

$$\text{Groups 2 and 3: } \lambda_{23} = \frac{14.17 - 15.25}{4.082} = \frac{-1.08}{4.082} = -0.26$$

$$\text{Groups 2 and 4: } \lambda_{24} = \frac{14.17 - 4.33}{4.082} = \frac{9.84}{4.082} = 2.41$$

$$\text{Groups 3 and 4: } \lambda_{34} = \frac{15.25 - 4.33}{4.082} = \frac{10.92}{4.082} = 2.68$$

The critical value for $\alpha = 0.05$ is given by $z_{1-\alpha*}$, where

$$\alpha* = \frac{0.05}{4 \times 3} = 0.0042$$

From Table 3 we see that $\Phi(2.635) = 0.9958 = 1 - 0.0042$. Thus $z_{1-.0042} = z_{.9958} = 2.635$ is the critical value. Since $\lambda_{14}$ and $\lambda_{34}$ are greater than the critical value, it follows that Indomethicin (group 1) and Piroxicam (group 3) have significantly better anti-inflammatory properties than BW755C (group 4), whereas the other treatment comparisons are not statistically significant.

# ■ 12.7  TWO-WAY ANALYSIS OF VARIANCE— GENERAL MODEL

In Sections 12.1 through 12.5, we focused on the problem of looking at the relationship between pulmonary function and cigarette smoking as an illustration of the one-way analysis of variance. In this example we defined the groups by only one variable, cigarette smoking habit. In some instances, the groups being considered can be classified by two different variables and thus can be arranged in the form of an $r \times c$ contingency table. We would like to be able to look at the effects of each variable after controlling for the effects of the other variable. The latter type of data is usually analyzed using a technique known as the **two-way analysis of variance**.

**Table 12.8**

*Data illustrating the effects of oral contraceptive use and cigarette smoking in 1976 on serum cholesterol level in 1976*

| Cigarette smoking status | | OC Use | |
|---|---|---|---|
| | | Current OC user | Non-OC user |
| Current smokers | Mean | 206.15 | 188.58 |
| | sd | 38.32 | 29.62 |
| | n | 34 | 33 |
| Noncurrent smokers | Mean | 207.54 | 185.34 |
| | sd | 35.86 | 35.52 |
| | n | 28 | 38 |

**Example 12.23** ·**Cardiovascular Disease** Consider the data given in Table 12.8. We are interested in the effects of OC use and cigarette smoking on serum cholesterol level. The effects of OC use and cigarette smoking may be independent or they may be related or "interact" with each other. One approach to the problem would be to construct a two-way ANOVA model predicting serum cholesterol level as a function of OC use and cigarette smoking. ■

---

**Definition 12.10**

An **interaction effect** between two variables is defined as one in which the effect of one variable depends on the level of the other variable. ■

**Example 12.24** *Cardiovascular Disease* Suppose hypothetically that OC users have serum cholesterol levels that are 20 mg% higher than those of 1976 non-OC users. Suppose, however, that among the subgroup of women who are cigarette smokers, there is a 40 mg% difference in serum cholesterol levels between those women who are and who are not OC users. Correspondingly, among the subgroup of women who are nonsmokers, there is a 10 mg% difference in serum cholesterol levels between those who are and who are not OC users. This relationship would be an example of an interaction effect between OC use and cigarette smoking on serum cholesterol levels. ■

The general model for the two-way analysis of variance is given as follows:

**12.21** *Two-Way Analysis of Variance—General Model*

$$y_{ijk} = \mu + \alpha_i + \beta_j + \gamma_{ij} + e$$

where

$y_{ijk}$ is the serum cholesterol of the $k$th woman in the $i$th cigarette smoking group and the $j$th OC use group

$\mu$ is a constant

$\alpha_i$ is a constant representing the effect of cigarette smoking

$\beta_j$ is a constant representing the effect of OC use

$\gamma_{ij}$ is a constant representing the interaction effect between cigarette smoking and OC use

$e$ is an error term, which is assumed to be normally distributed with mean 0 and variance $\sigma^2$

By convention,

$$\sum_{i=1}^{r} \alpha_i = \sum_{j=1}^{c} \beta_j = 0, \qquad \sum_{j=1}^{c} \gamma_{ij} = 0 \qquad \text{for all } i$$

$$\sum_{i=1}^{r} \gamma_{ij} = 0 \qquad \text{for all } j$$

Thus, from **(12.21)** we have that $y_{ijk}$ is normally distributed with mean $\mu + \alpha_i + \beta_j + \gamma_{ij}$ and variance $\sigma^2$.

# ■ 12.8 HYPOTHESIS TESTING IN TWO-WAY ANOVA

Let us denote the mean serum cholesterol for the $i$th row and $j$th column by $\bar{y}_{ij}$, the mean cholesterol for the $i$th row by $\bar{y}_{i.}$, the mean cholesterol for the $j$th column by $\bar{y}_{.j}$, and the overall mean by $\bar{y}_{..}$. We can represent the deviation of an individual observation from the overall mean as follows:

**12.22**
$$y_{ijk} - \bar{y}_{..} = (y_{ijk} - \bar{y}_{ij}) + (\bar{y}_{i.} - \bar{y}_{..}) + (\bar{y}_{.j} - \bar{y}_{..}) + (\bar{y}_{ij} - \bar{y}_{i.} - \bar{y}_{.j} + \bar{y}_{..})$$

**Definition 12.11**

The first term on the right-hand side $(y_{ijk} - \bar{y}_{ij})$ represents the deviation of an individual observation from the group mean for that observation. This expression is an indication of *within-group variability* and will be defined as the **error term**. ■

**Definition 12.12**

The second term on the right-hand side $(\bar{y}_{i.} - \bar{y}_{..})$ represents the deviation of the mean of the $i$th row from the overall mean and is defined as the **row effect**.

**Definition 12.13**

The third term on the right-hand side $(\bar{y}_{.j} - \bar{y}_{..})$ represents the deviation of the mean of the $j$th column from the overall mean and is defined as the **column effect**. ■

**Definition 12.14**

The fourth term on the right-hand side

$$(\bar{y}_{ij} - \bar{y}_{i.} - \bar{y}_{.j} + \bar{y}_{..}) = (\bar{y}_{ij} - \bar{y}_{i.}) - (\bar{y}_{.j} - \bar{y}_{..})$$

represents the deviation of the column effect in the $i$th row $(\bar{y}_{ij} - \bar{y}_{i.})$ from the overall column effect $(\bar{y}_{.j} - \bar{y}_{..})$ and is defined as the **interaction effect**. ■

We would like to test the following hypotheses concerning these data:

1. Test for the presence of row effects: $H_0$: all $\alpha_i = 0$ vs. $H_1$: at least one $\alpha_i \neq 0$. This is a test for the effect of cigarette smoking on serum cholesterol levels after controlling for the effect of OC use.

2. Test for the presence of column effects: $H_0$: all $\beta_j = 0$ vs. $H_1$: at least one $\beta_j \neq 0$. This is a test for the effect of OC use on serum cholesterol levels after controlling for the effect of cigarette smoking.

3. Test for the presence of interaction effects: $H_0$: all $\gamma_{ij} = 0$ vs. $H_1$: at least one $\gamma_{ij} \neq 0$. This is a test of whether or not there is a differential effect of OC use among different cigarette smoking groups. For example, OC use may only have an effect on serum cholesterol among women who are smokers.

## □ 12.8.1 The Method of Unweighted Means

**Definition 12.15**

We define the **total sum of squares** (total SS) for two-way ANOVA as the sum of $(y_{ijk} - \bar{y}_{..})^2$ over all observations over all samples. In symbols,

$$\text{Total SS} = \sum_{i=1}^{r} \sum_{j=1}^{c} \sum_{k=1}^{n_{ij}} (y_{ijk} - \bar{y}_{..})^2$$ ∎

We would like to decompose the total sum of squares into separate components that represent row, column, and interaction effects and perform exact significance tests based on these components. This strategy is only possible here under special circumstances, either when the number of observations is the same in each row and column combination or when the number of observations in each column within any particular row is proportional to the total number of observations in that column.

**Example 12.25**     If we refer to the data in Table 12.8, we see that the number of observations is different for each row and column combination. Furthermore, the proportionality assumption does not hold, since there are 62 observations in the first column (34 + 28) out of a total of 133 observations (34 + 33 + 28 + 38), or 46.6%, whereas in the first row there are 34 out of 67 observations in the first column, or 50.7%. ∎

Since these conditions rarely occur in practice, except in designed experiments, we will not assume that they exist. Instead, we will use an approximate test procedure known as the **method of unweighted means**, which does not make such strong assumptions for the number of observations in specific rows and columns. However, this test procedure is only valid if the number of observations in different row-column combinations is not too different. We will make this condition more precise by stating that there should not be more than a *twofold variation* in the number of observations in the $rc$ row-column combinations.

**12.23**   *Method of Unweighted Means for the Two-Way ANOVA*

If we wish to test for row, column, and interaction effects for the two-way ANOVA and $n_{ij}$ = the number of units in the $i$th row and $j$th column, then:

1. Compute the Row Sum of Squares (Row SS)

$$\frac{\sum_{i=1}^{r} y_{i\cdot}^{*2}}{c} - \frac{y_{..}^{*2}}{rc}$$

where

$$y_{i\cdot}^{*} = \sum_{j=1}^{c} \bar{y}_{ij}$$

$$y_{..}^{*} = \sum_{i=1}^{r} \sum_{j=1}^{c} \bar{y}_{ij}$$

2. Compute the Row Mean Square (Row MS) = Row SS/$(r-1)$.
3. Compute the Column Sum of Squares (Column SS)

$$\frac{\sum_{j=1}^{c} y_{\cdot j}^{*2}}{r} - \frac{y_{..}^{*2}}{rc}$$

where

$$y_{\cdot j}^{*} = \sum_{i=1}^{r} \bar{y}_{ij}$$

4. Compute the Column Mean Square (Column MS) = Column SS/$(c - 1)$.

5. Compute the Interaction Sum of Squares (Interaction SS)

$$\sum_{i=1}^{r} \sum_{j=1}^{c} \bar{y}_{ij}^2 - \frac{y_{..}^{*2}}{rc} - \text{Row SS} - \text{Column SS}$$

6. Compute the Interaction Mean Square (Interaction MS)

$$\text{Interaction SS}/[(r - 1)(c - 1)]$$

7. Compute the Error Mean Square (Error MS)

$$\sum_{i=1}^{r} \sum_{j=1}^{c} (n_{ij} - 1)s_{ij}^2/[(n - rc)n_h] = \left[ \sum_{i=1}^{r} \sum_{j=1}^{c} \sum_{k=1}^{n_{ij}} y_{ijk}^2 - \sum_{i=1}^{r} \sum_{j=1}^{c} \frac{y_{ij.}^{*2}}{n_{ij}} \right] / [(n - rc)n_h]$$

where

$$y_{ij.}^* = \sum_{k=1}^{n_{ij}} y_{ijk}, \quad n = \sum_{i=1}^{r} \sum_{j=1}^{c} n_{ij}$$

and $n_h$ is defined by

$$\frac{1}{n_h} = \left( \sum_{i=1}^{r} \sum_{j=1}^{c} 1/n_{ij} \right) / rc$$

8. We perform a test for **row effects** ($H_0$: all $\alpha_i = 0$ vs. $H_1$: at least one $\alpha_i \neq 0$) as follows:
(a)  We compute the test statistic

$$\lambda_{\text{ROW}} = \text{Row MS/Error MS}$$

which follows an $F_{r-1,n-rc}$ distribution under $H_0$.
(b)  For a level $\alpha$ test, if

$$\lambda_{\text{ROW}} > F_{r-1,n-rc,1-\alpha}$$

then we reject $H_0$; if

$$\lambda_{\text{ROW}} \leqslant F_{r-1,n-rc,1-\alpha}$$

then we accept $H_0$.
(c)  The exact $p$-value $= p_{\text{ROW}}$ is given by the area to the right of $\lambda_{\text{ROW}}$ under an $F_{r-1,n-rc}$ distribution $= Pr(F_{r-1,n-rc} > \lambda_{\text{ROW}})$.

9. We perform a test for **column effects** ($H_0$: all $\beta_j = 0$ vs. $H_1$: at least one $\beta_j \neq 0$) as follows:
(a)  We compute the test statistic

$$\lambda_{\text{COLUMN}} = \text{Column MS/Error MS}$$

which follows an $F_{c-1,n-rc}$ distribution under $H_0$.
(b)  If

$$\lambda_{\text{COLUMN}} > F_{c-1,n-rc,1-\alpha}$$

then we reject $H_0$; if

$$\lambda_{\text{COLUMN}} \leqslant F_{c-1,n-rc,1-\alpha}$$

then we accept $H_0$.

(c) The exact $p$-value $= p_{\text{COLUMN}}$ is given by the area to the right of $\lambda_{\text{COLUMN}}$ under an $F_{c-1,n-rc}$ distribution $= Pr(F_{c-1,n-rc} > \lambda_{\text{COLUMN}})$.

*10* We perform a test for **interaction effects** ($H_0$: all $\gamma_{ij} = 0$ vs. $H_1$: at least one $\gamma_{ij} \neq 0$) as follows:

(a) We compute the test statistic

$$\lambda_{\text{INT}} = \text{Interaction MS/Error MS}$$

which follows an $F_{(r-1)\times(c-1),n-rc}$ distribution under $H_0$.

(b) If

$$\lambda_{\text{INT}} > F_{(r-1)\times(c-1),n-rc,1-\alpha}$$

then we reject $H_0$; if

$$\lambda_{\text{INT}} \leqslant F_{(r-1)\times(c-1),n-rc,1-\alpha}$$

then we accept $H_0$.

(c) The exact $p$-value $= p_{\text{INT}}$ is given by the area to the right of $\lambda_{\text{INT}}$ under an $F_{(r-1)\times(c-1),n-rc}$ distribution $= Pr(F_{(r-1)\times(c-1),n-rc} > \lambda_{\text{INT}})$.

*11.* This test should be used only if there is no more than a twofold variation in the number of observations in the $rc$ row-column combinations.

The results can be displayed in the form of an ANOVA table, as shown in Table 12.9.

---

*Example 12.26*     ***Cardiovascular Disease*** Apply the method of unweighted means to the cholesterol data in Table 12.8 to assess the effects of cigarette smoking, OC use, and the interaction of these effects on cholesterol levels.

*Solution*     We first check the validity of using the method of unweighted means on these data. The maximum variation in the number of observations in particular cells is from 28 to 38. Since $38/28 = 1.36 < 2$, if follows from rule 11 in **(12.23)** that this method is valid for these data.
We now compute

$$y_{1.}^* = 206.15 + 188.58 = 394.73$$

$$y_{2.}^* = 207.54 + 185.34 = 392.88$$

$$y_{.1}^* = 206.15 + 207.54 = 413.69$$

$$y_{.2}^* = 188.58 + 185.34 = 373.92$$

$$y_{..}^* = 206.15 + 188.58 + 207.54 + 185.34 = 787.61$$

We then have

*1.* Row SS $= \dfrac{(394.73)^2 + (392.88)^2}{2} - \dfrac{(787.61)^2}{4}$

$= 155{,}083.234 - 155{,}082.378$

$= 0.856$

**Table 12.9** ANOVA table for method of unweighted means

| Source of variation | SS | df | MS | F Statistic | p-value |
|---|---|---|---|---|---|
| Row | $\sum\limits_{i=1}^{r} \dfrac{y_{i\cdot\cdot}^{*2}}{c} - \dfrac{y_{\cdot\cdot\cdot}^{*2}}{rc}$ | $r - 1$ | $SS/(r-1)$ | $\lambda_{\text{ROW}} = \dfrac{\text{Row MS}}{\text{Error MS}}$ | $\Pr(F_{r-1,n-rc} > \lambda_{\text{ROW}})$ |
| Column | $\sum\limits_{j=1}^{c} \dfrac{y_{\cdot j\cdot}^{*2}}{r} - \dfrac{y_{\cdot\cdot\cdot}^{*2}}{rc}$ | $c - 1$ | $SS/(c-1)$ | $\lambda_{\text{COLUMN}} = \dfrac{\text{Column MS}}{\text{Error MS}}$ | $\Pr(F_{c-1,n-rc} > \lambda_{\text{COLUMN}})$ |
| Interaction | $\sum\limits_{i=1}^{r}\sum\limits_{j=1}^{c} \bar{y}_{ij}^{2} - \dfrac{y_{\cdot\cdot\cdot}^{*2}}{rc}$ <br> $-$ Row SS $-$ Column SS | $(r-1)(c-1)$ | $SS/[(r-1)(c-1)]$ | $\lambda_{\text{INT}} = \dfrac{\text{Interaction MS}}{\text{Error MS}}$ | $\Pr[F_{(r-1)\times(c-1),n-rc} > \lambda_{\text{INT}}]$ |
| Error | $\dfrac{\sum\limits_{i=1}^{r}\sum\limits_{j=1}^{c} \dfrac{(n_{ij}-1)s_{ij}^{2}}{(n-rc)n_{h}}}{} $ <br> $= \dfrac{\sum\limits_{i=1}^{r}\sum\limits_{j=1}^{c}\sum\limits_{k=1}^{n_{ij}} y_{ijk}^{2} - \sum\limits_{i=1}^{r}\sum\limits_{j=1}^{c} y_{ij\cdot}^{*2}}{(n-rc)n_{h}}$ | $n - rc$ | | | |

*2.* Row MS = Row SS/1 = 0.856

*3.* Column SS $= \dfrac{(413.69)^2 + (373.92)^2}{2} - \dfrac{(787.61)^2}{4}$

$$= 155,477.791 - 155,082.378$$

$$= 395.413$$

*4.* Column MS = Column SS/1 = 395.413

*5.* Interaction SS $= (206.15)^2 + (188.58)^2 + (207.54)^2 + (185.34)^2$

$$- \dfrac{(787.61)^2}{4} - \text{Row SS} - \text{Column SS}$$

$$= 155,484.006 - 155,082.378 - 0.856 - 395.413$$

$$= 5.359$$

*6.* Interaction MS = Interaction SS/$(1 \times 1)$ = 5.359

*7.* We now compute the Error MS. We first need to compute $n_h$. We have

$$1/n_h = \left[\left(\frac{1}{34} + \frac{1}{33} + \frac{1}{28} + \frac{1}{38}\right)\bigg/4\right] = 0.03044$$

and

$$n_h = \frac{1}{0.03044} = 32.85$$

Thus,

Error MS $= [33(38.32)^2 + 32(29.62)^2 + 27(35.86)^2 + 37(35.52)^2]/[(133 - 4)32.85]$

$$= 157,935.134/[(129)(32.85)] = 37.27$$

*8.* $\lambda_{\text{ROW}} = 0.856/37.27 = 0.02 \sim F_{1,129}, \quad p > 0.05$

*9.* $\lambda_{\text{COLUMN}} = 395.413/37.27$

$$= 10.61 \sim F_{1,129}, \quad 0.001 < p < 0.005$$

*10.* $\lambda_{\text{INT}} = 5.359/37.27 = 0.14 \sim F_{1,129}, \quad p > 0.05$

These results are displayed in Table 12.10. Thus, there are significant column effects, but nonsignificant row and interaction effects. This result implies that there are significant

**Table 12.10**

ANOVA table for cholesterol data in Table 12.8

| Source of variation | SS | df | MS | F Statistic | p-value |
|---|---|---|---|---|---|
| Cigarette smoking | 0.856 | 1 | 0.856 | 0.02 | NS |
| OC use | 395.413 | 1 | 395.413 | 10.61 | 0.001 < p < 0.005 |
| Cigarette smoking × OC use | 5.359 | 1 | 5.359 | 0.14 | NS |
| Error | | 129 | 37.27 | | |

differences in cholesterol levels by OC use groups but no significant differences in cholesterol by cigarette smoking groups. Furthermore, there are no significant interaction effects, which implies that the differences in cholesterol levels by OC use is the same for those who are or who are not cigarette smokers. Thus, a reasonable interpretation of the data might be that current OC use is associated with elevated cholesterol levels, but current cigarette smoking is not.  ■

A key assumption with this test is that there is not too much variation in the number of observations for specific row-column combinations. If this criterion is not met, then the method of unweighted means is not valid, and a more exact test based on multiple regression methods must be used. (See Kleinbaum and Kupper for a description of these methods [2].)

Finally, we note that the data in Table 12.8 could have been analyzed separately for the effects of cigarette smoking and OC use on serum cholesterol levels using either several two-sample *t* tests or several one-way ANOVAs. The advantage of using the two-way ANOVA for this and other similar problems is that we can look at the effect of one variable *after controlling for the effect of the other variable.* Thus, a two-way ANOVA can be thought of as a type of multiple regression in which both variables are controlled simultaneously, whereas performing several one-way ANOVAs can be thought of as doing several simple linear regressions. If the two variables under study are closely related to each other, then the results from these two approaches can be very different, and the two-way ANOVA is preferred.

# ■ *12.9 SUMMARY*

In this chapter we studied **analysis of variance** methods. These methods enable us to relate outcome variables that are either continuous or ordinal to the levels of one or more categorical independent variables. If we are only considering a single categorical independent variable and our dependent variable is normally distributed, then **one-way analysis of variance (ANOVA)** methods are appropriate. Using these methods, we can test the hypothesis that the mean level of the dependent variable is different for different groups defined by the categorical variable. We can also identify which specific groups are different using *t* **tests** if we have planned our comparisons in advance or **multiple comparison methods** if we have not. If our dependent variable is ordinal or if it is far from being normally distributed, then a nonparametric analogue of one-way ANOVA is appropriate, namely, the **Kruskal–Wallis test.**

If our data are simultaneously stratified by two categorical variables, each of which we wish to simultaneously relate to a normally distributed outcome variable, then **two-way ANOVA methods** are appropriate. In this regard the **method of unweighted means** was introduced as a suitable method of analysis if the numbers of observations in the strata defined by the categorical variables are not that different. If our data are stratified by more than two categorical variables, then we can employ **higher-way ANOVA methods,** which are extensions of the methods in this chapter. Finally, all analysis of variance problems mentioned previously are actually special cases of multiple regression and can be solved using

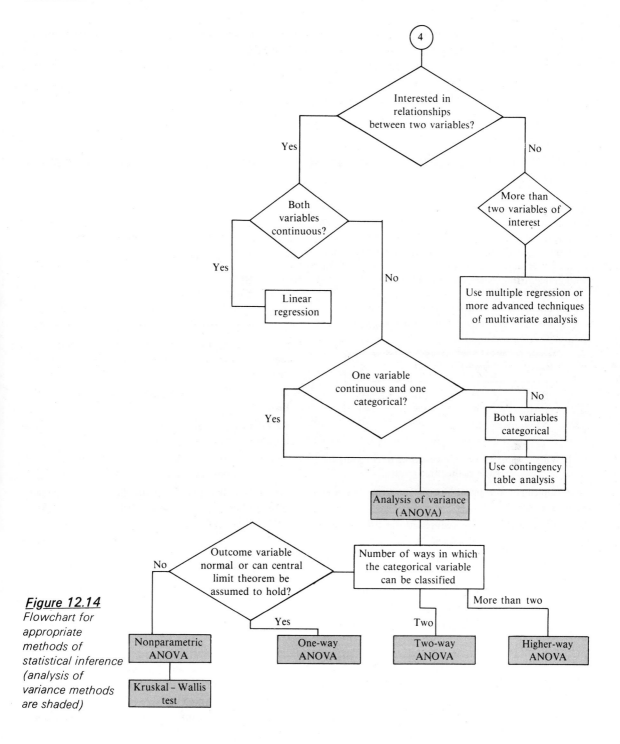

**Figure 12.14**
*Flowchart for appropriate methods of statistical inference (analysis of variance methods are shaded)*

the multiple regression methods introduced in Chapter 11. Despite this option, many researchers prefer to use ANOVA methods because the conceptualization and computations are easier, although this choice is a matter of taste. The general methodology discussed here is summarized in the flowchart on the preceding page and in the back of the book.

# Problems

### Nutrition, Arthritis

A comparison was made of the protein intake among three groups of premenopausal women: (1) women eating a standard American diet (STD), (2) women eating a lacto-ovo-vegetarian diet (LAC), and (3) women eating a strict vegetarian diet (VEG). The mean $\pm 1$ sd for protein intake (mg) is presented in Table 12.11.

**Table 12.11** *Protein intake (mg) among three dietary groups of premenopausal women*

| Group | Mean | sd | n |
|-------|------|----|----|
| STD | 74 | 16 | 10 |
| LAC | 56 | 16 | 10 |
| VEG | 55 | 9 | 10 |

**12.1** What parametric procedure can we use to compare the underlying variances of the three groups?

**12.2** Implement the procedure in Problem 12.1 and report a *p*-value.

**12.3** What parametric procedure can we use to compare the underlying means of the three groups?

**12.4** Implement the procedure in Problem 12.3 using the critical value method.

**12.5** Compare the underlying means of each specific pair of groups using the *t* test methodology.

**12.6** Suppose that in the general population 70% of vegetarians are lactovegetarians, whereas 30% are strict vegetarians. Perform a statistical procedure to test if the contrast $L = 0.7\bar{y}_2 + 0.3\bar{y}_3 - \bar{y}_1$ is significantly different from 0. What does this contrast mean?

Similar data was collected for postmenopausal women in Table 12.12.

**12.7** Perform a statistical procedure to compare the variances of the three groups using the critical value method.

**Table 12.12** *Protein intake (mg) among three dietary groups of premenopausal women*

| Group | Mean | sd | n |
|-------|------|----|----|
| STD | 75 | 9 | 10 |
| LAC | 57 | 13 | 10 |
| VEG | 47 | 17 | 6 |

**12.8** Perform a statistical procedure to compare the means of the three groups using the critical value method.

**12.9** What is the *p*-value from the test performed in Problem 12.8?

**12.10** Compare the means of each specific pair of groups using the *t* test methodology.

**12.11** Perform the test indicated in Problem 12.6 for the postmenopausal women in Table 12.12.

**12.12** Find the upper 5% point of the studentized range statistic based on three means, where the within MS is based on 18 degrees of freedom.

**12.13** Find the upper 1% point of the studentized range statistic based on five means, where the within MS is based on 30 degrees of freedom.

**12.14** Calculate the studentized range statistic for the group of three means in Table 12.11.

**12.15** Using the data in Table 12.11, perform a multiple comparisons procedure to identify which specific underlying means are different.

**12.16** Calculate the studentized range statistic for the group of three means in Table 12.12.

**12.17** Using the data in Table 12.12, perform a multiple comparisons procedure to identify which specific underlying means are different.

### Pulmonary Disease

Twenty-two young asthmatic volunteers were studied to

assess the short-term effects of sulfur dioxide ($SO_2$) exposure under various conditions [4]. The baseline data in Table 12.13 were presented regarding bronchial reactivity to $SO_2$ stratified by lung function (as defined by $FEV_1/FVC$) at screening.

*Table 12.13* *Relationship of bronchial reactivity to $SO_2$ (cm $H_2O/s$) grouped by lung function at screening among 22 asthmatic volunteers*

| Group A FEV$_1$/FVC ⩽74% | Group B FEV$_1$/FVC 75–84% | Group C FEV$_1$/FVC ⩾ 85% |
|---|---|---|
| 20.8 | 7.5 | 9.2 |
| 4.1 | 7.5 | 2.0 |
| 30.0 | 11.9 | 2.5 |
| 24.7 | 4.5 | 6.1 |
| 13.8 | 3.1 | 7.5 |
| | 8.0 | |
| | 4.7 | |
| | 28.1 | |
| | 10.3 | |
| | 10.0 | |
| | 5.1 | |
| | 2.2 | |

(Reprinted with permission of the *American Review of Respiratory Disease* **131(2)**: 221–225, 1985.)

**12.18** Suppose we do not wish to assume normality. What nonparametric test can we use to compare the three groups?

**12.19** Implement the test in Problem 12.18 and report a *p*-value.

Refer to Tables 12.11 and 12.12.

**12.20** Suppose we wish to simultaneously look at the effects of dietary group and menopausal status on protein intake. What statistical procedure can we use?

**12.21** Implement the procedure in Problem 12.20. Discuss the significance of the effects of diet group and menopausal status.

**12.22** Is there a significant interaction effect between menopausal status and dietary group?

**12.23** What does an interaction effect mean in Problem 12.22?

*Cardiovascular Disease*
Some recent reports in the literature have noted that

there is an inverse relationship between moderate alcohol consumption and cholesterol levels. To test this hypothesis, a questionnaire is administered to a group of workers at a particular company as to their alcohol consumption, and blood samples are taken to measure their cholesterol levels. The workers are subdivided into those who report no alcohol consumption, those who drink ⩽2 oz of alcohol, and those who drink more than 2 oz of alcohol on an average day. The 23 nondrinkers had average cholesterol levels of 205.6 with a standard deviation of 25.3. The 15 light drinkers had average cholesterol levels of 182.7 with a standard deviation of 21.9. The 12 heavy drinkers had average cholesterol levels of 199.8 with a standard deviation of 30.3.

**12.24** Is a one-way or two-way ANOVA appropriate here?

**12.25** Test the hypothesis that there is an overall difference in underlying mean cholesterol levels among these three groups.

**12.26** Use the method of multiple comparisons to test for significant differences in cholesterol levels between each pair of groups.

*Hypertension*
A recent phenomenon is the emergence of the automated blood pressure device, which has appeared in many banks, drug stores, and other public places. A study was conducted to assess the comparability of the machine readings with those of the standard cuff [5]. Readings were taken using both the machine and the standard cuff at four separate locations. The results are given in Table 12.14. Suppose we wish to test if the mean difference between the machine and the standard cuff is consistent over the four locations (i.e., if the bias is comparable over all four locations).

**12.27** Is a one-way or two-way ANOVA appropriate here?

**12.28** Perform Bartlett's test for homogeneity of variance.

**12.29** Test if the mean difference is consistent over all four locations.

**12.30** Why was it necessary to perform Bartlett's test in Problem 12.28 before performing the test in Problem 12.29?

*Cardiovascular Disease*
Physical activity has been shown to have beneficial effects on cardiovascular disease outcomes. As part of a study of physical activity assessment methodology, the number of hours of sleep, light activity, moderate activity,

**Table 12.14** *Mean bp and difference between machine and human readings at four locations*

| Location | Systolic bp machine (mm Hg) | | | Systolic bp standard cuff (mm Hg) | | | Systolic bp machine minus systolic bp standard cuff (mm Hg) | | |
|---|---|---|---|---|---|---|---|---|---|
| | Mean | sd | n | Mean | sd | n | Mean | sd | n |
| A | 142.5 | 21.0 | 98 | 142.0 | 18.1 | 98 | 0.5 | 11.2 | 98 |
| B | 134.1 | 22.5 | 84 | 133.6 | 23.2 | 84 | 0.5 | 12.1 | 84 |
| C | 147.9 | 20.3 | 98 | 133.9 | 18.3 | 98 | 14.0 | 11.7 | 98 |
| D | 135.4 | 16.7 | 62 | 128.5 | 19.0 | 62 | 6.9 | 13.6 | 62 |

(Reprinted with permission of the American Heart Association. *Hypertension* **2(2)**: 221–227, 1980.)

**Table 12.15** *Hours per week of moderate activity for men by age*

| Age group | | | | | | | | | | | |
|---|---|---|---|---|---|---|---|---|---|---|---|
| 20–34 | | | 35–49 | | | 50–64 | | | 65–74 | | |
| **Mean** | **sd** | **n** | **Mean** | **sd** | **n** | **Mean** | **sd** | **n** | **Mean** | **sd** | **n** |
| 8.1 | 10.4 | 487 | 9.7 | 10.2 | 233 | 7.9 | 10.2 | 191 | 5.8 | 10.3 | 82 |

(Reprinted with permission of the *American Journal of Epidemiology* **121(1)**: 91–106, 1985.)

hard activity, and very hard activity was computed for each person in the study [6]. These categories were defined in terms of levels of energy, or MET, where MET = ratio of working metabolic rate to resting metabolic rate. Using this classification, sleep = 1 MET; light activity = 1.1–2.9 MET; moderate activity = 3.0–5.0 MET; hard activity = 5.1–6.9 MET; very hard activity $\geq$ 7.0 MET. In Table 12.15 we present data relating the number of hours of moderate activity per week to age for males.

**12.31** What is the appropriate method of analysis to test for the effect of age on the number of hours of moderate activity per week?

**12.32** Perform the test mentioned in Problem 12.31 and report a *p*-value.

**12.33** Comment on which specific age groups are different based on the data in Table 12.15.

**12.34** Perform a test for whether or not there is a general trend for increasing or decreasing amounts of moderate activity by age based on the data in Table 12.15.

### Psychiatry

For the purpose of identifying older nondemented persons with early signs of senile dementia, a Mental Function Index was constructed based on three short tests of cognitive function. In Table 12.16, we present the data relating the Mental Function Index at baseline to clinical status determined independently at baseline and follow-up, with a median follow-up period of 959 days [7].

**12.35** What test procedure can we use to test for significant differences between groups?

**12.36** Perform the test mentioned in Problem 12.35 and report appropriate *p*-values identifying differences between specific groups.

### Gastroenterology

A recent study was performed focusing on the protein concentration of duodenal secretions from patients with cystic fibrosis [8]. Table 12.17 provides data relating protein concentration to pancreatic function as measured by trypsin secretion.

*Table 12.16* Relationship between clinical status at baseline and follow-up (median follow-up period of 959 days) to mean Mental Function Index at baseline

| Clinical status | | | | |
|---|---|---|---|---|
| Baseline | Follow-up | Mean | sd | n |
| Normal | Unchanged | 0.04 | 0.11 | 27 |
| Normal | Questionably or mildly affected | 0.22 | 0.17 | 9 |
| Questionably affected | Progressed | 0.43 | 0.35 | 7 |
| Definitely affected | Progressed | 0.76 | 0.58 | 10 |

(Reprinted with permission of the *American Journal of Epidemiology* **121**(1): 91–106, 1985.)

*12.37* If we do not wish to assume normality for these distributions, then what statistical procedure can we use to compare the three groups?

*12.38* Perform the test mentioned in Problem 12.37 and report a *p*-value.

### Obstetrics

The birthweight of an infant has been hypothesized to be associated with the smoking status of the mother during the first trimester of pregnancy. We test this hypothesis by recording the birthweights of infants and the smoking status of the mother during pregnancy for all mothers who register at the prenatal clinic at a particular hospital within a 1-month period. The mothers are divided into four groups according to smoking habit, and the sample of birthweights in pounds within each group is given as follows:

Group 1: Mother is a nonsmoker (NON):

7.5   6.2   6.9   7.4   9.2   8.3   7.6

Group 2: Mother is an exsmoker (smoked at some time prior to pregnancy but not during pregnancy) (EX):

5.8   7.3   8.2   7.1   7.8

Group 3: Mother is a current smoker and smokes less than 1 pack per day (CUR < 1):

5.9   6.2   5.8   4.7   8.3   7.2   6.2

Group 4: Mother is a current smoker and smokes greater than or equal to 1 pack per day (CUR ≥ 1):

6.2   6.8   5.7   4.9   6.2   7.1   5.8   5.4

*Table 12.17* Relationship between protein concentration (mg/mL) of duodenal secretions to pancreatic function as measured by trypsin secretion [u/(kg/hr)]

| | Trypsin secretion [u/(kg/hr)] | | | | |
|---|---|---|---|---|---|
| ≤ 50 | | 51–1000 | | > 1000 | |
| Subject number | Protein concentration | Subject number | Protein concentration | Subject number | Protein concentration |
| 1 | 1.7 | 1 | 1.4 | 1 | 2.9 |
| 2 | 2.0 | 2 | 2.4 | 2 | 3.8 |
| 3 | 2.0 | 3 | 2.4 | 3 | 4.4 |
| 4 | 2.2 | 4 | 3.3 | 4 | 4.7 |
| 5 | 4.0 | 5 | 4.4 | 5 | 5.0 |
| 6 | 4.0 | 6 | 4.7 | 6 | 5.6 |
| 7 | 5.0 | 7 | 6.7 | 7 | 7.4 |
| 8 | 6.7 | 8 | 7.6 | 8 | 9.4 |
| 9 | 7.8 | 9 | 9.5 | 9 | 10.3 |
| | | 10 | 11.7 | | |

(Reprinted with permission of the *New England Journal of Medicine* **312**(6): 329–334, 1985.)

**Table 12.18** *Reduction in fever for patients getting different doses of aspirin*

| Drug | | Mean (°F) | sd (°F) | n |
|------|------|-----------|---------|---|
| Drug A | 2.0, 1.6, 2.1, 0.6, 1.3 | 1.52 | 0.61 | 5 |
| Drug B | 0.5, 1.2, 0.3, 0.2, −0.4 | 0.36 | 0.58 | 5 |
| Drug C | 1.1, −1.0, −0.2, +0.2, +0.3 | 0.08 | 0.77 | 5 |
| Overall | | 0.65 | | 15 |

**12.39** Should a one-way or two-way ANOVA be used on these data?

**12.40** Test for the homogeneity of the variances in the four samples.

**12.41** Are the mean birthweights different overall in the four groups?

**12.42** Test for all differences between each pair of groups and summarize your results using a $t$ test procedure.

**12.43** Perform the same tests as in Problem 12.42 using the method of multiple comparisons.

**12.44** Are there any differences between the results in Problems 12.42 and 12.43?

**12.45** Suppose we assume that smokers of $\geq 1$ pack per day smoke an average of 1.3 packs per day, whereas smokers of $<1$ pack per day smoke an average of 0.5 pack per day. Use the method of linear contrasts to test if the amount of current cigarette consumption among *ever* smokers is significantly related to birthweight.

*Pharmacology*

Suppose we wish to test the relative effects of three drugs (A, B, C) on the reduction of fever. Drug A is 100% aspirin; drug B is 50% aspirin and 50% other compounds; drug C is 25% aspirin and 75% other compounds. We prescribe the drugs to children aged 5–14 entering the outpatient ward of a hospital complaining of the "flu," with fever of 100.0°F to 100.9°F. We assign the drugs in time sequence order; that is, the first patient gets drug A, the second drug B, the third drug C, the fourth drug A, and so forth, until we have a set of 15 patients. We then telephone the parents 4 hours after administration of the drug and note the reduction in fever. The results are given in Table 12.18. We assume that the timing of prescribing the drugs (i.e., when it is prescribed during the day) is irrelevant to the reduction in fever.

**12.46** What are the appropriate null and alternative hypotheses to test whether or not all three drugs are equally effective?

**12.47** Test for the homogeneity of variances in the three groups.

**12.48** Perform the significance test in Problem 12.46.

**12.49** Summarize the differences in treatment effects between the three drugs using the method of multiple comparisons.

**12.50** Use nonparametric methods to test for significant differences among groups. Identify which groups are significantly different.

**12.51** Compare your results for this problem using parametric and nonparametric methods? Which do you think is the more appropriate method here?

*Pulmonary Function*

In the same study referred to in Example 12.1, the authors also obtained other measures of pulmonary function on the 1050 men. In particular, the FEV data on these men are presented in Table 12.19.

**Table 12.19** *FEV data for smoking and nonsmoking males in the White and Froeb study [1]*

| Group number (i) | Group name | Mean FEV (l) | sd FEV (l) | $n_i$ |
|------------------|------------|--------------|------------|-------|
| 1 | NS | 3.72 | 0.65 | 200 |
| 2 | PS | 3.54 | 0.61 | 200 |
| 3 | NI | 3.56 | 0.76 | 50 |
| 4 | LS | 3.49 | 0.62 | 200 |
| 5 | MS | 3.08 | 0.61 | 200 |
| 6 | HS | 2.77 | 0.60 | 200 |
| Overall | | 3.331 | | 1050 |

(Reprinted with permission of *The New England Journal of Medicine* **302(13)**: 720–723, 1980.)

**12.52** Test for the homogeneity of variances in the six groups.

**12.53** Are the mean FEVs different overall in the six groups?

**Table 12.20** FEV (l) by age and height for boys ages 10–15

| Age | | Height | | | |
|-----|-----|-----|-----|-----|-----|
| | | 1st Quartile | 2nd Quartile | 3rd Quartile | 4th Quartile |
| 10–11 | Mean | 3.30 | 3.47 | 3.60 | 3.66 |
| | sd | 0.83 | 0.59 | 0.64 | 0.75 |
| | n | 17 | 18 | 12 | 21 |
| 12–13 | Mean | 3.38 | 3.52 | 3.79 | 3.80 |
| | sd | 0.50 | 0.92 | 0.73 | 0.64 |
| | n | 16 | 18 | 20 | 22 |
| 14–15 | Mean | 3.52 | 3.83 | 3.81 | 4.06 |
| | sd | 0.74 | 0.68 | 0.78 | 0.63 |
| | n | 15 | 21 | 20 | 18 |

**12.54** Analyze the data for between-group differences using the conventional $t$ test procedure.

**12.55** Analyze the data for between-group differences using a multiple comparisons procedure.

### Pulmonary Disease

To study the effects of parental smoking on children, 218 children 10–15 years of age are assessed. One problem is that lung function is believed to be influenced by age and height. Thus, these factors may have to be corrected for before looking at the effect of parental smoking. We explore this question by subdividing the children in each 2-year age group into height quartiles, with the first quartile of children having the smallest height and the fourth quartile the largest height. The data are given for boys in Table 12.20.

**12.56** Is a one-way or two-way ANOVA appropriate here?

**12.57** Are there significant differences in FEV by age? Report a $p$-value.

**12.58** Are there significant differences in FEV by height quartile? Report a $p$-value.

**12.59** Are the differences by height found in Problem 12.58 consistent over all age groups?

### Hypertension

Some common strategies for treating hypertensive patients by nonpharmacologic methods include (1) weight reduction and (2) trying to get the patient to relax more by meditational or other techniques. Suppose we evaluate these strategies by establishing four groups of hypertensive patients who receive the following types of nonpharmacologic therapy:

**Group I:**    Patients receive counseling for both weight reduction and meditation.

**Group II:**   Patients receive counseling for weight reduction but not for meditation.

**Group III:**  Patients receive counseling for meditation but not for weight reduction.

**Group IV:**   Patients receive no counseling at all.

Suppose that 20 hypertensive patients are assigned at random to each of the four groups, and the change in diastolic blood pressure is noted in these patients after a 1-month period. The results are given in Table 12.21.

**12.60** Is a one-way or two-way ANOVA appropriate here?

**12.61** Analyze if counseling for weight reduction is having a significant effect in reducing blood pressure.

**Table 12.21** Change in diastolic blood pressure for four groups of hypertensive patients who receive different kinds of nonpharmacologic therapy

| Group | Mean change in diastolic bp (baseline − follow up) (mm Hg) | sd change | n |
|-------|-----|-----|-----|
| I | 8.6 | 6.2 | 20 |
| II | 5.3 | 5.4 | 20 |
| III | 4.9 | 7.0 | 20 |
| IV | 1.1 | 6.5 | 20 |

**12.62** Analyze if meditation instruction has a significant effect in reducing blood pressure.

**12.63** Is there any relationship between the effects of weight reduction counseling and meditation counseling on blood pressure reduction. That is, does weight reduction counseling work better for people who receive meditational counseling or for people who do not receive meditational counseling, or is there no difference in effect between these two subgroups?

**12.64** Reanalyze the data in Table 8.15 (page 274) using **analysis of variance** methods to test if there are significant differences overall among the three groups.

**12.65** Test for which specific groups are different using the $t$ test methodology in this chapter (if appropriate).

**12.66** What is the difference in your conclusions between the methods used in Problems 12.64 and 12.65 and the $t$ test procedures in Chapter 8?

*Hypertension*
An instructor in health education wants to familiarize her students with the measurement of blood pressure. Each student in the class is given a portable blood pressure machine to take home. Readings are to be taken for 10 consecutive days, with one reading on each arm. Some of the goals of this study are to investigate (1) if there is a difference in blood pressure between the first and second readings and (2) if there is a difference in blood pressure between the left and right arms. For this purpose, on day 1 the first reading is taken on the left arm and the second reading on the right arm; on day 2 the first reading is taken on the right arm and the second reading on the left arm; on day 3 the day 1 schedule is used; on day 4 the day 2 schedule is used; and so forth. This protocol is followed for 10 consecutive days. The data are given in Table 12.22 for one student from the class.

**12.67** Why was it important to change the arm measured first on alternate days?

**12.68** Test for whether or not there are significant differences between the first and second readings. (Assume that there are no day effects, i.e., that blood pressures are comparable on different days.)

**12.69** Test for whether or not there are significant differences between the left and right arms. (Assume that there are no day effects i.e., that blood pressures are comparable on different days.)

**12.70** Some previous literature reports that blood pressure tends to decline the more times it is measured. Average the results over the left and right arms within a given day. Using these data, perform a test to study this phenomenon by relating the average blood pressure to the day of the study.

**Table 12.22** Systolic blood pressure recordings on 10 consecutive days by arm and order of readings

| Day | Left arm bp (mm Hg) | Left arm Reading order | Right arm bp (mm Hg) | Right arm Reading order |
|---|---|---|---|---|
| 1 | 98 | 1 | 99 | 2 |
| 2 | 93 | 2 | 102 | 1 |
| 3 | 100 | 1 | 98 | 2 |
| 4 | 100 | 2 | 99 | 1 |
| 5 | 96 | 1 | 100 | 2 |
| 6 | 100 | 2 | 95 | 1 |
| 7 | 90 | 1 | 98 | 2 |
| 8 | 93 | 2 | 102 | 1 |
| 9 | 91 | 1 | 92 | 2 |
| 10 | 94 | 2 | 90 | 1 |

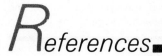

# References

[1] White, J. R. and Froeb, H. F. (1980) "Small-Airways Dysfunction in Nonsmokers Chronically Exposed to Tobacco Smoke," *New England Journal of Medicine* **302(13)**: 720–723.

[2] Kleinbaum, D. and Kupper, L. (1978) *Applied Regression Analysis and Other Multivariable Methods* (Boston: Duxbury Press).

[3] Abelson, M. B., Kliman, G. H., Butrus, S. I., and Weston, J. H. (1983) "Modulation of Arachidonic Acid in the Rabbit Conjunctiva: Predominance of the Cyclo-Oxygenase Pathway." Presented at the Annual Spring Meeting of the Association for Research in Vision and Ophthalmology, Sarasota, Florida, May 2–6, 1983.

[4] Linn, W. S., Shamoo, D. A., Anderson, K. R., Whynot, J. D., Avol, E. L., and Hackney, J. D. (1985) "Effects of Heat and Humidity on the Responses of Exercising Asthmatics to Sulfur Dioxide Exposure," *American Review of Respiratory Disease* **131(2)**: 221–225.

[5] Polk, B. F., Rosner, B., Feudo, R., and Van Denburgh, M. (1980) "An Evaluation of the Vita Stat Automatic Blood Pressure Measuring Device," *Hypertension* **2(2)**: 221–227.

[6] Sallis, J. F., Haskell, W. L., Wood, P. D., Fortmann, S. P., Rogers, T., Blair, S. N., and Paffenbarger, R. S. Jr. (1985) "Physical Activity Assessment Methodology in the Five-City Project," *American Journal of Epidemiology* **121(1)**: 91–106.

[ 7 ] Pfeffer, R. I., Kurosaki, T. T., Chance, J. M., Filos, S., and Bates, D. (1984) "Use of the Mental Function Index in Older Adults: Reliability, Validity and Measurement of Change Over Time," *American Journal of Epidemiology* **120(6)**: 922–935.

[8] Kopelman, H., Durie, P., Gaskin, K., Weizman, Z., and Forstner, G. (1985) "Pancreatic Fluid Secretion and Protein Hyperconcentration in Cystic Fibrosis," *New England Journal of Medicine* **312(6)**: 329–334.

# Table 1

Table 1

**Table 1** Exact binomial probabilities $Pr(X = k) = \binom{n}{k} p^k q^{n-k}$

| n | k | 0.05 | 0.10 | 0.15 | 0.20 | 0.25 | 0.30 | 0.35 | 0.40 | 0.45 | 0.50 |
|---|---|------|------|------|------|------|------|------|------|------|------|
| 2 | 0 | 0.9025 | 0.8100 | 0.7225 | 0.6400 | 0.5625 | 0.4900 | 0.4225 | 0.3600 | 0.3025 | 0.2500 |
|   | 1 | 0.0950 | 0.1800 | 0.2550 | 0.3200 | 0.3750 | 0.4200 | 0.4550 | 0.4800 | 0.4950 | 0.5000 |
|   | 2 | 0.0025 | 0.0100 | 0.0225 | 0.0400 | 0.0625 | 0.0900 | 0.1225 | 0.1600 | 0.2025 | 0.2500 |
| 3 | 0 | 0.8574 | 0.7290 | 0.6141 | 0.5120 | 0.4219 | 0.3430 | 0.2746 | 0.2160 | 0.1664 | 0.1250 |
|   | 1 | 0.1354 | 0.2430 | 0.3251 | 0.3840 | 0.4219 | 0.4410 | 0.4436 | 0.4320 | 0.4084 | 0.3750 |
|   | 2 | 0.0071 | 0.0270 | 0.0574 | 0.0960 | 0.1406 | 0.1890 | 0.2389 | 0.2880 | 0.3341 | 0.3750 |
|   | 3 | 0.0001 | 0.0010 | 0.0034 | 0.0080 | 0.0156 | 0.0270 | 0.0429 | 0.0640 | 0.0911 | 0.1250 |
| 4 | 0 | 0.8145 | 0.6561 | 0.5220 | 0.4096 | 0.3164 | 0.2401 | 0.1785 | 0.1296 | 0.0915 | 0.0625 |
|   | 1 | 0.1715 | 0.2916 | 0.3685 | 0.4096 | 0.4219 | 0.4116 | 0.3845 | 0.3456 | 0.2995 | 0.2500 |
|   | 2 | 0.0135 | 0.0486 | 0.0975 | 0.1536 | 0.2109 | 0.2646 | 0.3105 | 0.3456 | 0.3675 | 0.3750 |
|   | 3 | 0.0005 | 0.0036 | 0.0115 | 0.0256 | 0.0469 | 0.0756 | 0.1115 | 0.1536 | 0.2005 | 0.2500 |
|   | 4 | 0.0000 | 0.0001 | 0.0005 | 0.0016 | 0.0039 | 0.0081 | 0.0150 | 0.0256 | 0.0410 | 0.0625 |
| 5 | 0 | 0.7738 | 0.5905 | 0.4437 | 0.3277 | 0.2373 | 0.1681 | 0.1160 | 0.0778 | 0.0503 | 0.0313 |
|   | 1 | 0.2036 | 0.3280 | 0.3915 | 0.4096 | 0.3955 | 0.3602 | 0.3124 | 0.2592 | 0.2059 | 0.1563 |
|   | 2 | 0.0214 | 0.0729 | 0.1382 | 0.2048 | 0.2637 | 0.3087 | 0.3364 | 0.3456 | 0.3369 | 0.3125 |
|   | 3 | 0.0011 | 0.0081 | 0.0244 | 0.0512 | 0.0879 | 0.1323 | 0.1811 | 0.2304 | 0.2757 | 0.3125 |
|   | 4 | 0.0000 | 0.0004 | 0.0022 | 0.0064 | 0.0146 | 0.0283 | 0.0488 | 0.0768 | 0.1128 | 0.1563 |
|   | 5 | 0.0000 | 0.0000 | 0.0001 | 0.0003 | 0.0010 | 0.0024 | 0.0053 | 0.0102 | 0.0185 | 0.0313 |
| 6 | 0 | 0.7351 | 0.5314 | 0.3771 | 0.2621 | 0.1780 | 0.1176 | 0.0754 | 0.0467 | 0.0277 | 0.0156 |
|   | 1 | 0.2321 | 0.3543 | 0.3993 | 0.3932 | 0.3560 | 0.3025 | 0.2437 | 0.1866 | 0.1359 | 0.0938 |
|   | 2 | 0.0305 | 0.0984 | 0.1762 | 0.2458 | 0.2966 | 0.3241 | 0.3280 | 0.3110 | 0.2780 | 0.2344 |
|   | 3 | 0.0021 | 0.0146 | 0.0415 | 0.0819 | 0.1318 | 0.1852 | 0.2355 | 0.2765 | 0.3032 | 0.3125 |
|   | 4 | 0.0001 | 0.0012 | 0.0055 | 0.0154 | 0.0330 | 0.0595 | 0.0951 | 0.1382 | 0.1861 | 0.2344 |
|   | 5 | 0.0000 | 0.0001 | 0.0004 | 0.0015 | 0.0044 | 0.0102 | 0.0205 | 0.0369 | 0.0609 | 0.0938 |
|   | 6 | 0.0000 | 0.0000 | 0.0000 | 0.0001 | 0.0002 | 0.0007 | 0.0018 | 0.0041 | 0.0083 | 0.0156 |
| 7 | 0 | 0.6983 | 0.4783 | 0.3206 | 0.2097 | 0.1335 | 0.0824 | 0.0490 | 0.0280 | 0.0152 | 0.0078 |
|   | 1 | 0.2573 | 0.3720 | 0.3960 | 0.3670 | 0.3115 | 0.2471 | 0.1848 | 0.1306 | 0.0872 | 0.0547 |
|   | 2 | 0.0406 | 0.1240 | 0.2097 | 0.2753 | 0.3115 | 0.3177 | 0.2985 | 0.2613 | 0.2140 | 0.1641 |
|   | 3 | 0.0036 | 0.0230 | 0.0617 | 0.1147 | 0.1730 | 0.2269 | 0.2679 | 0.2903 | 0.2918 | 0.2734 |
|   | 4 | 0.0002 | 0.0026 | 0.0109 | 0.0287 | 0.0577 | 0.0972 | 0.1442 | 0.1935 | 0.2388 | 0.2734 |

**Table 1**  Exact Binomial Probabilities                                    *491*

**Table 1**  *(Continued)*

| n | k | 0.05 | 0.10 | 0.15 | 0.20 | 0.25 | 0.30 | 0.35 | 0.40 | 0.45 | 0.50 |
|---|---|------|------|------|------|------|------|------|------|------|------|
|   | 5 | 0.0000 | 0.0002 | 0.0012 | 0.0043 | 0.0115 | 0.0250 | 0.0466 | 0.0774 | 0.1172 | 0.1641 |
|   | 6 | 0.0000 | 0.0000 | 0.0001 | 0.0004 | 0.0013 | 0.0036 | 0.0084 | 0.0172 | 0.0320 | 0.0547 |
|   | 7 | 0.0000 | 0.0000 | 0.0000 | 0.0000 | 0.0001 | 0.0002 | 0.0006 | 0.0016 | 0.0037 | 0.0078 |
| 8 | 0 | 0.6634 | 0.4305 | 0.2725 | 0.1678 | 0.1001 | 0.0576 | 0.0319 | 0.0168 | 0.0084 | 0.0039 |
|   | 1 | 0.2793 | 0.3826 | 0.3847 | 0.3355 | 0.2670 | 0.1977 | 0.1373 | 0.0896 | 0.0548 | 0.0313 |
|   | 2 | 0.0515 | 0.1488 | 0.2376 | 0.2936 | 0.3115 | 0.2965 | 0.2587 | 0.2090 | 0.1569 | 0.1094 |
|   | 3 | 0.0054 | 0.0331 | 0.0839 | 0.1468 | 0.2076 | 0.2541 | 0.2786 | 0.2787 | 0.2568 | 0.2188 |
|   | 4 | 0.0004 | 0.0046 | 0.0185 | 0.0459 | 0.0865 | 0.1361 | 0.1875 | 0.2322 | 0.2627 | 0.2734 |
|   | 5 | 0.0000 | 0.0004 | 0.0026 | 0.0092 | 0.0231 | 0.0467 | 0.0808 | 0.1239 | 0.1719 | 0.2188 |
|   | 6 | 0.0000 | 0.0000 | 0.0002 | 0.0011 | 0.0038 | 0.0100 | 0.0217 | 0.0413 | 0.0703 | 0.1094 |
|   | 7 | 0.0000 | 0.0000 | 0.0000 | 0.0001 | 0.0004 | 0.0012 | 0.0033 | 0.0079 | 0.0164 | 0.0313 |
|   | 8 | 0.0000 | 0.0000 | 0.0000 | 0.0000 | 0.0000 | 0.0001 | 0.0002 | 0.0007 | 0.0017 | 0.0039 |
| 9 | 0 | 0.6302 | 0.3874 | 0.2316 | 0.1342 | 0.0751 | 0.0404 | 0.0207 | 0.0101 | 0.0046 | 0.0020 |
|   | 1 | 0.2985 | 0.3874 | 0.3679 | 0.3020 | 0.2253 | 0.1556 | 0.1004 | 0.0605 | 0.0339 | 0.0176 |
|   | 2 | 0.0629 | 0.1722 | 0.2597 | 0.3020 | 0.3003 | 0.2668 | 0.2162 | 0.1612 | 0.1110 | 0.0703 |
|   | 3 | 0.0077 | 0.0446 | 0.1069 | 0.1762 | 0.2336 | 0.2668 | 0.2716 | 0.2508 | 0.2119 | 0.1641 |
|   | 4 | 0.0006 | 0.0074 | 0.0283 | 0.0661 | 0.1168 | 0.1715 | 0.2194 | 0.2508 | 0.2600 | 0.2461 |
|   | 5 | 0.0000 | 0.0008 | 0.0050 | 0.0165 | 0.0389 | 0.0735 | 0.1181 | 0.1672 | 0.2128 | 0.2461 |
|   | 6 | 0.0000 | 0.0001 | 0.0006 | 0.0028 | 0.0087 | 0.0210 | 0.0424 | 0.0743 | 0.1160 | 0.1641 |
|   | 7 | 0.0000 | 0.0000 | 0.0000 | 0.0003 | 0.0012 | 0.0039 | 0.0098 | 0.0212 | 0.0407 | 0.0703 |
|   | 8 | 0.0000 | 0.0000 | 0.0000 | 0.0000 | 0.0001 | 0.0004 | 0.0013 | 0.0035 | 0.0083 | 0.0176 |
|   | 9 | 0.0000 | 0.0000 | 0.0000 | 0.0000 | 0.0000 | 0.0000 | 0.0001 | 0.0003 | 0.0008 | 0.0020 |
| 10 | 0 | 0.5987 | 0.3487 | 0.1969 | 0.1074 | 0.0563 | 0.0282 | 0.0135 | 0.0060 | 0.0025 | 0.0010 |
|   | 1 | 0.3151 | 0.3874 | 0.3474 | 0.2684 | 0.1877 | 0.1211 | 0.0725 | 0.0403 | 0.0207 | 0.0098 |
|   | 2 | 0.0746 | 0.1937 | 0.2759 | 0.3020 | 0.2816 | 0.2335 | 0.1757 | 0.1209 | 0.0763 | 0.0439 |
|   | 3 | 0.0105 | 0.0574 | 0.1298 | 0.2013 | 0.2503 | 0.2668 | 0.2522 | 0.2150 | 0.1665 | 0.1172 |
|   | 4 | 0.0010 | 0.0112 | 0.0401 | 0.0881 | 0.1460 | 0.2001 | 0.2377 | 0.2508 | 0.2384 | 0.2051 |
|   | 5 | 0.0001 | 0.0015 | 0.0085 | 0.0264 | 0.0584 | 0.1029 | 0.1536 | 0.2007 | 0.2340 | 0.2461 |
|   | 6 | 0.0000 | 0.0001 | 0.0012 | 0.0055 | 0.0162 | 0.0368 | 0.0689 | 0.1115 | 0.1596 | 0.2051 |
|   | 7 | 0.0000 | 0.0000 | 0.0001 | 0.0008 | 0.0031 | 0.0090 | 0.0212 | 0.0425 | 0.0746 | 0.1172 |
|   | 8 | 0.0000 | 0.0000 | 0.0000 | 0.0001 | 0.0004 | 0.0014 | 0.0043 | 0.0106 | 0.0229 | 0.0439 |
|   | 9 | 0.0000 | 0.0000 | 0.0000 | 0.0000 | 0.0000 | 0.0001 | 0.0005 | 0.0016 | 0.0042 | 0.0098 |
|   | 10 | 0.0000 | 0.0000 | 0.0000 | 0.0000 | 0.0000 | 0.0000 | 0.0000 | 0.0001 | 0.0003 | 0.0010 |
| 11 | 0 | 0.5688 | 0.3138 | 0.1673 | 0.0859 | 0.0422 | 0.0198 | 0.0088 | 0.0036 | 0.0014 | 0.0005 |
|   | 1 | 0.3293 | 0.3835 | 0.3248 | 0.2362 | 0.1549 | 0.0932 | 0.0518 | 0.0266 | 0.0125 | 0.0054 |
|   | 2 | 0.0867 | 0.2131 | 0.2866 | 0.2953 | 0.2581 | 0.1998 | 0.1395 | 0.0887 | 0.0513 | 0.0269 |
|   | 3 | 0.0137 | 0.0710 | 0.1517 | 0.2215 | 0.2581 | 0.2568 | 0.2254 | 0.1774 | 0.1259 | 0.0806 |
|   | 4 | 0.0014 | 0.0158 | 0.0536 | 0.1107 | 0.1721 | 0.2201 | 0.2428 | 0.2365 | 0.2060 | 0.1611 |
|   | 5 | 0.0001 | 0.0025 | 0.0132 | 0.0388 | 0.0803 | 0.1321 | 0.1830 | 0.2207 | 0.2360 | 0.2256 |
|   | 6 | 0.0000 | 0.0003 | 0.0023 | 0.0097 | 0.0268 | 0.0566 | 0.0985 | 0.1471 | 0.1931 | 0.2256 |
|   | 7 | 0.0000 | 0.0000 | 0.0003 | 0.0017 | 0.0064 | 0.0173 | 0.0379 | 0.0701 | 0.1128 | 0.1611 |
|   | 8 | 0.0000 | 0.0000 | 0.0000 | 0.0002 | 0.0011 | 0.0037 | 0.0102 | 0.0234 | 0.0462 | 0.0806 |
|   | 9 | 0.0000 | 0.0000 | 0.0000 | 0.0000 | 0.0001 | 0.0005 | 0.0018 | 0.0052 | 0.0126 | 0.0269 |
|   | 10 | 0.0000 | 0.0000 | 0.0000 | 0.0000 | 0.0000 | 0.0000 | 0.0002 | 0.0007 | 0.0021 | 0.0054 |
|   | 11 | 0.0000 | 0.0000 | 0.0000 | 0.0000 | 0.0000 | 0.0000 | 0.0000 | 0.0000 | 0.0002 | 0.0005 |

**Table 1** *(Continued)*

| n | k | 0.05 | 0.10 | 0.15 | 0.20 | 0.25 | 0.30 | 0.35 | 0.40 | 0.45 | 0.50 |
|---|---|------|------|------|------|------|------|------|------|------|------|
| 12 | 0 | 0.5404 | 0.2824 | 0.1422 | 0.0687 | 0.0317 | 0.0138 | 0.0057 | 0.0022 | 0.0008 | 0.0002 |
|    | 1 | 0.3413 | 0.3766 | 0.3012 | 0.2062 | 0.1267 | 0.0712 | 0.0368 | 0.0174 | 0.0075 | 0.0029 |
|    | 2 | 0.0988 | 0.2301 | 0.2924 | 0.2835 | 0.2323 | 0.1678 | 0.1088 | 0.0639 | 0.0339 | 0.0161 |
|    | 3 | 0.0173 | 0.0852 | 0.1720 | 0.2362 | 0.2581 | 0.2397 | 0.1954 | 0.1419 | 0.0923 | 0.0537 |
|    | 4 | 0.0021 | 0.0213 | 0.0683 | 0.1329 | 0.1936 | 0.2311 | 0.2367 | 0.2128 | 0.1700 | 0.1208 |
|    | 5 | 0.0002 | 0.0038 | 0.0193 | 0.0532 | 0.1032 | 0.1585 | 0.2039 | 0.2270 | 0.2225 | 0.1934 |
|    | 6 | 0.0000 | 0.0005 | 0.0040 | 0.0155 | 0.0401 | 0.0792 | 0.1281 | 0.1766 | 0.2124 | 0.2256 |
|    | 7 | 0.0000 | 0.0000 | 0.0006 | 0.0033 | 0.0115 | 0.0291 | 0.0591 | 0.1009 | 0.1489 | 0.1934 |
|    | 8 | 0.0000 | 0.0000 | 0.0001 | 0.0005 | 0.0024 | 0.0078 | 0.0199 | 0.0420 | 0.0762 | 0.1208 |
|    | 9 | 0.0000 | 0.0000 | 0.0000 | 0.0001 | 0.0004 | 0.0015 | 0.0048 | 0.0125 | 0.0277 | 0.0537 |
|    | 10 | 0.0000 | 0.0000 | 0.0000 | 0.0000 | 0.0000 | 0.0002 | 0.0008 | 0.0025 | 0.0068 | 0.0161 |
|    | 11 | 0.0000 | 0.0000 | 0.0000 | 0.0000 | 0.0000 | 0.0000 | 0.0001 | 0.0003 | 0.0010 | 0.0029 |
|    | 12 | 0.0000 | 0.0000 | 0.0000 | 0.0000 | 0.0000 | 0.0000 | 0.0000 | 0.0000 | 0.0001 | 0.0002 |
| 13 | 0 | 0.5133 | 0.2542 | 0.1209 | 0.0550 | 0.0238 | 0.0097 | 0.0037 | 0.0013 | 0.0004 | 0.0001 |
|    | 1 | 0.3512 | 0.3672 | 0.2774 | 0.1787 | 0.1029 | 0.0540 | 0.0259 | 0.0113 | 0.0045 | 0.0016 |
|    | 2 | 0.1109 | 0.2448 | 0.2937 | 0.2680 | 0.2059 | 0.1388 | 0.0836 | 0.0453 | 0.0220 | 0.0095 |
|    | 3 | 0.0214 | 0.0997 | 0.1900 | 0.2457 | 0.2517 | 0.2181 | 0.1651 | 0.1107 | 0.0660 | 0.0349 |
|    | 4 | 0.0028 | 0.0277 | 0.0838 | 0.1535 | 0.2097 | 0.2337 | 0.2222 | 0.1845 | 0.1350 | 0.0873 |
|    | 5 | 0.0003 | 0.0055 | 0.0266 | 0.0691 | 0.1258 | 0.1803 | 0.2154 | 0.2214 | 0.1989 | 0.1571 |
|    | 6 | 0.0000 | 0.0008 | 0.0063 | 0.0230 | 0.0559 | 0.1030 | 0.1546 | 0.1968 | 0.2169 | 0.2095 |
|    | 7 | 0.0000 | 0.0001 | 0.0011 | 0.0058 | 0.0186 | 0.0442 | 0.0833 | 0.1312 | 0.1775 | 0.2095 |
|    | 8 | 0.0000 | 0.0000 | 0.0001 | 0.0011 | 0.0047 | 0.0142 | 0.0336 | 0.0656 | 0.1089 | 0.1571 |
|    | 9 | 0.0000 | 0.0000 | 0.0000 | 0.0001 | 0.0009 | 0.0034 | 0.0101 | 0.0243 | 0.0495 | 0.0873 |
|    | 10 | 0.0000 | 0.0000 | 0.0000 | 0.0000 | 0.0001 | 0.0006 | 0.0022 | 0.0065 | 0.0162 | 0.0349 |
|    | 11 | 0.0000 | 0.0000 | 0.0000 | 0.0000 | 0.0000 | 0.0001 | 0.0003 | 0.0012 | 0.0036 | 0.0095 |
|    | 12 | 0.0000 | 0.0000 | 0.0000 | 0.0000 | 0.0000 | 0.0000 | 0.0000 | 0.0001 | 0.0005 | 0.0016 |
|    | 13 | 0.0000 | 0.0000 | 0.0000 | 0.0000 | 0.0000 | 0.0000 | 0.0000 | 0.0000 | 0.0000 | 0.0001 |
| 14 | 0 | 0.4877 | 0.2288 | 0.1028 | 0.0440 | 0.0178 | 0.0068 | 0.0024 | 0.0008 | 0.0002 | 0.0001 |
|    | 1 | 0.3593 | 0.3559 | 0.2539 | 0.1539 | 0.0832 | 0.0407 | 0.0181 | 0.0073 | 0.0027 | 0.0009 |
|    | 2 | 0.1229 | 0.2570 | 0.2912 | 0.2501 | 0.1802 | 0.1134 | 0.0634 | 0.0317 | 0.0141 | 0.0056 |
|    | 3 | 0.0259 | 0.1142 | 0.2056 | 0.2501 | 0.2402 | 0.1943 | 0.1366 | 0.0845 | 0.0462 | 0.0222 |
|    | 4 | 0.0037 | 0.0349 | 0.0998 | 0.1720 | 0.2202 | 0.2290 | 0.2022 | 0.1549 | 0.1040 | 0.0611 |
|    | 5 | 0.0004 | 0.0078 | 0.0352 | 0.0860 | 0.1468 | 0.1963 | 0.2178 | 0.2066 | 0.1701 | 0.1222 |
|    | 6 | 0.0000 | 0.0013 | 0.0093 | 0.0322 | 0.0734 | 0.1262 | 0.1759 | 0.2066 | 0.2088 | 0.1833 |
|    | 7 | 0.0000 | 0.0002 | 0.0019 | 0.0092 | 0.0280 | 0.0618 | 0.1082 | 0.1574 | 0.1952 | 0.2095 |
|    | 8 | 0.0000 | 0.0000 | 0.0003 | 0.0020 | 0.0082 | 0.0232 | 0.0510 | 0.0918 | 0.1398 | 0.1833 |
|    | 9 | 0.0000 | 0.0000 | 0.0000 | 0.0003 | 0.0018 | 0.0066 | 0.0183 | 0.0408 | 0.0762 | 0.1222 |
|    | 10 | 0.0000 | 0.0000 | 0.0000 | 0.0000 | 0.0003 | 0.0014 | 0.0049 | 0.0136 | 0.0312 | 0.0611 |
|    | 11 | 0.0000 | 0.0000 | 0.0000 | 0.0000 | 0.0000 | 0.0002 | 0.0010 | 0.0033 | 0.0093 | 0.0222 |
|    | 12 | 0.0000 | 0.0000 | 0.0000 | 0.0000 | 0.0000 | 0.0000 | 0.0001 | 0.0005 | 0.0019 | 0.0056 |
|    | 13 | 0.0000 | 0.0000 | 0.0000 | 0.0000 | 0.0000 | 0.0000 | 0.0000 | 0.0001 | 0.0002 | 0.0009 |
|    | 14 | 0.0000 | 0.0000 | 0.0000 | 0.0000 | 0.0000 | 0.0000 | 0.0000 | 0.0000 | 0.0000 | 0.0001 |
| 15 | 0 | 0.4633 | 0.2059 | 0.0874 | 0.0352 | 0.0134 | 0.0047 | 0.0016 | 0.0005 | 0.0001 | 0.0000 |
|    | 1 | 0.3658 | 0.3432 | 0.2312 | 0.1319 | 0.0668 | 0.0305 | 0.0126 | 0.0047 | 0.0016 | 0.0005 |
|    | 2 | 0.1348 | 0.2669 | 0.2856 | 0.2309 | 0.1559 | 0.0916 | 0.0476 | 0.0219 | 0.0090 | 0.0032 |
|    | 3 | 0.0307 | 0.1285 | 0.2184 | 0.2501 | 0.2252 | 0.1700 | 0.1110 | 0.0634 | 0.0318 | 0.0139 |

*Table 1* Exact Binomial Probabilities

493

## Table 1 (Continued)

| n | k | 0.05 | 0.10 | 0.15 | 0.20 | 0.25 | 0.30 | 0.35 | 0.40 | 0.45 | 0.50 |
|---|---|------|------|------|------|------|------|------|------|------|------|
|   | 4 | 0.0049 | 0.0428 | 0.1156 | 0.1876 | 0.2252 | 0.2186 | 0.1792 | 0.1268 | 0.0780 | 0.0417 |
|   | 5 | 0.0006 | 0.0105 | 0.0449 | 0.1032 | 0.1651 | 0.2061 | 0.2123 | 0.1859 | 0.1404 | 0.0916 |
|   | 6 | 0.0000 | 0.0019 | 0.0132 | 0.0430 | 0.0917 | 0.1472 | 0.1906 | 0.2066 | 0.1914 | 0.1527 |
|   | 7 | 0.0000 | 0.0003 | 0.0030 | 0.0138 | 0.0393 | 0.0811 | 0.1319 | 0.1771 | 0.2013 | 0.1964 |
|   | 8 | 0.0000 | 0.0000 | 0.0005 | 0.0035 | 0.0131 | 0.0348 | 0.0710 | 0.1181 | 0.1647 | 0.1964 |
|   | 9 | 0.0000 | 0.0000 | 0.0001 | 0.0007 | 0.0034 | 0.0116 | 0.0298 | 0.0612 | 0.1048 | 0.1527 |
|   | 10 | 0.0000 | 0.0000 | 0.0000 | 0.0001 | 0.0007 | 0.0030 | 0.0096 | 0.0245 | 0.0515 | 0.0916 |
|   | 11 | 0.0000 | 0.0000 | 0.0000 | 0.0000 | 0.0001 | 0.0006 | 0.0024 | 0.0074 | 0.0191 | 0.0417 |
|   | 12 | 0.0000 | 0.0000 | 0.0000 | 0.0000 | 0.0000 | 0.0001 | 0.0004 | 0.0016 | 0.0052 | 0.0139 |
|   | 13 | 0.0000 | 0.0000 | 0.0000 | 0.0000 | 0.0000 | 0.0000 | 0.0001 | 0.0003 | 0.0010 | 0.0032 |
|   | 14 | 0.0000 | 0.0000 | 0.0000 | 0.0000 | 0.0000 | 0.0000 | 0.0000 | 0.0000 | 0.0001 | 0.0005 |
|   | 15 | 0.0000 | 0.0000 | 0.0000 | 0.0000 | 0.0000 | 0.0000 | 0.0000 | 0.0000 | 0.0000 | 0.0000 |
| 16 | 0 | 0.4401 | 0.1853 | 0.0743 | 0.0281 | 0.0100 | 0.0033 | 0.0010 | 0.0003 | 0.0001 | 0.0000 |
|   | 1 | 0.3706 | 0.3294 | 0.2097 | 0.1126 | 0.0535 | 0.0228 | 0.0087 | 0.0030 | 0.0009 | 0.0002 |
|   | 2 | 0.1463 | 0.2745 | 0.2775 | 0.2111 | 0.1336 | 0.0732 | 0.0353 | 0.0150 | 0.0056 | 0.0018 |
|   | 3 | 0.0359 | 0.1423 | 0.2285 | 0.2463 | 0.2079 | 0.1465 | 0.0888 | 0.0468 | 0.0215 | 0.0085 |
|   | 4 | 0.0061 | 0.0514 | 0.1311 | 0.2001 | 0.2252 | 0.2040 | 0.1553 | 0.1014 | 0.0572 | 0.0278 |
|   | 5 | 0.0008 | 0.0137 | 0.0555 | 0.1201 | 0.1802 | 0.2099 | 0.2008 | 0.1623 | 0.1123 | 0.0667 |
|   | 6 | 0.0001 | 0.0028 | 0.0180 | 0.0550 | 0.1101 | 0.1649 | 0.1982 | 0.1983 | 0.1684 | 0.1222 |
|   | 7 | 0.0000 | 0.0004 | 0.0045 | 0.0197 | 0.0524 | 0.1010 | 0.1524 | 0.1889 | 0.1969 | 0.1746 |
|   | 8 | 0.0000 | 0.0001 | 0.0009 | 0.0055 | 0.0197 | 0.0487 | 0.0923 | 0.1417 | 0.1812 | 0.1964 |
|   | 9 | 0.0000 | 0.0000 | 0.0001 | 0.0012 | 0.0058 | 0.0185 | 0.0442 | 0.0840 | 0.1318 | 0.1746 |
|   | 10 | 0.0000 | 0.0000 | 0.0000 | 0.0002 | 0.0014 | 0.0056 | 0.0167 | 0.0392 | 0.0755 | 0.1222 |
|   | 11 | 0.0000 | 0.0000 | 0.0000 | 0.0000 | 0.0002 | 0.0013 | 0.0049 | 0.0142 | 0.0337 | 0.0667 |
|   | 12 | 0.0000 | 0.0000 | 0.0000 | 0.0000 | 0.0000 | 0.0002 | 0.0011 | 0.0040 | 0.0115 | 0.0278 |
|   | 13 | 0.0000 | 0.0000 | 0.0000 | 0.0000 | 0.0000 | 0.0000 | 0.0002 | 0.0008 | 0.0029 | 0.0085 |
|   | 14 | 0.0000 | 0.0000 | 0.0000 | 0.0000 | 0.0000 | 0.0000 | 0.0000 | 0.0001 | 0.0005 | 0.0018 |
|   | 15 | 0.0000 | 0.0000 | 0.0000 | 0.0000 | 0.0000 | 0.0000 | 0.0000 | 0.0000 | 0.0001 | 0.0002 |
|   | 16 | 0.0000 | 0.0000 | 0.0000 | 0.0000 | 0.0000 | 0.0000 | 0.0000 | 0.0000 | 0.0000 | 0.0000 |
| 17 | 0 | 0.4181 | 0.1668 | 0.0631 | 0.0225 | 0.0075 | 0.0023 | 0.0007 | 0.0002 | 0.0000 | 0.0000 |
|   | 1 | 0.3741 | 0.3150 | 0.1893 | 0.0957 | 0.0426 | 0.0169 | 0.0060 | 0.0019 | 0.0005 | 0.0001 |
|   | 2 | 0.1575 | 0.2800 | 0.2673 | 0.1914 | 0.1136 | 0.0581 | 0.0260 | 0.0102 | 0.0035 | 0.0010 |
|   | 3 | 0.0415 | 0.1556 | 0.2359 | 0.2393 | 0.1893 | 0.1245 | 0.0701 | 0.0341 | 0.0144 | 0.0052 |
|   | 4 | 0.0076 | 0.0605 | 0.1457 | 0.2093 | 0.2209 | 0.1868 | 0.1320 | 0.0796 | 0.0411 | 0.0182 |
|   | 5 | 0.0010 | 0.0175 | 0.0668 | 0.1361 | 0.1914 | 0.2081 | 0.1849 | 0.1379 | 0.0875 | 0.0472 |
|   | 6 | 0.0001 | 0.0039 | 0.0236 | 0.0680 | 0.1276 | 0.1784 | 0.1991 | 0.1839 | 0.1432 | 0.0944 |
|   | 7 | 0.0000 | 0.0007 | 0.0065 | 0.0267 | 0.0668 | 0.1201 | 0.1685 | 0.1927 | 0.1841 | 0.1484 |
|   | 8 | 0.0000 | 0.0001 | 0.0014 | 0.0084 | 0.0279 | 0.0644 | 0.1134 | 0.1606 | 0.1883 | 0.1855 |
|   | 9 | 0.0000 | 0.0000 | 0.0003 | 0.0021 | 0.0093 | 0.0276 | 0.0611 | 0.1070 | 0.1540 | 0.1855 |
|   | 10 | 0.0000 | 0.0000 | 0.0000 | 0.0004 | 0.0025 | 0.0095 | 0.0263 | 0.0571 | 0.1008 | 0.1484 |
|   | 11 | 0.0000 | 0.0000 | 0.0000 | 0.0001 | 0.0005 | 0.0026 | 0.0090 | 0.0242 | 0.0525 | 0.0944 |
|   | 12 | 0.0000 | 0.0000 | 0.0000 | 0.0000 | 0.0001 | 0.0006 | 0.0024 | 0.0081 | 0.0215 | 0.0472 |
|   | 13 | 0.0000 | 0.0000 | 0.0000 | 0.0000 | 0.0000 | 0.0001 | 0.0005 | 0.0021 | 0.0068 | 0.0182 |
|   | 14 | 0.0000 | 0.0000 | 0.0000 | 0.0000 | 0.0000 | 0.0000 | 0.0001 | 0.0004 | 0.0016 | 0.0052 |
|   | 15 | 0.0000 | 0.0000 | 0.0000 | 0.0000 | 0.0000 | 0.0000 | 0.0000 | 0.0001 | 0.0003 | 0.0010 |
|   | 16 | 0.0000 | 0.0000 | 0.0000 | 0.0000 | 0.0000 | 0.0000 | 0.0000 | 0.0000 | 0.0000 | 0.0001 |
|   | 17 | 0.0000 | 0.0000 | 0.0000 | 0.0000 | 0.0000 | 0.0000 | 0.0000 | 0.0000 | 0.0000 | 0.0000 |

**Table 1**    (Continued)

| n | k | 0.05 | 0.10 | 0.15 | 0.20 | 0.25 | 0.30 | 0.35 | 0.40 | 0.45 | 0.50 |
|---|---|------|------|------|------|------|------|------|------|------|------|
| 18 | 0 | 0.3972 | 0.1501 | 0.0536 | 0.0180 | 0.0056 | 0.0016 | 0.0004 | 0.0001 | 0.0000 | 0.0000 |
|    | 1 | 0.3763 | 0.3002 | 0.1704 | 0.0811 | 0.0338 | 0.0126 | 0.0042 | 0.0012 | 0.0003 | 0.0001 |
|    | 2 | 0.1683 | 0.2835 | 0.2556 | 0.1723 | 0.0958 | 0.0458 | 0.0190 | 0.0069 | 0.0022 | 0.0006 |
|    | 3 | 0.0473 | 0.1680 | 0.2406 | 0.2297 | 0.1704 | 0.1046 | 0.0547 | 0.0246 | 0.0095 | 0.0031 |
|    | 4 | 0.0093 | 0.0700 | 0.1592 | 0.2153 | 0.2130 | 0.1681 | 0.1104 | 0.0614 | 0.0291 | 0.0117 |
|    | 5 | 0.0014 | 0.0218 | 0.0787 | 0.1507 | 0.1988 | 0.2017 | 0.1664 | 0.1146 | 0.0666 | 0.0327 |
|    | 6 | 0.0002 | 0.0052 | 0.0301 | 0.0816 | 0.1436 | 0.1873 | 0.1941 | 0.1655 | 0.1181 | 0.0708 |
|    | 7 | 0.0000 | 0.0010 | 0.0091 | 0.0350 | 0.0820 | 0.1376 | 0.1792 | 0.1892 | 0.1657 | 0.1214 |
|    | 8 | 0.0000 | 0.0002 | 0.0022 | 0.0120 | 0.0376 | 0.0811 | 0.1327 | 0.1734 | 0.1864 | 0.1669 |
|    | 9 | 0.0000 | 0.0000 | 0.0004 | 0.0033 | 0.0139 | 0.0386 | 0.0794 | 0.1284 | 0.1694 | 0.1855 |
|    | 10 | 0.0000 | 0.0000 | 0.0001 | 0.0008 | 0.0042 | 0.0149 | 0.0385 | 0.0771 | 0.1248 | 0.1669 |
|    | 11 | 0.0000 | 0.0000 | 0.0000 | 0.0001 | 0.0010 | 0.0046 | 0.0151 | 0.0374 | 0.0742 | 0.1214 |
|    | 12 | 0.0000 | 0.0000 | 0.0000 | 0.0000 | 0.0002 | 0.0012 | 0.0047 | 0.0145 | 0.0354 | 0.0708 |
|    | 13 | 0.0000 | 0.0000 | 0.0000 | 0.0000 | 0.0000 | 0.0002 | 0.0012 | 0.0045 | 0.0134 | 0.0327 |
|    | 14 | 0.0000 | 0.0000 | 0.0000 | 0.0000 | 0.0000 | 0.0000 | 0.0002 | 0.0011 | 0.0039 | 0.0117 |
|    | 15 | 0.0000 | 0.0000 | 0.0000 | 0.0000 | 0.0000 | 0.0000 | 0.0000 | 0.0002 | 0.0009 | 0.0031 |
|    | 16 | 0.0000 | 0.0000 | 0.0000 | 0.0000 | 0.0000 | 0.0000 | 0.0000 | 0.0000 | 0.0001 | 0.0006 |
|    | 17 | 0.0000 | 0.0000 | 0.0000 | 0.0000 | 0.0000 | 0.0000 | 0.0000 | 0.0000 | 0.0000 | 0.0001 |
|    | 18 | 0.0000 | 0.0000 | 0.0000 | 0.0000 | 0.0000 | 0.0000 | 0.0000 | 0.0000 | 0.0000 | 0.0000 |
| 19 | 0 | 0.3774 | 0.1351 | 0.0456 | 0.0144 | 0.0042 | 0.0011 | 0.0003 | 0.0001 | 0.0000 | 0.0000 |
|    | 1 | 0.3774 | 0.2852 | 0.1529 | 0.0685 | 0.0268 | 0.0093 | 0.0029 | 0.0008 | 0.0002 | 0.0000 |
|    | 2 | 0.1787 | 0.2852 | 0.2428 | 0.1540 | 0.0803 | 0.0358 | 0.0138 | 0.0046 | 0.0013 | 0.0003 |
|    | 3 | 0.0533 | 0.1796 | 0.2428 | 0.2182 | 0.1517 | 0.0869 | 0.0422 | 0.0175 | 0.0062 | 0.0018 |
|    | 4 | 0.0112 | 0.0798 | 0.1714 | 0.2182 | 0.2023 | 0.1491 | 0.0909 | 0.0467 | 0.0203 | 0.0074 |
|    | 5 | 0.0018 | 0.0266 | 0.0907 | 0.1636 | 0.2023 | 0.1916 | 0.1468 | 0.0933 | 0.0497 | 0.0222 |
|    | 6 | 0.0002 | 0.0069 | 0.0374 | 0.0955 | 0.1574 | 0.1916 | 0.1844 | 0.1451 | 0.0949 | 0.0518 |
|    | 7 | 0.0000 | 0.0014 | 0.0122 | 0.0443 | 0.0974 | 0.1525 | 0.1844 | 0.1797 | 0.1443 | 0.0961 |
|    | 8 | 0.0000 | 0.0002 | 0.0032 | 0.0166 | 0.0487 | 0.0981 | 0.1489 | 0.1797 | 0.1771 | 0.1442 |
|    | 9 | 0.0000 | 0.0000 | 0.0007 | 0.0051 | 0.0198 | 0.0514 | 0.0980 | 0.1464 | 0.1771 | 0.1762 |
|    | 10 | 0.0000 | 0.0000 | 0.0001 | 0.0013 | 0.0066 | 0.0220 | 0.0528 | 0.0976 | 0.1449 | 0.1762 |
|    | 11 | 0.0000 | 0.0000 | 0.0000 | 0.0003 | 0.0018 | 0.0077 | 0.0233 | 0.0532 | 0.0970 | 0.1442 |
|    | 12 | 0.0000 | 0.0000 | 0.0000 | 0.0000 | 0.0004 | 0.0022 | 0.0083 | 0.0237 | 0.0529 | 0.0961 |
|    | 13 | 0.0000 | 0.0000 | 0.0000 | 0.0000 | 0.0001 | 0.0005 | 0.0024 | 0.0085 | 0.0233 | 0.0518 |
|    | 14 | 0.0000 | 0.0000 | 0.0000 | 0.0000 | 0.0000 | 0.0001 | 0.0006 | 0.0024 | 0.0082 | 0.0222 |
|    | 15 | 0.0000 | 0.0000 | 0.0000 | 0.0000 | 0.0000 | 0.0000 | 0.0001 | 0.0005 | 0.0022 | 0.0074 |
|    | 16 | 0.0000 | 0.0000 | 0.0000 | 0.0000 | 0.0000 | 0.0000 | 0.0000 | 0.0001 | 0.0005 | 0.0018 |
|    | 17 | 0.0000 | 0.0000 | 0.0000 | 0.0000 | 0.0000 | 0.0000 | 0.0000 | 0.0000 | 0.0001 | 0.0003 |
|    | 18 | 0.0000 | 0.0000 | 0.0000 | 0.0000 | 0.0000 | 0.0000 | 0.0000 | 0.0000 | 0.0000 | 0.0000 |
|    | 19 | 0.0000 | 0.0000 | 0.0000 | 0.0000 | 0.0000 | 0.0000 | 0.0000 | 0.0000 | 0.0000 | 0.0000 |
| 20 | 0 | 0.3585 | 0.1216 | 0.0388 | 0.0115 | 0.0032 | 0.0008 | 0.0002 | 0.0000 | 0.0000 | 0.0000 |
|    | 1 | 0.3774 | 0.2702 | 0.1368 | 0.0576 | 0.0211 | 0.0068 | 0.0020 | 0.0005 | 0.0001 | 0.0000 |
|    | 2 | 0.1887 | 0.2852 | 0.2293 | 0.1369 | 0.0669 | 0.0278 | 0.0100 | 0.0031 | 0.0008 | 0.0002 |
|    | 3 | 0.0596 | 0.1901 | 0.2428 | 0.2054 | 0.1339 | 0.0716 | 0.0323 | 0.0123 | 0.0040 | 0.0011 |
|    | 4 | 0.0133 | 0.0898 | 0.1821 | 0.2182 | 0.1897 | 0.1304 | 0.0738 | 0.0350 | 0.0139 | 0.0046 |
|    | 5 | 0.0022 | 0.0319 | 0.1028 | 0.1746 | 0.2023 | 0.1789 | 0.1272 | 0.0746 | 0.0365 | 0.0148 |
|    | 6 | 0.0003 | 0.0089 | 0.0454 | 0.1091 | 0.1686 | 0.1916 | 0.1712 | 0.1244 | 0.0746 | 0.0370 |

**_Table 1_**  Exact Binomial Probabilities                                                             *495*

**_Table 1_**  (Continued)

| n | k | 0.05 | 0.10 | 0.15 | 0.20 | 0.25 | 0.30 | 0.35 | 0.40 | 0.45 | 0.50 |
|---|---|------|------|------|------|------|------|------|------|------|------|
| | 7 | 0.0000 | 0.0020 | 0.0160 | 0.0546 | 0.1124 | 0.1643 | 0.1844 | 0.1659 | 0.1221 | 0.0739 |
| | 8 | 0.0000 | 0.0004 | 0.0046 | 0.0222 | 0.0609 | 0.1144 | 0.1614 | 0.1797 | 0.1623 | 0.1201 |
| | 9 | 0.0000 | 0.0001 | 0.0011 | 0.0074 | 0.0271 | 0.0654 | 0.1158 | 0.1597 | 0.1771 | 0.1602 |
| | 10 | 0.0000 | 0.0000 | 0.0002 | 0.0020 | 0.0099 | 0.0308 | 0.0686 | 0.1171 | 0.1593 | 0.1762 |
| | 11 | 0.0000 | 0.0000 | 0.0000 | 0.0005 | 0.0030 | 0.0120 | 0.0336 | 0.0710 | 0.1185 | 0.1602 |
| | 12 | 0.0000 | 0.0000 | 0.0000 | 0.0001 | 0.0008 | 0.0039 | 0.0136 | 0.0355 | 0.0727 | 0.1201 |
| | 13 | 0.0000 | 0.0000 | 0.0000 | 0.0000 | 0.0002 | 0.0010 | 0.0045 | 0.0146 | 0.0366 | 0.0739 |
| | 14 | 0.0000 | 0.0000 | 0.0000 | 0.0000 | 0.0000 | 0.0002 | 0.0012 | 0.0049 | 0.0150 | 0.0370 |
| | 15 | 0.0000 | 0.0000 | 0.0000 | 0.0000 | 0.0000 | 0.0000 | 0.0003 | 0.0013 | 0.0049 | 0.0148 |
| | 16 | 0.0000 | 0.0000 | 0.0000 | 0.0000 | 0.0000 | 0.0000 | 0.0000 | 0.0003 | 0.0013 | 0.0046 |
| | 17 | 0.0000 | 0.0000 | 0.0000 | 0.0000 | 0.0000 | 0.0000 | 0.0000 | 0.0000 | 0.0002 | 0.0011 |
| | 18 | 0.0000 | 0.0000 | 0.0000 | 0.0000 | 0.0000 | 0.0000 | 0.0000 | 0.0000 | 0.0000 | 0.0002 |
| | 19 | 0.0000 | 0.0000 | 0.0000 | 0.0000 | 0.0000 | 0.0000 | 0.0000 | 0.0000 | 0.0000 | 0.0000 |
| | 20 | 0.0000 | 0.0000 | 0.0000 | 0.0000 | 0.0000 | 0.0000 | 0.0000 | 0.0000 | 0.0000 | 0.0000 |

# Table 2

**Table 2** Exact Poisson Probabilities $Pr(X = k) = \dfrac{e^{-\mu}\mu^k}{k!}$

| | | | | | $\mu$ | | | | | |
|---|---|---|---|---|---|---|---|---|---|---|
| $k$ | 0.5 | 1.0 | 1.5 | 2.0 | 2.5 | 3.0 | 3.5 | 4.0 | 4.5 | 5.0 |
| 0 | 0.6065 | 0.3679 | 0.2231 | 0.1353 | 0.0821 | 0.0498 | 0.0302 | 0.0183 | 0.0111 | 0.0067 |
| 1 | 0.3033 | 0.3679 | 0.3347 | 0.2707 | 0.2052 | 0.1494 | 0.1057 | 0.0733 | 0.0500 | 0.0337 |
| 2 | 0.0758 | 0.1839 | 0.2510 | 0.2707 | 0.2565 | 0.2240 | 0.1850 | 0.1465 | 0.1125 | 0.0842 |
| 3 | 0.0126 | 0.0613 | 0.1255 | 0.1804 | 0.2138 | 0.2240 | 0.2158 | 0.1954 | 0.1687 | 0.1404 |
| 4 | 0.0016 | 0.0153 | 0.0471 | 0.0902 | 0.1336 | 0.1680 | 0.1888 | 0.1954 | 0.1898 | 0.1755 |
| 5 | 0.0002 | 0.0031 | 0.0141 | 0.0361 | 0.0668 | 0.1008 | 0.1322 | 0.1563 | 0.1708 | 0.1755 |
| 6 | 0.0000 | 0.0005 | 0.0035 | 0.0120 | 0.0278 | 0.0504 | 0.0771 | 0.1042 | 0.1281 | 0.1462 |
| 7 | 0.0000 | 0.0001 | 0.0008 | 0.0034 | 0.0099 | 0.0216 | 0.0385 | 0.0595 | 0.0824 | 0.1044 |
| 8 | 0.0000 | 0.0000 | 0.0001 | 0.0009 | 0.0031 | 0.0081 | 0.0169 | 0.0298 | 0.0463 | 0.0653 |
| 9 | 0.0000 | 0.0000 | 0.0000 | 0.0002 | 0.0009 | 0.0027 | 0.0066 | 0.0132 | 0.0232 | 0.0363 |
| 10 | 0.0000 | 0.0000 | 0.0000 | 0.0000 | 0.0002 | 0.0008 | 0.0023 | 0.0053 | 0.0104 | 0.0181 |
| 11 | 0.0000 | 0.0000 | 0.0000 | 0.0000 | 0.0000 | 0.0002 | 0.0007 | 0.0019 | 0.0043 | 0.0082 |
| 12 | 0.0000 | 0.0000 | 0.0000 | 0.0000 | 0.0000 | 0.0001 | 0.0002 | 0.0006 | 0.0016 | 0.0034 |
| 13 | 0.0000 | 0.0000 | 0.0000 | 0.0000 | 0.0000 | 0.0000 | 0.0001 | 0.0002 | 0.0006 | 0.0013 |
| 14 | 0.0000 | 0.0000 | 0.0000 | 0.0000 | 0.0000 | 0.0000 | 0.0000 | 0.0001 | 0.0002 | 0.0005 |
| 15 | 0.0000 | 0.0000 | 0.0000 | 0.0000 | 0.0000 | 0.0000 | 0.0000 | 0.0000 | 0.0001 | 0.0002 |
| 16 | 0.0000 | 0.0000 | 0.0000 | 0.0000 | 0.0000 | 0.0000 | 0.0000 | 0.0000 | 0.0000 | 0.0000 |

| | | | | | $\mu$ | | | | | |
|---|---|---|---|---|---|---|---|---|---|---|
| $k$ | 5.5 | 6.0 | 6.5 | 7.0 | 7.5 | 8.0 | 8.5 | 9.0 | 9.5 | 10.0 |
| 0 | 0.0041 | 0.0025 | 0.0015 | 0.0009 | 0.0006 | 0.0003 | 0.0002 | 0.0001 | 0.0001 | 0.0000 |
| 1 | 0.0225 | 0.0149 | 0.0098 | 0.0064 | 0.0041 | 0.0027 | 0.0017 | 0.0011 | 0.0007 | 0.0005 |
| 2 | 0.0618 | 0.0446 | 0.0318 | 0.0223 | 0.0156 | 0.0107 | 0.0074 | 0.0050 | 0.0034 | 0.0023 |
| 3 | 0.1133 | 0.0892 | 0.0688 | 0.0521 | 0.0389 | 0.0286 | 0.0208 | 0.0150 | 0.0107 | 0.0076 |
| 4 | 0.1558 | 0.1339 | 0.1118 | 0.0912 | 0.0729 | 0.0573 | 0.0443 | 0.0337 | 0.0254 | 0.0189 |
| 5 | 0.1714 | 0.1606 | 0.1454 | 0.1277 | 0.1094 | 0.0916 | 0.0752 | 0.0607 | 0.0483 | 0.0378 |
| 6 | 0.1571 | 0.1606 | 0.1575 | 0.1490 | 0.1367 | 0.1221 | 0.1066 | 0.0911 | 0.0764 | 0.0631 |

**Table 2** Exact Poisson Probabilities

*497*

**Table 2** (Continued)

| | | | | | $\mu$ | | | | | |
|---|---|---|---|---|---|---|---|---|---|---|
| k | 5.5 | 6.0 | 6.5 | 7.0 | 7.5 | 8.0 | 8.5 | 9.0 | 9.5 | 10.0 |
| 7 | 0.1234 | 0.1377 | 0.1462 | 0.1490 | 0.1465 | 0.1396 | 0.1294 | 0.1171 | 0.1037 | 0.0901 |
| 8 | 0.0849 | 0.1033 | 0.1188 | 0.1304 | 0.1373 | 0.1396 | 0.1375 | 0.1318 | 0.1232 | 0.1126 |
| 9 | 0.0519 | 0.0688 | 0.0858 | 0.1014 | 0.1144 | 0.1241 | 0.1299 | 0.1318 | 0.1300 | 0.1251 |
| 10 | 0.0285 | 0.0413 | 0.0558 | 0.0710 | 0.0858 | 0.0993 | 0.1104 | 0.1186 | 0.1235 | 0.1251 |
| 11 | 0.0143 | 0.0225 | 0.0330 | 0.0452 | 0.0585 | 0.0722 | 0.0853 | 0.0970 | 0.1067 | 0.1137 |
| 12 | 0.0065 | 0.0113 | 0.0179 | 0.0263 | 0.0366 | 0.0481 | 0.0604 | 0.0728 | 0.0844 | 0.0948 |
| 13 | 0.0028 | 0.0052 | 0.0089 | 0.0142 | 0.0211 | 0.0296 | 0.0395 | 0.0504 | 0.0617 | 0.0729 |
| 14 | 0.0011 | 0.0022 | 0.0041 | 0.0071 | 0.0113 | 0.0169 | 0.0240 | 0.0324 | 0.0419 | 0.0521 |
| 15 | 0.0004 | 0.0009 | 0.0018 | 0.0033 | 0.0057 | 0.0090 | 0.0136 | 0.0194 | 0.0265 | 0.0347 |
| 16 | 0.0001 | 0.0003 | 0.0007 | 0.0014 | 0.0026 | 0.0045 | 0.0072 | 0.0109 | 0.0157 | 0.0217 |
| 17 | 0.0000 | 0.0001 | 0.0003 | 0.0006 | 0.0012 | 0.0021 | 0.0036 | 0.0058 | 0.0088 | 0.0128 |
| 18 | 0.0000 | 0.0000 | 0.0001 | 0.0002 | 0.0005 | 0.0009 | 0.0017 | 0.0029 | 0.0046 | 0.0071 |
| 19 | 0.0000 | 0.0000 | 0.0000 | 0.0001 | 0.0002 | 0.0004 | 0.0008 | 0.0014 | 0.0023 | 0.0037 |
| 20 | 0.0000 | 0.0000 | 0.0000 | 0.0000 | 0.0001 | 0.0002 | 0.0003 | 0.0006 | 0.0011 | 0.0019 |
| 21 | 0.0000 | 0.0000 | 0.0000 | 0.0000 | 0.0000 | 0.0001 | 0.0001 | 0.0003 | 0.0005 | 0.0009 |
| 22 | 0.0000 | 0.0000 | 0.0000 | 0.0000 | 0.0000 | 0.0000 | 0.0001 | 0.0001 | 0.0002 | 0.0004 |
| 23 | 0.0000 | 0.0000 | 0.0000 | 0.0000 | 0.0000 | 0.0000 | 0.0000 | 0.0000 | 0.0001 | 0.0002 |
| 24 | 0.0000 | 0.0000 | 0.0000 | 0.0000 | 0.0000 | 0.0000 | 0.0000 | 0.0000 | 0.0000 | 0.0001 |
| 25 | 0.0000 | 0.0000 | 0.0000 | 0.0000 | 0.0000 | 0.0000 | 0.0000 | 0.0000 | 0.0000 | 0.0000 |

| | | | | | $\mu$ | | | | | |
|---|---|---|---|---|---|---|---|---|---|---|
| k | 10.5 | 11.0 | 11.5 | 12.0 | 12.5 | 13.0 | 13.5 | 14.0 | 14.5 | 15.0 |
| 0 | 0.0000 | 0.0000 | 0.0000 | 0.0000 | 0.0000 | 0.0000 | 0.0000 | 0.0000 | 0.0000 | 0.0000 |
| 1 | 0.0003 | 0.0002 | 0.0001 | 0.0001 | 0.0000 | 0.0000 | 0.0000 | 0.0000 | 0.0000 | 0.0000 |
| 2 | 0.0015 | 0.0010 | 0.0007 | 0.0004 | 0.0003 | 0.0002 | 0.0001 | 0.0001 | 0.0001 | 0.0000 |
| 3 | 0.0053 | 0.0037 | 0.0026 | 0.0018 | 0.0012 | 0.0008 | 0.0006 | 0.0004 | 0.0003 | 0.0002 |
| 4 | 0.0139 | 0.0102 | 0.0074 | 0.0053 | 0.0038 | 0.0027 | 0.0019 | 0.0013 | 0.0009 | 0.0006 |
| 5 | 0.0293 | 0.0224 | 0.0170 | 0.0127 | 0.0095 | 0.0070 | 0.0051 | 0.0037 | 0.0027 | 0.0019 |
| 6 | 0.0513 | 0.0411 | 0.0325 | 0.0255 | 0.0197 | 0.0152 | 0.0115 | 0.0087 | 0.0065 | 0.0048 |
| 7 | 0.0769 | 0.0646 | 0.0535 | 0.0437 | 0.0353 | 0.0281 | 0.0222 | 0.0174 | 0.0135 | 0.0104 |
| 8 | 0.1009 | 0.0888 | 0.0769 | 0.0655 | 0.0551 | 0.0457 | 0.0375 | 0.0304 | 0.0244 | 0.0194 |
| 9 | 0.1177 | 0.1085 | 0.0982 | 0.0874 | 0.0765 | 0.0661 | 0.0563 | 0.0473 | 0.0394 | 0.0324 |
| 10 | 0.1236 | 0.1194 | 0.1129 | 0.1048 | 0.0956 | 0.0859 | 0.0760 | 0.0663 | 0.0571 | 0.0486 |
| 11 | 0.1180 | 0.1194 | 0.1181 | 0.1144 | 0.1087 | 0.1015 | 0.0932 | 0.0844 | 0.0753 | 0.0663 |
| 12 | 0.1032 | 0.1094 | 0.1131 | 0.1144 | 0.1132 | 0.1099 | 0.1049 | 0.0984 | 0.0910 | 0.0829 |
| 13 | 0.0834 | 0.0926 | 0.1001 | 0.1056 | 0.1089 | 0.1099 | 0.1089 | 0.1060 | 0.1014 | 0.0956 |
| 14 | 0.0625 | 0.0728 | 0.0822 | 0.0905 | 0.0972 | 0.1021 | 0.1050 | 0.1060 | 0.1051 | 0.1024 |
| 15 | 0.0438 | 0.0534 | 0.0630 | 0.0724 | 0.0810 | 0.0885 | 0.0945 | 0.0989 | 0.1016 | 0.1024 |
| 16 | 0.0287 | 0.0367 | 0.0453 | 0.0543 | 0.0633 | 0.0719 | 0.0798 | 0.0866 | 0.0920 | 0.0960 |
| 17 | 0.0177 | 0.0237 | 0.0306 | 0.0383 | 0.0465 | 0.0550 | 0.0633 | 0.0713 | 0.0785 | 0.0847 |
| 18 | 0.0104 | 0.0145 | 0.0196 | 0.0255 | 0.0323 | 0.0397 | 0.0475 | 0.0554 | 0.0632 | 0.0706 |
| 19 | 0.0057 | 0.0084 | 0.0119 | 0.0161 | 0.0213 | 0.0272 | 0.0337 | 0.0409 | 0.0483 | 0.0557 |
| 20 | 0.0030 | 0.0046 | 0.0068 | 0.0097 | 0.0133 | 0.0177 | 0.0228 | 0.0286 | 0.0350 | 0.0418 |

*Table 2*  (Continued)

|  | | | | | μ | | | | | |
|---|---|---|---|---|---|---|---|---|---|---|
| k | 10.5 | 11.0 | 11.5 | 12.0 | 12.5 | 13.0 | 13.5 | 14.0 | 14.5 | 15.0 |
| 21 | 0.0015 | 0.0024 | 0.0037 | 0.0055 | 0.0079 | 0.0109 | 0.0146 | 0.0191 | 0.0242 | 0.0299 |
| 22 | 0.0007 | 0.0012 | 0.0020 | 0.0030 | 0.0045 | 0.0065 | 0.0090 | 0.0121 | 0.0159 | 0.0204 |
| 23 | 0.0003 | 0.0006 | 0.0010 | 0.0016 | 0.0024 | 0.0037 | 0.0053 | 0.0074 | 0.0100 | 0.0133 |
| 24 | 0.0001 | 0.0003 | 0.0005 | 0.0008 | 0.0013 | 0.0020 | 0.0030 | 0.0043 | 0.0061 | 0.0083 |
| 25 | 0.0001 | 0.0001 | 0.0002 | 0.0004 | 0.0006 | 0.0010 | 0.0016 | 0.0024 | 0.0035 | 0.0050 |
| 26 | 0.0000 | 0.0000 | 0.0001 | 0.0002 | 0.0003 | 0.0005 | 0.0008 | 0.0013 | 0.0020 | 0.0029 |
| 27 | 0.0000 | 0.0000 | 0.0000 | 0.0001 | 0.0001 | 0.0002 | 0.0004 | 0.0007 | 0.0011 | 0.0016 |
| 28 | 0.0000 | 0.0000 | 0.0000 | 0.0000 | 0.0001 | 0.0001 | 0.0002 | 0.0003 | 0.0005 | 0.0009 |
| 29 | 0.0000 | 0.0000 | 0.0000 | 0.0000 | 0.0000 | 0.0001 | 0.0001 | 0.0002 | 0.0003 | 0.0004 |
| 30 | 0.0000 | 0.0000 | 0.0000 | 0.0000 | 0.0000 | 0.0000 | 0.0000 | 0.0001 | 0.0001 | 0.0002 |
| 31 | 0.0000 | 0.0000 | 0.0000 | 0.0000 | 0.0000 | 0.0000 | 0.0000 | 0.0000 | 0.0001 | 0.0001 |
| 32 | 0.0000 | 0.0000 | 0.0000 | 0.0000 | 0.0000 | 0.0000 | 0.0000 | 0.0000 | 0.0000 | 0.0001 |
| 33 | 0.0000 | 0.0000 | 0.0000 | 0.0000 | 0.0000 | 0.0000 | 0.0000 | 0.0000 | 0.0000 | 0.0000 |

|  | | | | | μ | | | | | |
|---|---|---|---|---|---|---|---|---|---|---|
| k | 15.5 | 16.0 | 16.5 | 17.0 | 17.5 | 18.0 | 18.5 | 19.0 | 19.5 | 20.0 |
| 0 | 0.0000 | 0.0000 | 0.0000 | 0.0000 | 0.0000 | 0.0000 | 0.0000 | 0.0000 | 0.0000 | 0.0000 |
| 1 | 0.0000 | 0.0000 | 0.0000 | 0.0000 | 0.0000 | 0.0000 | 0.0000 | 0.0000 | 0.0000 | 0.0000 |
| 2 | 0.0000 | 0.0000 | 0.0000 | 0.0000 | 0.0000 | 0.0000 | 0.0000 | 0.0000 | 0.0000 | 0.0000 |
| 3 | 0.0001 | 0.0001 | 0.0001 | 0.0000 | 0.0000 | 0.0000 | 0.0000 | 0.0000 | 0.0000 | 0.0000 |
| 4 | 0.0004 | 0.0003 | 0.0002 | 0.0001 | 0.0001 | 0.0001 | 0.0000 | 0.0000 | 0.0000 | 0.0000 |
| 5 | 0.0014 | 0.0010 | 0.0007 | 0.0005 | 0.0003 | 0.0002 | 0.0002 | 0.0001 | 0.0001 | 0.0001 |
| 6 | 0.0036 | 0.0026 | 0.0019 | 0.0014 | 0.0010 | 0.0007 | 0.0005 | 0.0004 | 0.0003 | 0.0002 |
| 7 | 0.0079 | 0.0060 | 0.0045 | 0.0034 | 0.0025 | 0.0019 | 0.0014 | 0.0010 | 0.0007 | 0.0005 |
| 8 | 0.0153 | 0.0120 | 0.0093 | 0.0072 | 0.0055 | 0.0042 | 0.0031 | 0.0024 | 0.0018 | 0.0013 |
| 9 | 0.0264 | 0.0213 | 0.0171 | 0.0135 | 0.0107 | 0.0083 | 0.0065 | 0.0050 | 0.0038 | 0.0029 |
| 10 | 0.0409 | 0.0341 | 0.0281 | 0.0230 | 0.0186 | 0.0150 | 0.0120 | 0.0095 | 0.0074 | 0.0058 |
| 11 | 0.0577 | 0.0496 | 0.0422 | 0.0355 | 0.0297 | 0.0245 | 0.0201 | 0.0164 | 0.0132 | 0.0106 |
| 12 | 0.0745 | 0.0661 | 0.0580 | 0.0504 | 0.0432 | 0.0368 | 0.0310 | 0.0259 | 0.0214 | 0.0176 |
| 13 | 0.0888 | 0.0814 | 0.0736 | 0.0658 | 0.0582 | 0.0509 | 0.0441 | 0.0378 | 0.0322 | 0.0271 |
| 14 | 0.0983 | 0.0930 | 0.0868 | 0.0800 | 0.0728 | 0.0655 | 0.0583 | 0.0514 | 0.0448 | 0.0387 |
| 15 | 0.1016 | 0.0992 | 0.0955 | 0.0906 | 0.0849 | 0.0786 | 0.0719 | 0.0650 | 0.0582 | 0.0516 |
| 16 | 0.0984 | 0.0992 | 0.0985 | 0.0963 | 0.0929 | 0.0884 | 0.0831 | 0.0772 | 0.0710 | 0.0646 |
| 17 | 0.0897 | 0.0934 | 0.0956 | 0.0963 | 0.0956 | 0.0936 | 0.0904 | 0.0863 | 0.0814 | 0.0760 |
| 18 | 0.0773 | 0.0830 | 0.0876 | 0.0909 | 0.0929 | 0.0936 | 0.0930 | 0.0911 | 0.0882 | 0.0844 |
| 19 | 0.0630 | 0.0699 | 0.0761 | 0.0814 | 0.0856 | 0.0887 | 0.0905 | 0.0911 | 0.0905 | 0.0888 |
| 20 | 0.0489 | 0.0559 | 0.0628 | 0.0692 | 0.0749 | 0.0798 | 0.0837 | 0.0866 | 0.0883 | 0.0888 |
| 21 | 0.0361 | 0.0426 | 0.0493 | 0.0560 | 0.0624 | 0.0684 | 0.0738 | 0.0783 | 0.0820 | 0.0846 |
| 22 | 0.0254 | 0.0310 | 0.0370 | 0.0433 | 0.0496 | 0.0560 | 0.0620 | 0.0676 | 0.0727 | 0.0769 |
| 23 | 0.0171 | 0.0216 | 0.0265 | 0.0320 | 0.0378 | 0.0438 | 0.0499 | 0.0559 | 0.0616 | 0.0669 |
| 24 | 0.0111 | 0.0144 | 0.0182 | 0.0226 | 0.0275 | 0.0328 | 0.0385 | 0.0442 | 0.0500 | 0.0557 |
| 25 | 0.0069 | 0.0092 | 0.0120 | 0.0154 | 0.0193 | 0.0237 | 0.0285 | 0.0336 | 0.0390 | 0.0446 |
| 26 | 0.0041 | 0.0057 | 0.0076 | 0.0101 | 0.0130 | 0.0164 | 0.0202 | 0.0246 | 0.0293 | 0.0343 |

*Table 2* Exact Poisson Probabilities                                                                                499

*Table 2* (Continued)

| | | | | | | $\mu$ | | | | | |
| k | 15.5 | 16.0 | 16.5 | 17.0 | 17.5 | 18.0 | 18.5 | 19.0 | 19.5 | 20.0 |
|---|---|---|---|---|---|---|---|---|---|---|
| 27 | 0.0023 | 0.0034 | 0.0047 | 0.0063 | 0.0084 | 0.0109 | 0.0139 | 0.0173 | 0.0211 | 0.0254 |
| 28 | 0.0013 | 0.0019 | 0.0028 | 0.0038 | 0.0053 | 0.0070 | 0.0092 | 0.0117 | 0.0147 | 0.0181 |
| 29 | 0.0007 | 0.0011 | 0.0016 | 0.0023 | 0.0032 | 0.0044 | 0.0058 | 0.0077 | 0.0099 | 0.0125 |
| 30 | 0.0004 | 0.0006 | 0.0009 | 0.0013 | 0.0019 | 0.0026 | 0.0036 | 0.0049 | 0.0064 | 0.0083 |
| 31 | 0.0002 | 0.0003 | 0.0005 | 0.0007 | 0.0010 | 0.0015 | 0.0022 | 0.0030 | 0.0040 | 0.0054 |
| 32 | 0.0001 | 0.0001 | 0.0002 | 0.0004 | 0.0006 | 0.0009 | 0.0012 | 0.0018 | 0.0025 | 0.0034 |
| 33 | 0.0000 | 0.0001 | 0.0001 | 0.0002 | 0.0003 | 0.0005 | 0.0007 | 0.0010 | 0.0015 | 0.0020 |
| 34 | 0.0000 | 0.0000 | 0.0001 | 0.0001 | 0.0002 | 0.0002 | 0.0004 | 0.0006 | 0.0008 | 0.0012 |
| 35 | 0.0000 | 0.0000 | 0.0000 | 0.0000 | 0.0001 | 0.0001 | 0.0002 | 0.0003 | 0.0005 | 0.0007 |
| 36 | 0.0000 | 0.0000 | 0.0000 | 0.0000 | 0.0000 | 0.0001 | 0.0001 | 0.0002 | 0.0003 | 0.0004 |
| 37 | 0.0000 | 0.0000 | 0.0000 | 0.0000 | 0.0000 | 0.0000 | 0.0001 | 0.0001 | 0.0001 | 0.0002 |
| 38 | 0.0000 | 0.0000 | 0.0000 | 0.0000 | 0.0000 | 0.0000 | 0.0000 | 0.0000 | 0.0001 | 0.0001 |
| 39 | 0.0000 | 0.0000 | 0.0000 | 0.0000 | 0.0000 | 0.0000 | 0.0000 | 0.0000 | 0.0000 | 0.0001 |
| 40 | 0.0000 | 0.0000 | 0.0000 | 0.0000 | 0.0000 | 0.0000 | 0.0000 | 0.0000 | 0.0000 | 0.0000 |

# Table 3

## Table 3 The Normal Distribution

$$A(x) = \Phi(k) = \Pr(X \le x) \qquad f(x) = \frac{1}{\sqrt{2\pi}} e^{(-1/2)x^2}$$

(A)

$$B(x) = 1 - \Phi(x) = \Pr(X > x) \qquad f(x) = \frac{1}{\sqrt{2\pi}} e^{(-1/2)x^2}$$

(B)

$$C(x) = \Pr(0 \le X \le x) \qquad f(x) = \frac{1}{\sqrt{2\pi}} e^{(-1/2)x^2}$$

(C)

$$D(x) = \Pr(-x \le X \le x) \qquad f(x) = \frac{1}{\sqrt{2\pi}} e^{(-1/2)x^2}$$

(D)

| x | A* | B† | C‡ | D§ | x | A | B | C | D |
|---|---|---|---|---|---|---|---|---|---|
| 0.0 | 0.5000 | 0.5000 | 0.0 | 0.0 | 0.32 | 0.6255 | 0.3745 | 0.1255 | 0.2510 |
| 0.01 | 0.5040 | 0.4960 | 0.0040 | 0.0080 | 0.33 | 0.6293 | 0.3707 | 0.1293 | 0.2586 |
| 0.02 | 0.5080 | 0.4920 | 0.0080 | 0.0160 | 0.34 | 0.6331 | 0.3669 | 0.1331 | 0.2661 |
| 0.03 | 0.5120 | 0.4880 | 0.0120 | 0.0239 | 0.35 | 0.6368 | 0.3632 | 0.1368 | 0.2737 |
| 0.04 | 0.5160 | 0.4840 | 0.0160 | 0.0319 | 0.36 | 0.6406 | 0.3594 | 0.1406 | 0.2812 |
| 0.05 | 0.5199 | 0.4801 | 0.0199 | 0.0399 | 0.37 | 0.6443 | 0.3557 | 0.1443 | 0.2886 |
| 0.06 | 0.5239 | 0.4761 | 0.0239 | 0.0478 | 0.38 | 0.6480 | 0.3520 | 0.1480 | 0.2961 |
| 0.07 | 0.5279 | 0.4721 | 0.0279 | 0.0558 | 0.39 | 0.6517 | 0.3483 | 0.1517 | 0.3035 |
| 0.08 | 0.5319 | 0.4681 | 0.0319 | 0.0638 | 0.40 | 0.6554 | 0.3446 | 0.1554 | 0.3108 |
| 0.09 | 0.5359 | 0.4641 | 0.0359 | 0.0717 | 0.41 | 0.6591 | 0.3409 | 0.1591 | 0.3182 |
| 0.10 | 0.5398 | 0.4602 | 0.0398 | 0.0797 | 0.42 | 0.6628 | 0.3372 | 0.1628 | 0.3255 |
| 0.11 | 0.5438 | 0.4562 | 0.0438 | 0.0876 | 0.43 | 0.6664 | 0.3336 | 0.1664 | 0.3328 |
| 0.12 | 0.5478 | 0.4522 | 0.0478 | 0.0955 | 0.44 | 0.6700 | 0.3300 | 0.1700 | 0.3401 |
| 0.13 | 0.5517 | 0.4483 | 0.0517 | 0.1034 | 0.45 | 0.6736 | 0.3264 | 0.1736 | 0.3473 |
| 0.14 | 0.5557 | 0.4443 | 0.0557 | 0.1113 | 0.46 | 0.6772 | 0.3228 | 0.1772 | 0.3545 |
| 0.15 | 0.5596 | 0.4404 | 0.0596 | 0.1192 | 0.47 | 0.6808 | 0.3192 | 0.1808 | 0.3616 |
| 0.16 | 0.5636 | 0.4364 | 0.0636 | 0.1271 | 0.48 | 0.6844 | 0.3156 | 0.1844 | 0.3688 |
| 0.17 | 0.5675 | 0.4325 | 0.0675 | 0.1350 | 0.49 | 0.6879 | 0.3121 | 0.1879 | 0.3759 |
| 0.18 | 0.5714 | 0.4286 | 0.0714 | 0.1428 | 0.50 | 0.6915 | 0.3085 | 0.1915 | 0.3829 |
| 0.19 | 0.5753 | 0.4247 | 0.0753 | 0.1507 | 0.51 | 0.6950 | 0.3050 | 0.1950 | 0.3899 |
| 0.20 | 0.5793 | 0.4207 | 0.0793 | 0.1585 | 0.52 | 0.6985 | 0.3015 | 0.1985 | 0.3969 |
| 0.21 | 0.5832 | 0.4168 | 0.0832 | 0.1663 | 0.53 | 0.7019 | 0.2981 | 0.2019 | 0.4039 |
| 0.22 | 0.5871 | 0.4129 | 0.0871 | 0.1741 | 0.54 | 0.7054 | 0.2946 | 0.2054 | 0.4108 |
| 0.23 | 0.5910 | 0.4090 | 0.0910 | 0.1819 | 0.55 | 0.7088 | 0.2912 | 0.2088 | 0.4177 |
| 0.24 | 0.5948 | 0.4052 | 0.0948 | 0.1897 | 0.56 | 0.7123 | 0.2877 | 0.2123 | 0.4245 |
| 0.25 | 0.5987 | 0.4013 | 0.0987 | 0.1974 | 0.57 | 0.7157 | 0.2843 | 0.2157 | 0.4313 |
| 0.26 | 0.6026 | 0.3974 | 0.1026 | 0.2051 | 0.58 | 0.7190 | 0.2810 | 0.2190 | 0.4381 |
| 0.27 | 0.6064 | 0.3936 | 0.1064 | 0.2128 | 0.59 | 0.7224 | 0.2776 | 0.2224 | 0.4448 |
| 0.28 | 0.6103 | 0.3897 | 0.1103 | 0.2205 | 0.60 | 0.7257 | 0.2743 | 0.2257 | 0.4515 |
| 0.29 | 0.6141 | 0.3859 | 0.1141 | 0.2282 | 0.61 | 0.7291 | 0.2709 | 0.2291 | 0.4581 |
| 0.30 | 0.6179 | 0.3821 | 0.1179 | 0.2358 | 0.62 | 0.7324 | 0.2676 | 0.2324 | 0.4647 |
| 0.31 | 0.6217 | 0.3783 | 0.1217 | 0.2434 | 0.63 | 0.7357 | 0.2643 | 0.2357 | 0.4713 |

*Table 3*  The Normal Distribution                                                                501

**Table 3**  *(Continued)*

| x | A* | B† | C‡ | D§ | x | A | B | C | D |
|---|----|----|----|----|---|---|---|---|---|
| 0.64 | 0.7389 | 0.2611 | 0.2389 | 0.4778 | 1.10 | 0.8643 | 0.1357 | 0.3643 | 0.7287 |
| 0.65 | 0.7422 | 0.2578 | 0.2422 | 0.4843 | 1.11 | 0.8665 | 0.1335 | 0.3665 | 0.7330 |
| 0.66 | 0.7454 | 0.2546 | 0.2454 | 0.4907 | 1.12 | 0.8686 | 0.1314 | 0.3686 | 0.7373 |
| 0.67 | 0.7486 | 0.2514 | 0.2486 | 0.4971 | 1.13 | 0.8708 | 0.1292 | 0.3708 | 0.7415 |
| 0.68 | 0.7517 | 0.2483 | 0.2517 | 0.5035 | 1.14 | 0.8729 | 0.1271 | 0.3729 | 0.7457 |
| 0.69 | 0.7549 | 0.2451 | 0.2549 | 0.5098 | 1.15 | 0.8749 | 0.1251 | 0.3749 | 0.7499 |
| 0.70 | 0.7580 | 0.2420 | 0.2580 | 0.5161 | 1.16 | 0.8770 | 0.1230 | 0.3770 | 0.7540 |
| 0.71 | 0.7611 | 0.2389 | 0.2611 | 0.5223 | 1.17 | 0.8790 | 0.1210 | 0.3790 | 0.7580 |
| 0.72 | 0.7642 | 0.2358 | 0.2642 | 0.5285 | 1.18 | 0.8810 | 0.1190 | 0.3810 | 0.7620 |
| 0.73 | 0.7673 | 0.2327 | 0.2673 | 0.5346 | 1.19 | 0.8830 | 0.1170 | 0.3830 | 0.7660 |
| 0.74 | 0.7703 | 0.2297 | 0.2703 | 0.5407 | 1.20 | 0.8849 | 0.1151 | 0.3849 | 0.7699 |
| 0.75 | 0.7734 | 0.2266 | 0.2734 | 0.5467 | 1.21 | 0.8869 | 0.1131 | 0.3869 | 0.7737 |
| 0.76 | 0.7764 | 0.2236 | 0.2764 | 0.5527 | 1.22 | 0.8888 | 0.1112 | 0.3888 | 0.7775 |
| 0.77 | 0.7793 | 0.2207 | 0.2793 | 0.5587 | 1.23 | 0.8907 | 0.1093 | 0.3907 | 0.7813 |
| 0.78 | 0.7823 | 0.2177 | 0.2823 | 0.5646 | 1.24 | 0.8925 | 0.1075 | 0.3925 | 0.7850 |
| 0.79 | 0.7852 | 0.2148 | 0.2852 | 0.5705 | 1.25 | 0.8944 | 0.1056 | 0.3944 | 0.7887 |
| 0.80 | 0.7881 | 0.2119 | 0.2881 | 0.5763 | 1.26 | 0.8962 | 0.1038 | 0.3962 | 0.7923 |
| 0.81 | 0.7910 | 0.2090 | 0.2910 | 0.5821 | 1.27 | 0.8980 | 0.1020 | 0.3980 | 0.7959 |
| 0.82 | 0.7939 | 0.2061 | 0.2939 | 0.5878 | 1.28 | 0.8997 | 0.1003 | 0.3997 | 0.7995 |
| 0.83 | 0.7967 | 0.2033 | 0.2967 | 0.5935 | 1.29 | 0.9015 | 0.0985 | 0.4015 | 0.8029 |
| 0.84 | 0.7995 | 0.2005 | 0.2995 | 0.5991 | 1.30 | 0.9032 | 0.0968 | 0.4032 | 0.8064 |
| 0.85 | 0.8023 | 0.1977 | 0.3023 | 0.6047 | 1.31 | 0.9049 | 0.0951 | 0.4049 | 0.8098 |
| 0.86 | 0.8051 | 0.1949 | 0.3051 | 0.6102 | 1.32 | 0.9066 | 0.0934 | 0.4066 | 0.8132 |
| 0.87 | 0.8078 | 0.1922 | 0.3078 | 0.6157 | 1.33 | 0.9082 | 0.0918 | 0.4082 | 0.8165 |
| 0.88 | 0.8106 | 0.1894 | 0.3106 | 0.6211 | 1.34 | 0.9099 | 0.0901 | 0.4099 | 0.8198 |
| 0.89 | 0.8133 | 0.1867 | 0.3133 | 0.6265 | 1.35 | 0.9115 | 0.0885 | 0.4115 | 0.8230 |
| 0.90 | 0.8159 | 0.1841 | 0.3159 | 0.6319 | 1.36 | 0.9131 | 0.0869 | 0.4131 | 0.8262 |
| 0.91 | 0.8186 | 0.1814 | 0.3186 | 0.6372 | 1.37 | 0.9147 | 0.0853 | 0.4147 | 0.8293 |
| 0.92 | 0.8212 | 0.1788 | 0.3212 | 0.6424 | 1.38 | 0.9162 | 0.0838 | 0.4162 | 0.8324 |
| 0.93 | 0.8238 | 0.1762 | 0.3238 | 0.6476 | 1.39 | 0.9177 | 0.0823 | 0.4177 | 0.8355 |
| 0.94 | 0.8264 | 0.1736 | 0.3264 | 0.6528 | 1.40 | 0.9192 | 0.0808 | 0.4192 | 0.8385 |
| 0.95 | 0.8289 | 0.1711 | 0.3289 | 0.6579 | 1.41 | 0.9207 | 0.0793 | 0.4207 | 0.8415 |
| 0.96 | 0.8315 | 0.1685 | 0.3315 | 0.6629 | 1.42 | 0.9222 | 0.0778 | 0.4222 | 0.8444 |
| 0.97 | 0.8340 | 0.1660 | 0.3340 | 0.6680 | 1.43 | 0.9236 | 0.0764 | 0.4236 | 0.8473 |
| 0.98 | 0.8365 | 0.1635 | 0.3365 | 0.6729 | 1.44 | 0.9251 | 0.0749 | 0.4251 | 0.8501 |
| 0.99 | 0.8389 | 0.1611 | 0.3389 | 0.6778 | 1.45 | 0.9265 | 0.0735 | 0.4265 | 0.8529 |
| 1.00 | 0.8413 | 0.1587 | 0.3413 | 0.6827 | 1.46 | 0.9279 | 0.0721 | 0.4279 | 0.8557 |
| 1.01 | 0.8438 | 0.1562 | 0.3438 | 0.6875 | 1.47 | 0.9292 | 0.0708 | 0.4292 | 0.8584 |
| 1.02 | 0.8461 | 0.1539 | 0.3461 | 0.6923 | 1.48 | 0.9306 | 0.0694 | 0.4306 | 0.8611 |
| 1.03 | 0.8485 | 0.1515 | 0.3485 | 0.6970 | 1.49 | 0.9319 | 0.0681 | 0.4319 | 0.8638 |
| 1.04 | 0.8508 | 0.1492 | 0.3508 | 0.7017 | 1.50 | 0.9332 | 0.0668 | 0.4332 | 0.8664 |
| 1.05 | 0.8531 | 0.1469 | 0.3531 | 0.7063 | 1.51 | 0.9345 | 0.0655 | 0.4345 | 0.8690 |
| 1.06 | 0.8554 | 0.1446 | 0.3554 | 0.7109 | 1.52 | 0.9357 | 0.0643 | 0.4357 | 0.8715 |
| 1.07 | 0.8577 | 0.1423 | 0.3577 | 0.7154 | 1.53 | 0.9370 | 0.0630 | 0.4370 | 0.8740 |
| 1.08 | 0.8599 | 0.1401 | 0.3599 | 0.7199 | 1.54 | 0.9382 | 0.0618 | 0.4382 | 0.8764 |
| 1.09 | 0.8621 | 0.1379 | 0.3621 | 0.7243 | 1.55 | 0.9394 | 0.0606 | 0.4394 | 0.8789 |

**Table 3**   (Continued)

| x | A* | B† | C‡ | D§ | x | A | B | C | D |
|---|---|---|---|---|---|---|---|---|---|
| 1.56 | 0.9406 | 0.0594 | 0.4406 | 0.8812 | 2.03 | 0.9788 | 0.0212 | 0.4788 | 0.9576 |
| 1.57 | 0.9418 | 0.0582 | 0.4418 | 0.8836 | 2.04 | 0.9793 | 0.0207 | 0.4793 | 0.9586 |
| 1.58 | 0.9429 | 0.0571 | 0.4429 | 0.8859 | 2.05 | 0.9798 | 0.0202 | 0.4798 | 0.9596 |
| 1.59 | 0.9441 | 0.0559 | 0.4441 | 0.8882 | 2.06 | 0.9803 | 0.0197 | 0.4803 | 0.9606 |
| 1.60 | 0.9452 | 0.0548 | 0.4452 | 0.8904 | 2.07 | 0.9808 | 0.0192 | 0.4808 | 0.9615 |
| 1.61 | 0.9463 | 0.0537 | 0.4463 | 0.8926 | 2.08 | 0.9812 | 0.0188 | 0.4812 | 0.9625 |
| 1.62 | 0.9474 | 0.0526 | 0.4474 | 0.8948 | 2.09 | 0.9817 | 0.0183 | 0.4817 | 0.9634 |
| 1.63 | 0.9484 | 0.0516 | 0.4484 | 0.8969 | 2.10 | 0.9821 | 0.0179 | 0.4821 | 0.9643 |
| 1.64 | 0.9495 | 0.0505 | 0.4495 | 0.8990 | 2.11 | 0.9826 | 0.0174 | 0.4826 | 0.9651 |
| 1.65 | 0.9505 | 0.0495 | 0.4505 | 0.9011 | 2.12 | 0.9830 | 0.0170 | 0.4830 | 0.9660 |
| 1.66 | 0.9515 | 0.0485 | 0.4515 | 0.9031 | 2.13 | 0.9834 | 0.0166 | 0.4834 | 0.9668 |
| 1.67 | 0.9525 | 0.0475 | 0.4525 | 0.9051 | 2.14 | 0.9838 | 0.0162 | 0.4838 | 0.9676 |
| 1.68 | 0.9535 | 0.0465 | 0.4535 | 0.9070 | 2.15 | 0.9842 | 0.0158 | 0.4842 | 0.9684 |
| 1.69 | 0.9545 | 0.0455 | 0.4545 | 0.9090 | 2.16 | 0.9846 | 0.0154 | 0.4846 | 0.9692 |
| 1.70 | 0.9554 | 0.0446 | 0.4554 | 0.9109 | 2.17 | 0.9850 | 0.0150 | 0.4850 | 0.9700 |
| 1.71 | 0.9564 | 0.0436 | 0.4564 | 0.9127 | 2.18 | 0.9854 | 0.0146 | 0.4854 | 0.9707 |
| 1.72 | 0.9573 | 0.0427 | 0.4573 | 0.9146 | 2.19 | 0.9857 | 0.0143 | 0.4857 | 0.9715 |
| 1.73 | 0.9582 | 0.0418 | 0.4582 | 0.9164 | 2.20 | 0.9861 | 0.0139 | 0.4861 | 0.9722 |
| 1.74 | 0.9591 | 0.0409 | 0.4591 | 0.9181 | 2.21 | 0.9864 | 0.0136 | 0.4864 | 0.9729 |
| 1.75 | 0.9599 | 0.0401 | 0.4599 | 0.9199 | 2.22 | 0.9868 | 0.0132 | 0.4868 | 0.9736 |
| 1.76 | 0.9608 | 0.0392 | 0.4608 | 0.9216 | 2.23 | 0.9871 | 0.0129 | 0.4871 | 0.9743 |
| 1.77 | 0.9616 | 0.0384 | 0.4616 | 0.9233 | 2.24 | 0.9875 | 0.0125 | 0.4875 | 0.9749 |
| 1.78 | 0.9625 | 0.0375 | 0.4625 | 0.9249 | 2.25 | 0.9878 | 0.0122 | 0.4878 | 0.9756 |
| 1.79 | 0.9633 | 0.0367 | 0.4633 | 0.9265 | 2.26 | 0.9881 | 0.0119 | 0.4881 | 0.9762 |
| 1.80 | 0.9641 | 0.0359 | 0.4641 | 0.9281 | 2.27 | 0.9884 | 0.0116 | 0.4884 | 0.9768 |
| 1.81 | 0.9649 | 0.0351 | 0.4649 | 0.9297 | 2.28 | 0.9887 | 0.0113 | 0.4887 | 0.9774 |
| 1.82 | 0.9656 | 0.0344 | 0.4656 | 0.9312 | 2.29 | 0.9890 | 0.0110 | 0.4890 | 0.9780 |
| 1.83 | 0.9664 | 0.0336 | 0.4664 | 0.9327 | 2.30 | 0.9893 | 0.0107 | 0.4893 | 0.9786 |
| 1.84 | 0.9671 | 0.0329 | 0.4671 | 0.9342 | 2.31 | 0.9896 | 0.0104 | 0.4896 | 0.9791 |
| 1.85 | 0.9678 | 0.0322 | 0.4678 | 0.9357 | 2.32 | 0.9898 | 0.0102 | 0.4898 | 0.9797 |
| 1.86 | 0.9686 | 0.0314 | 0.4686 | 0.9371 | 2.33 | 0.9901 | 0.0099 | 0.4901 | 0.9802 |
| 1.87 | 0.9693 | 0.0307 | 0.4693 | 0.9385 | 2.34 | 0.9904 | 0.0096 | 0.4904 | 0.9807 |
| 1.88 | 0.9699 | 0.0301 | 0.4699 | 0.9399 | 2.35 | 0.9906 | 0.0094 | 0.4906 | 0.9812 |
| 1.89 | 0.9706 | 0.0294 | 0.4706 | 0.9412 | 2.36 | 0.9909 | 0.0091 | 0.4909 | 0.9817 |
| 1.90 | 0.9713 | 0.0287 | 0.4713 | 0.9426 | 2.37 | 0.9911 | 0.0089 | 0.4911 | 0.9822 |
| 1.91 | 0.9719 | 0.0281 | 0.4719 | 0.9439 | 2.38 | 0.9913 | 0.0087 | 0.4913 | 0.9827 |
| 1.92 | 0.9726 | 0.0274 | 0.4726 | 0.9451 | 2.39 | 0.9916 | 0.0084 | 0.4916 | 0.9832 |
| 1.93 | 0.9732 | 0.0268 | 0.4732 | 0.9464 | 2.40 | 0.9918 | 0.0082 | 0.4918 | 0.9836 |
| 1.94 | 0.9738 | 0.0262 | 0.4738 | 0.9476 | 2.41 | 0.9920 | 0.0080 | 0.4920 | 0.9840 |
| 1.95 | 0.9744 | 0.0256 | 0.4744 | 0.9488 | 2.42 | 0.9922 | 0.0078 | 0.4922 | 0.9845 |
| 1.96 | 0.9750 | 0.0250 | 0.4750 | 0.9500 | 2.43 | 0.9925 | 0.0075 | 0.4925 | 0.9849 |
| 1.97 | 0.9756 | 0.0244 | 0.4756 | 0.9512 | 2.44 | 0.9927 | 0.0073 | 0.4927 | 0.9853 |
| 1.98 | 0.9761 | 0.0239 | 0.4761 | 0.9523 | 2.45 | 0.9929 | 0.0071 | 0.4929 | 0.9857 |
| 1.99 | 0.9767 | 0.0233 | 0.4767 | 0.9534 | 2.46 | 0.9931 | 0.0069 | 0.4931 | 0.9861 |
| 2.00 | 0.9772 | 0.0228 | 0.4772 | 0.9545 | 2.47 | 0.9932 | 0.0068 | 0.4932 | 0.9865 |
| 2.01 | 0.9778 | 0.0222 | 0.4778 | 0.9556 | 2.48 | 0.9934 | 0.0066 | 0.4934 | 0.9869 |
| 2.02 | 0.9783 | 0.0217 | 0.4783 | 0.9566 | 2.49 | 0.9936 | 0.0064 | 0.4936 | 0.9872 |

**Table 3**   The Normal Distribution                                        *503*

**Table 3**   *(Continued)*

| x | A* | B† | C‡ | D§ | x | A | B | C | D |
|------|--------|--------|--------|--------|------|--------|--------|--------|--------|
| 2.50 | 0.9938 | 0.0062 | 0.4938 | 0.9876 | 2.97 | 0.9985 | 0.0015 | 0.4985 | 0.9970 |
| 2.51 | 0.9940 | 0.0060 | 0.4940 | 0.9879 | 2.98 | 0.9986 | 0.0014 | 0.4986 | 0.9971 |
| 2.52 | 0.9941 | 0.0059 | 0.4941 | 0.9883 | 2.99 | 0.9986 | 0.0014 | 0.4986 | 0.9972 |
| 2.53 | 0.9943 | 0.0057 | 0.4943 | 0.9886 | 3.00 | 0.9987 | 0.0013 | 0.4987 | 0.9973 |
| 2.54 | 0.9945 | 0.0055 | 0.4945 | 0.9889 | 3.01 | 0.9987 | 0.0013 | 0.4987 | 0.9974 |
| 2.55 | 0.9946 | 0.0054 | 0.4946 | 0.9892 | 3.02 | 0.9987 | 0.0013 | 0.4987 | 0.9975 |
| 2.56 | 0.9948 | 0.0052 | 0.4948 | 0.9895 | 3.03 | 0.9988 | 0.0012 | 0.4988 | 0.9976 |
| 2.57 | 0.9949 | 0.0051 | 0.4949 | 0.9898 | 3.04 | 0.9988 | 0.0012 | 0.4988 | 0.9976 |
| 2.58 | 0.9951 | 0.0049 | 0.4951 | 0.9901 | 3.05 | 0.9989 | 0.0011 | 0.4989 | 0.9977 |
| 2.59 | 0.9952 | 0.0048 | 0.4952 | 0.9904 | 3.06 | 0.9989 | 0.0011 | 0.4989 | 0.9978 |
| 2.60 | 0.9953 | 0.0047 | 0.4953 | 0.9907 | 3.07 | 0.9989 | 0.0011 | 0.4989 | 0.9979 |
| 2.61 | 0.9955 | 0.0045 | 0.4955 | 0.9909 | 3.08 | 0.9990 | 0.0010 | 0.4990 | 0.9979 |
| 2.62 | 0.9956 | 0.0044 | 0.4956 | 0.9912 | 3.09 | 0.9990 | 0.0010 | 0.4990 | 0.9980 |
| 2.63 | 0.9957 | 0.0043 | 0.4957 | 0.9915 | 3.10 | 0.9990 | 0.0010 | 0.4990 | 0.9981 |
| 2.64 | 0.9959 | 0.0041 | 0.4959 | 0.9917 | 3.11 | 0.9991 | 0.0009 | 0.4991 | 0.9981 |
| 2.65 | 0.9960 | 0.0040 | 0.4960 | 0.9920 | 3.12 | 0.9991 | 0.0009 | 0.4991 | 0.9982 |
| 2.66 | 0.9961 | 0.0039 | 0.4961 | 0.9922 | 3.13 | 0.9991 | 0.0009 | 0.4991 | 0.9983 |
| 2.67 | 0.9962 | 0.0038 | 0.4962 | 0.9924 | 3.14 | 0.9992 | 0.0008 | 0.4992 | 0.9983 |
| 2.68 | 0.9963 | 0.0037 | 0.4963 | 0.9926 | 3.15 | 0.9992 | 0.0008 | 0.4992 | 0.9984 |
| 2.69 | 0.9964 | 0.0036 | 0.4964 | 0.9929 | 3.16 | 0.9992 | 0.0008 | 0.4992 | 0.9984 |
| 2.70 | 0.9965 | 0.0035 | 0.4965 | 0.9931 | 3.17 | 0.9992 | 0.0008 | 0.4992 | 0.9985 |
| 2.71 | 0.9966 | 0.0034 | 0.4966 | 0.9933 | 3.18 | 0.9993 | 0.0007 | 0.4993 | 0.9985 |
| 2.72 | 0.9967 | 0.0033 | 0.4967 | 0.9935 | 3.19 | 0.9993 | 0.0007 | 0.4993 | 0.9986 |
| 2.73 | 0.9968 | 0.0032 | 0.4968 | 0.9937 | 3.20 | 0.9993 | 0.0007 | 0.4993 | 0.9986 |
| 2.74 | 0.9969 | 0.0031 | 0.4969 | 0.9939 | 3.21 | 0.9993 | 0.0007 | 0.4993 | 0.9987 |
| 2.75 | 0.9970 | 0.0030 | 0.4970 | 0.9940 | 3.22 | 0.9994 | 0.0006 | 0.4994 | 0.9987 |
| 2.76 | 0.9971 | 0.0029 | 0.4971 | 0.9942 | 3.23 | 0.9994 | 0.0006 | 0.4994 | 0.9988 |
| 2.77 | 0.9972 | 0.0028 | 0.4972 | 0.9944 | 3.24 | 0.9994 | 0.0006 | 0.4994 | 0.9988 |
| 2.78 | 0.9973 | 0.0027 | 0.4973 | 0.9946 | 3.25 | 0.9994 | 0.0006 | 0.4994 | 0.9988 |
| 2.79 | 0.9974 | 0.0026 | 0.4974 | 0.9947 | 3.26 | 0.9994 | 0.0006 | 0.4994 | 0.9989 |
| 2.80 | 0.9974 | 0.0026 | 0.4974 | 0.9949 | 3.27 | 0.9995 | 0.0005 | 0.4995 | 0.9989 |
| 2.81 | 0.9975 | 0.0025 | 0.4975 | 0.9950 | 3.28 | 0.9995 | 0.0005 | 0.4995 | 0.9990 |
| 2.82 | 0.9976 | 0.0024 | 0.4976 | 0.9952 | 3.29 | 0.9995 | 0.0005 | 0.4995 | 0.9990 |
| 2.83 | 0.9977 | 0.0023 | 0.4977 | 0.9953 | 3.30 | 0.9995 | 0.0005 | 0.4995 | 0.9990 |
| 2.84 | 0.9977 | 0.0023 | 0.4977 | 0.9955 | 3.31 | 0.9995 | 0.0005 | 0.4995 | 0.9991 |
| 2.85 | 0.9978 | 0.0022 | 0.4978 | 0.9956 | 3.32 | 0.9995 | 0.0005 | 0.4995 | 0.9991 |
| 2.86 | 0.9979 | 0.0021 | 0.4979 | 0.9958 | 3.33 | 0.9996 | 0.0004 | 0.4996 | 0.9991 |
| 2.87 | 0.9979 | 0.0021 | 0.4979 | 0.9959 | 3.34 | 0.9996 | 0.0004 | 0.4996 | 0.9992 |
| 2.88 | 0.9980 | 0.0020 | 0.4980 | 0.9960 | 3.35 | 0.9996 | 0.0004 | 0.4996 | 0.9992 |
| 2.89 | 0.9981 | 0.0019 | 0.4981 | 0.9961 | 3.36 | 0.9996 | 0.0004 | 0.4996 | 0.9992 |
| 2.90 | 0.9981 | 0.0019 | 0.4981 | 0.9963 | 3.37 | 0.9996 | 0.0004 | 0.4996 | 0.9992 |
| 2.91 | 0.9982 | 0.0018 | 0.4982 | 0.9964 | 3.38 | 0.9996 | 0.0004 | 0.4996 | 0.9993 |
| 2.92 | 0.9982 | 0.0018 | 0.4982 | 0.9965 | 3.39 | 0.9997 | 0.0003 | 0.4997 | 0.9993 |
| 2.93 | 0.9983 | 0.0017 | 0.4983 | 0.9966 | 3.40 | 0.9997 | 0.0003 | 0.4997 | 0.9993 |
| 2.94 | 0.9984 | 0.0016 | 0.4984 | 0.9967 | 3.41 | 0.9997 | 0.0003 | 0.4997 | 0.9993 |
| 2.95 | 0.9984 | 0.0016 | 0.4984 | 0.9968 | 3.42 | 0.9997 | 0.0003 | 0.4997 | 0.9994 |
| 2.96 | 0.9985 | 0.0015 | 0.4985 | 0.9969 | 3.43 | 0.9997 | 0.0003 | 0.4997 | 0.9994 |

**Table 3**   (Continued)

| x | A* | B† | C‡ | D§ | x | A | B | C | D |
|---|---|---|---|---|---|---|---|---|---|
| 3.44 | 0.9997 | 0.0003 | 0.4997 | 0.9994 | 3.72 | 0.9999 | 0.0001 | 0.4999 | 0.9998 |
| 3.45 | 0.9997 | 0.0003 | 0.4997 | 0.9994 | 3.73 | 0.9999 | 0.0001 | 0.4999 | 0.9998 |
| 3.46 | 0.9997 | 0.0003 | 0.4997 | 0.9995 | 3.74 | 0.9999 | 0.0001 | 0.4999 | 0.9998 |
| 3.47 | 0.9997 | 0.0003 | 0.4997 | 0.9995 | 3.75 | 0.9999 | 0.0001 | 0.4999 | 0.9998 |
| 3.48 | 0.9997 | 0.0003 | 0.4997 | 0.9995 | 3.76 | 0.9999 | 0.0001 | 0.4999 | 0.9998 |
| 3.49 | 0.9998 | 0.0002 | 0.4998 | 0.9995 | 3.77 | 0.9999 | 0.0001 | 0.4999 | 0.9998 |
| 3.50 | 0.9998 | 0.0002 | 0.4998 | 0.9995 | 3.78 | 0.9999 | 0.0001 | 0.4999 | 0.9998 |
| 3.51 | 0.9998 | 0.0002 | 0.4998 | 0.9996 | 3.79 | 0.9999 | 0.0001 | 0.4999 | 0.9998 |
| 3.52 | 0.9998 | 0.0002 | 0.4998 | 0.9996 | 3.80 | 0.9999 | 0.0001 | 0.4999 | 0.9999 |
| 3.53 | 0.9998 | 0.0002 | 0.4998 | 0.9996 | 3.81 | 0.9999 | 0.0001 | 0.4999 | 0.9999 |
| 3.54 | 0.9998 | 0.0002 | 0.4998 | 0.9996 | 3.82 | 0.9999 | 0.0001 | 0.4999 | 0.9999 |
| 3.55 | 0.9998 | 0.0002 | 0.4998 | 0.9996 | 3.83 | 0.9999 | 0.0001 | 0.4999 | 0.9999 |
| 3.56 | 0.9998 | 0.0002 | 0.4998 | 0.9996 | 3.84 | 0.9999 | 0.0001 | 0.4999 | 0.9999 |
| 3.57 | 0.9998 | 0.0002 | 0.4998 | 0.9996 | 3.85 | 0.9999 | 0.0001 | 0.4999 | 0.9999 |
| 3.58 | 0.9998 | 0.0002 | 0.4998 | 0.9997 | 3.86 | 0.9999 | 0.0001 | 0.4999 | 0.9999 |
| 3.59 | 0.9998 | 0.0002 | 0.4998 | 0.9997 | 3.87 | 0.9999 | 0.0001 | 0.4999 | 0.9999 |
| 3.60 | 0.9998 | 0.0002 | 0.4998 | 0.9997 | 3.88 | 0.9999 | 0.0001 | 0.4999 | 0.9999 |
| 3.61 | 0.9998 | 0.0002 | 0.4998 | 0.9997 | 3.89 | 0.9999 | 0.0001 | 0.4999 | 0.9999 |
| 3.62 | 0.9999 | 0.0001 | 0.4999 | 0.9997 | 3.90 | 1.0000 | 0.0000 | 0.5000 | 0.9999 |
| 3.63 | 0.9999 | 0.0001 | 0.4999 | 0.9997 | 3.91 | 1.0000 | 0.0000 | 0.5000 | 0.9999 |
| 3.64 | 0.9999 | 0.0001 | 0.4999 | 0.9997 | 3.92 | 1.0000 | 0.0000 | 0.5000 | 0.9999 |
| 3.65 | 0.9999 | 0.0001 | 0.4999 | 0.9997 | 3.93 | 1.0000 | 0.0000 | 0.5000 | 0.9999 |
| 3.66 | 0.9999 | 0.0001 | 0.4999 | 0.9997 | 3.94 | 1.0000 | 0.0000 | 0.5000 | 0.9999 |
| 3.67 | 0.9999 | 0.0001 | 0.4999 | 0.9998 | 3.95 | 1.0000 | 0.0000 | 0.5000 | 0.9999 |
| 3.68 | 0.9999 | 0.0001 | 0.4999 | 0.9998 | 3.96 | 1.0000 | 0.0000 | 0.5000 | 0.9999 |
| 3.69 | 0.9999 | 0.0001 | 0.4999 | 0.9998 | 3.97 | 1.0000 | 0.0000 | 0.5000 | 0.9999 |
| 3.70 | 0.9999 | 0.0001 | 0.4999 | 0.9998 | 3.98 | 1.0000 | 0.0000 | 0.5000 | 0.9999 |
| 3.71 | 0.9999 | 0.0001 | 0.4999 | 0.9998 | 3.99 | 1.0000 | 0.0000 | 0.5000 | 0.9999 |

*$A(x) = \Phi(x) = Pr(X \leqslant x)$, where $X$ is a standard normal distribution.
†$B(x) = 1 - \Phi(x) = Pr(X > x)$, where $X$ is a standard normal distribution.
‡$C(x) = Pr(0 \leqslant X \leqslant x)$, where $X$ is a standard normal distribution.
§$D(x) = Pr(-x \leqslant X \leqslant x)$, where $X$ is a standard normal distribution.

# Table 4

**Table 4** *Table of 1000 random digits*

| | | | | | | | | | |
|---|---|---|---|---|---|---|---|---|---|
| 01 | 32924 | 22324 | 18125 | 09077 | 26 | 96772 | 16443 | 39877 | 04653 |
| 02 | 54632 | 90374 | 94143 | 49295 | 27 | 52167 | 21038 | 14338 | 01395 |
| 03 | 88720 | 43035 | 97081 | 83373 | 28 | 69644 | 37198 | 00028 | 98195 |
| 04 | 21727 | 11904 | 41513 | 31653 | 29 | 71011 | 62004 | 81712 | 87536 |
| 05 | 80985 | 70799 | 57975 | 69282 | 30 | 31217 | 75877 | 85366 | 55500 |
| 06 | 40412 | 58826 | 94868 | 52632 | 31 | 64990 | 98735 | 02999 | 35521 |
| 07 | 43918 | 56807 | 75218 | 46077 | 32 | 48417 | 23569 | 59307 | 46550 |
| 08 | 26513 | 47480 | 77410 | 47741 | 33 | 07900 | 65059 | 48592 | 44087 |
| 09 | 18164 | 35784 | 44255 | 30124 | 34 | 74526 | 32601 | 24482 | 16981 |
| 10 | 39446 | 01375 | 75264 | 51173 | 35 | 51056 | 04402 | 58353 | 37332 |
| 11 | 16638 | 04680 | 98617 | 90298 | 36 | 39005 | 93458 | 63143 | 21817 |
| 12 | 16872 | 94749 | 44012 | 48884 | 37 | 67883 | 76343 | 78155 | 67733 |
| 13 | 65419 | 87092 | 78596 | 91512 | 38 | 06014 | 60999 | 87226 | 36071 |
| 14 | 05207 | 36702 | 56804 | 10498 | 39 | 93147 | 88766 | 04148 | 42471 |
| 15 | 78807 | 79243 | 13729 | 81222 | 40 | 01099 | 95731 | 47622 | 13294 |
| 16 | 69341 | 79028 | 64253 | 80447 | 41 | 89252 | 01201 | 58138 | 13809 |
| 17 | 41871 | 17566 | 61200 | 15994 | 42 | 41766 | 57239 | 50251 | 64675 |
| 18 | 25758 | 04625 | 43226 | 32986 | 43 | 92736 | 77800 | 81996 | 45646 |
| 19 | 06604 | 94486 | 40174 | 10742 | 44 | 45118 | 36600 | 68977 | 68831 |
| 20 | 82259 | 56512 | 48945 | 18183 | 45 | 73457 | 01579 | 00378 | 70197 |
| 21 | 07895 | 37090 | 50627 | 71320 | 46 | 49465 | 85251 | 42914 | 17277 |
| 22 | 59836 | 71148 | 42320 | 67816 | 47 | 15745 | 37285 | 23768 | 39302 |
| 23 | 57133 | 76610 | 89104 | 30481 | 48 | 28760 | 81331 | 78265 | 60690 |
| 24 | 76964 | 57126 | 87174 | 61025 | 49 | 82193 | 32787 | 70451 | 91141 |
| 25 | 27694 | 17145 | 32439 | 68245 | 50 | 89664 | 50242 | 12382 | 39379 |

# Table 5

**Table 5** Percentage points of the t distribution $(t_{d,p})^*$

| Degrees of freedom, d | p | | | | | | | | |
|---|---|---|---|---|---|---|---|---|---|
| | 0.75 | 0.8 | 0.85 | 0.9 | 0.95 | 0.975 | 0.99 | 0.995 | 0.9995 |
| 1 | 1.000 | 1.376 | 1.963 | 3.078 | 6.314 | 12.706 | 31.821 | 63.657 | 636.619 |
| 2 | 0.816 | 1.061 | 1.386 | 1.886 | 2.920 | 4.303 | 6.965 | 9.925 | 31.598 |
| 3 | 0.765 | 0.978 | 1.250 | 1.638 | 2.353 | 3.182 | 4.541 | 5.841 | 12.924 |
| 4 | 0.741 | 0.941 | 1.190 | 1.533 | 2.132 | 2.776 | 3.747 | 4.604 | 8.610 |
| 5 | 0.727 | 0.920 | 1.156 | 1.476 | 2.015 | 2.571 | 3.365 | 4.032 | 6.869 |
| 6 | 0.718 | 0.906 | 1.134 | 1.440 | 1.943 | 2.447 | 3.143 | 3.707 | 5.959 |
| 7 | 0.711 | 0.896 | 1.119 | 1.415 | 1.895 | 2.365 | 2.998 | 3.499 | 5.408 |
| 8 | 0.706 | 0.889 | 1.108 | 1.397 | 1.860 | 2.306 | 2.896 | 3.355 | 5.041 |
| 9 | 0.703 | 0.883 | 1.100 | 1.383 | 1.833 | 2.262 | 2.821 | 3.250 | 4.781 |
| 10 | 0.700 | 0.879 | 1.093 | 1.372 | 1.812 | 2.228 | 2.764 | 3.169 | 4.587 |
| 11 | 0.697 | 0.876 | 1.088 | 1.363 | 1.796 | 2.201 | 2.718 | 3.106 | 4.437 |
| 12 | 0.695 | 0.873 | 1.083 | 1.356 | 1.782 | 2.179 | 2.681 | 3.055 | 4.318 |
| 13 | 0.694 | 0.870 | 1.079 | 1.350 | 1.771 | 2.160 | 2.650 | 3.012 | 4.221 |
| 14 | 0.692 | 0.868 | 1.076 | 1.345 | 1.761 | 2.145 | 2.624 | 2.977 | 4.140 |
| 15 | 0.691 | 0.866 | 1.074 | 1.341 | 1.753 | 2.131 | 2.602 | 2.947 | 4.073 |
| 16 | 0.690 | 0.865 | 1.071 | 1.337 | 1.746 | 2.120 | 2.583 | 2.921 | 4.015 |
| 17 | 0.689 | 0.863 | 1.069 | 1.333 | 1.740 | 2.110 | 2.567 | 2.898 | 3.965 |
| 18 | 0.688 | 0.862 | 1.067 | 1.330 | 1.734 | 2.101 | 2.552 | 2.878 | 3.922 |
| 19 | 0.688 | 0.861 | 1.066 | 1.328 | 1.729 | 2.093 | 2.539 | 2.861 | 3.883 |
| 20 | 0.687 | 0.860 | 1.064 | 1.325 | 1.725 | 2.086 | 2.528 | 2.845 | 3.850 |
| 21 | 0.686 | 0.859 | 1.063 | 1.323 | 1.721 | 2.080 | 2.518 | 2.831 | 3.819 |
| 22 | 0.686 | 0.858 | 1.061 | 1.321 | 1.717 | 2.074 | 2.508 | 2.819 | 3.792 |
| 23 | 0.685 | 0.858 | 1.060 | 1.319 | 1.714 | 2.069 | 2.500 | 2.807 | 3.767 |
| 24 | 0.685 | 0.857 | 1.059 | 1.318 | 1.711 | 2.064 | 2.492 | 2.797 | 3.745 |
| 25 | 0.684 | 0.856 | 1.058 | 1.316 | 1.708 | 2.060 | 2.485 | 2.787 | 3.725 |
| 26 | 0.684 | 0.856 | 1.058 | 1.315 | 1.706 | 2.056 | 2.479 | 2.779 | 3.707 |
| 27 | 0.684 | 0.855 | 1.057 | 1.314 | 1.703 | 2.052 | 2.473 | 2.771 | 3.690 |
| 28 | 0.683 | 0.855 | 1.056 | 1.313 | 1.701 | 2.048 | 2.467 | 2.763 | 3.674 |

***Table 5*** *Percentage Points of the t Distribution ($t_{d, p}$)* 507

***Table 5*** *(Continued)*

| Degrees of freedom, $d$ | $p$ | | | | | | | | |
|---|---|---|---|---|---|---|---|---|---|
| | 0.75 | 0.8 | 0.85 | 0.9 | 0.95 | 0.975 | 0.99 | 0.995 | 0.9995 |
| 29 | 0.683 | 0.854 | 1.055 | 1.311 | 1.699 | 2.045 | 2.462 | 2.756 | 3.659 |
| 30 | 0.683 | 0.854 | 1.055 | 1.310 | 1.697 | 2.042 | 2.457 | 2.750 | 3.646 |
| 40 | 0.681 | 0.851 | 1.050 | 1.303 | 1.684 | 2.021 | 2.423 | 2.704 | 3.551 |
| 60 | 0.679 | 0.848 | 1.046 | 1.296 | 1.671 | 2.000 | 2.390 | 2.660 | 3.460 |
| 120 | 0.677 | 0.845 | 1.041 | 1.289 | 1.658 | 1.980 | 2.358 | 2.617 | 3.373 |
| ∞ | 0.674 | 0.842 | 1.036 | 1.282 | 1.645 | 1.960 | 2.326 | 2.576 | 3.291 |

*The $p$th percentile of a $t$ distribution with $d$ degrees of freedom.
(Table 5 is taken from Table III of Fisher and Yates: "Statistical Tables for Biological, Agricultural and Medical Research," published by Longman Group Ltd., London (previously published by Oliver and Boyd Ltd., Edinburgh) and by permission of the authors and publishers.)

# Table 6

**Table 6** Percentage points of the chi-square distribution ($\chi^2_{d,p}$) §

| d | 0.005 | 0.01 | 0.025 | 0.05 | 0.10 | 0.25 | 0.50 | 0.75 | 0.90 | 0.95 | 0.975 | 0.99 | 0.995 | 0.999 |
|---|---|---|---|---|---|---|---|---|---|---|---|---|---|---|
| 1 | $0.0^4393$* | $0.0^3157$† | $0.0^3982$‡ | 0.00393 | 0.02 | 0.10 | 0.45 | 1.32 | 2.71 | 3.84 | 5.02 | 6.63 | 7.88 | 10.83 |
| 2 | 0.0100 | 0.0201 | 0.0506 | 0.103 | 0.21 | 0.58 | 1.39 | 2.77 | 4.61 | 5.99 | 7.38 | 9.21 | 10.60 | 13.81 |
| 3 | 0.0717 | 0.115 | 0.216 | 0.352 | 0.58 | 1.21 | 2.37 | 4.11 | 6.25 | 7.81 | 9.35 | 11.34 | 12.84 | 16.27 |
| 4 | 0.207 | 0.297 | 0.484 | 0.711 | 1.06 | 1.92 | 3.36 | 5.39 | 7.78 | 9.49 | 11.14 | 13.28 | 14.86 | 18.47 |
| 5 | 0.412 | 0.554 | 0.831 | 1.15 | 1.61 | 2.67 | 4.35 | 6.63 | 9.24 | 11.07 | 12.83 | 15.09 | 16.75 | 20.52 |
| 6 | 0.676 | 0.872 | 1.24 | 1.64 | 2.20 | 3.45 | 5.35 | 7.84 | 10.64 | 12.59 | 14.45 | 16.81 | 18.55 | 22.46 |
| 7 | 0.989 | 1.24 | 1.69 | 2.17 | 2.83 | 4.25 | 6.35 | 9.04 | 12.02 | 14.07 | 16.01 | 18.48 | 20.28 | 24.32 |
| 8 | 1.34 | 1.65 | 2.18 | 2.73 | 3.49 | 5.07 | 7.34 | 10.22 | 13.36 | 15.51 | 17.53 | 20.09 | 21.95 | 26.12 |
| 9 | 1.73 | 2.09 | 2.70 | 3.33 | 4.17 | 5.90 | 8.34 | 11.39 | 14.68 | 16.92 | 19.02 | 21.67 | 23.59 | 27.88 |
| 10 | 2.16 | 2.56 | 3.25 | 3.94 | 4.87 | 6.74 | 9.34 | 12.55 | 15.99 | 18.31 | 20.48 | 23.21 | 25.19 | 29.59 |
| 11 | 2.60 | 3.05 | 3.82 | 4.57 | 5.58 | 7.58 | 10.34 | 13.70 | 17.28 | 19.68 | 21.92 | 24.72 | 26.76 | 31.26 |
| 12 | 3.07 | 3.57 | 4.40 | 5.23 | 6.30 | 8.44 | 11.34 | 14.85 | 18.55 | 21.03 | 23.34 | 26.22 | 28.30 | 32.91 |
| 13 | 3.57 | 4.11 | 5.01 | 5.89 | 7.04 | 9.30 | 12.34 | 15.98 | 19.81 | 22.36 | 24.74 | 27.69 | 29.82 | 34.53 |
| 14 | 4.07 | 4.66 | 5.63 | 6.57 | 7.79 | 10.17 | 13.34 | 17.12 | 21.06 | 23.68 | 26.12 | 29.14 | 31.32 | 36.12 |
| 15 | 4.60 | 5.23 | 6.27 | 7.26 | 8.55 | 11.04 | 14.34 | 18.25 | 22.31 | 25.00 | 27.49 | 30.58 | 32.80 | 37.70 |
| 16 | 5.14 | 5.81 | 6.91 | 7.96 | 9.31 | 11.91 | 15.34 | 19.37 | 23.54 | 26.30 | 28.85 | 32.00 | 34.27 | 39.25 |
| 17 | 5.70 | 6.41 | 7.56 | 8.67 | 10.09 | 12.79 | 16.34 | 20.49 | 24.77 | 27.59 | 30.19 | 33.41 | 35.72 | 40.79 |
| 18 | 6.26 | 7.01 | 8.23 | 9.39 | 10.86 | 13.68 | 17.34 | 21.60 | 25.99 | 28.87 | 31.53 | 34.81 | 37.16 | 42.31 |
| 19 | 6.84 | 7.63 | 8.91 | 10.12 | 11.65 | 14.56 | 18.34 | 22.72 | 27.20 | 30.14 | 32.85 | 36.19 | 38.58 | 43.82 |
| 20 | 7.43 | 8.26 | 9.59 | 10.85 | 12.44 | 15.45 | 19.34 | 23.83 | 28.41 | 31.41 | 34.17 | 37.57 | 40.00 | 45.32 |

| $d$ | | | | | | | | | | | | | | |
|---|---|---|---|---|---|---|---|---|---|---|---|---|---|---|
| 21 | 8.03 | 8.90 | 10.28 | 11.59 | 13.24 | 16.34 | 20.34 | 24.93 | 29.62 | 32.67 | 35.48 | 38.93 | 41.40 | 46.80 |
| 22 | 8.64 | 9.54 | 10.98 | 12.34 | 14.04 | 17.24 | 21.34 | 26.04 | 30.81 | 33.92 | 36.78 | 40.29 | 42.80 | 48.27 |
| 23 | 9.26 | 10.20 | 11.69 | 13.09 | 14.85 | 18.14 | 22.34 | 27.14 | 32.01 | 35.17 | 38.08 | 41.64 | 44.18 | 49.73 |
| 24 | 9.89 | 10.86 | 12.40 | 13.85 | 15.66 | 19.04 | 23.34 | 28.24 | 33.20 | 36.42 | 39.36 | 42.98 | 45.56 | 51.18 |
| 25 | 10.52 | 11.52 | 13.12 | 14.61 | 16.47 | 19.94 | 24.34 | 29.34 | 34.38 | 37.65 | 40.65 | 44.31 | 46.93 | 52.62 |
| 26 | 11.16 | 12.20 | 13.84 | 15.38 | 17.29 | 20.84 | 25.34 | 30.43 | 35.56 | 38.89 | 41.92 | 45.64 | 48.29 | 54.05 |
| 27 | 11.81 | 12.88 | 14.57 | 16.15 | 18.11 | 21.75 | 26.34 | 31.53 | 36.74 | 40.11 | 43.19 | 46.96 | 49.64 | 55.48 |
| 28 | 12.46 | 13.56 | 15.31 | 16.93 | 18.94 | 22.66 | 27.34 | 32.62 | 37.92 | 41.34 | 44.46 | 48.28 | 50.99 | 56.89 |
| 29 | 13.12 | 14.26 | 16.05 | 17.71 | 19.77 | 23.57 | 28.34 | 33.71 | 39.09 | 42.56 | 45.72 | 49.59 | 52.34 | 58.30 |
| 30 | 13.79 | 14.95 | 16.79 | 18.49 | 20.60 | 24.48 | 29.34 | 34.80 | 40.26 | 43.77 | 46.98 | 50.89 | 53.67 | 59.70 |
| 40 | 20.71 | 22.16 | 24.43 | 26.51 | 29.05 | 33.66 | 39.34 | 45.62 | 51.81 | 55.76 | 59.34 | 63.69 | 66.77 | 73.40 |
| 50 | 27.99 | 29.71 | 32.36 | 34.76 | 37.69 | 42.94 | 49.33 | 56.33 | 63.17 | 67.50 | 71.42 | 76.15 | 79.49 | 86.66 |
| 60 | 35.53 | 37.48 | 40.48 | 43.19 | 46.46 | 52.29 | 59.33 | 66.98 | 74.40 | 79.08 | 83.30 | 88.38 | 91.95 | 99.61 |
| 70 | 43.28 | 45.44 | 48.76 | 51.74 | 55.33 | 61.70 | 69.33 | 77.58 | 85.53 | 90.53 | 95.02 | 100.42 | 104.22 | 112.32 |
| 80 | 51.17 | 53.54 | 57.15 | 60.39 | 64.28 | 71.14 | 79.33 | 88.13 | 96.58 | 101.88 | 106.63 | 112.33 | 116.32 | 124.84 |
| 90 | 59.20 | 61.75 | 65.65 | 69.13 | 73.29 | 80.62 | 89.33 | 98.64 | 107.56 | 113.14 | 118.14 | 124.12 | 128.30 | 137.21 |
| 100 | 67.33 | 70.06 | 74.22 | 77.93 | 82.36 | 90.13 | 99.33 | 109.14 | 118.50 | 124.34 | 129.56 | 135.81 | 140.17 | 149.45 |

* = 0.0000393    † = 0.000157    ‡ = 0.000982    § $\chi^2_{d,p}$ = $p$th percentile of a $\chi^2$ distribution with $d$ degrees of freedom.

(Reproduced in part with permission of the Biometrika Trustees, from Table 3 of "Biometrika Tables for Statisticians," Volume II, edited by E. S. Pearson and H. O. Hartley, published for the Biometrika Trustees, Cambridge University Press, Cambridge, England, 1972.)

# Table 7

**Table 7a** _Exact two-sided 100% × (1 − α) confidence limits for binomial proportions (α = 0.05)_

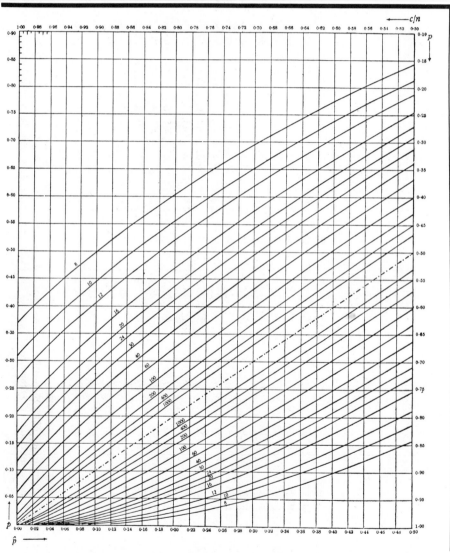

510

**Table 7b**   *Exact two-sided 100% × (1 − α) confidence limits for binomial proportions (α = 0.01)*

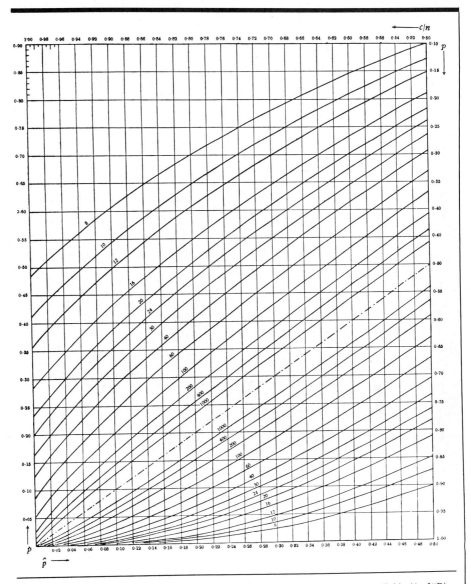

(These tables have been reproduced with permission of the Biometrika Trustees, from Table 41 of "Biometrika Tables for Statisticians," 3rd Edition, Volume II, Published for the Biometrika Trustees, Cambridge University Press, Cambridge, England, 1966.)

# Table 8

**Table 8**  *Percentage points of the F distribution ($F_{d_1, d_2, p}$)*

| df for denominator, $d_2$ | p | df for numerator, $d_1$ | | | | | | | | | | |
|---|---|---|---|---|---|---|---|---|---|---|---|---|
| | | 1 | 2 | 3 | 4 | 5 | 6 | 7 | 8 | 12 | 24 | ∞ |
| 1 | 0.90 | 39.86 | 49.50 | 53.59 | 55.83 | 57.24 | 58.20 | 58.91 | 59.44 | 60.71 | 62.00 | 63.33 |
| | 0.95 | 161.4 | 199.5 | 215.7 | 224.6 | 230.2 | 234.0 | 236.8 | 238.9 | 243.9 | 249.1 | 254.3 |
| | 0.975 | 647.8 | 799.5 | 864.2 | 899.6 | 921.8 | 937.1 | 948.2 | 956.7 | 976.7 | 997.2 | 1018. |
| | 0.99 | 4052. | 5000. | 5403. | 5625. | 5764. | 5859. | 5928. | 5981. | 6106. | 6235. | 6366. |
| | 0.995 | 16211. | 20000. | 21615. | 22500. | 23056. | 23437. | 23715. | 23925. | 24426. | 24940. | 25464. |
| | 0.999 | 405280. | 500000. | 540380. | 562500. | 576400. | 585940. | 592870. | 598140. | 610670. | 623500. | 636620. |
| 2 | 0.90 | 8.53 | 9.00 | 9.16 | 9.24 | 9.29 | 9.33 | 9.35 | 9.37 | 9.41 | 9.45 | 9.49 |
| | 0.95 | 18.51 | 19.00 | 19.16 | 19.25 | 19.30 | 19.33 | 19.35 | 19.37 | 19.41 | 19.45 | 19.50 |
| | 0.975 | 38.51 | 39.00 | 39.17 | 39.25 | 39.30 | 39.33 | 39.36 | 39.37 | 39.42 | 39.46 | 39.50 |
| | 0.99 | 98.50 | 99.00 | 99.17 | 99.25 | 99.30 | 99.33 | 99.36 | 99.37 | 99.42 | 99.46 | 99.50 |
| | 0.995 | 198.5 | 199.0 | 199.2 | 199.2 | 199.3 | 199.3 | 199.4 | 199.4 | 199.4 | 199.5 | 199.5 |
| | 0.999 | 998.5 | 999.0 | 999.2 | 999.2 | 999.3 | 999.3 | 999.4 | 999.4 | 999.4 | 999.5 | 999.5 |
| 3 | 0.90 | 5.54 | 5.46 | 5.39 | 5.34 | 5.31 | 5.28 | 5.27 | 5.25 | 5.22 | 5.18 | 5.13 |
| | 0.95 | 10.13 | 9.55 | 9.28 | 9.12 | 9.01 | 8.94 | 8.89 | 8.85 | 8.74 | 8.64 | 8.53 |
| | 0.975 | 17.44 | 16.04 | 15.44 | 15.10 | 14.88 | 14.74 | 14.62 | 14.54 | 14.34 | 14.12 | 13.90 |
| | 0.99 | 34.12 | 30.82 | 29.46 | 28.71 | 28.24 | 27.91 | 27.67 | 27.49 | 27.05 | 26.60 | 26.13 |
| | 0.995 | 55.55 | 49.80 | 47.47 | 46.20 | 45.39 | 44.84 | 44.43 | 44.13 | 43.39 | 42.62 | 41.83 |
| | 0.999 | 167.00 | 148.5 | 141.1 | 137.1 | 134.6 | 132.8 | 131.6 | 130.6 | 128.3 | 125.9 | 123.5 |
| 4 | 0.90 | 4.54 | 4.32 | 4.19 | 4.11 | 4.05 | 4.01 | 3.98 | 3.95 | 3.90 | 3.83 | 3.76 |
| | 0.95 | 7.71 | 6.94 | 6.59 | 6.39 | 6.26 | 6.16 | 6.09 | 6.04 | 5.91 | 5.77 | 5.63 |
| | 0.975 | 12.22 | 10.65 | 9.98 | 9.60 | 9.36 | 9.20 | 9.07 | 8.98 | 8.75 | 8.51 | 8.26 |
| | 0.99 | 21.20 | 18.00 | 16.69 | 15.98 | 15.52 | 15.21 | 14.98 | 14.80 | 14.37 | 13.93 | 13.46 |
| | 0.995 | 31.33 | 26.28 | 24.26 | 23.16 | 22.46 | 21.98 | 21.62 | 21.35 | 20.70 | 20.03 | 19.32 |
| | 0.999 | 74.14 | 61.25 | 56.18 | 53.44 | 51.71 | 50.53 | 49.66 | 49.00 | 47.41 | 45.77 | 44.05 |

| | | | | | | | | | | | | |
|---|---|---|---|---|---|---|---|---|---|---|---|---|
| 5 | 0.90 | 4.06 | 3.78 | 3.62 | 3.52 | 3.45 | 3.40 | 3.37 | 3.34 | 3.27 | 3.19 | 3.10 |
| | 0.95 | 6.61 | 5.79 | 5.41 | 5.19 | 5.05 | 4.95 | 4.88 | 4.82 | 4.68 | 4.53 | 4.36 |
| | 0.975 | 10.01 | 8.43 | 7.76 | 7.39 | 7.15 | 6.98 | 6.85 | 6.76 | 6.52 | 6.28 | 6.02 |
| | 0.99 | 16.26 | 13.27 | 12.06 | 11.39 | 10.97 | 10.67 | 10.46 | 10.29 | 9.89 | 9.47 | 9.02 |
| | 0.995 | 22.78 | 18.31 | 16.53 | 15.56 | 14.94 | 14.51 | 14.20 | 13.96 | 13.38 | 12.78 | 12.14 |
| | 0.999 | 47.18 | 37.12 | 33.20 | 31.09 | 29.75 | 28.83 | 28.16 | 27.65 | 26.42 | 25.13 | 23.79 |
| 6 | 0.90 | 3.78 | 3.46 | 3.29 | 3.18 | 3.11 | 3.05 | 3.01 | 2.98 | 2.90 | 2.82 | 2.72 |
| | 0.95 | 5.99 | 5.14 | 4.76 | 4.53 | 4.39 | 4.28 | 4.21 | 4.15 | 4.00 | 3.84 | 3.67 |
| | 0.975 | 8.81 | 7.26 | 6.60 | 6.23 | 5.99 | 5.82 | 5.70 | 5.60 | 5.37 | 5.12 | 4.85 |
| | 0.99 | 13.75 | 10.92 | 9.78 | 9.15 | 8.75 | 8.47 | 8.26 | 8.10 | 7.72 | 7.31 | 6.88 |
| | 0.995 | 18.64 | 14.54 | 12.92 | 12.03 | 11.46 | 11.07 | 10.79 | 10.57 | 10.03 | 9.47 | 8.88 |
| | 0.999 | 35.51 | 27.00 | 23.70 | 21.92 | 20.80 | 20.03 | 19.46 | 19.03 | 17.99 | 16.90 | 15.75 |
| 7 | 0.90 | 3.59 | 3.26 | 3.07 | 2.96 | 2.88 | 2.83 | 2.78 | 2.75 | 2.67 | 2.58 | 2.47 |
| | 0.95 | 5.59 | 4.74 | 4.35 | 4.12 | 3.97 | 3.87 | 3.79 | 3.73 | 3.57 | 3.41 | 3.23 |
| | 0.975 | 8.07 | 6.54 | 5.89 | 5.52 | 5.29 | 5.12 | 4.99 | 4.90 | 4.67 | 4.42 | 4.14 |
| | 0.99 | 12.25 | 9.55 | 8.45 | 7.85 | 7.46 | 7.19 | 6.99 | 6.84 | 6.47 | 6.07 | 5.65 |
| | 0.995 | 16.24 | 12.40 | 10.88 | 10.05 | 9.52 | 9.16 | 8.89 | 8.68 | 8.18 | 7.65 | 7.08 |
| | 0.999 | 29.25 | 21.69 | 18.77 | 17.20 | 16.21 | 15.52 | 15.02 | 14.63 | 13.71 | 12.73 | 11.70 |
| 8 | 0.90 | 3.46 | 3.11 | 2.92 | 2.81 | 2.73 | 2.67 | 2.62 | 2.59 | 2.50 | 2.40 | 2.29 |
| | 0.95 | 5.32 | 4.46 | 4.07 | 3.84 | 3.69 | 3.58 | 3.50 | 3.44 | 3.28 | 3.12 | 2.93 |
| | 0.975 | 7.57 | 6.06 | 5.42 | 5.05 | 4.82 | 4.65 | 4.53 | 4.43 | 4.20 | 3.95 | 3.67 |
| | 0.99 | 11.26 | 8.65 | 7.59 | 7.01 | 6.63 | 6.37 | 6.18 | 6.03 | 5.67 | 5.28 | 4.86 |
| | 0.995 | 14.69 | 11.04 | 9.60 | 8.81 | 8.30 | 7.95 | 7.69 | 7.50 | 7.01 | 6.50 | 5.95 |
| | 0.999 | 25.42 | 18.49 | 15.83 | 14.39 | 13.49 | 12.86 | 12.40 | 12.04 | 11.19 | 10.30 | 9.33 |
| 9 | 0.90 | 3.36 | 3.01 | 2.81 | 2.69 | 2.61 | 2.55 | 2.51 | 2.47 | 2.38 | 2.28 | 2.16 |
| | 0.95 | 5.12 | 4.26 | 3.86 | 3.63 | 3.48 | 3.37 | 3.29 | 3.23 | 3.07 | 2.90 | 2.71 |
| | 0.975 | 7.21 | 5.71 | 5.08 | 4.72 | 4.48 | 4.32 | 4.20 | 4.10 | 3.87 | 3.61 | 3.33 |
| | 0.99 | 10.56 | 8.02 | 6.99 | 6.42 | 6.06 | 5.80 | 5.61 | 5.47 | 5.11 | 4.73 | 4.31 |
| | 0.995 | 13.61 | 10.11 | 8.72 | 7.96 | 7.47 | 7.13 | 6.88 | 6.69 | 6.23 | 5.73 | 5.19 |
| | 0.999 | 22.86 | 16.39 | 13.90 | 12.56 | 11.71 | 11.13 | 10.70 | 10.37 | 9.57 | 8.72 | 7.81 |
| 10 | 0.90 | 3.29 | 2.92 | 2.73 | 2.61 | 2.52 | 2.46 | 2.41 | 2.38 | 2.28 | 2.18 | 2.06 |
| | 0.95 | 4.96 | 4.10 | 3.71 | 3.48 | 3.33 | 3.22 | 3.14 | 3.07 | 2.91 | 2.74 | 2.54 |
| | 0.975 | 6.94 | 5.46 | 4.83 | 4.47 | 4.24 | 4.07 | 3.95 | 3.85 | 3.62 | 3.37 | 3.08 |
| | 0.99 | 10.04 | 7.56 | 6.55 | 5.99 | 5.64 | 5.39 | 5.20 | 5.06 | 4.71 | 4.33 | 3.91 |
| | 0.995 | 12.83 | 9.43 | 8.08 | 7.34 | 6.87 | 6.54 | 6.30 | 6.12 | 5.66 | 5.17 | 4.64 |
| | 0.999 | 21.04 | 14.91 | 12.55 | 11.28 | 10.48 | 9.93 | 9.52 | 9.20 | 8.45 | 7.64 | 6.76 |

**Table 8** (Continued)

| df for denominator, $d_2$ | $p$ | 1 | 2 | 3 | 4 | 5 | 6 | 7 | 8 | 12 | 24 | ∞ |
|---|---|---|---|---|---|---|---|---|---|---|---|---|
| | | | | | | | | df for numerator, $d_1$ | | | | |
| 12 | 0.90 | 3.18 | 2.81 | 2.61 | 2.48 | 2.39 | 2.33 | 2.28 | 2.24 | 2.15 | 2.04 | 1.90 |
| | 0.95 | 4.75 | 3.89 | 3.49 | 3.26 | 3.11 | 3.00 | 2.91 | 2.85 | 2.69 | 2.51 | 2.30 |
| | 0.975 | 6.55 | 5.10 | 4.47 | 4.12 | 3.89 | 3.73 | 3.61 | 3.51 | 3.28 | 3.02 | 2.72 |
| | 0.99 | 9.33 | 6.93 | 5.95 | 5.41 | 5.06 | 4.82 | 4.64 | 4.50 | 4.16 | 3.78 | 3.36 |
| | 0.995 | 11.75 | 8.51 | 7.23 | 6.52 | 6.07 | 5.76 | 5.52 | 5.35 | 4.91 | 4.43 | 3.90 |
| | 0.999 | 18.64 | 12.97 | 10.80 | 9.63 | 8.89 | 8.38 | 8.00 | 7.71 | 7.00 | 6.25 | 5.42 |
| 14 | 0.90 | 3.10 | 2.73 | 2.52 | 2.39 | 2.31 | 2.24 | 2.19 | 2.15 | 2.05 | 1.94 | 1.80 |
| | 0.95 | 4.60 | 3.74 | 3.34 | 3.11 | 2.96 | 2.85 | 2.76 | 2.70 | 2.53 | 2.35 | 2.13 |
| | 0.975 | 6.30 | 4.86 | 4.24 | 3.89 | 3.66 | 3.50 | 3.38 | 3.29 | 3.05 | 2.79 | 2.49 |
| | 0.99 | 8.86 | 6.51 | 5.56 | 5.04 | 4.69 | 4.46 | 4.28 | 4.14 | 3.80 | 3.43 | 3.00 |
| | 0.995 | 11.06 | 7.92 | 6.68 | 6.00 | 5.56 | 5.26 | 5.03 | 4.86 | 4.43 | 3.96 | 3.44 |
| | 0.999 | 17.14 | 11.78 | 9.73 | 8.62 | 7.92 | 7.44 | 7.08 | 6.80 | 6.13 | 5.41 | 4.60 |
| 16 | 0.90 | 3.05 | 2.67 | 2.46 | 2.33 | 2.24 | 2.18 | 2.13 | 2.09 | 1.99 | 1.87 | 1.72 |
| | 0.95 | 4.49 | 3.63 | 3.24 | 3.01 | 2.85 | 2.74 | 2.66 | 2.59 | 2.42 | 2.24 | 2.01 |
| | 0.975 | 6.12 | 4.69 | 4.08 | 3.73 | 3.50 | 3.34 | 3.22 | 3.12 | 2.89 | 2.63 | 2.32 |
| | 0.99 | 8.53 | 6.23 | 5.29 | 4.77 | 4.44 | 4.20 | 4.03 | 3.89 | 3.55 | 3.18 | 2.75 |
| | 0.995 | 10.58 | 7.51 | 6.30 | 5.64 | 5.21 | 4.91 | 4.69 | 4.52 | 4.10 | 3.64 | 3.11 |
| | 0.999 | 16.12 | 10.97 | 9.01 | 7.94 | 7.27 | 6.80 | 6.46 | 6.19 | 5.55 | 4.85 | 4.06 |
| 18 | 0.90 | 3.01 | 2.62 | 2.42 | 2.29 | 2.20 | 2.13 | 2.08 | 2.04 | 1.93 | 1.81 | 1.66 |
| | 0.95 | 4.41 | 3.55 | 3.16 | 2.93 | 2.77 | 2.66 | 2.58 | 2.51 | 2.34 | 2.15 | 1.92 |
| | 0.975 | 5.98 | 4.56 | 3.95 | 3.61 | 3.38 | 3.22 | 3.10 | 3.01 | 2.77 | 2.50 | 2.19 |
| | 0.99 | 8.29 | 6.01 | 5.09 | 4.58 | 4.25 | 4.01 | 3.84 | 3.71 | 3.37 | 3.00 | 2.57 |
| | 0.995 | 10.22 | 7.21 | 6.03 | 5.37 | 4.96 | 4.66 | 4.44 | 4.28 | 3.86 | 3.40 | 2.87 |
| | 0.999 | 15.38 | 10.39 | 8.49 | 7.46 | 6.81 | 6.35 | 6.02 | 5.76 | 5.13 | 4.45 | 3.67 |
| 20 | 0.90 | 2.97 | 2.59 | 2.38 | 2.25 | 2.16 | 2.09 | 2.04 | 2.00 | 1.89 | 1.77 | 1.61 |
| | 0.95 | 4.35 | 3.49 | 3.10 | 2.87 | 2.71 | 2.60 | 2.51 | 2.45 | 2.28 | 2.08 | 1.84 |
| | 0.975 | 5.87 | 4.46 | 3.86 | 3.51 | 3.29 | 3.13 | 3.01 | 2.91 | 2.68 | 2.41 | 2.09 |
| | 0.99 | 8.10 | 5.85 | 4.94 | 4.43 | 4.10 | 3.87 | 3.70 | 3.56 | 3.23 | 2.86 | 2.42 |
| | 0.995 | 9.94 | 6.99 | 5.82 | 5.17 | 4.76 | 4.47 | 4.26 | 4.09 | 3.68 | 3.22 | 2.69 |
| | 0.999 | 14.82 | 9.95 | 8.10 | 7.10 | 6.46 | 6.02 | 5.69 | 5.44 | 4.82 | 4.15 | 3.38 |

| $d_2$ | $p$ | | | | | | | | | | | |
|---|---|---|---|---|---|---|---|---|---|---|---|---|
| 30 | 0.90 | 2.88 | 2.49 | 2.28 | 2.14 | 2.05 | 1.98 | 1.93 | 1.88 | 1.77 | 1.64 | 1.46 |
| | 0.95 | 4.17 | 3.32 | 2.92 | 2.69 | 2.53 | 2.42 | 2.33 | 2.27 | 2.09 | 1.89 | 1.62 |
| | 0.975 | 5.57 | 4.18 | 3.59 | 3.25 | 3.03 | 2.87 | 2.75 | 2.65 | 2.41 | 2.14 | 1.79 |
| | 0.99 | 7.56 | 5.39 | 4.51 | 4.02 | 3.70 | 3.47 | 3.30 | 3.17 | 2.84 | 2.47 | 2.01 |
| | 0.995 | 9.18 | 6.35 | 5.24 | 4.62 | 4.23 | 3.95 | 3.74 | 3.58 | 3.18 | 2.73 | 2.18 |
| | 0.999 | 13.29 | 8.77 | 7.05 | 6.12 | 5.53 | 5.12 | 4.82 | 4.58 | 4.00 | 3.36 | 2.59 |
| 40 | 0.90 | 2.84 | 2.44 | 2.23 | 2.09 | 2.00 | 1.93 | 1.87 | 1.83 | 1.71 | 1.57 | 1.38 |
| | 0.95 | 4.08 | 3.23 | 2.84 | 2.61 | 2.45 | 2.34 | 2.25 | 2.18 | 2.00 | 1.79 | 1.51 |
| | 0.975 | 5.42 | 4.05 | 3.46 | 3.13 | 2.90 | 2.74 | 2.62 | 2.53 | 2.29 | 2.01 | 1.64 |
| | 0.99 | 7.31 | 5.18 | 4.31 | 3.83 | 3.51 | 3.29 | 3.12 | 2.99 | 2.66 | 2.29 | 1.80 |
| | 0.995 | 8.83 | 6.07 | 4.98 | 4.37 | 3.99 | 3.71 | 3.51 | 3.35 | 2.95 | 2.50 | 1.93 |
| | 0.999 | 12.61 | 8.25 | 6.59 | 5.70 | 5.13 | 4.73 | 4.44 | 4.21 | 3.64 | 3.01 | 2.23 |
| 60 | 0.90 | 2.79 | 2.39 | 2.18 | 2.04 | 1.95 | 1.87 | 1.82 | 1.77 | 1.66 | 1.51 | 1.29 |
| | 0.95 | 4.00 | 3.15 | 2.76 | 2.53 | 2.37 | 2.25 | 2.17 | 2.10 | 1.92 | 1.70 | 1.39 |
| | 0.975 | 5.29 | 3.93 | 3.34 | 3.01 | 2.79 | 2.63 | 2.51 | 2.41 | 2.17 | 1.88 | 1.48 |
| | 0.99 | 7.08 | 4.98 | 4.13 | 3.65 | 3.34 | 3.12 | 2.95 | 2.82 | 2.50 | 2.12 | 1.60 |
| | 0.995 | 8.49 | 5.80 | 4.73 | 4.14 | 3.76 | 3.49 | 3.29 | 3.13 | 2.74 | 2.29 | 1.69 |
| | 0.999 | 11.97 | 7.77 | 6.17 | 5.31 | 4.76 | 4.37 | 4.09 | 3.86 | 3.32 | 2.69 | 1.89 |
| 120 | 0.90 | 2.75 | 2.35 | 2.13 | 1.99 | 1.90 | 1.82 | 1.77 | 1.72 | 1.60 | 1.45 | 1.19 |
| | 0.95 | 3.92 | 3.07 | 2.68 | 2.45 | 2.29 | 2.17 | 2.09 | 2.02 | 1.83 | 1.61 | 1.25 |
| | 0.975 | 5.15 | 3.80 | 3.23 | 2.89 | 2.67 | 2.52 | 2.39 | 2.30 | 2.05 | 1.76 | 1.31 |
| | 0.99 | 6.85 | 4.79 | 3.95 | 3.48 | 3.17 | 2.96 | 2.79 | 2.66 | 2.34 | 1.95 | 1.38 |
| | 0.995 | 8.18 | 5.54 | 4.50 | 3.92 | 3.55 | 3.28 | 3.09 | 2.93 | 2.54 | 2.09 | 1.43 |
| | 0.999 | 11.38 | 7.32 | 5.78 | 4.95 | 4.42 | 4.04 | 3.77 | 3.55 | 3.02 | 2.40 | 1.54 |
| ∞ | 0.90 | 2.71 | 2.30 | 2.08 | 1.94 | 1.85 | 1.77 | 1.72 | 1.67 | 1.55 | 1.38 | 1.00 |
| | 0.95 | 3.84 | 3.00 | 2.60 | 2.37 | 2.21 | 2.10 | 2.01 | 1.94 | 1.75 | 1.52 | 1.00 |
| | 0.975 | 5.02 | 3.69 | 3.12 | 2.79 | 2.57 | 2.41 | 2.29 | 2.19 | 1.94 | 1.64 | 1.00 |
| | 0.99 | 6.63 | 4.61 | 3.78 | 3.32 | 3.02 | 2.80 | 2.64 | 2.51 | 2.18 | 1.79 | 1.00 |
| | 0.995 | 7.88 | 5.30 | 4.28 | 3.72 | 3.35 | 3.09 | 2.90 | 2.74 | 2.36 | 1.90 | 1.00 |
| | 0.999 | 10.83 | 6.91 | 5.42 | 4.62 | 4.10 | 3.74 | 3.47 | 3.27 | 2.74 | 2.13 | 1.00 |

*$F_{d_1,d_2,p}$ = $p$th percentile of an F distribution with $d_1$ and $d_2$ degrees of freedom.
(This table has been reproduced in part with the permission of the Biometrika Trustees, from "Biometrika Tables for Statisticians," Volume II, edited by E. S. Pearson and H. O. Hartley, published for the Biometrika Trustees, Cambridge University Press, Cambridge, England, 1972.)

# Table 9

**Table 9** *Two-tailed critical values for the Wilcoxon sign rank test*

| | 0.10 | | 0.05 | | 0.02 | | 0.01 | |
|---|---|---|---|---|---|---|---|---|
| n* | Lower | Upper | Lower | Upper | Lower | Upper | Lower | Upper |
| 1 | — | | — | | — | | — | |
| 2 | — | | — | | — | | — | |
| 3 | — | | — | | — | | — | |
| 4 | — | | — | | — | | — | |
| 5 | 0 | 15 | — | | — | | — | |
| 6 | 2 | 19 | 0 | 21 | — | | — | |
| 7 | 3 | 25 | 2 | 26 | 0 | 28 | — | |
| 8 | 5 | 31 | 3 | 33 | 1 | 35 | 0 | 36 |
| 9 | 8 | 37 | 5 | 40 | 3 | 42 | 1 | 44 |
| 10 | 10 | 45 | 8 | 47 | 5 | 50 | 3 | 52 |
| 11 | 13 | 53 | 10 | 56 | 7 | 59 | 5 | 61 |
| 12 | 17 | 61 | 13 | 65 | 9 | 69 | 7 | 71 |
| 13 | 21 | 70 | 17 | 74 | 12 | 79 | 9 | 82 |
| 14 | 25 | 80 | 21 | 84 | 15 | 90 | 12 | 93 |
| 15 | 30 | 90 | 25 | 95 | 19 | 101 | 15 | 105 |

*n = number of untied pairs.

(Figures from "Documenta Geigy Scientific Tables," 6th Edition. Reprinted with the kind permission of CIBA-GEIGY Limited, Basle, Switzerland.)

# Table 10

*Table 10* Two-tailed critical values for the Wilcoxon rank sum test

## α = 0.10

| $n_2$ \ $n_1$ → | 4 $T_l$ | $T_r$ | 5 $T_l$ | $T_r$ | 6 $T_l$ | $T_r$ | 7 $T_l$ | $T_r$ | 8 $T_l$ | $T_r$ | 9 $T_l$ | $T_r$ |
|---|---|---|---|---|---|---|---|---|---|---|---|---|
| 4 | 11 | 25 | 17 | 33 | 24 | 42 | 32 | 52 | 41 | 63 | 51 | 75 |
| 5 | 12 | 28 | 19 | 36 | 26 | 46 | 34 | 57 | 44 | 68 | 54 | 81 |
| 6 | 13 | 31 | 20 | 40 | 28 | 50 | 36 | 62 | 46 | 74 | 57 | 87 |
| 7 | 14 | 34 | 21 | 44 | 29 | 55 | 39 | 66 | 49 | 79 | 60 | 93 |
| 8 | 15 | 37 | 23 | 47 | 31 | 59 | 41 | 71 | 51 | 85 | 63 | 99 |
| 9 | 16 | 40 | 24 | 51 | 33 | 63 | 43 | 76 | 54 | 90 | 66 | 105 |
| 10 | 17 | 43 | 26 | 54 | 35 | 67 | 45 | 81 | 56 | 96 | 69 | 111 |
| 11 | 18 | 46 | 27 | 58 | 37 | 71 | 47 | 86 | 59 | 101 | 72 | 117 |
| 12 | 19 | 49 | 28 | 62 | 38 | 76 | 49 | 91 | 62 | 106 | 75 | 123 |
| 13 | 20 | 52 | 30 | 65 | 40 | 80 | 52 | 95 | 64 | 112 | 78 | 129 |
| 14 | 21 | 55 | 31 | 69 | 42 | 84 | 54 | 100 | 67 | 117 | 81 | 135 |
| 15 | 22 | 58 | 33 | 72 | 44 | 88 | 56 | 105 | 69 | 123 | 84 | 141 |
| 16 | 24 | 60 | 34 | 76 | 46 | 92 | 58 | 110 | 72 | 128 | 87 | 147 |
| 17 | 25 | 63 | 35 | 80 | 47 | 97 | 61 | 114 | 75 | 133 | 90 | 153 |
| 18 | 26 | 66 | 37 | 83 | 49 | 101 | 63 | 119 | 77 | 139 | 93 | 159 |
| 19 | 27 | 69 | 38 | 87 | 51 | 105 | 65 | 124 | 80 | 144 | 96 | 165 |
| 20 | 28 | 72 | 40 | 90 | 53 | 109 | 67 | 129 | 83 | 149 | 99 | 171 |
| 21 | 29 | 75 | 41 | 94 | 55 | 113 | 69 | 134 | 85 | 155 | 102 | 177 |
| 22 | 30 | 78 | 43 | 97 | 57 | 117 | 72 | 138 | 88 | 160 | 105 | 183 |
| 23 | 31 | 81 | 44 | 101 | 58 | 122 | 74 | 143 | 90 | 166 | 108 | 189 |
| 24 | 32 | 84 | 45 | 105 | 60 | 126 | 76 | 148 | 93 | 171 | 111 | 195 |
| 25 | 33 | 87 | 47 | 108 | 62 | 130 | 78 | 153 | 96 | 176 | 114 | 201 |

## α = 0.05

| $n_2$ \ $n_1$ → | 4 $T_l$ | $T_r$ | 5 $T_l$ | $T_r$ | 6 $T_l$ | $T_r$ | 7 $T_l$ | $T_r$ | 8 $T_l$ | $T_r$ | 9 $T_l$ | $T_r$ |
|---|---|---|---|---|---|---|---|---|---|---|---|---|
| 4 | 10 | 26 | 16 | 34 | 23 | 43 | 31 | 53 | 40 | 64 | 49 | 77 |
| 5 | 11 | 29 | 17 | 38 | 24 | 48 | 33 | 58 | 42 | 70 | 52 | 83 |
| 6 | 12 | 32 | 18 | 42 | 26 | 52 | 34 | 64 | 44 | 76 | 55 | 89 |
| 7 | 13 | 35 | 20 | 45 | 27 | 57 | 36 | 69 | 46 | 82 | 57 | 96 |
| 8 | 14 | 38 | 21 | 49 | 29 | 61 | 38 | 74 | 49 | 87 | 60 | 102 |
| 9 | 14 | 42 | 22 | 53 | 31 | 65 | 40 | 79 | 51 | 93 | 62 | 109 |
| 10 | 15 | 45 | 23 | 57 | 32 | 70 | 42 | 84 | 53 | 99 | 65 | 115 |
| 11 | 16 | 48 | 24 | 61 | 34 | 74 | 44 | 89 | 55 | 105 | 68 | 121 |
| 12 | 17 | 51 | 26 | 64 | 35 | 79 | 46 | 94 | 58 | 110 | 71 | 127 |
| 13 | 18 | 54 | 27 | 68 | 37 | 83 | 48 | 99 | 60 | 116 | 73 | 134 |
| 14 | 19 | 57 | 28 | 72 | 38 | 88 | 50 | 104 | 62 | 122 | 76 | 140 |
| 15 | 20 | 60 | 29 | 76 | 40 | 92 | 52 | 109 | 65 | 127 | 79 | 146 |
| 16 | 21 | 63 | 30 | 80 | 42 | 96 | 54 | 114 | 67 | 133 | 82 | 152 |
| 17 | 21 | 67 | 32 | 83 | 43 | 101 | 56 | 119 | 70 | 138 | 84 | 159 |
| 18 | 22 | 70 | 33 | 87 | 45 | 105 | 58 | 124 | 72 | 144 | 87 | 165 |
| 19 | 23 | 73 | 34 | 91 | 46 | 110 | 60 | 129 | 74 | 150 | 90 | 171 |
| 20 | 24 | 76 | 35 | 95 | 48 | 114 | 62 | 134 | 77 | 155 | 93 | 177 |
| 21 | 25 | 79 | 37 | 98 | 50 | 118 | 64 | 139 | 79 | 161 | 95 | 184 |
| 22 | 26 | 82 | 38 | 102 | 51 | 123 | 66 | 144 | 81 | 167 | 98 | 190 |
| 23 | 27 | 85 | 39 | 106 | 53 | 127 | 68 | 149 | 84 | 172 | 101 | 196 |
| 24 | 27 | 89 | 40 | 110 | 54 | 132 | 70 | 154 | 86 | 178 | 104 | 202 |
| 25 | 28 | 92 | 42 | 113 | 56 | 136 | 72 | 159 | 89 | 183 | 107 | 208 |

## Table 10 (Continued)

### α = 0.02

| $n_2$ \ $n_1 \rightarrow$ | 4 ($T_l$–$T_r$) | 5 ($T_l$–$T_r$) | 6 ($T_l$–$T_r$) | 7 ($T_l$–$T_r$) | 8 ($T_l$–$T_r$) | 9 ($T_l$–$T_r$) |
|---|---|---|---|---|---|---|
| 4 | — — | 15–35 | 22–44 | 29–55 | 38–66 | 48–78 |
| 5 | 10–30 | 16–39 | 23–49 | 31–60 | 40–72 | 50–85 |
| 6 | 11–33 | 17–43 | 24–54 | 32–66 | 42–78 | 52–92 |
| 7 | 11–37 | 18–47 | 25–59 | 34–71 | 43–85 | 54–99 |
| 8 | 12–40 | 19–51 | 27–63 | 35–77 | 45–91 | 56–106 |
| 9 | 13–43 | 20–55 | 28–68 | 37–82 | 47–97 | 59–112 |
| 10 | 13–47 | 21–59 | 29–73 | 39–87 | 49–103 | 61–119 |
| 11 | 14–50 | 22–63 | 30–78 | 40–93 | 51–109 | 63–126 |
| 12 | 15–53 | 23–67 | 32–82 | 42–98 | 53–115 | 66–132 |
| 13 | 15–57 | 24–71 | 33–87 | 44–103 | 56–120 | 68–139 |
| 14 | 16–60 | 25–75 | 34–92 | 45–109 | 58–126 | 71–145 |
| 15 | 17–63 | 26–79 | 36–96 | 47–114 | 60–132 | 73–152 |
| 16 | 17–67 | 27–83 | 37–101 | 49–119 | 62–138 | 76–158 |
| 17 | 18–70 | 28–87 | 39–105 | 51–124 | 64–144 | 78–165 |
| 18 | 19–73 | 29–91 | 40–110 | 52–130 | 66–150 | 81–171 |
| 19 | 19–77 | 30–95 | 41–115 | 54–135 | 68–156 | 83–178 |
| 20 | 20–80 | 31–99 | 43–119 | 56–140 | 70–162 | 85–185 |
| 21 | 21–83 | 32–103 | 44–124 | 58–145 | 72–168 | 88–191 |
| 22 | 21–87 | 33–107 | 45–129 | 59–151 | 74–174 | 90–198 |
| 23 | 22–90 | 34–111 | 47–133 | 61–156 | 76–180 | 93–204 |
| 24 | 23–93 | 35–115 | 48–138 | 63–161 | 78–186 | 95–211 |
| 25 | 23–97 | 36–119 | 50–142 | 64–167 | 81–191 | 98–217 |

### α = 0.01

| $n_2$ \ $n_1 \rightarrow$ | 4 ($T_l$–$T_r$) | 5 ($T_l$–$T_r$) | 6 ($T_l$–$T_r$) | 7 ($T_l$–$T_r$) | 8 ($T_l$–$T_r$) | 9 ($T_l$–$T_r$) |
|---|---|---|---|---|---|---|
| 4 | — | — | 21–45 | 28–56 | 37–67 | 46–80 |
| 5 | — | 15–40 | 22–50 | 29–62 | 38–74 | 48–87 |
| 6 | 10–34 | 16–44 | 23–55 | 31–67 | 40–80 | 50–94 |
| 7 | 10–38 | 16–49 | 24–60 | 32–73 | 42–86 | 52–101 |
| 8 | 11–41 | 17–53 | 25–65 | 34–78 | 43–93 | 54–108 |
| 9 | 11–45 | 18–57 | 26–70 | 35–84 | 45–99 | 56–115 |
| 10 | 12–48 | 19–61 | 27–75 | 37–89 | 47–105 | 58–122 |
| 11 | 12–52 | 20–65 | 28–80 | 38–95 | 49–111 | 61–128 |
| 12 | 13–55 | 21–69 | 30–84 | 40–100 | 51–117 | 63–135 |
| 13 | 13–59 | 22–73 | 31–89 | 41–106 | 53–123 | 65–142 |
| 14 | 14–62 | 22–78 | 32–94 | 43–111 | 54–130 | 67–149 |
| 15 | 15–65 | 23–82 | 33–99 | 44–117 | 56–136 | 69–156 |
| 16 | 15–69 | 24–86 | 34–104 | 46–122 | 58–142 | 72–162 |
| 17 | 16–72 | 25–90 | 36–108 | 47–128 | 60–148 | 74–169 |
| 18 | 16–76 | 26–94 | 37–113 | 49–133 | 62–154 | 76–176 |
| 19 | 17–79 | 27–98 | 38–118 | 50–139 | 64–160 | 78–183 |
| 20 | 18–82 | 28–102 | 39–123 | 52–144 | 66–166 | 81–189 |
| 21 | 18–86 | 29–106 | 40–128 | 53–150 | 68–172 | 83–196 |
| 22 | 19–89 | 29–111 | 42–132 | 55–155 | 70–178 | 85–203 |
| 23 | 19–93 | 30–115 | 43–137 | 57–160 | 71–185 | 88–209 |
| 24 | 20–96 | 31–119 | 44–142 | 58–166 | 73–191 | 90–216 |
| 25 | 20–100 | 32–123 | 45–147 | 60–171 | 75–197 | 92–223 |

**Table 10** (Continued)

### α = 0.10

| $n_2$ \ $n_1$ → | 4 $T_l$–$T_r$ | 5 $T_l$–$T_r$ | 6 $T_l$–$T_r$ | 7 $T_l$–$T_r$ | 8 $T_l$–$T_r$ | 9 $T_l$–$T_r$ |
|---|---|---|---|---|---|---|
| 26 | 34–90 | 48–112 | 64–134 | 81–157 | 98–182 | 117–207 |
| 27 | 35–93 | 50–115 | 66–138 | 83–162 | 101–187 | 120–213 |
| 28 | 36–96 | 51–119 | 67–143 | 85–167 | 103–193 | 123–219 |
| 29 | 37–99 | 53–122 | 69–147 | 87–172 | 106–198 | 126–225 |
| 30 | 38–102 | 54–126 | 71–151 | 89–177 | 109–203 | 129–231 |
| 31 | 39–105 | 55–130 | 73–155 | 92–181 | 111–209 | 132–237 |
| 32 | 40–108 | 57–133 | 75–159 | 94–186 | 114–214 | 135–243 |
| 33 | 41–111 | 58–137 | 77–163 | 96–191 | 117–219 | 138–249 |
| 34 | 42–114 | 60–140 | 78–168 | 98–196 | 119–225 | 141–255 |
| 35 | 43–117 | 61–144 | 80–172 | 100–201 | 122–230 | 144–261 |
| 36 | 44–120 | 62–148 | 82–176 | 102–206 | 124–236 | 148–266 |
| 37 | 45–123 | 64–151 | 84–180 | 105–210 | 127–241 | 151–272 |
| 38 | 46–126 | 65–155 | 85–185 | 107–215 | 130–246 | 154–278 |
| 39 | 47–129 | 67–158 | 87–189 | 109–220 | 132–252 | 157–284 |
| 40 | 48–132 | 68–162 | 89–193 | 111–225 | 135–257 | 160–290 |
| 41 | 49–135 | 69–166 | 91–197 | 114–229 | 138–262 | 163–296 |
| 42 | 50–138 | 71–169 | 93–201 | 116–234 | 140–268 | 166–302 |
| 43 | 51–141 | 72–173 | 95–205 | 118–239 | 143–273 | 169–308 |
| 44 | 52–144 | 74–176 | 96–210 | 120–244 | 146–278 | 172–314 |
| 45 | 53–147 | 75–180 | 98–214 | 123–248 | 148–284 | 175–320 |
| 46 | 55–149 | 77–183 | 100–218 | 125–253 | 151–289 | 178–326 |
| 47 | 56–152 | 78–187 | 102–222 | 127–258 | 154–294 | 181–332 |
| 48 | 57–155 | 79–191 | 104–226 | 129–263 | 156–300 | 184–338 |
| 49 | 58–158 | 81–194 | 106–230 | 132–267 | 159–305 | 187–344 |
| 50 | 59–161 | 82–198 | 107–235 | 134–272 | 162–310 | 190–350 |

### α = 0.05

| $n_2$ \ $n_1$ → | 4 $T_l$–$T_r$ | 5 $T_l$–$T_r$ | 6 $T_l$–$T_r$ | 7 $T_l$–$T_r$ | 8 $T_l$–$T_r$ | 9 $T_l$–$T_r$ |
|---|---|---|---|---|---|---|
| 26 | 29–95 | 43–117 | 58–140 | 74–164 | 91–189 | 109–215 |
| 27 | 30–98 | 44–121 | 59–145 | 76–169 | 93–195 | 112–221 |
| 28 | 31–101 | 45–125 | 61–149 | 78–174 | 96–200 | 115–227 |
| 29 | 32–104 | 47–128 | 63–153 | 80–179 | 98–206 | 118–233 |
| 30 | 33–107 | 48–132 | 64–158 | 82–184 | 101–211 | 121–239 |
| 31 | 34–110 | 49–136 | 66–162 | 84–189 | 103–217 | 123–246 |
| 32 | 34–114 | 50–140 | 67–167 | 86–194 | 106–222 | 126–252 |
| 33 | 35–117 | 52–143 | 69–171 | 88–199 | 108–228 | 129–258 |
| 34 | 36–120 | 53–147 | 71–175 | 90–204 | 110–234 | 132–264 |
| 35 | 37–123 | 54–151 | 72–180 | 92–209 | 113–239 | 135–270 |
| 36 | 38–126 | 55–155 | 74–184 | 94–214 | 115–245 | 137–277 |
| 37 | 39–129 | 57–158 | 76–188 | 96–219 | 117–251 | 140–283 |
| 38 | 40–132 | 58–162 | 77–193 | 98–224 | 120–256 | 143–289 |
| 39 | 41–135 | 59–166 | 79–197 | 100–229 | 122–262 | 146–295 |
| 40 | 41–139 | 60–170 | 80–202 | 102–234 | 125–267 | 149–301 |
| 41 | 42–142 | 61–174 | 82–206 | 104–239 | 127–273 | 151–308 |
| 42 | 43–145 | 63–177 | 84–210 | 106–244 | 129–279 | 154–314 |
| 43 | 44–148 | 64–181 | 85–215 | 108–249 | 132–284 | 157–320 |
| 44 | 45–151 | 65–185 | 87–219 | 110–254 | 134–290 | 160–326 |
| 45 | 46–154 | 66–189 | 88–224 | 112–259 | 137–295 | 163–332 |
| 46 | 47–157 | 68–192 | 90–228 | 114–264 | 139–301 | 165–339 |
| 47 | 48–160 | 69–196 | 92–232 | 116–269 | 141–307 | 168–345 |
| 48 | 48–164 | 70–200 | 93–237 | 118–274 | 144–312 | 171–351 |
| 49 | 49–167 | 71–204 | 95–241 | 120–279 | 146–318 | 174–357 |
| 50 | 50–170 | 73–207 | 97–245 | 122–284 | 149–323 | 177–363 |

*Table 10* (Continued)

|  | α = 0.02 | | | | | | α = 0.01 | | | | | |
|---|---|---|---|---|---|---|---|---|---|---|---|---|
| $n_2$ \ $n_1 \rightarrow$ | 4 | 5 | 6 | 7 | 8 | 9 | 4 | 5 | 6 | 7 | 8 | 9 |
|  | $T_l$–$T_r$ | $T_l$–$T_r$ | $T_l$–$T_r$ | $T_l$–$T_r$ | $T_l$–$T_r$ | $T_l$–$T_r$ | $T_l$–$T_r$ | $T_l$–$T_r$ | $T_l$–$T_r$ | $T_l$–$T_r$ | $T_l$–$T_r$ | $T_l$–$T_r$ |
| **26** | 24–100 | 37–123 | 51–147 | 66–172 | 83–197 | 100–224 | 21–103 | 33–127 | 46–152 | 61–177 | 77–203 | 94–230 |
| 27 | 25–103 | 38–127 | 52–152 | 68–177 | 85–203 | 103–230 | 22–106 | 34–131 | 48–156 | 63–182 | 79–209 | 97–236 |
| 28 | 26–106 | 39–131 | 54–156 | 70–182 | 87–209 | 105–237 | 22–110 | 35–135 | 49–161 | 64–188 | 81–215 | 99–243 |
| 29 | 26–110 | 40–135 | 55–161 | 71–188 | 89–215 | 108–243 | 23–113 | 36–139 | 50–166 | 66–193 | 83–221 | 101–250 |
| **30** | 27–113 | 41–139 | 56–166 | 73–193 | 91–221 | 110–250 | 23–117 | 37–143 | 51–171 | 68–198 | 85–227 | 103–257 |
| 31 | 28–116 | 42–143 | 58–170 | 75–198 | 93–227 | 112–257 | 24–120 | 37–148 | 53–175 | 68–204 | 87–233 | 106–263 |
| 32 | 28–120 | 43–147 | 59–175 | 77–203 | 95–233 | 115–263 | 24–124 | 38–152 | 54–180 | 71–209 | 89–239 | 108–270 |
| 33 | 29–123 | 44–151 | 61–179 | 78–209 | 97–239 | 117–270 | 25–127 | 39–156 | 55–185 | 72–215 | 90–246 | 110–277 |
| 34 | 30–126 | 45–155 | 62–184 | 79–215 | 99–245 | 120–276 | 26–130 | 40–160 | 56–190 | 73–221 | 92–252 | 112–284 |
| **35** | 30–130 | 46–159 | 63–189 | 81–220 | 101–251 | 122–283 | 26–134 | 41–164 | 57–195 | 75–226 | 94–258 | 114–291 |
| 36 | 31–133 | 47–163 | 65–193 | 83–225 | 103–257 | 125–289 | 27–137 | 42–168 | 58–200 | 76–232 | 96–264 | 117–297 |
| 37 | 32–136 | 48–167 | 66–198 | 84–231 | 105–263 | 127–296 | 28–140 | 43–172 | 60–204 | 78–237 | 98–270 | 119–304 |
| 38 | 32–140 | 49–171 | 67–203 | 86–236 | 107–269 | 129–303 | 28–144 | 44–176 | 61–209 | 79–243 | 100–276 | 121–311 |
| 39 | 33–143 | 50–175 | 69–207 | 88–241 | 109–275 | 132–309 | 29–147 | 45–180 | 62–214 | 81–248 | 102–282 | 123–318 |
| **40** | 34–146 | 51–179 | 70–212 | 90–246 | 111–281 | 134–316 | 29–151 | 46–184 | 63–219 | 82–254 | 103–289 | 126–324 |
| 41 | 34–150 | 52–183 | 72–216 | 91–252 | 113–287 | 137–322 | 30–154 | 46–189 | 65–223 | 84–259 | 105–295 | 128–331 |
| 42 | 35–153 | 53–187 | 73–221 | 93–257 | 116–292 | 139–329 | 31–157 | 47–193 | 66–228 | 85–265 | 107–301 | 130–338 |
| 43 | 35–157 | 54–191 | 74–226 | 95–262 | 118–298 | 142–335 | 31–161 | 48–197 | 67–233 | 87–270 | 109–307 | 133–344 |
| 44 | 36–160 | 55–195 | 76–230 | 97–267 | 120–304 | 144–342 | 32–164 | 49–201 | 68–238 | 88–276 | 111–313 | 135–351 |
| **45** | 37–163 | 56–199 | 77–235 | 98–273 | 122–310 | 147–348 | 32–168 | 50–205 | 69–243 | 90–281 | 113–319 | 137–358 |
| 46 | 37–167 | 57–203 | 78–240 | 100–278 | 124–316 | 149–355 | 33–171 | 51–209 | 71–247 | 91–287 | 115–325 | 139–365 |
| 47 | 38–170 | 58–207 | 80–244 | 102–283 | 126–322 | 152–361 | 34–174 | 52–213 | 72–252 | 93–292 | 117–331 | 142–371 |
| 48 | 39–173 | 59–211 | 81–249 | 103–289 | 128–328 | 154–368 | 34–178 | 53–217 | 73–257 | 95–297 | 118–338 | 144–378 |
| 49 | 39–177 | 60–215 | 82–254 | 105–294 | 130–334 | 157–374 | 35–181 | 54–221 | 74–262 | 96–303 | 120–344 | 146–385 |
| **50** | 40–180 | 61–219 | 84–258 | 107–299 | 132–340 | 159–381 | 36–184 | 55–225 | 76–266 | 98–308 | 122–350 | 148–392 |

$n_1$ = minimum of the two sample sizes.
$n_2$ = maximum of the two sample sizes.
$T_l$ = lower critical value for the rank sum in the first sample.
$T_r$ = upper critical value for the rank sum in the first sample.

(The data of this table are reproduced with permission from *Documenta Geigy Scientific Tables*, 6th Ed., pp. 124–127, Geigy Pharmaceuticals, Division of Geigy Chemical Corporation, Ardsley, N.Y. Figures from "Documenta Geigy Scientific Tables," 6th Edition. Reprinted with the kind permission of CIBA-GEIGY Limited, Basle, Switzerland.)

# Table 11

**Table 11**  *Fisher's z transformation*

| r | z | r | z | r | z |
|------|-------|------|-------|------|-------|
| 0.00 | 0.000 |      |       |      |       |
| 0.01 | 0.010 | 0.41 | 0.436 | 0.81 | 1.127 |
| 0.02 | 0.020 | 0.42 | 0.448 | 0.82 | 1.157 |
| 0.03 | 0.030 | 0.43 | 0.460 | 0.83 | 1.188 |
| 0.04 | 0.040 | 0.44 | 0.472 | 0.84 | 1.221 |
| 0.05 | 0.050 | 0.45 | 0.485 | 0.85 | 1.256 |
| 0.06 | 0.060 | 0.46 | 0.497 | 0.86 | 1.293 |
| 0.07 | 0.070 | 0.47 | 0.510 | 0.87 | 1.333 |
| 0.08 | 0.080 | 0.48 | 0.523 | 0.88 | 1.376 |
| 0.09 | 0.090 | 0.49 | 0.536 | 0.89 | 1.422 |
| 0.10 | 0.100 | 0.50 | 0.549 | 0.90 | 1.472 |
| 0.11 | 0.110 | 0.51 | 0.563 | 0.91 | 1.528 |
| 0.12 | 0.121 | 0.52 | 0.576 | 0.92 | 1.589 |
| 0.13 | 0.131 | 0.53 | 0.590 | 0.93 | 1.658 |
| 0.14 | 0.141 | 0.54 | 0.604 | 0.94 | 1.738 |
| 0.15 | 0.151 | 0.55 | 0.618 | 0.95 | 1.832 |
| 0.16 | 0.161 | 0.56 | 0.633 | 0.96 | 1.946 |
| 0.17 | 0.172 | 0.57 | 0.648 | 0.97 | 2.092 |
| 0.18 | 0.182 | 0.58 | 0.662 | 0.98 | 2.298 |
| 0.19 | 0.192 | 0.59 | 0.678 | 0.99 | 2.647 |
| 0.20 | 0.203 | 0.60 | 0.693 |      |       |
| 0.21 | 0.213 | 0.61 | 0.709 |      |       |
| 0.22 | 0.224 | 0.62 | 0.725 |      |       |
| 0.23 | 0.234 | 0.63 | 0.741 |      |       |
| 0.24 | 0.245 | 0.64 | 0.758 |      |       |
| 0.25 | 0.255 | 0.65 | 0.775 |      |       |
| 0.26 | 0.266 | 0.66 | 0.793 |      |       |
| 0.27 | 0.277 | 0.67 | 0.811 |      |       |
| 0.28 | 0.288 | 0.68 | 0.829 |      |       |
| 0.29 | 0.299 | 0.69 | 0.848 |      |       |
| 0.30 | 0.310 | 0.70 | 0.867 |      |       |
| 0.31 | 0.321 | 0.71 | 0.887 |      |       |
| 0.32 | 0.332 | 0.72 | 0.908 |      |       |
| 0.33 | 0.343 | 0.73 | 0.929 |      |       |
| 0.34 | 0.354 | 0.74 | 0.950 |      |       |
| 0.35 | 0.365 | 0.75 | 0.973 |      |       |
| 0.36 | 0.377 | 0.76 | 0.996 |      |       |
| 0.37 | 0.388 | 0.77 | 1.020 |      |       |
| 0.38 | 0.400 | 0.78 | 1.045 |      |       |
| 0.39 | 0.412 | 0.79 | 1.071 |      |       |
| 0.40 | 0.424 | 0.80 | 1.099 |      |       |

# Table 12

Table 12

**Table 12** Two-tailed upper critical values for the Spearman rank correlation coefficient ($r_s$)

| | α | | | |
|---|---|---|---|---|
| n | 0.10 | 0.05 | 0.02 | 0.01 |
| 1 | — | — | — | — |
| 2 | — | — | — | — |
| 3 | — | — | — | — |
| 4 | 1.0 | — | — | — |
| 5 | 0.900 | 1.0 | 1.0 | — |
| 6 | 0.829 | 0.886 | 0.943 | 1.0 |
| 7 | 0.714 | 0.786 | 0.893 | 0.929 |
| 8 | 0.643 | 0.738 | 0.833 | 0.881 |
| 9 | 0.600 | 0.683 | 0.783 | 0.833 |

(The data for this table have been adapted with permission from Olds, E. G. (1938) "Distributions of Sums of Squares of Rank Differences for Small Numbers of Individuals," *Ann. Math. Statist.* **9**: 133–148.)

# Table 13

**Table 13** Upper $\alpha$ percentage points of the studentized range

$\alpha = 0.05$

| $d\dagger$ | $c^*$ | | | | | | | | | | | | | | | | | | |
|---|---|---|---|---|---|---|---|---|---|---|---|---|---|---|---|---|---|---|---|
| | 2 | 3 | 4 | 5 | 6 | 7 | 8 | 9 | 10 | 11 | 12 | 13 | 14 | 15 | 16 | 17 | 18 | 19 | 20 |
| 1 | 18.0 | 27.0 | 32.8 | 37.1 | 40.4 | 43.1 | 45.4 | 47.4 | 49.1 | 50.6 | 52.0 | 53.2 | 54.3 | 55.4 | 56.3 | 57.2 | 58.0 | 58.8 | 59.6 |
| 2 | 6.08 | 8.33 | 9.80 | 10.9 | 11.7 | 12.4 | 13.0 | 13.5 | 14.0 | 14.4 | 14.7 | 15.1 | 15.4 | 15.7 | 15.9 | 16.1 | 16.4 | 16.6 | 16.8 |
| 3 | 4.50 | 5.91 | 6.82 | 7.50 | 8.04 | 8.48 | 8.85 | 9.18 | 9.46 | 9.72 | 9.95 | 10.2 | 10.3 | 10.5 | 10.7 | 10.8 | 11.0 | 11.1 | 11.2 |
| 4 | 3.93 | 5.04 | 5.76 | 6.29 | 6.71 | 7.05 | 7.35 | 7.60 | 7.83 | 8.03 | 8.21 | 8.37 | 8.52 | 8.66 | 8.79 | 8.91 | 9.03 | 9.13 | 9.23 |
| 5 | 3.64 | 4.60 | 5.22 | 5.67 | 6.03 | 6.33 | 6.58 | 6.80 | 6.99 | 7.17 | 7.32 | 7.47 | 7.60 | 7.72 | 7.83 | 7.93 | 8.03 | 8.12 | 8.21 |
| 6 | 3.46 | 4.34 | 4.90 | 5.30 | 5.63 | 5.90 | 6.12 | 6.32 | 6.49 | 6.65 | 6.79 | 6.92 | 7.03 | 7.14 | 7.24 | 7.34 | 7.43 | 7.51 | 7.59 |
| 7 | 3.34 | 4.16 | 4.68 | 5.06 | 5.36 | 5.61 | 5.82 | 6.00 | 6.16 | 6.30 | 6.43 | 6.55 | 6.66 | 6.76 | 6.85 | 6.94 | 7.02 | 7.10 | 7.17 |
| 8 | 3.26 | 4.04 | 4.53 | 4.89 | 5.17 | 5.40 | 5.60 | 5.77 | 5.92 | 6.05 | 6.18 | 6.29 | 6.39 | 6.48 | 6.57 | 6.65 | 6.73 | 6.80 | 6.87 |
| 9 | 3.20 | 3.95 | 4.41 | 4.76 | 5.02 | 5.24 | 5.43 | 5.59 | 5.74 | 5.87 | 5.98 | 6.09 | 6.19 | 6.28 | 6.36 | 6.44 | 6.51 | 6.58 | 6.64 |
| 10 | 3.15 | 3.88 | 4.33 | 4.65 | 4.91 | 5.12 | 5.30 | 5.46 | 5.60 | 5.72 | 5.83 | 5.93 | 6.03 | 6.11 | 6.19 | 6.27 | 6.34 | 6.40 | 6.47 |
| 11 | 3.11 | 3.82 | 4.26 | 4.57 | 4.82 | 5.03 | 5.20 | 5.35 | 5.49 | 5.61 | 5.71 | 5.81 | 5.90 | 5.98 | 6.06 | 6.13 | 6.20 | 6.27 | 6.33 |
| 12 | 3.08 | 3.77 | 4.20 | 4.51 | 4.75 | 4.95 | 5.12 | 5.27 | 5.39 | 5.51 | 5.61 | 5.71 | 5.80 | 5.88 | 5.95 | 6.02 | 6.09 | 6.15 | 6.21 |
| 13 | 3.06 | 3.73 | 4.15 | 4.45 | 4.69 | 4.88 | 5.05 | 5.19 | 5.32 | 5.43 | 5.53 | 5.63 | 5.71 | 5.79 | 5.86 | 5.93 | 5.99 | 6.05 | 6.11 |
| 14 | 3.03 | 3.70 | 4.11 | 4.41 | 4.64 | 4.83 | 4.99 | 5.13 | 5.25 | 5.36 | 5.46 | 5.55 | 5.64 | 5.71 | 5.79 | 5.85 | 5.91 | 5.97 | 6.03 |
| 15 | 3.01 | 3.67 | 4.08 | 4.37 | 4.59 | 4.78 | 4.94 | 5.08 | 5.20 | 5.31 | 5.40 | 5.49 | 5.57 | 5.65 | 5.72 | 5.78 | 5.85 | 5.90 | 5.96 |
| 16 | 3.00 | 3.65 | 4.05 | 4.33 | 4.56 | 4.74 | 4.90 | 5.03 | 5.15 | 5.26 | 5.35 | 5.44 | 5.52 | 5.59 | 5.66 | 5.73 | 5.79 | 5.84 | 5.90 |
| 17 | 2.98 | 3.63 | 4.02 | 4.30 | 4.52 | 4.70 | 4.86 | 4.99 | 5.11 | 5.21 | 5.31 | 5.39 | 5.47 | 5.54 | 5.61 | 5.67 | 5.73 | 5.79 | 5.84 |
| 18 | 2.97 | 3.61 | 4.00 | 4.28 | 4.49 | 4.67 | 4.82 | 4.96 | 5.07 | 5.17 | 5.27 | 5.35 | 5.43 | 5.50 | 5.57 | 5.63 | 5.69 | 5.74 | 5.79 |
| 19 | 2.96 | 3.59 | 3.98 | 4.25 | 4.47 | 4.65 | 4.79 | 4.92 | 5.04 | 5.14 | 5.23 | 5.31 | 5.39 | 5.46 | 5.53 | 5.59 | 5.65 | 5.70 | 5.75 |
| 20 | 2.95 | 3.58 | 3.96 | 4.23 | 4.45 | 4.62 | 4.77 | 4.90 | 5.01 | 5.11 | 5.20 | 5.28 | 5.36 | 5.43 | 5.49 | 5.55 | 5.61 | 5.66 | 5.71 |
| 24 | 2.92 | 3.53 | 3.90 | 4.17 | 4.37 | 4.54 | 4.68 | 4.81 | 4.92 | 5.01 | 5.10 | 5.18 | 5.25 | 5.32 | 5.38 | 5.44 | 5.49 | 5.55 | 5.59 |
| 30 | 2.89 | 3.49 | 3.85 | 4.10 | 4.30 | 4.46 | 4.60 | 4.72 | 4.82 | 4.92 | 5.00 | 5.08 | 5.15 | 5.21 | 5.27 | 5.33 | 5.38 | 5.43 | 5.47 |
| 40 | 2.86 | 3.44 | 3.79 | 4.04 | 4.23 | 4.39 | 4.52 | 4.63 | 4.73 | 4.82 | 4.90 | 4.98 | 5.04 | 5.11 | 5.16 | 5.22 | 5.27 | 5.31 | 5.36 |
| 60 | 2.83 | 3.40 | 3.74 | 3.98 | 4.16 | 4.31 | 4.44 | 4.55 | 4.65 | 4.73 | 4.81 | 4.88 | 4.94 | 5.00 | 5.06 | 5.11 | 5.15 | 5.20 | 5.24 |
| 120 | 2.80 | 3.36 | 3.68 | 3.92 | 4.10 | 4.24 | 4.36 | 4.47 | 4.56 | 4.64 | 4.71 | 4.78 | 4.84 | 4.90 | 4.95 | 5.00 | 5.04 | 5.09 | 5.13 |
| $\infty$ | 2.77 | 3.31 | 3.63 | 3.86 | 4.03 | 4.17 | 4.29 | 4.39 | 4.47 | 4.55 | 4.62 | 4.68 | 4.74 | 4.80 | 4.85 | 4.89 | 4.93 | 4.97 | 5.01 |

**Table 13** (Continued)

α = 0.01

| d† | 2 | 3 | 4 | 5 | 6 | 7 | 8 | 9 | 10 | 11 | 12 | 13 | 14 | 15 | 16 | 17 | 18 | 19 | 20 |
|---|---|---|---|---|---|---|---|---|---|---|---|---|---|---|---|---|---|---|---|
| 1 | 90.0 | 135. | 164. | 186. | 202. | 216. | 227. | 237. | 246. | 253. | 260. | 266. | 272. | 277. | 282. | 286. | 290. | 294. | 298. |
| 2 | 14.0 | 19.0 | 22.3 | 24.7 | 26.6 | 28.2 | 29.5 | 30.7 | 31.7 | 32.6 | 33.4 | 34.1 | 34.8 | 35.4 | 36.0 | 36.5 | 37.0 | 37.5 | 37.9 |
| 3 | 8.26 | 10.6 | 12.2 | 13.3 | 14.2 | 15.0 | 15.6 | 16.2 | 16.7 | 17.1 | 17.5 | 17.9 | 18.2 | 18.5 | 18.8 | 19.1 | 19.3 | 19.5 | 19.8 |
| 4 | 6.51 | 8.12 | 9.17 | 9.96 | 10.6 | 11.1 | 11.5 | 11.9 | 12.3 | 12.6 | 12.8 | 13.1 | 13.3 | 13.5 | 13.7 | 13.9 | 14.1 | 14.2 | 14.4 |
| 5 | 5.70 | 6.98 | 7.80 | 8.42 | 8.91 | 9.32 | 9.67 | 9.97 | 10.2 | 10.5 | 10.7 | 10.9 | 11.1 | 11.2 | 11.4 | 11.6 | 11.7 | 11.8 | 11.9 |
| 6 | 5.24 | 6.33 | 7.03 | 7.56 | 7.97 | 8.32 | 8.61 | 8.87 | 9.10 | 9.30 | 9.48 | 9.65 | 9.81 | 9.95 | 10.1 | 10.2 | 10.3 | 10.4 | 10.5 |
| 7 | 4.95 | 5.92 | 6.54 | 7.01 | 7.37 | 7.68 | 7.94 | 8.17 | 8.37 | 8.55 | 8.71 | 8.86 | 9.00 | 9.12 | 9.24 | 9.35 | 9.46 | 9.55 | 9.65 |
| 8 | 4.75 | 5.64 | 6.20 | 6.62 | 6.96 | 7.24 | 7.47 | 7.68 | 7.86 | 8.03 | 8.18 | 8.31 | 8.44 | 8.55 | 8.66 | 8.76 | 8.85 | 8.94 | 9.03 |
| 9 | 4.60 | 5.43 | 5.96 | 6.35 | 6.66 | 6.91 | 7.13 | 7.33 | 7.49 | 7.65 | 7.78 | 7.91 | 8.03 | 8.13 | 8.23 | 8.33 | 8.41 | 8.49 | 8.57 |
| 10 | 4.48 | 5.27 | 5.77 | 6.14 | 6.43 | 6.67 | 6.87 | 7.05 | 7.21 | 7.36 | 7.49 | 7.60 | 7.71 | 7.81 | 7.91 | 7.99 | 8.08 | 8.15 | 8.23 |
| 11 | 4.39 | 5.15 | 5.62 | 5.97 | 6.25 | 6.48 | 6.67 | 6.84 | 6.99 | 7.13 | 7.25 | 7.36 | 7.46 | 7.56 | 7.65 | 7.73 | 7.81 | 7.88 | 7.95 |
| 12 | 4.32 | 5.05 | 5.50 | 5.84 | 6.10 | 6.32 | 6.51 | 6.67 | 6.81 | 6.94 | 7.06 | 7.17 | 7.26 | 7.36 | 7.44 | 7.52 | 7.59 | 7.66 | 7.73 |
| 13 | 4.26 | 4.96 | 5.40 | 5.73 | 5.98 | 6.19 | 6.37 | 6.53 | 6.67 | 6.79 | 6.90 | 7.01 | 7.10 | 7.19 | 7.27 | 7.35 | 7.42 | 7.48 | 7.55 |
| 14 | 4.21 | 4.89 | 5.32 | 5.63 | 5.88 | 6.08 | 6.26 | 6.41 | 6.54 | 6.66 | 6.77 | 6.87 | 6.96 | 7.05 | 7.13 | 7.20 | 7.27 | 7.33 | 7.39 |
| 15 | 4.17 | 4.84 | 5.25 | 5.56 | 5.80 | 5.99 | 6.16 | 6.31 | 6.44 | 6.55 | 6.66 | 6.76 | 6.84 | 6.93 | 7.00 | 7.07 | 7.14 | 7.20 | 7.26 |
| 16 | 4.13 | 4.79 | 5.19 | 5.49 | 5.72 | 5.92 | 6.08 | 6.22 | 6.35 | 6.46 | 6.56 | 6.66 | 6.74 | 6.82 | 6.90 | 6.97 | 7.03 | 7.09 | 7.15 |
| 17 | 4.10 | 4.74 | 5.14 | 5.43 | 5.66 | 5.85 | 6.01 | 6.15 | 6.27 | 6.38 | 6.48 | 6.57 | 6.66 | 6.73 | 6.81 | 6.87 | 6.94 | 7.00 | 7.05 |
| 18 | 4.07 | 4.70 | 5.09 | 5.38 | 5.60 | 5.79 | 5.94 | 6.08 | 6.20 | 6.31 | 6.41 | 6.50 | 6.58 | 6.65 | 6.73 | 6.79 | 6.85 | 6.91 | 6.96 |
| 19 | 4.05 | 4.67 | 5.05 | 5.33 | 5.55 | 5.73 | 5.89 | 6.02 | 6.14 | 6.25 | 6.34 | 6.43 | 6.51 | 6.58 | 6.65 | 6.72 | 6.78 | 6.84 | 6.89 |
| 20 | 4.02 | 4.64 | 5.02 | 5.29 | 5.51 | 5.69 | 5.84 | 5.97 | 6.09 | 6.19 | 6.28 | 6.37 | 6.45 | 6.52 | 6.59 | 6.65 | 6.71 | 6.77 | 6.82 |
| 24 | 3.96 | 4.55 | 4.91 | 5.17 | 5.37 | 5.54 | 5.69 | 5.81 | 5.92 | 6.02 | 6.11 | 6.19 | 6.26 | 6.33 | 6.39 | 6.45 | 6.51 | 6.56 | 6.61 |
| 30 | 3.89 | 4.45 | 4.80 | 5.05 | 5.24 | 5.40 | 5.54 | 5.65 | 5.76 | 5.85 | 5.93 | 6.01 | 6.08 | 6.14 | 6.20 | 6.26 | 6.31 | 6.36 | 6.41 |
| 40 | 3.82 | 4.37 | 4.70 | 4.93 | 5.11 | 5.26 | 5.39 | 5.50 | 5.60 | 5.69 | 5.76 | 5.83 | 5.90 | 5.96 | 6.02 | 6.07 | 6.12 | 6.16 | 6.21 |
| 60 | 3.76 | 4.28 | 4.59 | 4.82 | 4.99 | 5.13 | 5.25 | 5.36 | 5.45 | 5.53 | 5.60 | 5.67 | 5.73 | 5.78 | 5.84 | 5.89 | 5.93 | 5.97 | 6.01 |
| 120 | 3.70 | 4.20 | 4.50 | 4.71 | 4.87 | 5.01 | 5.12 | 5.21 | 5.30 | 5.37 | 5.44 | 5.50 | 5.56 | 5.61 | 5.66 | 5.71 | 5.75 | 5.79 | 5.83 |
| ∞ | 3.64 | 4.12 | 4.40 | 4.60 | 4.76 | 4.88 | 4.99 | 5.08 | 5.16 | 5.23 | 5.29 | 5.35 | 5.40 | 5.45 | 5.49 | 5.54 | 5.57 | 5.61 | 5.65 |

*c = number of means in the group of means considered.

†d = df for the Within MS.

(This table has been reproduced with permission of the Biometrika Trustees from "Biometrika Tables for Statisticians," Volume I, edited by E. S. Pearson and H. O. Hartley, published for the Biometrika Trustees, pp. 176–177, Cambridge University Press, Cambridge, England, 1959.)

# Table 14

**Table 14** Critical values for the Kruskal–Wallis test statistic (H) for selected sample sizes for k = 3

| | | | | α | | |
|---|---|---|---|---|---|---|
| $n_1$ | $n_2$ | $n_3$ | 0.10 | 0.05 | 0.02 | 0.01 |
| 1 | 1 | 2 | — | — | — | — |
| 1 | 1 | 3 | — | — | — | — |
| 1 | 1 | 4 | — | — | — | — |
| 1 | 1 | 5 | — | — | — | — |
| 1 | 2 | 2 | — | — | — | — |
| 1 | 2 | 3 | 4.286 | — | — | — |
| 1 | 2 | 4 | 4.500 | — | — | — |
| 1 | 2 | 5 | 4.200 | 5.000 | — | — |
| 1 | 3 | 3 | 4.571 | 5.143 | — | — |
| 1 | 3 | 4 | 4.056 | 5.389 | — | — |
| 1 | 3 | 5 | 4.018 | 4.960 | 6.400 | — |
| 1 | 4 | 4 | 4.167 | 4.967 | 6.667 | — |
| 1 | 4 | 5 | 3.987 | 4.986 | 6.431 | 6.954 |
| 1 | 5 | 5 | 4.109 | 5.127 | 6.146 | 7.309 |
| 2 | 2 | 2 | 4.571 | — | — | — |
| 2 | 2 | 3 | 4.500 | 4.714 | — | — |
| 2 | 2 | 4 | 4.500 | 5.333 | 6.000 | — |
| 2 | 2 | 5 | 4.373 | 5.160 | 6.000 | 6.533 |
| 2 | 3 | 3 | 4.694 | 5.361 | 6.250 | — |
| 2 | 3 | 4 | 4.511 | 5.444 | 6.144 | 6.444 |
| 2 | 3 | 5 | 4.651 | 5.251 | 6.294 | 6.909 |
| 2 | 4 | 4 | 4.554 | 5.454 | 6.600 | 7.036 |
| 2 | 4 | 5 | 4.541 | 5.273 | 6.541 | 7.204 |
| 2 | 5 | 5 | 4.623 | 5.338 | 6.469 | 7.392 |
| 3 | 3 | 3 | 5.067 | 5.689 | 6.489 | 7.200 |
| 3 | 3 | 4 | 4.709 | 5.791 | 6.564 | 7.000 |
| 3 | 3 | 5 | 4.533 | 5.648 | 6.533 | 7.079 |
| 3 | 4 | 4 | 4.546 | 5.598 | 6.712 | 7.212 |
| 3 | 4 | 5 | 4.549 | 5.656 | 6.703 | 7.477 |
| 3 | 5 | 5 | 4.571 | 5.706 | 6.866 | 7.622 |
| 4 | 4 | 4 | 4.654 | 5.692 | 6.962 | 7.654 |
| 4 | 4 | 5 | 4.668 | 5.657 | 6.976 | 7.760 |
| 4 | 5 | 5 | 4.523 | 5.666 | 7.000 | 7.903 |
| 5 | 5 | 5 | 4.580 | 5.780 | 7.220 | 8.000 |

(The data for this table have been adapted from Table F of *A Nonparametric Introduction to Statistics* by C. H. Kraft and C. Van Eeden, Macmillan, New York, 1968, with the permission of the publisher and the authors.)

# A nswers to Selected Problems

# C hapter 2

2.1–2.2 We have the following basic statistics (Table A.1).

2.3 We will use groups in increments of 100 g for heart weight and 10 kg for body weight. This yields the following frequency distributions and statistics (Tables A.2–A.4).

**Table A.1**  Basic statistics for left heart disease and normal males

|  | Left heart disease males | | Normal males | |
| --- | --- | --- | --- | --- |
|  | THW (g) | BW (kg) | THW (g) | BW (kg) |
| Sample size | 11 | 11 | 10 | 10 |
| Mean | 450 | 55.61 | 317 | 56.23 |
| Median | 450 | 54.6 | 305 | 56.15 |
| Variance | 19,415 | 133.44 | 2,217.78 | 133.13 |
| Standard deviation | 139.34 | 11.55 | 47.09 | 11.54 |
| Range | 475 | 34.2 | 160 | 34.4 |
| Coefficient of variation | 30.96% | 20.77% | 14.85% | 20.52% |

**Table A.2**  Frequency distribution for left heart disease males

| THW | | | BW | | |
| --- | --- | --- | --- | --- | --- |
| Interval | Midpoint | Frequency | Interval | Midpoint | Frequency |
| 200–299 | 249.5 | 1 | 40–49.9 | 44.95 | 3 |
| 300–399 | 349.5 | 3 | 50–59.9 | 54.95 | 5 |
| 400–499 | 449.5 | 5 | 60–69.9 | 64.95 | 1 |
| 500–599 | 549.5 | 0 | 70–79.9 | 74.95 | 2 |
| 600–699 | 649.5 | 1 | | | |
| 700–799 | 749.5 | 1 | | | |

*Table A.3* Frequency distribution for normal males

| | THW | | | BW | |
|---|---|---|---|---|---|
| *Interval* | *Midpoint* | *Frequency* | *Interval* | *Midpoint* | *Frequency* |
| 200–299 | 249.5 | 3 | 40–49.9 | 44.95 | 3 |
| 300–399 | 349.5 | 6 | 50–59.9 | 54.95 | 3 |
| 400–499 | 449.5 | 1 | 60–69.9 | 64.95 | 3 |
| | | | 70–79.9 | 74.95 | 1 |

*Table A.4* Grouped statistics for left heart disease and normal males

| | Left heart disease males | | Normal males | |
|---|---|---|---|---|
| | *THW* | *BW* | *THW* | *BW* |
| Grouped mean | 449.5 | 56.77 | 329.5 | 56.95 |
| Grouped variance | 20,000 | 116.4 | 4000 | 106.7 |
| Grouped standard deviation | 141.4 | 10.8 | 63.2 | 10.3 |

*2.4* We have the following histograms of the preceding variables (Figures A.1–A.4).

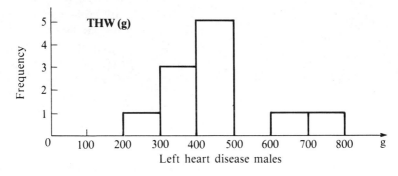

*Figure A.1*

Left heart disease males

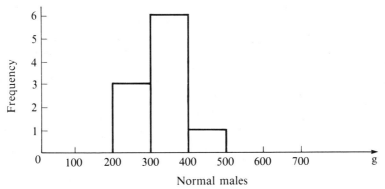

*Figure A.2*

Normal males

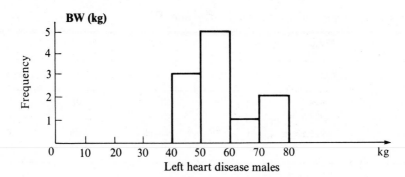

*Figure A.3*

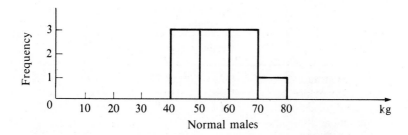

*Figure A.4*

**2.5** We have the following stem and leaf plots.

Total heart weight (g) (=STEM·LEAF × $10^2$)

| Left heart disease | | | | | | Normal | | | | | |
|---|---|---|---|---|---|---|---|---|---|---|---|
| **2** | 85 | | | | | **2** | 45 | 70 | 90 | | |
| **3** | 25 | 75 | 10 | | | **3** | 50 | 40 | 00 | 10 | 00 | 60 |
| **4** | 50 | 95 | 50 | 60 | 25 | **4** | 05 | | | | |
| **5** | | | | | | **5** | | | | | |
| **6** | 15 | | | | | **6** | | | | | |
| **7** | 60 | | | | | **7** | | | | | |

Body weight (kg) (=STEM·LEAF × $10^1$)

| Left heart disease | | | | | Normal | | | |
|---|---|---|---|---|---|---|---|---|
| **4** | 46 | 11 | 17 | | **4** | 08 | 75 | 05 |
| **5** | 46 | 03 | 81 | 15 | 97 | **5** | 33 | 12 | 90 |
| **6** | 13 | | | | **6** | 74 | 22 | 55 |
| **7** | 35 | 53 | | | **7** | 49 | | |

**2.6** From Problems 2.3, 2.4, and 2.5, it appears that body weight is comparable in the two groups, but heart weight is higher and more variable in the diseased group.

**2.7** There appears to be a positive relationship between THW and BW in the normal group. No relationship seems to exist in the diseased group. (See Figure A.5.)

**2.8** The principal differences between the groups are that the left heart disease males have larger and more variable heart weights than the normal males. However, the body weights of the two groups are comparable. Finally, there appears to be a relationship between total heart weight and body weight among normal males but not among diseased males.

**2.16–2.19** Changing the scale by a factor $c$ will multiply each data value $x_i$ by $c$, changing it to $cx_i$ (Figure A.6). Again the same individual's value will be at the median and the same individual's value will be at the mode, but these values will be multiplied by $c$. The geometric mean will be multiplied by $c$ also, as we can easily show:

$$\text{Geometric mean} = [(cx_1)(cx_2) \cdots (cx_n)]^{1/n}$$
$$= (c^n x_1 \cdot x_2 \cdots x_n)^{1/n}$$
$$= c(x_1 \cdot x_2 \cdots x_n)^{1/n}$$
$$= c \times \text{old geometric mean}$$

The range will also be multiplied by $c$.

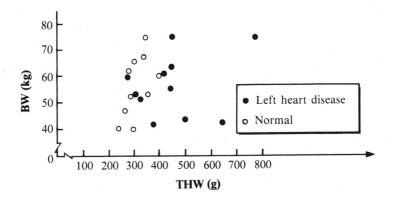

Figure A.5

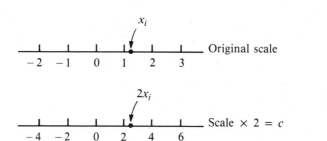

Figure A.6

# $C$hapter 3

**3.1** Yes

**3.2** No

**3.3** 0.3

**3.4** $A \cup C = \{\text{serum cholesterol} \leqslant 299\}$.

**3.5** $A \cap C = \{250 \leqslant \text{serum cholesterol} \leqslant 280\}$.

**3.6** $B \cup C = \{\text{serum cholesterol} \leqslant 280 \text{ or } \geqslant 300\}$.

**3.7** $B \cap C$ is the empty set; that is, it can never occur.

**3.8** Yes

**3.9** $\bar{B} = \{\text{serum cholesterol} < 300\}$. $Pr(\bar{B}) = 0.9$.

**3.25** 0.18

**3.26** 0.30

**3.30** 0.0167

**3.31** 180

**3.36** The probability that both siblings are affected is

$$\tfrac{1}{2} \times \tfrac{1}{2} = \tfrac{1}{4}$$

**3.37** The probability that exactly one sibling is affected is

$$(2)(\tfrac{1}{2}) \times (\tfrac{1}{2}) = \tfrac{1}{2}$$

**3.38** The probability that neither sibling will be affected is

$$\tfrac{1}{2} \times \tfrac{1}{2} = \tfrac{1}{4}$$

**3.39** The probability that the younger child is affected should not be influenced by whether or not the older child is affected. Thus, the probability of the younger child being affected remains at $\tfrac{1}{2}$.

**3.40** The events $A, B$ are independent because whether or not a child is affected does not influence the outcome for other children in the family.

**3.50** We use Bayes' theorem here. We will denote dominant by **DOM**, autosomal recessive by **AR**, and sex linked by **SL**. Let $A$ be the event that two male siblings are affected. We have

$Pr(DOM|A) =$

$$\frac{Pr(A|DOM) \times Pr(DOM)}{Pr(A|DOM)Pr(DOM) + Pr(A|AR)Pr(AR) + Pr(A|SL)Pr(SL)}$$

We also know that

$$Pr(DOM) = Pr(AR) = Pr(SL) = \tfrac{1}{3}$$

from the conditions stated in the problem. Thus, we have

$$Pr(DOM|A) = \frac{Pr(A|DOM)}{Pr(A|DOM) + Pr(A|AR) + Pr(A|SL)}$$

Finally, we know from Problems 3.36, 3.41, and 3.47 that

$$Pr(A|DOM) = \tfrac{1}{4} \qquad Pr(A|AR) = \tfrac{1}{16} \qquad Pr(A|SL) = \tfrac{1}{4}$$

Thus,

$$Pr(DOM|A) = \frac{1/4}{1/4 + 1/16 + 1/4} = \frac{1/4}{9/16} = \frac{4}{9}$$

Similarly,

$$Pr(AR|A) = \frac{Pr(A|AR)}{Pr(A|DOM) + Pr(A|AR) + Pr(A|SL)}$$

$$= \frac{1/16}{9/16} = \frac{1}{9}$$

$$Pr(SL|A) = \frac{Pr(A|SL)}{Pr(A|DOM) + Pr(A|AR) + Pr(A|SL)}$$

$$= \frac{1/4}{9/16} = \frac{4}{9}$$

Thus, the dominant and sex-linked modes of inheritance are the most likely, with the autosomal recessive mode being less likely.

**3.51** Let $B = \{$exactly one of two male siblings is affected$\}$. We have from Problems 3.37, 3.42, and 3.48 that

$$Pr(B|DOM) = \tfrac{1}{2} \qquad Pr(B|AR) = \tfrac{3}{8} \qquad Pr(B|SL) = \tfrac{1}{2}$$

Thus, we have from Bayes' theorem that

$$Pr(DOM|B) = \frac{Pr(B|DOM)}{Pr(B|DOM) + Pr(B|AR) + Pr(B|SL)}$$

$$= \frac{1/2}{1/2 + 3/8 + 1/2} = \frac{1/2}{11/8} = \frac{4}{11}$$

$$Pr(AR|B) = \frac{Pr(B|AR)}{Pr(B|DOM) + Pr(B|AR) + Pr(B|SL)}$$

$$= \frac{3/8}{11/8} = \frac{3}{11}$$

$$Pr(SL|B) = \frac{Pr(B|SL)}{Pr(B|DOM) + Pr(B|AR) + Pr(B|SL)}$$

$$= \frac{1/2}{11/8} = \frac{4}{11}$$

Here the three genetic types are about equally likely.

**3.52** Let $C = \{$both one male and one female sibling are affected$\}$. The sex of the siblings is only relevant for sex-linked disease. Thus, we have from Problems 3.36, 3.41, and 3.44 that

$$Pr(C|DOM) = \tfrac{1}{4} \qquad Pr(C|AR) = \tfrac{1}{16} \qquad Pr(C|SL) = 0$$

Thus,

$$Pr(DOM|C) = \frac{Pr(C|DOM)}{Pr(C|DOM) + Pr(C|AR) + Pr(C|SL)}$$

$$= \frac{1/4}{1/4 + 1/16} = \frac{1/4}{5/16} = \frac{4}{5}$$

$$Pr(AR|C) = \frac{Pr(C|AR)}{Pr(C|DOM) + Pr(C|AR) + Pr(C|SL)}$$

$$= \frac{1/16}{5/16} = \frac{1}{5}$$

$$Pr(SL|C) = 0$$

**3.53** Let $D = \{$male sibling affected, female sibling not affected$\}$. We have

$$Pr(D|DOM) = \tfrac{1}{2} \times \tfrac{1}{2} = \tfrac{1}{4} \qquad Pr(D|AR) = \tfrac{1}{4} \times \tfrac{3}{4} = \tfrac{3}{16}$$

$$Pr(D|SL) = \tfrac{1}{2} \times 1 = \tfrac{1}{2}$$

Notice that the event $D$ is not the same as the event that exactly one sibling is affected, since we are specifying which of the two siblings is affected. We have

$$Pr(DOM|D) = \frac{Pr(D|DOM)}{Pr(D|DOM) + Pr(D|AR) + Pr(D|SL)}$$

$$= \frac{1/4}{1/4 + 3/16 + 1/2} = \frac{1/4}{15/16} = \frac{4}{15}$$

$$Pr(AR|D) = \frac{Pr(D|AR)}{Pr(D|DOM)+Pr(D|AR)+Pr(D|SL)}$$

$$= \frac{3/16}{1/4+3/16+1/2} = \frac{3/16}{15/16} = \frac{1}{5}$$

$$Pr(SL|D) = \frac{Pr(D|SL)}{Pr(D|DOM)+Pr(D|AR)+Pr(D|SL)}$$

$$= \frac{1/2}{15/16} = \frac{8}{15}$$

Thus, in this situation the sex-linked mode of inheritance is the most likely.

### 3.55

$$Pr(LOW) = Pr(LOW \cap <20 \text{ weeks})$$
$$+ Pr(LOW \cap 20-27 \text{ weeks})$$
$$+ Pr(LOW \cap 28-36 \text{ weeks})$$
$$+ Pr(LOW \cap >36 \text{ weeks})$$

$$= Pr(LOW|<20 \text{ weeks})Pr(<20 \text{ weeks})$$
$$+ Pr(LOW|20-27 \text{ weeks})Pr(20-27 \text{ weeks})$$
$$+ Pr(LOW|28-36 \text{ weeks})Pr(28-36 \text{ weeks})$$
$$+ Pr(LOW|>36 \text{ weeks})Pr(>36 \text{ weeks})$$

$$= (0.540)(0.0004)+(0.813)(0.0059)$$
$$+(0.379)(0.0855)+(0.035)(0.9082)$$

$$= 0.069$$

**3.56** We can show the dependence of the events $\{\leqslant 27 \text{ weeks}\}$ and $\{LOW\}$ by showing that

$$Pr\{\leqslant 27 \text{ weeks} \cap LOW\} \neq Pr\{\leqslant 27 \text{ weeks}\} \times Pr\{LOW\}$$

We have

$$Pr\{\leqslant 27 \text{ weeks} \cap LOW\} = Pr\{LOW \cap <20 \text{ weeks}\}$$
$$+ Pr\{LOW \cap 20-27 \text{ weeks}\}$$

$$= 0.540(0.0004)+0.813(0.0059)$$

$$= 0.0050 \quad \text{(from Problem 3.55)}$$

Similarly, from Problem 3.55

$$Pr(LOW) = 0.069$$

$$Pr(\leqslant 27 \text{ weeks}) = 0.0004 + 0.0059 = 0.0063$$

Thus,

$$Pr(LOW) \times Pr(\leqslant 27 \text{ weeks})$$

$$= 0.00043 \approx \tfrac{1}{10} Pr\{\leqslant 27 \text{ weeks} \cap LOW\} = 0.0050$$

Thus, the two events are dependent.

**3.57** We must compute $Pr(\leqslant 36 \text{ weeks}|LOW)$. We use Bayes' theorem as follows:

$$Pr(\leqslant 36 \text{ weeks}|LOW)$$

$$= \frac{Pr(\leqslant 36 \text{ weeks} \cap LOW)}{Pr(LOW)}$$

$$= \frac{Pr(LOW \cap <20 \text{ weeks})+Pr(LOW \cap 20-27 \text{ weeks})}{Pr(LOW)} \frac{+ Pr(LOW \cap 28-36 \text{ weeks})}{}$$

$$= \frac{(0.540)(0.0004)+(0.813)(0.0059)+(0.379)(0.0855)}{0.069}$$

$$= \frac{0.0374}{0.069} = 0.542$$

# Chapter 4

**4.1** We have the distribution

| $x$ | 0 | 1 | 2 |
|---|---|---|---|
| $Pr(X = x)$ | 0.80 | 0.18 | 0.02 |

**4.2** 0.22

**4.3** 0.212

**4.4** We have the distribution

| $x$ | $< 0$ | $\geqslant 0, < 1$ | $\geqslant 1, < 2$ | $\geqslant 2$ |
|---|---|---|---|---|
| $F(x)$ | 0.00 | 0.80 | 0.98 | 1.00 |

*4.13* $50 \times 49 \times 48 \times 47 \times 46 = 2.543 \times 10^8$.

*4.14* $_{50}C_5 = 2.119 \times 10^6$.

*4.19* $X$ = number of hypertensives over a lifetime is binomially distributed with parameters $n = 20$, $p = 0.2$; that is,

$$Pr(X = x) = {}_{20}C_x(0.2)^x(0.8)^{20-x} \qquad x = 0, 1, \ldots, 20$$

or

| $x$ | $Pr(X = x)$ | $x$ | $Pr(X = x)$ |
|---|---|---|---|
| 0 | 0.0115 | 7 | 0.0546 |
| 1 | 0.0576 | 8 | 0.0222 |
| 2 | 0.1369 | 9 | 0.0074 |
| 3 | 0.2054 | 10 | 0.0020 |
| 4 | 0.2182 | 11 | 0.0005 |
| 5 | 0.1746 | 12 | 0.0001 |
| 6 | 0.1091 | 13–20 | 0.0000 |

*4.26* 0.1042

*4.27* 0.2148

*4.28* Expected value = 4.0; variance = 4.0.

*4.34* We approximate the distribution of the number of gonorrhea cases that occurred over a 3-month period by a Poisson distribution with parameter $\mu = np = 10,000 \times (50/100,000) = 5.0$. From the Poisson tables we compute

$$Pr(X \geqslant 10 | \mu = 5) = 0.0181 + 0.0082 + 0.0034 + 0.0013$$
$$+ 0.0005 + 0.0002$$
$$= 0.032$$

Thus, the number of gonorrhea cases in this county over this time period is unusual, since the probability of observing at least 10 cases is quite small.

*4.35* The probability that exactly 2 out of 50 men will die over a 3-year period is given by

$$\binom{50}{2}(0.1)^2(0.9)^{48}$$

The probability that not more than two men will die out of 50 = $Pr(X \leqslant 2)$ is given by

$$\sum_{k=0}^{2} \binom{50}{k}(0.1)^k(0.9)^{50-k}$$

We can evaluate this expression from the recursion rule

for binomial probabilities. We have

$$Pr(0) = (0.9)^{50} = 0.00515$$

$$Pr(1) = \frac{50}{1} \times \frac{0.1}{0.9} \times Pr(0) = 0.02861$$

$$Pr(2) = \frac{49}{2} \times \frac{0.1}{0.9} \times Pr(1) = 0.07788$$

Thus, $Pr(X \leqslant 2) = 0.00515 + 0.02861 + 0.07788 = 0.112$.

*4.54* The probability that a hypertensive is being treated appropriately and is complying with the treatment is

$Pr$(hypertensive is told he or she has high blood pressure)

$\times Pr$(adequately treated|told)

$\times Pr$(complying|adequately treated)

$= (\frac{1}{2})^3 = 0.125$

Thus, we want

$$Pr(X \geqslant 5) = 1 - Pr(X \leqslant 4)$$
$$= 1 - \sum_{k=0}^{4} \binom{10}{k}(0.125)^k(0.875)^{10-k}$$

$$Pr(0) = (\tfrac{7}{8})^{10} = 0.26308$$

$$Pr(1) = (\tfrac{10}{1})(\tfrac{1}{7})(0.26308) = 0.37583$$

$$Pr(2) = (\tfrac{9}{2})(\tfrac{1}{7})(0.37583) = 0.24161$$

$$Pr(3) = (\tfrac{8}{3})(\tfrac{1}{7})(0.24161) = 0.09204$$

$$Pr(4) = (\tfrac{7}{4})(\tfrac{1}{7})(0.09204) = 0.02301$$

Thus, $Pr(X \leqslant 4) = 0.996$, $Pr(X \geqslant 5) = 1 - 0.996 = 0.004$.

*4.55* $Pr$(hypertensive knows he or she has high blood pressure) = $\frac{1}{2}$. We want

$$Pr(X \geqslant 7) = \binom{10}{7}\left(\frac{1}{2}\right)^{10} + \binom{10}{8}\left(\frac{1}{2}\right)^{10} + \binom{10}{9}\left(\frac{1}{2}\right)^{10}$$
$$+ \binom{10}{10}\left(\frac{1}{2}\right)^{10}$$

We refer to the binomial tables (Table 1) with $n = 10$, $p = 0.50$ and find that

$$Pr(X = 10) = 0.0010$$

$$Pr(X = 9) = 0.0098$$

$$Pr(X = 8) = 0.0439$$

$$Pr(X = 7) = 0.1172$$

Thus, $Pr(X \geqslant 7) = 0.0010 + 0.0098 + 0.0439 + 0.1172 = 0.172$.

**4.56** If the rates are each decreased to 40%, then $(0.6)^3 = 0.216 = 21.6\%$ of hypertensives will be appropriately treated as opposed to $(0.5)^3 = 0.125 = 12.5\%$. Thus, if the current annual mortality rate for *untreated* hypertensives is $x$ and for *treated* hypertensives is $0.8x$, then the *current overall* mortality rate for hypertensives is

$$0.125(0.8x) + 0.875x = 0.975x$$

The *new overall mortality* rate would be

$$0.216(0.8x) + 0.784x = 0.957x$$

Thus, the ratio of the new mortality to the current mortality rate is

$$0.957x/0.975x = 0.982 = 98.2\%$$

Thus, the overall mortality rate among hypertensives would be reduced by 1.8%.

**4.60** We have

$$Pr(k \text{ positives}) = \binom{5}{k}(0.05)^k(0.95)^{5-k}$$

Thus,

$$Pr(1 \text{ or more} +) = 1 - Pr(0+)$$
$$Pr(0+) = (0.95)^5 = 0.77$$

Thus,

$$Pr(1 \text{ or more} +) = 0.23$$

**4.61** $Pr(3 \text{ or more} +) = 1 - Pr(2 \text{ or less} +)$

$$Pr(2 \text{ or less} +) = Pr(0) + Pr(1) + Pr(2)$$

$$Pr(0) = (0.95)^{100} = 0.0059$$

$$Pr(1) = \frac{100}{1}\left(\frac{0.05}{0.95}\right)Pr(0) = 0.0311$$

$$Pr(2) = \frac{99}{2}\left(\frac{0.05}{0.95}\right)Pr(1) = 0.0810$$

Hence, $Pr(2 \text{ or less} +) = 0.118$ and $Pr(3 \text{ or more} +) = 0.882$.

**4.62** We know that $X$ can only take on the values 0, 1, or 2.

$Pr(0) = Pr(2 \text{ negatives}) = Pr(\text{negative at time } 0)$
     $\times Pr(\text{negative at time 1|negative at time 0})$

     $= (0.95)(1 - 0.042) = (0.95)(0.958) = 0.910$

$Pr(1) = Pr(1 \text{ positive})$

     $= Pr(\text{negative at time } 0 \cap \text{positive at time 1})$
       $+ Pr(\text{positive at time } 0 \cap \text{negative at time 1})$

     $= Pr(\text{negative at time 0})$
       $\times Pr(\text{positive at time 1|negative at time 0})$
       $+ Pr(\text{positive at time 0})$
       $\times Pr(\text{negative at time 1|positive at time 0})$

     $= (0.95)(0.042) + (0.05)(0.80) = 0.080$

$Pr(2) = Pr(2 \text{ positives}) = Pr(\text{positive at time 0})$
     $\times Pr(\text{positive at time 1|positive at time 0})$

     $= (0.05)(0.20) = 0.010$

Thus, we have

| $X$ | $Pr(X)$ |
|---|---|
| 0 | 0.910 |
| 1 | 0.080 |
| 2 | 0.010 |

**4.63** Mean of $X = E[X] = 0(0.910) + 1(0.080) + 2(0.010) = 0.100$.

**4.64** Variance of $X = E[X^2] - E^2[X]$

$$E[X^2] = 0(0.910) + 1(0.080) + 4(0.010) = 0.120$$

$$Var(X) = 0.120 - (0.100)^2 = 0.110$$

**4.65** The probability of living to age 65 given that one is age 21 is given by

$$Pr = \frac{\ell_{22}}{\ell_{21}} \times \frac{\ell_{23}}{\ell_{22}} \times \cdots \times \frac{\ell_{64}}{\ell_{63}} \times \frac{\ell_{65}}{\ell_{64}} = \frac{\ell_{65}}{\ell_{21}} = \frac{64{,}177}{95{,}330}$$
$$= 0.673$$

**4.66** The probability of dying exactly between the ages of 56 and 57 given that one is age 21 in 1960 = the probability that one lives to age 56 and then dies before age 57:

$$\frac{\ell_{56}}{\ell_{21}} \times \left(1 - \frac{\ell_{57}}{\ell_{56}}\right) = \frac{79,783}{95,330} \times \left(1 - \frac{78,451}{79,783}\right)$$

$$= 0.8369 \times (1 - 0.9833) = 0.8369 \times 0.0167 = 0.014$$

**4.67** We first compute the probability of a single person dying before age 30 given that he or she is age 21 in 1960. This probability is given by

$$Pr = 1 - \frac{\ell_{30}}{\ell_{21}} = 1 - \frac{93,826}{95,330} = 1 - 0.984 = 0.016$$

We are now interested in the distribution of the number of deaths in 100 persons, which is a binomial distribution with parameters $n = 100$, $p = 0.016$. Thus, the probability of $k$ deaths is given by

$$Pr(k) = \binom{100}{k}(0.016)^k(0.984)^{100-k}$$

$$k = 0, 1, 2, \ldots, 100$$

We specifically want $Pr(k \geq 5) = 1 - Pr(k \leq 4)$. We use the recursion rule for binomial probabilities

$$Pr(0) = (0.984)^{100} = 0.1993$$

$$Pr(1) = \frac{100}{1}\left(\frac{0.016}{0.984}\right)(0.1993) = 0.3241$$

$$Pr(2) = \frac{99}{2}\left(\frac{0.016}{0.984}\right)(0.3241) = 0.2609$$

$$Pr(3) = \frac{98}{3}\left(\frac{0.016}{0.984}\right)(0.2609) = 0.1386$$

$$Pr(4) = \frac{97}{4}\left(\frac{0.016}{0.984}\right)(0.1386) = 0.0547$$

Thus,

$$Pr(k \leq 4) = 0.1993 + 0.3241 + 0.2609 + 0.1386 + 0.0547$$

$$= 0.978$$

$$Pr(k \geq 5) = 1 - 0.978 = 0.022$$

**4.69** We *cannot* answer the questions if we do not assume that the $P_x$'s remain constant. We would need current life tables for each succeeding year after 1960. For example, in computing the probability that someone will live to age 23 given that they are age 21 in 1960, we must multiply the probabilities that they will reach age 22 in 1961 by the probability that they will reach age 23 in 1962 given that they were age 22 in 1961. We must assume that the latter probability is the same as the probability that someone will reach age 23 in 1961 given that they were age 22 in 1960, which is not necessarily the case. This assumption is especially risky if we are considering events happening over a large number of years, since death rates have tended to go down. The probability that 65-year-old persons will live 1 extra year given that they were 65 in the year 2025 is likely to be quite different from the corresponding probability if they were 65 in the year 1960. Life tables that follow the *same* group of people over time are called *cohort* life tables as opposed to the *current* life table data given in this example. These cohort life tables are especially useful in providing baseline mortality data for epidemiologic studies of mortality in high-risk groups.

# *C*hapter 5

**5.1** 0.6915

**5.2** 0.3085

**5.3** 0.7745

**5.4** 0.0228

**5.5** 0.0440

**5.6** We have the table

| $x$ | $\Phi(x)$ | $x$ | $\Phi(x)$ |
|---|---|---|---|
| $-1.28$ | 0.10 | 0.25 | 0.60 |
| $-0.84$ | 0.20 | 0.52 | 0.70 |
| $-0.52$ | 0.30 | 0.84 | 0.80 |
| $-0.25$ | 0.40 | 1.28 | 0.90 |
| 0.00 | 0.50 | | |

**5.7** We have the table

| $x$ | $-0.67$ | $0.00$ | $0.67$ |
|---|---|---|---|
| $\Phi(x)$ | $0.25$ | $0.50$ | $0.75$ |

**5.19** 0.010

**5.20** The number of breast cancer cases ($X$) is binomially distributed with parameters $n = 10,000$, $p = 0.010$. We approximate this distribution by a normal distribution ($Y$) with mean $= np = 100$, variance $= npq = 99$. We have

$$Pr(X \geqslant 120) \approx Pr(Y \geqslant 119.5) = 1 - \Phi[(119.5 - 100)/\sqrt{99}]$$

$$= 1 - \Phi(1.96)$$

$$= 0.025$$

**5.24** If $X =$ birthweight, then $X \sim N(3400, 700^2)$. Thus,

$$Pr(X \leqslant 2500) = \Phi\left(\frac{2500 - 3400}{700}\right) = \Phi(-1.29)$$

$$= 1 - \Phi(1.29) = 1 - 0.9015 = 0.0985$$

**5.25**

$$Pr(X \leqslant 2000) = \Phi\left(\frac{2000 - 3400}{700}\right) = \Phi(-2.00)$$

$$= 1 - \Phi(2.00) = 1 - 0.9772 = 0.0228$$

**5.26** Let $X =$ number of low-birthweight deliveries. $X$ is binomially distributed with parameters $n = 3$, $p = 0.0985$. We wish to compute $Pr(X \geqslant 2)$. We have

$$Pr(X \geqslant 2) = \binom{3}{2}(0.0985)^2(0.9015) + \binom{3}{3}(0.0985)^3$$

$$= 0.0262 + 0.0010 = 0.0272$$

**5.29** Let $X$ be the number of persons positive for bacteriuria out of 1000. $X$ follows a binomial distribution with parameters $n = 1000$ and $p = 0.05$. We wish to compute $Pr(X \geqslant 50)$. We will approximate $X$ by a normal random variable $Y$ with mean $= 1000 \times 0.05 = 50$ and variance $= 1000 \times 0.05 \times 0.95 = 47.5$. We wish to compute

$$Pr(X \geqslant 50) \approx Pr(Y \geqslant 49.5) = 1 - \Phi\left(\frac{49.5 - 50}{\sqrt{47.5}}\right)$$

$$= 1 - \Phi(-0.07)$$

$$= \Phi(0.07) = 0.5279$$

**5.34** Let $X =$ serum cholesterol and $Y = \ln X$. We wish to compute

$$Pr(X \leqslant 150) = Pr(Y \leqslant \ln 150) = Pr(Y \leqslant 5.01)$$

$$= \Phi\left(\frac{5.01 - 5.39}{0.23}\right)$$

$$= \Phi(-1.65) = 1 - \Phi(1.65)$$

$$= 1 - 0.9505 = 0.0495$$

**5.35** We want

$$Pr(X \geqslant 250) = Pr(Y \geqslant \ln 250) = Pr(Y \geqslant 5.52)$$

$$= 1 - \Phi\left(\frac{5.52 - 5.39}{0.23}\right)$$

$$= 1 - \Phi(0.57) = 1 - 0.7157$$

$$= 0.2843$$

**5.36** We want

$$Pr(X \geqslant 300) = Pr(Y \geqslant \ln 300) = Pr(Y \geqslant 5.70)$$

$$= 1 - \Phi\left(\frac{5.70 - 5.39}{0.23}\right)$$

$$= 1 - \Phi(1.35) = 1 - 0.9115$$

$$= 0.0885$$

The proportion of the subpopulation with abnormally high levels, which this represents, is 0.0885/0.2843, or 31%.

**5.37** From Problem 5.36 we have 0.0885, or 9%.

**5.44** Suppose we sample $n$ persons for the study. The number of hypertensives $X$ ascertained from this procedure will be binomially distributed with parameters $n$ and $p = 0.10$. For large $n$ from the normal approximation to the binomial, it follows that we can approximate the distribution of $X$ by a normal distribution $Y$ with mean $0.1n$ and variance $n \times 0.1 \times 0.9 = 0.09n$. Thus, we want $n$ to be large enough so that $Pr(X \geqslant 100) = 0.8$. We have

$$Pr(X \geqslant 100) \approx Pr(Y \geqslant 99.5) = 1 - Pr(Y \leqslant 99.5)$$

$$= 1 - \Phi\left(\frac{99.5 - 0.1n}{\sqrt{0.09n}}\right) = 0.8$$

or

$$\Phi\left(\frac{99.5 - 0.1n}{\sqrt{0.09n}}\right) = 0.2$$

However, from the normal tables we have that $\Phi(0.84) = 0.8$ or $\Phi(-0.84) = 0.2$. Thus, we have

$$\frac{99.5 - 0.1n}{\sqrt{0.09n}} = -0.84 \quad \text{or}$$

$$99.5 - 0.1n = -0.84\sqrt{0.09n} \quad \text{or}$$

$$0.1n - 0.252\sqrt{n} - 99.5 = 0$$

If we substitute $z^2$ for $n$, we can rewrite this equation as $0.1z^2 - 0.252z - 99.5 = 0$. The solution of this quadratic equation is given by

$$z = \sqrt{n} = \frac{0.252 \pm \sqrt{(0.252)^2 + 4(99.5)(0.1)}}{2(0.1)}$$

$$= \frac{0.252 \pm \sqrt{39.864}}{0.2} = \frac{0.252 \pm 6.314}{0.2}$$

$$= -30.310 \quad \text{or} \quad 32.830$$

or $n = z^2 = (-30.310)^2$ or $(32.830)^2 = 918.70$ or $1077.81$. Since $n$ must be larger than $100/0.1 = 1000$, we have $n = 1077.81$, or 1078. Thus, we need to sample 1078 people to be 80% sure of recruiting 100 hypertensives.

**5.45** We use the same approach as in Problem 5.44. We want to find $n$ such that

$$Pr(Y \geqslant 99.5) = 1 - \Phi\left(\frac{99.5 - 0.1n}{\sqrt{0.09n}}\right) = 0.9 \quad \text{or}$$

$$\Phi\left(\frac{99.5 - 0.1n}{\sqrt{0.09n}}\right) = 0.1$$

From the normal tables we have that $\Phi(1.28) = 0.9$ or $\Phi(-1.28) = 0.1$. Thus, we have

$$\frac{99.5 - 0.1n}{\sqrt{0.09n}} = -1.28 \quad \text{or}$$

$$99.5 - 0.1n = -0.384\sqrt{n} \quad \text{or}$$

$$0.1n - 0.384\sqrt{n} - 99.5 = 0$$

We substitute $z^2$ for $n$ and obtain the quadratic equation

$$0.1z^2 - 0.384z - 99.5 = 0$$

The solution is given by

$$z = \frac{0.384 \pm \sqrt{(0.384)^2 + 4(0.1)(99.5)}}{2(0.1)}$$

$$= \frac{0.384 \pm \sqrt{39.947}}{0.2} = \frac{0.384 \pm 6.320}{0.2}$$

$$= -29.68 \quad \text{or} \quad 33.52$$

Thus,

$$n = z^2 = (-29.68)^2 = 880.90 \quad \text{or} \quad (33.52)^2 = 1123.59$$

We again use the root such that $n > 1000$, and thus $n = 1123.59$, or 1124 if rounded up to the nearest integer. Thus, we need to sample 1124 persons to be 90% sure of recruiting 100 hypertensives.

# *C*hapter 6

**6.1** We will label the treatments as A and B and will assign patients to treatment A if the random digit is from 0 to 4 inclusive and to treatment B if it is from 5 to 9 inclusive. Please note that this method is one among many possible randomization schemes we could use. We obtain the following treatment assignments if we start at the 28th row of the table.

| Patient number | Random digit | Treatment assignment |
|---|---|---|
| 1 | 6 | B |
| 2 | 9 | B |
| 3 | 6 | B |

| Patient number | Random digit | Treatment assignment |
|:---:|:---:|:---:|
| 4 | 4 | A |
| 5 | 4 | A |
| 6 | 3 | A |
| 7 | 7 | B |
| 8 | 1 | A |
| 9 | 9 | B |
| 10 | 8 | B |
| 11 | 0 | A |
| 12 | 0 | A |
| 13 | 0 | A |
| 14 | 2 | A |
| 15 | 8 | B |
| 16 | 9 | B |
| 17 | 8 | B |
| 18 | 1 | A |
| 19 | 9 | B |
| 20 | 5 | B |

**6.2** There are 9 patients assigned to treatment A and 11 patients assigned to treatment B. We would expect 10 patients in each treatment group.

**6.3** We will label the treatments as A, B, C, and D. Since 10 is not divisible by 4 but 100 is, we will use two random digits to generate the treatment assignments. If the number formed by two successive random digits is between 00 and 24, we will assign the patient to treatment A; if between 25 and 49, to treatment B; if between 50 and 74, to treatment C; if between 75 and 99, to treatment D. We obtain the following treatment assignments starting at the 12th row of the table.

| Patient number | Random digit | Treatment assignment |
|:---:|:---:|:---:|
| 1 | 16 | A |
| 2 | 87 | D |
| 3 | 29 | B |
| 4 | 47 | B |
| 5 | 49 | B |
| 6 | 44 | B |
| 7 | 01 | A |
| 8 | 24 | A |
| 9 | 88 | D |
| 10 | 84 | D |

| Patient number | Random digit | Treatment assignment |
|:---:|:---:|:---:|
| 11 | 65 | C |
| 12 | 41 | B |
| 13 | 98 | D |
| 14 | 70 | C |
| 15 | 92 | D |
| 16 | 78 | D |
| 17 | 59 | C |
| 18 | 69 | C |
| 19 | 15 | A |
| 20 | 12 | A |
| 21 | 05 | A |
| 22 | 20 | A |
| 23 | 73 | C |
| 24 | 67 | C |
| 25 | 02 | A |
| 26 | 56 | C |
| 27 | 80 | D |
| 28 | 41 | B |
| 29 | 04 | A |
| 30 | 98 | D |
| 31 | 78 | D |
| 32 | 80 | D |
| 33 | 77 | D |
| 34 | 92 | D |
| 35 | 43 | B |
| 36 | 13 | A |
| 37 | 72 | C |
| 38 | 98 | D |
| 39 | 12 | A |
| 40 | 22 | A |

**6.4** There are 12 patients assigned to treatment A, 7 patients to treatment B, 8 patients to treatment C, and 13 patients to treatment D. We would expect 10 patients to be assigned to each treatment group.

**6.11** 2.583.

**6.12** $-1.313$

**6.13** 0.711

**6.20** 9.24

**6.21** 11.34

**6.22** The upper 2.5 percentile $= \chi^2_{2,.975} = 7.38$. The lower 2.5 percentile $= \chi^2_{2,.025} = 0.0506$.

**6.23** We approximate the chi-square distribution with $n$ d.f. by a normal distribution with mean $n$ and variance

$2n$. Therefore, the upper and lower 2.5 percentiles are given by

$$140 \pm z_{.975}\sqrt{280}$$

$$= 140 \pm 1.96(16.733)$$

$$= 140 \pm 32.80$$

$$= 107.20 \text{ (lower 2.5 percentile), } 172.80 \text{ (upper } 2.5 \text{ percentile)}$$

**6.28** Case women, $\frac{89}{283} = 0.314$; control women, $\frac{640}{3833} = 0.167$

**6.29** A 95% confidence interval for case women is given by

$$0.314 \pm 1.96\sqrt{(0.314)(0.686)/283}$$

$$= 0.314 \pm 1.96(0.0276)$$

$$= 0.314 \pm 0.054$$

$$= (0.260, 0.368)$$

A 95% confidence interval for control women is given by

$$0.167 \pm 1.96\sqrt{(0.167)(0.833)/3833}$$

$$= 0.167 \pm 1.96(0.0060)$$

$$= 0.167 \pm 0.012$$

$$= (0.155, 0.179)$$

**6.44** sem $= 500/\sqrt{20} = 111.8$.

**6.45** The standard deviation is a measure of variability for the birthweight of *one* infant. The standard error of the mean is a measure of variability for the *mean* birthweight of a group of $n$ infants (in this case $n = 20$). The standard error will always be smaller than the standard deviation because a mean of more than one birthweight will be less variable in repeated samples than an individual birthweight.

**6.56** The best point estimate is $\hat{p} = 6/46 = 0.130$.

**6.57** If we use a normal approximation, then the lower confidence limit is

$$c_1 = \hat{p} - 1.96\sqrt{\frac{\hat{p}\hat{q}}{n}}$$

$$= 0.130 - 1.96\sqrt{\frac{(0.130)(0.870)}{46}} = 0.033$$

The upper confidence limit is

$$c_2 = \hat{p} + 1.96\sqrt{\frac{\hat{p}\hat{q}}{n}}$$

$$= 0.130 + 1.96\sqrt{\frac{(0.130)(0.870)}{46}} = 0.227$$

**6.58** Since 10% is within the 95% confidence interval, we would conclude that it is possible that the two drugs are equally effective (i.e., have the same failure rate).

**6.63** A 95% confidence interval is given by

$$\hat{p} \pm 1.96\sqrt{\hat{p}\hat{q}/n} = \frac{64}{750} \pm 1.96\sqrt{\left(\frac{64}{750}\right)\left(1 - \frac{64}{750}\right)\bigg/750}$$

$$= 0.085 \pm 1.96\sqrt{(0.085)(0.915)/750}$$

$$= 0.085 \pm 0.020$$

$$= (0.065, 0.105)$$

**6.64** The rate of 0.10 is compatible with these data, since it falls within the 95% confidence interval in Problem 6.63. Thus, we *cannot* conclude from these data that jogging 10 miles per week prevents death from cardiovascular disease.

**6.65** We assume that $x_1, \ldots, x_{25} \sim N(\mu, \sigma^2)$, where $\mu, \sigma^2$ are unknown, and find that $\bar{x} = 7.0$, $s^2 = 4.0$. Thus, a two-sided 95% confidence interval for the mean with unknown variance is given by

$$\left(\bar{x} - t_{n-1,.975}\frac{s}{\sqrt{n}}, \bar{x} + t_{n-1,.975}\frac{s}{\sqrt{n}}\right)$$

$$= [7.0 - 2.064(2)/5, 7.0 + 2.064(2)/5]$$

$$= (6.17, 7.83)$$

**6.66** A two-sided 99% confidence interval for the unknown variance $\sigma^2$ is given by

$$\left(\frac{(n-1)s^2}{\chi^2_{n-1,.995}}, \frac{(n-1)s^2}{\chi^2_{n-1,.005}}\right) = \left(\frac{24(4)}{45.56}, \frac{24(4)}{9.89}\right)$$

$$= (2.11, 9.71)$$

**6.67** The length of the 95% confidence interval in Problem 6.65 is given by

$$2t_{n-1,.975}\frac{s}{\sqrt{n}}$$

and we want $n$ large enough so that this value is 0.5. Thus,

$$2t_{n-1,.975}(2)/\sqrt{n} = 0.5 \quad \text{or}$$

$$\sqrt{n} = 8t_{n-1,.975}, \quad n = 64t_{n-1,.975}^2$$

For large $n$ we could assume $t_{n-1,.975} = z_{.975} = 1.96$. Thus, $n = 64(1.96)^2 = 245.9$, and an adequate sample size would be 246. We can improve on this estimate by using conventional $t$ tables, since we could establish by trial and error that $n > 121$, in which case

$$t_{n-1,.975} < t_{120,.975} = 1.98$$

Thus,

$$n < 64(1.98)^2 = 250.9$$

Thus, we know that $245.9 < n < 250.9$. A conservative estimate of the necessary sample size would be 251. We could improve on this estimate with more extensive $t$ tables, but this level of accuracy is probably adequate for an estimate of sample size.

**6.74** We are concerned here with the variability of two methods of measuring flow, a manual method and a digitizer method. We must construct a 95% confidence interval for

$$\sigma_{\text{manual differences}}$$

We have

$$s_{\text{diff}} = 0.0779, \quad n = 10$$

Our interval is given by

$$\left( \frac{(n-1)s^2}{\chi_{n-1,.975}^2}, \frac{(n-1)s^2}{\chi_{n-1,.025}^2} \right) = \left( \frac{9(0.0779)^2}{\chi_{9,.975}^2}, \frac{9(0.0779)^2}{\chi_{9,.025}^2} \right)$$

$$= \left( \frac{9(0.0779)^2}{19.02}, \frac{9(0.0779)^2}{2.70} \right)$$

$$= (0.0029, 0.0202)$$

So, our 95% confidence interval for

$$\sigma^2_{\text{manual}} = (0.0029, 0.0202)$$

and thus our 95% confidence for

$$\sigma_{\text{manual}} = (0.054, 0.142)$$

**6.75** We use the same method for the digitizer differences. We have that $s^2 = 0.00083$. Thus, the 95%

confidence interval is given by

$$\left( \frac{(n-1)s^2}{\chi_{9,.975}^2}, \frac{(n-1)s^2}{\chi_{9,.025}^2} \right) = \left( \frac{9(0.00083)}{19.02}, \frac{9(0.00083)}{2.70} \right)$$

$$= (0.00039, 0.00277)$$

Finally, the 95% confidence interval for

$$\sigma_{\text{dig}} = (0.020, 0.053)$$

**6.76** $d_i = |\text{manual diff}_i| = |\text{digitizer diff}_i|$. A 95% confidence interval for $\mu_d$ comes from the usual $t$ statistic formulation

$$\bar{d} \pm t_{9,.975}\left( \frac{s_d}{\sqrt{10}} \right) = 0.0440 \pm 2.262\left( \frac{0.0353}{\sqrt{10}} \right)$$

$$= (0.0187, 0.0693)$$

**6.77** The digitizer method appears to be significantly less variable than the manual method, as shown in Problem 6.76, since the 95% confidence interval for $\mu_d$ does not include 0.

**6.98** We can select the random samples in many

**Table A.5**  *Random numbers*

| | Sample point | | | | |
|---|---|---|---|---|---|
| Sample | 1 | 2 | 3 | 4 | 5 |
| 1 | 329 | 242 | 232 | 418 | 125 |
| 2 | 090 | 775 | 463 | 290 | 374 |
| 3 | 941 | 434 | 929 | 588 | 720 |
| 4 | 430 | 359 | 708 | 183 | 373 |
| 5 | 217 | 271 | 190 | 441 | 513 |
| 6 | 316 | 538 | 098 | 570 | 799 |

**Table A.6**  *Random samples of birthweights (oz)*

| | Sample point | | | | |
|---|---|---|---|---|---|
| Sample | 1 | 2 | 3 | 4 | 5 |
| 1 | 88 | 132 | 86 | 97 | 113 |
| 2 | 118 | 81 | 128 | 114 | 108 |
| 3 | 116 | 109 | 121 | 108 | 127 |
| 4 | 125 | 113 | 119 | 121 | 98 |
| 5 | 118 | 108 | 91 | 95 | 105 |
| 6 | 118 | 114 | 140 | 91 | 133 |

different ways. We will use the random numbers in Table 4, starting in row 1, where each unique set of 3 digits identifies a unique delivery in Table 6.2. The random numbers and corresponding random samples of birthweights are identified in Tables A.5 and A.6, respectively. The mean birthweights for the 6 samples are 103.2, 109.8, 116.2, 115.2, 103.4, and 119.2.

**6.99** The standard deviation is given by

$$s = \sqrt{\frac{\sum\limits_{i=1}^{n} x_i^2 - \left(\sum\limits_{i=1}^{n} x_i\right)^2 \Big/ n}{(n-1)}} = \sqrt{\frac{74,379.96 - (667)^2/6}{5}}$$

$$= 6.81$$

**6.100** The standard deviation from the collection of 6 third points is

$$\sqrt{\frac{80,463 - 6(685)^2/6}{5}} = 21.25.$$

**6.101** Theoretically, the standard deviation in Problem 6.99 is an expression of the variability of the mean of 5 sample points $= \sigma/\sqrt{5}$, whereas the standard deviation in Problem 6.100 is an expression of the variability of individual sample points $= \sigma$. Thus, we should approximately have

$$\frac{s \text{ in Problem } 6.100}{s \text{ in Problem } 6.99} \approx \sqrt{5} = 2.24$$

**6.102** Indeed,

$$\frac{s \text{ in Problem } 6.100}{s \text{ in Problem } 6.99} = \frac{21.25}{6.81} = 3.12$$

This result shows that the variability of individual sample points is far greater than that of the mean of 5 sample points.

# Chapter 7

**7.1** We test the hypothesis $H_0$: $\mu = 15 = \mu_0$ vs. $H_1$: $\mu < 15$. We reject $H_0$ if $\bar{x} < \mu_0 + z_\alpha\sigma/\sqrt{n} = 15 + z_{.05}(4)/\sqrt{10} = 15 - 1.645(4)/\sqrt{10} = 12.92$ and accept $H_0$ if $\bar{x} \geqslant 12.92$. Since $\bar{x} = 13 > 12.92$, we accept $H_0$ at the 5% level.

**7.2** The $p$-value is given by $\Phi[(\bar{x} - \mu_0)/(\sigma/\sqrt{n})] = \Phi[(13-15)/(4/\sqrt{10})] = \Phi(-2.0/1.265) = \Phi(-1.58) = 1 - \Phi(1.58) = 1 - 0.9429 = 0.057.$

**7.3** We test the hypothesis $H_0$: $\mu = 24 = \mu_0$ vs. $H_1$: $\mu < 24$. We reject $H_0$ if $\bar{x} < \mu_0 + z_\alpha\sigma/\sqrt{n} = 24 + z_{.01}(11)/\sqrt{8} = 24 - 2.326(11)/\sqrt{8} = 24 - 9.05 = 14.95$ and accept $H_0$ otherwise. Since $\bar{x} = 11 < 14.95$, we reject $H_0$ at the 1% level.

**7.4** The $p$-value is given by $\Phi[(\bar{x} - \mu_0)/(\sigma/\sqrt{n})] = \Phi[(11-24)/(11/\sqrt{8})] = \Phi(-13/3.889) = \Phi(-3.34) = 1 - \Phi(3.34) = 1 - 0.9996 = 0.0004.$

**7.5** Since we rejected $H_0$ at the 1% level in Problem 7.3, $p$ must be $<0.01$, which is indeed the case.

**7.6** The hypotheses to be tested are $H_0$: $\mu = 15$ vs. $H_1$: $\mu \neq 15$. This alternative is two sided in contrast to the one-sided alternative in Problem 7.1.

**7.7** The rejection region is given by $\bar{x} < \mu_0 + z_{\alpha/2}\sigma/\sqrt{n} = c_1$ or $\bar{x} > \mu_0 + z_{1-\alpha/2}\sigma/\sqrt{n} = c_2$. We have that

$c_1 = 15 + z_{.025}(4)/\sqrt{10} = 15 - 1.96(4)/\sqrt{10} = 15 - 2.48 = 12.52$, $c_2 = 15 + 2.48 = 17.48$. Since $\bar{x} = 13 > 12.52$, we accept $H_0$ using a two-sided test at the 5% level. The exact $p$-value is given by $2 \times \Phi[(\bar{x} - \mu_0)/(\sigma/\sqrt{n})] = 2 \times \Phi[(13-15)/(4/\sqrt{10})] = 2 \times \Phi(-2.0/1.265) = 2 \times \Phi(-1.58) = 2 \times [1 - \Phi(1.58)] = 2 \times (1 - 0.9429) = 0.114.$

**7.11** $p = 2 \times Pr(t_7 < -1.52) = 2 \times Pr(t_7 > 1.52)$. Since $t_{7,.9} = 1.415$, $t_{7,.95} = 1.895$, and $1.415 < 1.52 < 1.895$, it follows that $2 \times (1 - 0.95) < p < 2 \times (1 - 0.9)$, or $0.1 < p < 0.2$.

**7.14** We use a one-sample $t$ test. We have the test statistic $\lambda = (\bar{x} - \mu_0)/(s/\sqrt{n}) = (13 - 15)/(6/\sqrt{10}) = -2/1.897 = -1.05 \sim t_9$ under $H_0$. Since we are performing a two-sided test, we reject $H_0$ if $\lambda < t_{9,.025} = -2.262$ or $\lambda > t_{9,.975} = 2.262$ and accept $H_0$ otherwise. Since $-2.262 \leqslant -1.05 \leqslant 2.262$, it follows that we accept $H_0$. The exact $p$-value is given by $2 \times Pr(t_9 < [(\bar{x} - \mu_0)/(s/\sqrt{n})] = 2 \times Pr(t_9 < -1.05) = 2 \times Pr(t_9 > 1.05)$. Since $t_{9,.8} = 0.883$, $t_{9,.85} = 1.100$, and $0.883 < 1.05 < 1.100$, it follows that $2 \times (1 - 0.85) < p < 2 \times (1 - 0.8)$, or $0.3 < p < 0.4$.

**7.21** We wish to test the hypothesis $H_0$: $\mu = \mu_0$ vs. $H_1$: $\mu \neq \mu_0$. We use the following power formula:

Power $= \Phi[z_{\alpha/2} + |\mu_1 - \mu_0|\sqrt{n}/\sigma]$

$= \Phi(z_{.025} + 0.10\sqrt{100}/0.54)$

$= \Phi(-1.96 + 1.852)$

$= \Phi(-0.108)$

$= 1 - \Phi(0.108)$

$= 1 - 0.54 = 0.46$

Thus, the study has 46% power.

**7.22** We have

Power $= \Phi(z_{.025} + 0.20\sqrt{100}/0.54)$

$= \Phi(-1.96 + 3.704)$

$= \Phi(1.744)$

$= 0.96$

**7.23** The required sample size is given by

$$n = \frac{\sigma^2(z_{1-\alpha/2} + z_{1-\beta})^2}{(\mu_1 - \mu_0)^2}$$

$$= \frac{(0.54)^2(z_{.975} + z_{.80})^2}{(0.10)^2}$$

$$= 29.16(1.96 + 0.84)^2$$

$$= 228.6$$

Thus, we need to study 229 persons to achieve an 80% power.

**7.28** We wish to test the hypothesis $H_0: \sigma_1^2 = \sigma_0^2$ vs. $H_1: \sigma_1^2 \neq \sigma_0^2$. We will use the one-sample $\chi^2$ test for the variance of a normal distribution to test these hypotheses.

**7.29** We have the test statistic

$$\lambda = \frac{(n-1)s^2}{\sigma_0^2}$$

$$= \frac{19(15)^2}{(20)^2}$$

$$= 10.69 \sim \chi_{19}^2 \text{ under } H_0$$

Since $\chi_{19,.05}^2 = 10.12$, $\chi_{19,.10}^2 = 11.65$, and $10.12 < 10.69 < 11.65$, it follows that $2 \times 0.05 < p < 2 \times 0.10$, or $0.10 < p < 0.20$. Thus, there is no significant difference between the variances using the two methods.

**7.30** We test the hypothesis $H_0: \sigma^2 = \sigma_0^2 = (0.020)^2$ vs. $H_1: \sigma^2 \neq \sigma_0^2$. We reject $H_0$ if $s^2 < \sigma_0^2\chi_{n-1,\alpha/2}^2/(n-1) = c_1$ or $s^2 > \sigma_0^2\chi_{n-1,1-\alpha/2}^2/(n-1) = c_2$ and accept $H_0$ otherwise. We have

$$c_1 = (0.020)^2\chi_{19,.025}^2/19$$

$$= (0.020)^2(8.91)/19$$

$$= 0.000188$$

$$c_2 = (0.020)^2\chi_{19,.975}^2/19$$

$$= (0.020)^2(32.85)/19$$

$$= 0.000692$$

Since $s^2 = (0.016)^2 = 0.000256$ and $c_1 < s^2 < c_2$, it follows that we accept $H_0$ at the 5% level and conclude that the variances of the two methods are the same.

**7.31** We have the test statistic

$$\lambda = \frac{(n-1)s^2}{\sigma_0^2}$$

$$= \frac{(19)(0.000256)}{(0.000400)}$$

$$= 12.16 \sim \chi_{19}^2 \text{ under } H_0$$

Since $\chi_{19,.10}^2 = 11.65$, $\chi_{19,.25}^2 = 14.56$, and $11.65 < 12.16 < 14.56$, it follows that $2 \times 0.10 < p < 2 \times 0.25$, or $0.20 < p < 0.50$.

**7.41** We test the hypothesis $H_0: \mu = 130 = \mu_0$ vs. $H_1: \mu \neq 130$, where $\sigma$ is assumed to be 20 mm. We use the test statistic

$$\lambda = \frac{\bar{x} - \mu_0}{\sigma/\sqrt{n}} = \frac{135 - 130}{20/\sqrt{85}} = 2.30 \sim N(0, 1) \text{ under } H_0$$

Thus, the two-tailed $p$-value equals $2 \times [1 - \Phi(2.30)] = 2 \times (1 - 0.9893) = 0.021$. Therefore, there is a significant association between glaucoma and high blood pressure.

**7.42** Here we perform the one-sample $t$ test, since the standard deviation is not assumed known. We use the test statistic

$$\lambda = \frac{\bar{x} - \mu_0}{s/\sqrt{n}} = \frac{135 - 130}{22/\sqrt{85}} = 2.10 \sim t_{84} \text{ under } H_0$$

Since

$$t_{60,.975} = 2.000, \qquad t_{60,.99} = 2.390,$$

$$t_{120,.975} = 1.980, \qquad t_{120,.99} = 2.358$$

it follows that if we had 60 or 120 degrees of freedom, then

$$2 \times (1 - 0.99) < p < 2 \times (1 - 0.975) \qquad \text{or}$$

$$0.02 < p < 0.05$$

Since we have 84 degrees of freedom, we must also have $0.02 < p < 0.05$. Thus, there is a significant association between glaucoma and high blood pressure in this case as well.

**7.47** We use a one-sample test for binomial proportions. We have the hypotheses

$$H_0: p = p_0 = 0.3$$

$$H_1: p \neq p_0$$

Since

$$np_0q_0 = 200(0.3)(0.7) = 42 \geqslant 5$$

we can use the normal approximation. We use the test statistic

$$\lambda = \frac{\hat{p} - p_0}{\sqrt{\dfrac{p_0q_0}{n}}} = \frac{\frac{110}{200} - 0.3}{\sqrt{\dfrac{(0.3)(0.7)}{200}}} = \frac{0.55 - 0.3}{\sqrt{\dfrac{(0.3)(0.7)}{200}}} = 7.72$$

Since this statistic is distributed as $N(0, 1)$, we have that the $p$-value $= 2 \times [1 - \Phi(7.72)] \ll 0.001$. This result is very highly significant.

**7.48** We wish to test the hypothesis $H_0: p = p_0$ vs. $H_1: p > p_0$. A one-sided alternative is more appropriate here, since we wish to detect only if hair dyes increase the risk of breast cancer rather than decrease the risk.

**7.49** Since $np_0q_0 = 1000(0.007)(0.993) = 6.95 \geqslant 5$, we will use the normal test. We have the test statistic

$$\lambda = \frac{\hat{p} - p_0}{\sqrt{\dfrac{p_0q_0}{n}}}$$

$$= \frac{\frac{20}{1000} - 0.007}{\sqrt{\dfrac{0.007 \times 0.993}{1000}}} = \frac{0.013}{0.0026} = 5.00 \sim N(0, 1) \text{ under } H_0$$

The $p$-value is given by $p = 1 - \Phi(\lambda) = 1 - \Phi(5.00) < 0.001$. Thus, the results are very highly statistically significant, and we conclude that extensive occupational exposure to hair dyes significantly increases the risk of breast cancer.

**7.54** We wish to test the hypothesis $H_0: \mu = \mu_0 = 230$ vs. $H_1: \mu \neq \mu_0$, where $\sigma^2$ is assumed unknown. We use a one-sample $t$ test with test statistic

$$\lambda = \frac{\bar{x} - \mu_0}{s/\sqrt{n}} = \frac{175 - 230}{35/\sqrt{24}} = \frac{-55}{7.144} = -7.70 \sim t_{23}$$

Clearly, since $t_{23,.9995} = 3.767$ and $|\lambda| > 3.767$, it follows that $p < 2 \times 0.0005 = 0.001$.

**7.55** A two-sided 95% confidence interval for $\mu_0$ is given by

$$\bar{x} \pm t_{n-1,1-\alpha/2} \frac{s}{\sqrt{n}} = 175 \pm t_{23,.975} \left(\frac{35}{\sqrt{24}}\right)$$

$$= 175 \pm 2.069 \left(\frac{35}{\sqrt{24}}\right)$$

$$= 175 \pm 14.78 = (160.22, 189.78)$$

Since the 95% confidence interval does not contain 230, we can again conclude that the underlying cholesterol level for macrobiotics is significantly lower than 230.

**7.56** The hypothesis test tells us precisely how significant our results are ($p < 0.001$). The confidence interval gives us a range of values within which the true mean cholesterol for macrobiotics is likely to fall.

**7.60** We want to test the hypothesis $H_0: p = 0.10 = p_0$ vs. the alternative $H_1: p > 0.10$. We use the normal approximation test, since $np_0q_0 = 100(0.1)(0.9) = 9 \geqslant 5$. We have the test statistic

$$\lambda = \frac{(\hat{p} - p_0)}{\sqrt{\dfrac{p_0q_0}{n}}}$$

which should be distributed as $N(0, 1)$ under $H_0$. We have $\hat{p} = 0.13$, $p_0 = 0.10$, $n = 100$. Thus,

$$\lambda = \frac{(0.13 - 0.10)}{\sqrt{\dfrac{0.1(0.9)}{100}}} = \frac{0.03}{0.03} = 1.0$$

The $p$-value $= 1 - \Phi(1.0) = 1 - 0.8413 = 0.159$. This result is not significant using a one-sided hypothesis test at the 5% level, and we accept the null hypothesis. Thus, this finding is not indicative of anything about cholesterol, since it is quite possible that the underlying rate for this group of 100 men is 0.1.

**7.61** We perform the same test here with $n = 1000$. We have

$$\lambda = \frac{(\hat{p} - p_0)}{\sqrt{\frac{p_0 q_0}{n}}} = \frac{0.13 - 0.10}{\sqrt{\frac{0.1(0.9)}{1000}}} = \frac{0.03}{0.0095} = 3.16$$

We see from the normal tables that the one-sided $p$-value $= 1 - \Phi(3.16) < 0.001$. Thus, we reject the null hypothesis that $p = 0.1$ and accept the alternative that the underlying rate for the high cholesterol group is larger than 0.10.

**7.62** We refer to the sample size formula for one-sided alternatives given in **(7.37)**. We use $\alpha = 0.05$, $\beta = 1 - 0.80 = 0.20$, $p_0 = 0.10$, $q_0 = 0.90$, $p_1 = 0.13$, $q_1 = 0.87$.

We have

$$n = \frac{p_0 q_0 [z_{1-\alpha} + z_{1-\beta}\sqrt{(p_1 q_1)/(p_0 q_0)}]^2}{|p_1 - p_0|^2}$$

$$= \frac{(0.10)(0.90)[z_{0.95} + z_{0.80}\sqrt{(0.13)(0.87)/(0.10)(0.90)}]^2}{(0.13 - 0.10)^2}$$

$$= \frac{(0.09)(1.645 + 0.84\sqrt{1.257})^2}{0.0009}$$

$$= 100(1.645 + 0.942)^2$$

$$= 100(6.693)$$

$$= 669.3$$

Thus, we need 670 men in the sample to have an 80% chance of finding a significant difference using a one-sided test with $\alpha = 0.05$.

# Chapter 8

**8.1** We can use the paired $t$ test because each person is used as their own control.

**8.2** We have the test statistic

$$\lambda = \frac{\bar{d}}{s_d/\sqrt{n}}$$

$$= \frac{0.02}{0.04}$$

$$= 0.50 \sim t_{89} \text{ under } H_0$$

Since $0.50 < t_{120,.975} = 1.980 < t_{89,.975}$, it follows that we accept $H_0$ and there is no significant visual field loss over 1 year. Furthermore, since $0.50 < t_{120,.75} = 0.677 < t_{89,.75}$, it follows that $p > 2 \times (1 - 0.75) = 0.50$.

**8.3** We have the test statistic $\lambda = 0.08/0.05 = 1.60 \sim t_{89}$ under $H_0$. Since $1.60 < 1.980$, we accept $H_0$ and there is no significant visual field loss over 2 years. Furthermore, if we had 60 d.f., then since $t_{60,.9} = 1.296 < 1.60 < t_{60,.95} = 1.671$, it follows that $2 \times (1 - 0.95) < p < 2 \times (1 - 0.90)$, or $0.10 < p < 0.20$. Similarly, if we had 120 d.f., then since $t_{120,.9} = 1.289 < 1.60 < t_{120,.95} = 1.658$, it would also follow that $0.10 < p < 0.20$. Finally, since we have 89 d.f. and we reached the same decision with 60 or 120 d.f., then it follows that $0.10 < p < 0.20$.

**8.4** We have the test statistic $\lambda = 0.14/0.07 = 2.000$. The

critical value $= t_{89,.975} < t_{60,.975} = 2.000$. Since $\lambda >$ critical value, we reject $H_0$ at the 5% level. Since $2.000 < 2.358 = t_{120,.99} < t_{89,.99}$, it follows that $p > 2 \times (1 - 0.99) = 0.02$. Therefore, $0.02 < p < 0.05$.

**8.9** $F_{14,7,.025} = 1/F_{7,14,.975} = 1/3.38 = 0.296$.

**8.12** $F_{50,10,.025} = 1/F_{10,50,.975}$. This percentile is not given in the table; so we must use interpolation methods. The following 97.5 percentiles are given in the table.

|  | Numerator d.f. | |
|---|---|---|
|  | 8 | 12 |
| Denominator d.f. 40 | 2.53 | 2.29 |
| 60 | 2.41 | 2.17 |

We first compute $F_{10,40,.975}$ and $F_{10,60,.975}$ as follows:

$$F_{10,40,.975} = \frac{(1/10 - 1/12)(2.53) + (1/8 - 1/10)(2.29)}{(1/8 - 1/12)}$$

$$= \frac{(0.0167)(2.53) + (0.0250)(2.29)}{0.0417}$$

$$= 2.386$$

$$F_{10,60,.975} = \frac{(0.0167)(2.41) + (0.0250)(2.17)}{0.0417}$$

$$= 2.266$$

We now compute $F_{10,50,.975}$ by interpolation as follows:

$$F_{10,50,.975} = \frac{(1/50 - 1/60)(2.386) + (1/40 - 1/50)(2.266)}{(1/40 - 1/60)}$$

$$= \frac{(0.0033)(2.386) + (0.0050)(2.266)}{0.0083}$$

$$= 2.314$$

Finally,

$$F_{50,10,.025} = 1/2.314 = 0.432$$

**8.15** We test the hypothesis $H_0: \sigma_1^2 = \sigma_2^2$ vs. $H_1$: $\sigma_1^2 \neq \sigma_2^2$. We have the test statistic $\lambda = s_2^2/s_1^2 = (0.76/0.64)^2 = 1.410 \sim F_{39,24}$ under $H_0$. Since $\lambda < F_{\infty,30,.975} = 1.79 < F_{39,24,.975}$, it follows that we accept $H_0$ at the 5% level and conclude that there is no significant difference between the variances.

**8.16** Since we accepted $H_0$ in Problem 8.15, we should use the two-sample $t$ test for independent samples with equal variances.

**8.17** We first compute the pooled variance estimate:

$$s^2 = \frac{(n_1 - 1)s_1^2 + (n_2 - 1)s_2^2}{n_1 + n_2 - 2}$$

$$= \frac{24(0.64)^2 + 39(0.76)^2}{63}$$

$$= \frac{32.357}{63}$$

$$= 0.514$$

We compute the test statistic

$$\lambda = \frac{\bar{x}_1 - \bar{x}_2}{\sqrt{s^2(1/n_1 + 1/n_2)}}$$

$$= \frac{6.56 - 6.80}{\sqrt{0.514(1/25 + 1/40)}}$$

$$= \frac{-0.24}{0.183}$$

$$= -1.311$$

The critical value is given by $t_{63,.975} > t_{120,.975} = 1.980 > |\lambda|$. Therefore, we accept $H_0$ at the 5% level.

**8.18** The $p$-value is given by $2 \times Pr(t_{63} < -1.311) = 2 \times Pr(t_{63} > 1.311)$. If we had 60 $d.f.$, then since $t_{60,.9} = 1.296$, $t_{60,.95} = 1.671$, and $1.296 < 1.311 < 1.671$, it would follow that $2 \times (1 - 0.95) < p < 2 \times (1 - 0.9)$, or $0.10 < p < 0.20$. If we had 120 $d.f.$, then since $t_{120,.9} = 1.289$, $t_{120,.95} = 1.658$, and $1.289 < 1.311 < 1.658$, it would follow that $0.10 < p < 0.20$. Since we reach the same conclusion with either 60 or 120 $d.f.$ and $60 < 63 < 120$, it follows that $0.10 < p < 0.20$.

**8.19** The 95% confidence interval is given by $\bar{x}_1 - \bar{x}_2 \pm t_{63,.975}\sqrt{s^2(1/n_1 + 1/n_2)}$. We interpolate to obtain $t_{63,.975}$. We have

$$t_{63,.975} = \frac{(1/63 - 1/120)(2.000) + (1/60 - 1/63)(1.980)}{(1/60 - 1/120)}$$

$$= \frac{(0.0075)(2.000) + (0.0008)(1.980)}{0.0083}$$

$$= 1.998$$

Therefore, the 95% confidence interval is given by $-0.24 \pm 1.998(0.183) = -0.24 \pm 0.366 = (-0.61, 0.13)$.

**8.33** We have the sample size formula

$$n = \frac{(\sigma_1^2 + \sigma_2^2)(z_{1-\alpha/2} + z_{1-\beta})^2}{\Delta^2}$$

$$= \frac{[(0.64^2 + 0.76^2)(z_{.975} + z_{.80})^2]}{(0.24)^2}$$

$$= \frac{0.9872(1.96 + 0.84)^2}{0.0576}$$

$$= 134.4$$

Thus, we need to recruit 135 girls in each group or 270 girls in total.

**8.34** We use the sample size formula

$$n = \frac{(0.64^2 + 0.76^2)(z_{.95} + z_{.80})^2}{(0.24)^2}$$

$$= \frac{(0.9872)(1.645 + 0.84)^2}{0.0576}$$

$$= 105.8$$

Thus, we need to recruit 106 girls in each group or 212 girls in total using a one-sided test.

**8.35** We use the following sample size formula for the below-poverty-level group (group 1)

$$n_1 = \frac{(\sigma_1^2 + \sigma_2^2/2)(z_{1-\alpha/2} + z_{1-\beta})^2}{\Delta^2}$$

$$= \frac{(0.64^2 + 0.76^2/2)(z_{.975} + z_{.80})^2}{0.24^2}$$

$$= \frac{(0.6984)(1.96 + 0.84)^2}{0.0576}$$

$$= 95.1$$

Thus, we need to recruit 96 women in the below-poverty-level group and $2 \times 96 = 192$ women in the above-poverty-level group.

**8.41** We have the following basic statistics for total heart weight (THW) and body weight (BW) in the two groups

***Table A.7*** *Total heart weight and body weight in diseased and normal males*

| | Left heart disease | | | Normals | | |
|---|---|---|---|---|---|---|
| | Mean | sd | n | Mean | sd | n |
| THW | 450.0 | 139.34 | 11 | 317.0 | 47.09 | 10 |
| BW | 55.61 | 11.55 | 11 | 56.23 | 11.54 | 10 |

**THW** We perform the $F$ test for the equality of two variances as follows:

$$\lambda = s_1^2/s_2^2 = (139.34/47.09)^2 = 8.76 \sim F_{10,9} \text{ under } H_0$$

We have

$$F_{10,9,.995} < F_{8,9,.995} = 6.69 < \lambda$$

Thus, the p-value for $\lambda$ is $<2(0.005) = 0.01$, and the variances are significantly different. We must use the $t$ test with unequal variances. We have the following test statistic:

$$\lambda = \frac{\bar{x}_1 - \bar{x}_2}{\sqrt{\dfrac{s_1^2}{n_1} + \dfrac{s_2^2}{n_2}}} = \frac{450.0 - 317.0}{\sqrt{\dfrac{(139.34)^2}{11} + \dfrac{(47.09)^2}{10}}} = \frac{133.0}{44.57} = 2.98$$

We must compute the appropriate $df(d')$. We have

$$d' = \frac{\left[\dfrac{139.34^2}{11} + \dfrac{47.09^2}{10}\right]^2}{\left(\dfrac{139.34^2}{11}\right)^2 \Big/ 10 + \left(\dfrac{47.09^2}{10}\right)^2 \Big/ 9}$$

$$= \frac{3,947,392}{317,006} = 12.45$$

Thus, we have 12 *df.* Since $|\lambda| > t_{12,.975} = 2.179$, it follows that we reject $H_0$ at the 5% level.

**8.42 BW** We again perform the $F$ test for the equality of two variances. We have

$$\lambda = s_1^2/s_2^2 = (11.55/11.54)^2 = 1.002 \sim F_{10,9}$$

which is clearly not statistically significant. We therefore use the $t$ test with equal variances. We have

$$s^2 = \frac{(n_1 - 1)s_1^2 + (n_2 - 1)s_2^2}{n_1 + n_2 - 2} = \frac{10(11.55)^2 + 9(11.54)^2}{19}$$

$$= 133.29$$

$$\lambda = \frac{\bar{x}_1 - \bar{x}_2}{\sqrt{s^2\left(\dfrac{1}{n_1} + \dfrac{1}{n_2}\right)}} = \frac{55.61 - 56.23}{\sqrt{133.29\left(\dfrac{1}{11} + \dfrac{1}{10}\right)}} = \frac{-0.62}{5.044}$$

$$= -0.12 \sim t_{19}$$

which is not statistically significant. Thus, there is no significant difference in body weight between the two groups.

**8.47** The distinction between a one-sided and two-sided test in this case is that for a one-sided test we would test the hypothesis $H_0$: $\mu_1 = \mu_2$ vs. $H_1$: $\mu_1 > \mu_2$ or, alternatively, $H_0$: $\mu_1 = \mu_2$ vs. $H_1$: $\mu_1 < \mu_2$, where $\mu_1$ represents mean systolic bp sitting upright and $\mu_2$ represents mean systolic bp lying down. For a two-sided test we would test the hypothesis $H_0$: $\mu_1 = \mu_2$ vs. $H_1$: $\mu_1 \neq \mu_2$.

**8.48** A two-sided test is appropriate here, since we have no preconceived notions as to the relative orderings of $\mu_1$ and $\mu_2$ and would be equally interested in the outcomes $\mu_1 < \mu_2$ and $\mu_1 > \mu_2$.

**8.49** Since each person is serving as his or her own control, we are dealing with highly dependent samples and must use the paired $t$ test. We test the hypothesis $H_0$: $\mu_d = 0$ vs. $H_1$: $\mu_d \neq 0$, where $d_i =$ sitting bp $-$ lying bp for the $i$th person and $d_1 \sim N(\mu_d, \sigma_d^2)$. We have the following set of within-pair differences: $-12, -6, +2,$

$-8, -8, 0, -12, +4, 0, -16$. We compute the test statistic

$$\lambda = \bar{d}/(s_d/\sqrt{n}) = -5.60/(6.786/\sqrt{10}) = -5.60/2.146$$

$$= -2.61.$$

Under $H_0, \lambda \sim t_9$ and we have from Table 5 that $t_{9,.975} = 2.262 < |\lambda|$.

$$t_{9,.975} = 2.262 \qquad t_{9,.99} = 2.821$$

Therefore, we would reject $H_0$ at the 5% level and accept the hypothesis that the position affects bp, with the upright position having the lower blood pressure.

**8.50** Since $t_{.99} = 2.821 > |\lambda|$, we have $0.02 < p < 0.05$.

**8.51** We test the hypotheses $H_0: \mu_d = 0$ vs. $H_1: \mu_d \neq 0$, where $\mu_d$ represents the mean difference in 1-hour concentration (drug A − drug B) in a specific person. We use a paired $t$ test to test these hypotheses. We cannot use an independent samples $t$ test in this case, since the two samples are from the same people and are not independent.

**8.52** The assumption behind this test is that $d_i$ = difference in 1-hour concentration for the $i$th person is normally distributed with mean $\mu_d$ and variance $\sigma_d^2$.

**8.53** We have the $d_i$ in Table A.8.

**Table A.8** *Difference in 1-hour urine concentration between type A and type B aspirin*

| Person (i) | 1 | 2 | 3 | 4 | 5 | 6 | 7 | 8 | 9 | 10 |
|---|---|---|---|---|---|---|---|---|---|---|
| $d_i$ | 2 | 6 | 3 | 7 | 0 | −2 | 2 | 6 | 5 | 7 |

It follows that $\bar{d} = 3.60$, $s_d = 3.098$. Thus,

$$\lambda = \bar{d}/(s_d/\sqrt{n}) = 3.60/(3.098/\sqrt{10}) = 3.60/0.980 = 3.67 \sim t_9$$

Since $t_{9,.995} = 3.250$, $t_{9,.9995} = 4.781$ based on a two-sided test, it follows that $0.001 < p < 0.01$, and we reject $H_0$ and conclude that aspirin A has a significantly higher concentration in urine specimens than aspirin B does.

**8.54** The best point estimate is $\bar{d} = 3.60$ mg%.

**8.55** A 95% confidence interval is given by

$$\bar{d} \pm t_{9,.975}(s_d/\sqrt{10}) = 3.60 \pm 2.262(3.098)/\sqrt{10}$$

$$= (1.38, 5.82)$$

**8.56** If the test result had been significant at the 5%

level, then the confidence interval would have excluded 0; otherwise, it would have included 0. The former possibility is what actually occurred.

**8.70** We wish to test the hypotheses $H_0: \sigma_1^2 = \sigma_2^2$ vs. $H_1: \sigma_1^2 \neq \sigma_2^2$. We use the $F$ test with test statistic

$$\lambda = \frac{s_1^2}{s_2^2} = \left(\frac{7.3}{2.7}\right)^2 = 7.31 \sim F_{39,39} \text{ under } H_0$$

Since $F_{39,39,.975} < F_{24,30,.975} = 2.14 < \lambda$, it follows that $p < 0.05$, and the variances (and thus the standard deviations) of the two groups are significantly different.

**8.71** We wish to test the hypothesis $H_0: \mu_1 = \mu_2$, $\sigma_1^2 \neq \sigma_2^2$ vs. $H_1: \mu_1 \neq \mu_2$, $\sigma_1^2 \neq \sigma_2^2$. We use the two-sample $t$ test with unequal variances because we rejected $H_0$ in Problem 8.70. We have the test statistic

$$\lambda = \frac{\bar{x}_1 - \bar{x}_2}{\sqrt{\dfrac{s_1^2}{n_1} + \dfrac{s_2^2}{n_2}}} = \frac{11.6 - 6.9}{\sqrt{\dfrac{(7.3)^2}{40} + \dfrac{(2.7)^2}{40}}} = \frac{4.7}{1.231} = 3.82$$

We compute the appropriate $df$ ($d'$) as follows:

$$d' = \frac{\left(\dfrac{7.3^2}{40} + \dfrac{2.7^2}{40}\right)^2}{\left(\dfrac{7.3^2}{40}\right)^2 \Big/ 39 + \left(\dfrac{2.7^2}{40}\right)^2 \Big/ 39}$$

$$= \frac{2.294}{0.046} = 49.9$$

Thus, we have 49 $df$. Since $\lambda = 3.82 > t_{40,.975} = 2.021 > t_{49,.975}$, it follows that $p < 0.05$ and we reject $H_0$ at the 5% level. Thus, there is a significant difference between the CO concentrations in the two working environments.

**8.72** The standard deviations of the two groups were significantly different in Problem 8.70, and thus we had to use a two-sample $t$ test with *unequal* variances. If the standard deviations were not significantly different, then we would have used a two-sample $t$ test with *equal* variances.

**8.98** The hypotheses to be tested are $H_0: \mu_d = 0$ vs. $H_1: \mu_d > 0$, where $\mu_d$ = underlying mean change in temperature within a specific patient after taking aspirin. We choose a one-sided alternative here, since it is only plausible that aspirin could reduce temperature.

**8.99** A type I error here is the probability of declaring that aspirin reduces temperature given that it, in fact, has no effect on temperature.

**8.100** The power of the test vs. this alternative is the probability of declaring that aspirin reduces temperature given that the underlying mean reduction in temperature is 1 degree.

**8.101** The power would increase because the alternative mean is further away from 0.

**8.102** We will perform a paired $t$ test to test the hypotheses in Problem 8.98. We have the set of within-pair differences given in Table A.9. It follows that $\bar{d} = 1.75$, $s_d = 0.869$.

The paired $t$ statistic is given by

$$\lambda = \frac{\bar{d}}{(s_d/\sqrt{n})} = \frac{1.75}{(0.869/\sqrt{12})} = \frac{1.75}{0.251} = 6.97 \sim t_{11}$$

under $H_0$

*Table A.9* The temperature reduction 1-hour after taking aspirin for 12 5-year-old girls

| $i$ | $d_i$ | $i$ | $d_i$ |
|---|---|---|---|
| 1 | +2.8 | 7 | +1.5 |
| 2 | +3.1 | 8 | +3.0 |
| 3 | +1.7 | 9 | +2.1 |
| 4 | +1.9 | 10 | +1.2 |
| 5 | +1.4 | 11 | +0.6 |
| 6 | +0.5 | 12 | +1.2 |

Since $t_{11,.9995} = 4.437$, the one-tailed $p$-value $< 0.0005$, indicating that aspirin intake has a very highly significant effect on reducing temperature.

# *C*hapter 9

**9.1** We use the sign test. If we ignore the persons who have remained the same, then 27 persons have either improved or declined. Thus, we can use the normal theory version of the test. We have that $C$ = number of patients improved = 20, $n = 27$. We reject $H_0$ if either

$$C > \frac{n}{2} + \frac{1}{2} + z_{1-\alpha/2}\sqrt{n/4} = c_2 \qquad \text{or}$$

$$C < \frac{n}{2} - \frac{1}{2} - z_{1-\alpha/2}\sqrt{n/4} = c_1$$

and accept $H_0$ otherwise. We have that $\alpha = 0.05$. Therefore,

$$c_2 = \frac{27}{2} + \frac{1}{2} + z_{.975}\sqrt{27/4}$$

$$= 14 + 1.96(2.598)$$

$$= 14 + 5.09$$

$$= 19.09$$

$$c_1 = 14 - 5.09$$

$$= 8.91$$

Since $C = 20 > 19.09$, we reject $H_0$ at the 5% level. The exact $p$-value is given by

$$p = 2 \times \left[ 1 - \Phi\left( \frac{|C - n/2| - 0.5}{\sqrt{n/4}} \right) \right]$$

$$= 2 \times \left[ 1 - \Phi\left( \frac{|20 - 27/2| - 0.5}{\sqrt{27/4}} \right) \right]$$

$$= 2 \times \left[ 1 - \left( \frac{6.5 - 0.5}{2.598} \right) \right]$$

$$= 2 \times \left[ 1 - \Phi\left( \frac{6.0}{2.598} \right) \right]$$

$$= 2 \times (1 - 0.9896)$$

$$= 0.021$$

**9.2** In the subgroup of patients with better visual acuity, 13 patients have either improved or declined. Thus, we must use the exact binomial test. We have $C = 8$, $n = 13$. We refer to the exact binomial tables under $n = 13$, $p = 0.5$ to compute

$$p = 2 \times \sum_{k=8}^{13} \binom{13}{k}\left(\frac{1}{2}\right)^{13}$$

$$= 2 \times (0.1571 + 0.0873 + 0.0349 + 0.0095$$
$$+ 0.0016 + 0.0001)$$

$$= 2 \times 0.2905$$

$$= 0.581$$

Thus, there is no significant change in VA in the sub-group of patients with VA 20/40 or better.

**9.3** Fourteen patients who have either improved or declined. Thus, we again must use the exact binomial test. We have $C = 12, n = 14$. We refer to the exact binomial tables under $n = 14, p = 0.5$ to compute

$$p = 2 \times \sum_{k=12}^{14} \binom{14}{k}\left(\frac{1}{2}\right)^{14}$$

$$= 2 \times (0.0056 + 0.0009 + 0.0001)$$

$$= 2 \times 0.0066$$

$$= 0.013$$

Thus, the visual acuity of persons with VA of 20/50 or worse at baseline has significantly improved.

**9.8** The Wilcoxon sign rank test.

**9.9** We first rank the data by absolute value of the change score ($d_i$) as follows:

$$= \frac{|175 - 138| - 0.5}{\sqrt{1081 - \dfrac{210 + 336 + 990}{2}}}$$

$$= \frac{36.5}{\sqrt{1081 - 768}}$$

$$= \frac{36.5}{17.692}$$

$$= 2.063 \sim N(0, 1) \text{ under } H_0$$

The $p$-value is obtained from

$$p = 2 \times [1 - \Phi(2.063)]$$

$$= 2 \times (1 - 0.9805)$$

$$= 0.039$$

Thus, the periodontal status of the patients has significantly improved over time.

| $|d_i|$ | Negative $d_i$ | Frequency | Positive $d_i$ | Frequency | Total frequency | Range of ranks | Average rank |
|---|---|---|---|---|---|---|---|
| 3 | $-3$ | 2 | 3 | 4 | 6 | 1–6 | 3.5 |
| 2 | $-2$ | 2 | 2 | 5 | 7 | 7–13 | 10.0 |
| 1 | $-1$ | 4 | 1 | 6 | 10 | 14–23 | 18.5 |
| | | 8 | | 15 | 23 | | |
| 0 | 0 | 5 | | | | | |

Since there are 23 untied pairs, we can use the normal theory test. We have that the rank sum of the positive differences ($R_1$) $= 4 \times 3.5 + 5 \times 10.0 + 6 \times 18.5 = 175.0$. The test statistic is given by

$$T = \frac{\left|R_1 - \dfrac{n(n + 1)}{4}\right| - 0.5}{\sqrt{\dfrac{n(n + 1)(2n + 1)}{24} - \sum_{i=1}^{g}\dfrac{(t_i^3 - t_i)}{2}}}$$

$$= \frac{\left|175 - \dfrac{23(24)}{4}\right| - 0.5}{\sqrt{\dfrac{23(24)(47)}{24} - \dfrac{(6^3 - 6) + (7^3 - 7) + (10^3 - 10)}{2}}}$$

**9.12** We must use the exact tables for the sign rank test, since the number of untied pairs is less than 16. We refer to Table 9 under $n = 15$ and note that the upper critical value for $\alpha = 0.10 = 90$, whereas the upper and lower critical values for $\alpha = 0.05$ are 95 and 25, respectively. Since $R_1 = 90 \geqslant 90$ and $25 < 90 < 95$, we have $0.05 \leqslant p < 0.10$ using a two-sided test.

**9.15** We can use the normal theory test, since $\min(n_1, n_2) = 12 \geqslant 10$. We have the test statistic

$$T = \frac{\left|R_1 - \dfrac{n_1(n_1 + n_2 + 1)}{2}\right| - 0.5}{\sqrt{\dfrac{n_1 n_2(n_1 + n_2 + 1)}{12}}}$$

$$= \frac{\left|220 - \dfrac{12(28)}{2}\right| - 0.5}{\sqrt{\dfrac{12(15)(28)}{12}}}$$

$$= \frac{|220 - 168| - 0.5}{20.494}$$

$$= \frac{52.0 - 0.5}{20.494}$$

$$= \frac{51.5}{20.494}$$

$$= 2.513 \sim N(0, 1) \text{ under } H_0$$

The $p$-value is given by

$$p = 2 \times [1 - \Phi(2.513)]$$

$$= 2 \times (1 - 0.9940)$$

$$= 0.012$$

Thus, there is a significant difference between the two groups.

**9.22** The distribution of length of stay in a hospital is notoriously very skewed and far from being normal. This is due to the relatively short stays of most patients and the very long stays of a relatively small number of patients. To use the $t$ test, we would have to assume underlying normality of the length-of-stay distribution or at the very least that mean length of stay ($\bar{x}$) was normally distributed for moderate sample sizes, which is unlikely to be the case here.

**9.23** We can instead use the Wilcoxon rank sum test to test if the median length of stay is significantly different in the two hospitals. We first rank the length of stay in the combined sample, as given in Table A.10.

Next we compute the rank sum for hospital 1 as follows:

$$R_1 = 1.0 + 2.0 + 3.5 + 5.0 + 6.0 + 7.0 + 9.0 + 10.0$$
$$+ 11.0 + 13.5 + 15.5 = 83.5$$

**Table A.10** *Data layout for length-of-stay data for Wilcoxon rank sum test*

| Value | Frequency, hospital 1 | Frequency, hospital 2 | Total frequency | Rank range | Average rank |
|-------|-----------------------|-----------------------|-----------------|------------|--------------|
| 5 | 1 | 0 | 1 | 1 | 1.0 |
| 8 | 1 | 0 | 1 | 2 | 2.0 |
| 10 | 1 | 1 | 2 | 3–4 | 3.5 |
| 13 | 1 | 0 | 1 | 5 | 5.0 |
| 21 | 1 | 0 | 1 | 6 | 6.0 |
| 26 | 1 | 0 | 1 | 7 | 7.0 |
| 27 | 0 | 1 | 1 | 8 | 8.0 |
| 29 | 1 | 0 | 1 | 9 | 9.0 |
| 32 | 1 | 0 | 1 | 10 | 10.0 |
| 33 | 1 | 0 | 1 | 11 | 11.0 |
| 35 | 0 | 1 | 1 | 12 | 12.0 |
| 44 | 1 | 1 | 2 | 13–14 | 13.5 |
| 60 | 1 | 1 | 2 | 15–16 | 15.5 |
| 68 | 0 | 1 | 1 | 17 | 17.0 |
| 73 | 0 | 1 | 1 | 18 | 18.0 |
| 76 | 0 | 1 | 1 | 19 | 19.0 |
| 86 | 0 | 1 | 1 | 20 | 20.0 |
| 87 | 0 | 1 | 1 | 21 | 21.0 |
| 96 | 0 | 1 | 1 | 22 | 22.0 |
| 125 | 0 | 1 | 1 | 23 | 23.0 |
| 238 | 0 | 1 | 1 | 24 | 24.0 |
| Total | 11 | 13 | 24 | | |

We will assume that $R_1$ is normally distributed. Under $H_0$ we know that

$$E(R_1) = n_1(n_1 + n_2 + 1)/2 = 11(25)/2 = 137.5$$

$$Var(R_1) = \frac{n_1 n_2}{12}\left[n_1 + n_2 + 1 - \frac{\sum\limits_{i=1}^{q} t_i(t_i^2 - 1)}{(n_1 + n_2)(n_1 + n_2 - 1)}\right]$$

$$= \frac{11(13)}{12}\left[25 - \frac{2(3) + 2(3) + 2(3)}{24(23)}\right]$$

$$= 297.528$$

$$sd(R_1) = 17.249$$

Thus, we compute the test statistic

$$T = (|R_1 - E(R_1)| - 0.5)/sd(R_1)$$

$$= (|83.5 - 137.5| - 0.5)/17.249$$

$$= 53.5/17.249$$

$$= 3.10 \sim N(0, 1)$$

The two-sided $p$-value is given by

$$2 \times [1 - \Phi(3.10)] = 2 \times (1 - 0.9990) = 0.002$$

Thus, there is a significant difference in length of stay between the two hospitals, with hospital 2 patients staying longer. We would have to assess the patient characteristics in the two hospitals before concluding that this difference was due to procedural variations between the two hospitals.

**9.37** The hypotheses being tested are $H_0$: median duration of effusion of breast-fed babies = median duration of effusion of bottle-fed babies vs. $H_1$: median duration of effusion of breast-fed babies < median duration of effusion of bottle-fed babies.

**9.38** A nonparametric test would be useful because the distribution of duration of effusion is very skewed and the assumptions about normality of the underlying distribution are very unlikely to hold.

**9.39** The Wilcoxon sign rank test should be used here because the breast- and bottle-fed babies are matched on age, sex, socioeconomic status, and type of medications and thus form two paired samples.

**9.40** We apply the sign rank test to these data. We first compute the difference $(d_i)$ in duration of effusion between

**Table A.11** *Difference in duration of effusion between breast-fed and bottle-fed babies*

| $i$ | $d_i$ | $i$ | $d_i$ |
|-----|-------|-----|-------|
| 1 | +2 | 13 | +13 |
| 2 | −24 | 14 | −1 |
| 3 | −4 | 15 | −9 |
| 4 | −158 | 16 | +2 |
| 5 | +1 | 17 | −1 |
| 6 | −5 | 18 | −12 |
| 7 | −165 | 19 | −12 |
| 8 | 0 | 20 | −2 |
| 9 | −18 | 21 | −1 |
| 10 | −59 | 22 | +3 |
| 11 | −169 | 23 | +6 |
| 12 | −17 | 24 | +5 |

the breast- and bottle-fed babies in the matched pairs, as given in Table A.11.

We now separate the positive and negative differences and order the differences by absolute value (Table A.12).

We then count the number of persons with the same absolute value and assign an average rank to each absolute value, as shown in Table A.12. Since the number of nonzero differences $= 23 \geqslant 16$, we can use the normal approximation test in **(9.5)**. We compute the rank sum of the positive differences as follows:

$$R_1 = 1(2.5) + 2(6.0) + 1(8.0) + 1(10.5) + 1(12.0) + 1(16.0)$$

$$= 61$$

The expected value and variance of the rank sum are given as follows:

$$E(R_1) = \frac{n(n+1)}{4} = \frac{23(24)}{4} = 138$$

$$Var(R_1) = \frac{n(n+1)(2n+1)}{24} - \frac{\sum\limits_{i=1}^{g}(t_i^3 - t_i)}{2}$$

$$= \frac{23(24)(47)}{24} - \frac{(4^3 - 4) + (3^3 - 3) + (2^3 - 2) + (2^3 - 2)}{2}$$

$$= 1081 - \frac{96}{2} = 1033$$

$$sd(R_1) = 32.14$$

**Table A.12** *Data layout for duration of effusion for Wilcoxon sign rank test*

| $\|d_i\|$ | Negative $d_i$ | $f_i$ | Positive $d_i$ | $f_i$ | Number of persons with same absolute value | Range of ranks | Average rank |
|---|---|---|---|---|---|---|---|
| 169 | $-169$ | 1 | 169 | 0 | 1 | 23 | 23.0 |
| 165 | $-165$ | 1 | 165 | 0 | 1 | 22 | 22.0 |
| 158 | $-158$ | 1 | 158 | 0 | 1 | 21 | 21.0 |
| 59 | $-59$ | 1 | 59 | 0 | 1 | 20 | 20.0 |
| 24 | $-24$ | 1 | 24 | 0 | 1 | 19 | 19.0 |
| 18 | $-18$ | 1 | 18 | 0 | 1 | 18 | 18.0 |
| 17 | $-17$ | 1 | 17 | 0 | 1 | 17 | 17.0 |
| 13 | $-13$ | 0 | 13 | 1 | 1 | 16 | 16.0 |
| 12 | $-12$ | 2 | 12 | 0 | 2 | 14–15 | 14.5 |
| 9 | $-9$ | 1 | 9 | 0 | 1 | 13 | 13.0 |
| 6 | $-6$ | 0 | 6 | 1 | 1 | 12 | 12.0 |
| 5 | $-5$ | 1 | 5 | 1 | 2 | 10–11 | 10.5 |
| 4 | $-4$ | 1 | 4 | 0 | 1 | 9 | 9.0 |
| 3 | $-3$ | 0 | 3 | 1 | 1 | 8 | 8.0 |
| 2 | $-2$ | 1 | 2 | 2 | 3 | 5–7 | 6.0 |
| 1 | $-1$ | 3 | 1 | 1 | 4 | 1–4 | 2.5 |
| 0 | 0 | 1 | | | | | |

The test statistic is then obtained from

$$T = \frac{|61 - 138| - 1/2}{32.14} = 2.38 \sim N(0, 1) \text{ under } H_0$$

It follows that

$$p = 1 - \Phi(2.38) = 1 - 0.9913 = 0.009$$

Thus, breast-fed babies have significantly shorter effusions than bottle-fed babies do.

**9.49** A nonparametric statistical test would be useful because we cannot numerically quantify the change in redness or itching but can only assess which eye has improved more.

**9.50** The degree of redness or itching is probably similar in two eyes of the same person at baseline. Thus, this procedure would eliminate the substantial between-person variability that can occur if the drug were administered to one group of people and the placebo to another group.

**9.51** The sign test should be used here because we are comparing two paired samples consisting of alternate eyes from the same people and we only know which eye

did better but not how much better.

**9.52** We find that there are 5 +'s and 11 −'s for redness. Since there are $<20$ nonzero differences, we must use the exact test. In particular, the $p$-value is given by

$$p = 2 \times \sum_{k=0}^{5} \binom{16}{k}\left(\frac{1}{2}\right)^{16}$$

From the binomial tables (Table 1) using $n = 16$, $p = 0.50$, we have

$$Pr(0) = 0.0000 \qquad Pr(1) = 0.0002$$

$$Pr(2) = 0.0018 \qquad Pr(3) = 0.0085$$

$$Pr(4) = 0.0278 \qquad Pr(5) = 0.0667$$

Thus,

$$p = 2 \times (0.0000 + 0.0002 + 0.0018 + 0.0085 +$$

$$+ 0.0278 + 0.0667)$$

$$= 0.210$$

Thus, there is no significant difference in redness between the two sets of treated eyes.

**9.53** We find that there are 12 +'s and 3 −'s for itching. We again use the exact test, calculated from the binomial tables, with the *p*-value given by

$$p = 2 \times \sum_{k=0}^{3} \binom{15}{k}\left(\frac{1}{2}\right)^{15}$$

$$= 2 \times (0.0000 + 0.0005 + 0.0032 + 0.0139)$$

$$= 0.035$$

Thus, there is a significant difference in itching between the drug-treated and placebo-treated eyes. This is what we expect, since drug A is only supposed to be effective against itching.

**9.54** For redness there are 22 +'s and 3 0's. We can use the sign test using the normal approximation, since we have 22 untied pairs. The test statistic is given by

$$\lambda = \frac{\left|C - \dfrac{n}{2}\right| - 0.5}{\sqrt{\dfrac{n}{4}}} = \frac{|22 - 11| - 0.5}{\sqrt{\dfrac{22}{4}}} = \frac{10.5}{2.345}$$

$$= 4.48 \sim N(0, 1) \text{ under } H_0$$

The *p*-value is

$$2 \times [1 - \Phi(\lambda)] = 2 \times [1 - \Phi(4.48)] < 0.001$$

There is clearly overwhelming evidence that drug B is effective against redness.

**9.55** For itching there are 7 +'s and 6 −'s. We use the exact binomial version of the sign test. The *p*-value is obtained from the binomial tables as follows:

$$p = 2 \times \sum_{k=0}^{6} \binom{13}{k}\left(\frac{1}{2}\right)^{13}$$

$$= 2 \times (0.0001 + 0.0016 + 0.0095 + 0.0349$$
$$+ 0.0873 + 0.1571 + 0.2095)$$

$$= 1.0$$

There is clearly no significant difference in itching between treated and untreated eyes with drug B. These results are again consistent with our expectations for drug B, which is only supposed to be effective against redness.

**9.56** For redness there are 23 +'s and 2 0's. This result is even more extreme than that in Problem 9.54, and if we use the sign test with the normal approximation, we surely will find $p < 0.001$. Thus, the combination drug is very effective vs. redness.

**9.57** For itching there are 14 +'s and 3 −'s. We use the exact binomial version of the sign test as follows:

$$p = 2 \times \sum_{k=0}^{3} \binom{17}{k}\left(\frac{1}{2}\right)^{17}$$

$$= 2 \times (0.0000 + 0.0001 + 0.0010 + 0.0052)$$

$$= 0.013$$

Thus, the combination drug is significantly better than the placebo for itching as well, but not as strongly as for redness.

**9.58** The results of the three experiments agree with our prior hypotheses. Indeed, drug A is significantly better than the placebo for itching ($p = 0.035$) but not for redness; drug B is significantly better than the placebo for redness ($p < 0.001$) but not for itching; the combination drug is significantly better than the placebo for both redness ($p < 0.001$) and itching ($p = 0.013$).

# *C*hapter 10

**10.1** We wish to test the hypothesis $H_0: p_1 = p_2$ vs. $H_1: p_1 \neq p_2$. We have the test statistic

$$\lambda = \frac{\hat{p}_1 - \hat{p}_2}{\sqrt{\hat{p}\hat{q}(1/n_1 + 1/n_2)}}$$

where $\hat{p}_1 = 9/199 = 0.0452$, $\hat{p}_2 = 13/97 = 0.1340$, $\hat{p} = (9 + 13)/(199 + 97) = 22/296 = 0.0743$, $\hat{q} = 1 - \hat{p} =$ 0.9257. We have

$$\lambda = \frac{0.0452 - 0.1340}{\sqrt{(0.0743)(0.9257)(1/199 + 1/97)}}$$

$$= \frac{-0.0888}{0.0325}$$

$$= -2.7323 \sim N(0, 1) \text{ under } H_0$$

Since $\lambda < -1.96$, we reject $H_0$ at the 5% level.

**10.2** The observed table is given by

**12-month mortality status**

|  | Dead | Alive |  |
|---|---|---|---|
| Streptokinase | 9 | 190 | 199 |
| Control | 13 | 84 | 97 |
|  | 22 | 274 | 296 |

The expected cell counts are obtained from the row and column margins as follows:

$$E_{11} = \frac{199 \times 22}{296} = 14.79$$

$$E_{12} = \frac{199 \times 274}{296} = 184.21$$

$$E_{21} = \frac{97 \times 22}{296} = 7.21$$

$$E_{22} = \frac{97 \times 274}{296} = 89.79$$

These values can be displayed in the following expected table:

**12-month mortality status**

|  | Dead | Alive |  |
|---|---|---|---|
| Streptokinase | 14.79 | 184.21 | 199 |
| Control | 7.21 | 89.79 | 97 |
|  | 22 | 274 | 296 |

**10.3** We compute the Yates-corrected chi-square statistic as follows:

$$T = \frac{(|9 - 14.79| - 0.5)^2}{14.79} + \cdots + \frac{(|84 - 89.79| - 0.5)^2}{89.79}$$

$$= \frac{5.29^2}{14.79} + \cdots + \frac{5.29^2}{89.79}$$

$$= 1.892 + 0.152 + 3.881 + 0.312$$

$$= 6.24 \sim \chi_1^2 \text{ under } H_0$$

Since $\chi^2_{1,.95} = 3.84 < T$, we reject $H_0$ at the 5% level.

**10.4** The decisions reached in Problems 10.1 and 10.3 were the same (reject $H_0$ at the 5% level). If we had used a chi-square test without continuity correction, the results would have been identical, since $T = (5.79)^2/14.79 + \cdots + (5.79)^2/89.79 = 7.47 = (2.7323)^2 = \lambda^2$ and we get exactly the same $p$-value whether we compare $\lambda$ to a $N(0, 1)$ distribution or $T = \lambda^2$ to a $\chi_1^2$ distribution.

**10.21** We form the following observed $2 \times 2$ table:

**12-month mortality status**

|  | Dead | Alive |  |
|---|---|---|---|
| Streptokinase | 2 | 13 | 15 |
| Control | 4 | 15 | 19 |
|  | 6 | 28 | 34 |

The smallest expected value $= E_{11} = (15 \times 6)/34 = 2.65 < 5$. Thus, we must use Fisher's exact test.

**10.22**

| 0 | 15 | | 1 | 14 | | 2 | 13 | | 3 | 12 |
|---|---|---|---|---|---|---|---|---|---|---|
| 6 | 13 | | 5 | 14 | | 4 | 15 | | 3 | 16 |

| 4 | 11 | | 5 | 10 | | 6 | 9 |
|---|---|---|---|---|---|---|---|
| 2 | 17 | | 1 | 18 | | 0 | 19 |

**10.23** We use the recursion rule as follows:

$$Pr(0) = 1 \times Pr(0)$$

$$Pr(1) = \frac{6 \times 15}{1 \times 14} Pr(0) = 6.429 Pr(0)$$

$$Pr(2) = \frac{5 \times 14}{2 \times 15} Pr(1) = 15.001 Pr(0)$$

$$Pr(3) = \frac{4 \times 13}{3 \times 16} Pr(2) = 16.251 Pr(0)$$

$$Pr(4) = \frac{3 \times 12}{4 \times 17} Pr(3) = 8.603 Pr(0)$$

$$Pr(5) = \frac{2 \times 11}{5 \times 18} Pr(4) = 2.103 Pr(0)$$

$$Pr(6) = \frac{1 \times 10}{6 \times 19} Pr(5) = 0.184 Pr(0)$$

Thus,

$$Pr(0) \times (1 + 6.429 + \cdots + 0.184) = 1$$

or

$$Pr(0) \times (49.571) = 1$$

or

$$Pr(0) = \frac{1}{49.571} = 0.0202$$

Furthermore,

$$Pr(1) = 0.130, \qquad Pr(2) = 0.303, \qquad Pr(3) = 0.328,$$

$$Pr(4) = 0.174, \qquad Pr(5) = 0.042, \qquad Pr(6) = 0.004$$

**10.24** Our table is the "2" table. Therefore, the two-tailed $p$-value is given by

$$p = 2 \times \min[Pr(0) + Pr(1) + Pr(2),$$
$$Pr(2) + Pr(3) + \cdots + Pr(7)]$$

$$= 2 \times \min(0.453, 0.851)$$

$$= 2 \times 0.453 = 0.906$$

Clearly, there is no significant difference in 12-month mortality status between the two treatment groups for females.

**10.29** 87

**10.30** 13

**10.31** Since there are less than 20 discordant pairs, we must use the exact binomial version of McNemar's test. We refer to the exact binomial tables (Table 1) with $n = 13$, $p = 0.50$ to evaluate

$$p = 2 \times \sum_{k=9}^{13} {}_{13}C_k (1/2)^{13}$$

$$= 2 \times (0.0873 + 0.0349 + 0.0095 + 0.0016 + 0.0001)$$

$$= 2 \times 0.1334$$

$$= 0.267$$

Therefore, there is no significant difference between the effectiveness of the two drugs for males.

**10.41** We wish to test the hypothesis $H_0: p_A = p_B$ vs. $H_1: p_A \neq p_B$, where

$$p_A = Pr(\text{first born child has asthma in a type A family})$$

$$p_B = Pr(\text{first born child has asthma in a type B family})$$

We have the following observed and expected $2 \times 2$ tables (Tables A.13 and A.14). We will use the $\chi^2$ test for $2 \times 2$ tables, since the expected table has no *expected* value $< 5$. We have the following Yates-corrected chi-square statistic

$$T = \frac{(|15 - 6.3| - 0.5)^2}{6.3} + \cdots + \frac{(|196 - 187.3| - 0.5)^2}{187.3}$$

$$= 17.04 \sim \chi_1^2$$

### Table A.13

|  |  | Observed asthma status of first-born child | | |
|---|---|---|---|---|
|  |  | + | − | |
| Type of family | A | 15 | 85 | 100 |
|  | B | 4 | 196 | 200 |
|  |  | 19 | 281 | 300 |

### Table A.14

|  |  | Expected asthma status of first-born child | | |
|---|---|---|---|---|
|  |  | + | − | |
| Type of family | A | 6.3 | 93.7 | 100 |
|  | B | 12.7 | 187.3 | 200 |
|  |  | 19.0 | 281.0 | 300 |

+ = asthma
− = no asthma

The *p*-value for this result is $<0.001$, since

$$\chi^2_{1,.999} = 10.83 < 17.04$$

Thus, there is a highly significant association between the type of family and the asthma status of the children.

*10.42* We have the following $2 \times 2$ table (Table A.15).

*Table A.15*

|                | Nonasthmatic respiratory disease status + | − | |
|----------------|------|------|-----|
| Type of family A | 3 | 97 | 100 |
| B | 2 | 198 | 200 |
| | 5 | 295 | 300 |

+ = nonasthmatic respiratory disease
− = no nonasthmatic respiratory disease

There are two expected values $<5$; in particular,

$$E_{11} = \frac{5(100)}{300} = 1.7 \qquad E_{21} = \frac{5(200)}{300} = 3.3$$

Thus, we must use Fisher's exact test to analyze this table. We write all possible tables with the same margins as the observed table, as follows:

| 0 | 100 |
|---|-----|
| 5 | 195 |

| 1 | 99 |
|---|-----|
| 4 | 196 |

| 2 | 98 |
|---|-----|
| 3 | 197 |

| 3 | 97 |
|---|-----|
| 2 | 198 |

| 4 | 96 |
|---|-----|
| 1 | 199 |

| 5 | 95 |
|---|-----|
| 0 | 200 |

We use the recursion rule to compute the probability of each table. We have

$$Pr(0) = 1 \times Pr(0)$$

$$Pr(1) = Pr(0) \times \frac{5 \times 100}{1 \times 196} = 2.551 Pr(0)$$

$$Pr(2) = Pr(1) \times \frac{4 \times 99}{2 \times 197} = 2.564 Pr(0)$$

$$Pr(3) = Pr(2) \times \frac{3 \times 98}{3 \times 198} = 1.269 Pr(0)$$

$$Pr(4) = Pr(3) \times \frac{2 \times 97}{4 \times 199} = 0.309 Pr(0)$$

$$Pr(5) = Pr(4) \times \frac{1 \times 96}{5 \times 200} = 0.030 Pr(0)$$

Thus,

$$Pr(0)(1 + 2.551 + 2.564 + 1.269 + 0.309 + 0.030) = 1$$

$$Pr(0) = \frac{1}{7.723} = 0.1295$$

$$Pr(1) = 0.330$$

$$Pr(2) = 0.332$$

$$Pr(3) = 0.164$$

$$Pr(4) = 0.040$$

$$Pr(5) = 0.004$$

Thus, since the observed table is the "3" table, the two-tailed *p*-value is given by

$$2 \times \min(0.164 + 0.040 + 0.004, 0.164 + 0.332 + 0.330$$
$$+ 0.1295) = 2 \times 0.208 = 0.416$$

The results are not statistically significant and indicate that there is no significant difference in the prevalence of nonasthmatic respiratory disease among households in which the parents do or do not have asthma.

*10.45* We have the following observed table (Table A.16).

*Table A.16* Association between Oracon use and endometrial cancer

|          | Use Oracon Yes | No | |
|----------|------|------|-----|
| Cases | 6 | 111 | 117 |
| Controls | 8 | 387 | 395 |
| | 14 | 498 | 512 |

The smallest expected value $= 14 \times 117/512 = 3.20 < 5$. Thus, we must use Fisher's exact test to analyze this table. We construct all tables with the same row and column margins as the observed table:

| 0 | 117 |
|---|-----|
| 14 | 381 |

| 1 | 116 |
|---|-----|
| 13 | 382 |

| 2 | 115 |
|---|-----|
| 12 | 383 |

| 3 | 114 |
|---|-----|
| 11 | 384 |

| 4 | 113 |
|---|-----|
| 10 | 385 |

| 5 | 112 |
|---|-----|
| 9 | 386 |

| 6 | 111 |
|---|-----|
| 8 | 387 |

| 7 | 110 |
|---|-----|
| 7 | 388 |

| 8 | 109 |
|---|-----|
| 6 | 389 |

| 9 | 108 |
|---|-----|
| 5 | 390 |

| 10 | 107 |
|----|-----|
| 4 | 391 |

| 11 | 106 |
|----|-----|
| 3 | 392 |

| 12 | 105 |
|----|-----|
| 2 | 393 |

| 13 | 104 |
|----|-----|
| 1 | 394 |

| 14 | 103 |
|----|-----|
| 0 | 395 |

We use the recursion rule to compute the exact probability of each table. We have

$$Pr(0) = 1 \, Pr(0)$$

$$Pr(1) = \frac{14 \times 117}{1 \times 382} Pr(0) = 4.288 Pr(0)$$

$$Pr(2) = \frac{13 \times 116}{2 \times 383} Pr(1) = 8.442 Pr(0)$$

$$Pr(3) = \frac{12 \times 115}{3 \times 384} Pr(2) = 10.113 Pr(0)$$

$$Pr(4) = \frac{11 \times 114}{4 \times 385} Pr(3) = 8.235 Pr(0)$$

$$Pr(5) = \frac{10 \times 113}{5 \times 386} Pr(4) = 4.822 Pr(0)$$

$$Pr(6) = \frac{9 \times 112}{6 \times 387} Pr(5) = 2.093 Pr(0)$$

$$Pr(7) = \frac{8 \times 111}{7 \times 388} Pr(6) = 0.684 Pr(0)$$

$$Pr(8) = \frac{7 \times 110}{8 \times 389} Pr(7) = 0.169 Pr(0)$$

$$Pr(9) = \frac{6 \times 109}{9 \times 390} Pr(8) = 0.031 Pr(0)$$

$$Pr(10) = \frac{5 \times 108}{10 \times 391} Pr(9) = 0.0043 Pr(0)$$

$$Pr(11) = \frac{4 \times 107}{11 \times 392} Pr(10) = 0.00043 Pr(0)$$

$$Pr(12) = \frac{3 \times 106}{12 \times 393} Pr(11) = 0.000029 Pr(0)$$

$$Pr(13) = \frac{2 \times 105}{13 \times 394} Pr(12) = 1.2 \times 10^{-6} Pr(0)$$

$$Pr(14) = \frac{1 \times 104}{14 \times 395} Pr(13) = 2.3 \times 10^{-8} Pr(0)$$

Thus,

$$Pr(0)(1 + 4.288 + \cdots + 2.3 \times 10^{-8}) = 1$$

or

$$Pr(0) = \frac{1}{39.882} = 0.0251$$

It follows that

$$Pr(1) = 0.108$$

$$Pr(2) = 0.212$$

$$Pr(3) = 0.254$$

$$Pr(4) = 0.207$$

$$Pr(5) = 0.121$$

$$Pr(6) = 0.053$$

$$Pr(7) = 0.017$$

$$Pr(8) = 0.004$$

$$Pr(9) = 0.001$$

$$Pr(10) = 1.1 \times 10^{-4}$$

$$Pr(11) = 1.1 \times 10^{-5}$$

$$Pr(12) = 7.3 \times 10^{-7}$$

$$Pr(13) = 3.0 \times 10^{-8}$$

$$Pr(14) = 5.8 \times 10^{-10}$$

The observed table is the "6" table. Thus, the one-tailed *p*-value is given by

$$\sum_{i=6}^{14} Pr(i) = 0.053 + 0.017 + \cdots + 5.8 \times 10^{-10} = 0.075$$

and the two-tailed *p*-value is given by

$$2 \times \min\left[ \sum_{i=0}^{6} Pr(i), \sum_{i=6}^{14} Pr(i) \right] = 2 \times \min(0.980, 0.075)$$

$$= 2(0.075) = 0.150.$$

Thus, there is no significant association between the use of Oracon and the development of endometrial cancer. These results differ from those in the article, in which the authors reported a significant association between these two variables. One explanation is that the authors found this significant association after adjusting for age and certain other variables, whereas our results are unadjusted.

**10.51** We have the following 2 × 2 contingency table (Table A.17).

*Table A.17*

| Community | Disease status + | − | |
|---|---|---|---|
| A | 5 | 99,995 | 100,000 |
| B | 1 | 199,999 | 200,000 |
| | 6 | 299,994 | 300,000 |

We form the expected table as follows:

| 2.0 | 99,998 |
|---|---|
| 4.0 | 199,996 |

Since two of the four cells have expected values <5, we must use Fisher's exact test rather than the $\chi^2$ test. We thus form the following seven tables:

| 0 | 100,000 |
|---|---|
| 6 | 199,994 |

| 1 | 99,999 |
|---|---|
| 5 | 199,995 |

| 2 | 99,998 |
|---|---|
| 4 | 199,996 |

| 3 | 99,997 |
|---|---|
| 3 | 199,997 |

| 4 | 99,996 |
|---|---|
| 2 | 199,998 |

| 5 | 99,995 |
|---|---|
| 1 | 199,999 |

| 6 | 99,994 |
|---|---|
| 0 | 200,000 |

We have

$$Pr(0) = 1.00Pr(0)$$

$$Pr(1) = \frac{6 \times 100,000}{1 \times 199,995} Pr(0) = 3.000Pr(0)$$

$$Pr(2) = \frac{5 \times 99,999}{2 \times 199,996} Pr(1) = 3.750Pr(0)$$

$$Pr(3) = \frac{4 \times 99,998}{3 \times 199,997} Pr(2) = 2.500Pr(0)$$

$$Pr(4) = \frac{3 \times 99,997}{4 \times 199,998} Pr(3) = 0.937Pr(0)$$

$$Pr(5) = \frac{2 \times 99,996}{5 \times 199,999} Pr(4) = 0.187Pr(0)$$

$$Pr(6) = \frac{1 \times 99,995}{6 \times 200,000} Pr(5) = 0.016Pr(0)$$

Thus, $Pr(0)(1 + 3.000 + 3.750 + 2.500 + 0.937 + 0.187 + 0.016) = 1$

$$Pr(0) = 0.0878$$

$$Pr(1) = 0.263$$

$$Pr(2) = 0.329$$

$$Pr(3) = 0.220$$

$$Pr(4) = 0.082$$

$$Pr(5) = 0.016$$

$$Pr(6) = 0.001$$

The one-sided $p$-value associated with the "5" table is $0.016 + 0.001 = 0.017$. The two-sided $p$-value is 0.034. Thus, there is a significant difference in the incidence rates.

**10.55** The samples are not independent; so we use McNemar's test. We have the following distribution of matched pairs (Table A.18).

**Table A.18** *Association between computer and attending physician diagnoses*

|  |  | Computer + | Computer − |  |
|---|---|---|---|---|
| Attending physician | + | 48 | 2 | 50 |
| | − | 20 | 9930 | 9950 |
| | | 68 | 9932 | 10,000 |

We have

$$n_A = 2 \qquad n_B = 20 \qquad n_D = 22$$

Since $n_D/4 \geqslant 5$, we can use the normal approximation. We have, under $H_0$,

$$S = \frac{\left(\left|n_A - \frac{n_D}{2}\right| - \frac{1}{2}\right)^2}{\frac{n_D}{4}} = \frac{\left(|2 - 11| - \frac{1}{2}\right)^2}{5.5} = 13.14 \sim x_1^2$$

Since $\chi_{1,.999}^2 = 10.83 < 13.14 = S$, it follows that $p < 0.001$. The computer seems more likely to diagnose this type of viral infection than the attending physician.

**10.61** A two-sample test is needed here, since we are comparing samples of men who survived and died, respectively, from a first heart attack.

**10.62** We have the following observed table (Table A.19). The smallest expected value is

$$\frac{40 \times 100}{200} = 20 \geqslant 5$$

Thus, we can use the $\chi^2$ test for $2 \times 2$ contingency tables here.

**Table A.19** *Observed table relating sudden death from a first heart attack and previous physical activity*

|  |  | Physical activity Active | Inactive |  |
|---|---|---|---|---|
| Mortality status | Survived | 30 | 70 | 100 |
| | Died | 10 | 90 | 100 |
| | | 40 | 160 | 200 |

**10.63** The test statistic is given by

$$T = \frac{n\left[|ad - bc| - \frac{n}{2}\right]^2}{(a+b)(c+d)(a+c)(b+d)}$$

$$= \frac{200(|30 \times 90 - 10 \times 70| - 100)^2}{(100)(100)(40)(160)}$$

$$= \frac{200(1900)^2}{(100)(100)(40)(160)}$$

$$= 11.28 \sim \chi_1^2 \text{ under } H_0$$

Since $\chi_{1,.999}^2 = 10.83 < T$, it follows that $p < 0.001$, and we can conclude that there is a significant association between physical activity and survival of an MI.

**10.64** The odds ratio in favor of prior physical activity for MI survivors vs. MI deceased is given by

$$\widehat{OR} = \frac{30 \times 90}{70 \times 10}$$

$$= \frac{2700}{700}$$

$$= 3.86$$

**10.65** We use the test-based method to obtain 95% confidence limits. The 95% confidence interval is given by $(OR_1, OR_2)$, where

$$OR_1 = \widehat{OR}^{1-(1.96/\sqrt{T}}$$

$$= 3.86^{1-(1.96/\sqrt{11.28})}$$

$$= 3.86^{1-0.58}$$

$$= 3.86^{0.42}$$

$$= 1.76$$

$$OR_2 = \hat{OR}^{1+(1.96/\sqrt{T})}$$

$$= 3.86^{1+0.58}$$

$$= 3.86^{1.58}$$

$$= 8.45$$

Thus, $(1.76, 8.45)$ is a 95% confidence interval for $OR$. This interval excludes 1, as it must, since our $p$-value is less than 0.05.

*10.70* This is a classic example illustrating the use of McNemar's test for correlated proportions. We have two groups of patients, one receiving lithium and one receiving placebo, but the two groups are matched on age, sex, and clinical condition and thus represent dependent samples. Let a type A discordant pair be a pair of persons such that the lithium member of the pair has a manic depressive episode and the placebo member does not. Let a type B discordant pair be a pair of persons such that the placebo member of the pair has a manic depressive episode and the lithium member does not. Let $p =$ probability that a discordant pair is of type A. Then we wish to test the hypothesis

$$H_0: p = \tfrac{1}{2} \text{ vs. } H_1: p \neq \tfrac{1}{2}$$

*10.71* There are 2 type A discordant pairs and 10 type B discordant pairs, giving a total of 12 discordant pairs. Since $npq = 12(\tfrac{1}{2})(\tfrac{1}{2}) = 3 < 5$, we *cannot* assume that the normal approximation to the binomial holds and we must use an exact binomial test. Under $H_0$: we have

$$Pr(k \text{ type A discordant pairs}) = \binom{12}{k}\left(\frac{1}{2}\right)^{12}$$

In particular, from Table 1 we have

$$Pr(k \leqslant 2) = \left(\frac{1}{2}\right)^{12}\left[\binom{12}{0} + \binom{12}{1} + \binom{12}{2}\right]$$

$$= 0.0002 + 0.0029 + 0.0161 = 0.0192$$

Since we are performing a two-sided test, we have

$$p = 2 \times 0.0192 = 0.038$$

Thus, we reject $H_0$ and conclude that the placebo patients are more likely to have manic depressive episodes when the results differ in the two members of a pair.

*10.76* We set up a $2 \times 2$ contingency table to display the data (Table A.20).

We use the chi-square test for trend, as outlined in **(10.20)**. In this regard we use scores $1, 2, \ldots, k$ for the $k$ groups. We compute the test statistic $T_1 = A^2/B$, where

$$A = \left(\sum_{i=1}^{k} x_i S_i\right) - x\left(\sum_{i=1}^{k} n_i S_i\right)\Big/N$$

$$= [20(1) + 14(2) + \cdots + 13(5)]$$

$$- \frac{92[256(1) + 710(2) + \cdots + 1292(5)]}{5374}$$

$$= 266 - \frac{92 \times 19{,}252}{5374}$$

$$= 266 - 329.58$$

$$= -63.58$$

**Table A.20** *Observed table relating age to 3-year survival for cancer of the pancreas*

| | | Age group | | | | | |
|---|---|---|---|---|---|---|---|
| | | < 45 | 45–54 | 55–64 | 65–74 | 75 + | Total |
| **Outcome** | Survive | 20 | 14 | 27 | 18 | 13 | 92 |
| | Die | 236 | 696 | 1321 | 1750 | 1279 | 5282 |
| | | 256 | 710 | 1348 | 1768 | 1292 | 5374 |
| | Survival rates | 0.08 | 0.02 | 0.02 | 0.01 | 0.01 | 0.017 |

$$B = \bar{p}\bar{q}\left[\left(\sum_{i=1}^{k} n_i S_i^2\right) - \left(\sum_{i=1}^{k} n_i S_i\right)^2 \Big/ N\right]$$

$$= \frac{92}{5374} \times \frac{5282}{5374}$$

$$\times \left[256(1^2) + 710(2^2) + \cdots + 1292(5^2) - \frac{19,252^2}{5374}\right]$$

$$= 0.0168(75,816 - 68,969.02)$$

$$= 0.0168 \times 6846.98$$

$$= 115.03$$

Thus,

$$T_1 = \frac{(-63.58)^2}{115.03} = 35.14 \sim \chi_1^2$$

Since $\chi_{1,.999}^2 = 10.83$, it follows that $p < 0.001$. Thus, there is a highly significant inverse relationship between 3-year survival and age.

**10.92** The data are in the form of a $2 \times 2$ table, so that the chi-square test may be an appropriate method of analysis if the expected cell counts are large enough. The smallest expected value is given by $(12 \times 22)/50 = 5.28 > 5$. Thus, this is a reasonable method of analysis.

**10.93** The observed table is given as Table A.21.

**Table A.21** *Association of working status and health status*

|  | III | Well |  |
|---|---|---|---|
| Worked | 10 | 12 | 22 |
| Did not work | 2 | 26 | 28 |
|  | 12 | 38 | 50 |

We compute the following chi-square statistic:

$$\lambda = \frac{n\left(|ad - bc| - \dfrac{n}{2}\right)^2}{(a + b)(c + d)(a + c)(b + d)}$$

$$= \frac{50(|10 \times 26 - 2 \times 12| - 25)^2}{(22)(28)(12)(38)}$$

$$= \frac{50(211)^2}{(22)(28)(12)(38)} = 7.92 \sim \chi_1^2$$

Referring to our $\chi^2$ tables, we find that

$$\chi_{1,.995}^2 = 7.88, \quad \chi_{1,.999}^2 = 10.83$$

Thus, $0.001 < p < 0.005$. The authors found a chi-square of 7.8, $p = 0.01$, and thus our results are somewhat more significant than those claimed in the article.

**10.94** The $t$ test is *not* a reasonable test to use in comparing binomial proportions from two independent samples. We instead should use either the chi-square test for $2 \times 2$ tables with large expected values or Fisher's exact test for tables with small expected values.

**10.95** We have the following $2 \times 2$ table (Table A.22).

**Table A.22** *Association of salad consumption and health status*

|  |  | III | Well |  |
|---|---|---|---|---|
| Ate salad | Yes | 25 | 8 | 33 |
|  | No | 3 | 6 | 9 |
|  |  | 28 | 14 | 42 |

The smallest expected value $= (14 \times 9)/42 = 3.0 < 5$, which implies that we must use Fisher's exact test. We first rearrange the table so that the smaller row total is in row 1 and the smaller column total is in column 1, as in Table A.23.

**Table A.23**

|  |  | Well | III |  |
|---|---|---|---|---|
| Ate salad | No | 6 | 3 | 9 |
|  | Yes | 8 | 25 | 33 |
|  |  | 14 | 28 |  |

We now enumerate all tables with the same row and column margins as follows:

| 0 | 9 |
|---|---|
| 14 | 19 |

| 1 | 8 |
|---|---|
| 13 | 20 |

| 2 | 7 |
|---|---|
| 12 | 21 |

| 3 | 6 |
|---|---|
| 11 | 22 |

| 4 | 5 |
|---|---|
| 10 | 23 |

| 5 | 4 |
|---|---|
| 9 | 24 |

| 6 | 3 |
|---|---|
| 8 | 25 |

| 7 | 2 |
|---|---|
| 7 | 26 |

| 8 | 1 |
|---|---|
| 6 | 27 |

| 9 | 0 |
|---|---|
| 5 | 28 |

We now use the recursion rule to compute the exact probability of each table. We have

$$Pr(0) = 1\ Pr(0)$$

$$Pr(1) = \frac{14 \times 9}{1 \times 20} Pr(0) = 6.300\ Pr(0)$$

$$Pr(2) = \frac{13 \times 8}{2 \times 21} Pr(1) = 15.600\ Pr(0)$$

$$Pr(3) = \frac{12 \times 7}{3 \times 22} Pr(2) = 19.855\ Pr(0)$$

$$Pr(4) = \frac{11 \times 6}{4 \times 23} Pr(3) = 14.244\ Pr(0)$$

$$Pr(5) = \frac{10 \times 5}{5 \times 24} Pr(4) = 5.935\ Pr(0)$$

$$Pr(6) = \frac{9 \times 4}{6 \times 25} Pr(5) = 1.424\ Pr(0)$$

$$Pr(7) = \frac{8 \times 3}{7 \times 26} Pr(6) = 0.188\ Pr(0)$$

$$Pr(8) = \frac{7 \times 2}{8 \times 27} Pr(7) = 0.012\ Pr(0)$$

$$Pr(9) = \frac{6 \times 1}{9 \times 28} Pr(8) = 0.00029\ Pr(0)$$

Thus,

$$Pr(0)(1 + 6.300 + 15.600 + 19.855 + 14.244 + 5.935 + 1.424 + 0.188 + 0.012 + 0.00029) = 1$$

or

$$Pr(0) = \frac{1}{64.558} = 0.0155.$$

$$Pr(1) = 0.098$$

$$Pr(2) = 0.242$$

$$Pr(3) = 0.308$$

$$Pr(4) = 0.221$$

$$Pr(5) = 0.092$$

$$Pr(6) = 0.022$$

$$Pr(7) = 0.003$$

$$Pr(8) = 0.0002$$

$$Pr(9) = 4.50 \times 10^{-6}$$

Since our observed table is the "6" table, the two-sided *p*-value is given by

$$p = 2 \times \min\left[\sum_{i=0}^{6} Pr(i), \sum_{i=6}^{9} Pr(i)\right]$$

$$= 2 \times \min(0.999, 0.0252) = 0.050$$

Thus, the results are on the margin of being statistically significant ($p = 0.05$) as opposed to the *p*-value of 0.01 given in the paper.

# Chapter 11

*11.1* We have that

$$L_{xx} = \sum x_i^2 - \frac{(\sum x_i)^2}{n}$$

$$= 54{,}749 - \frac{(1137)^2}{27}$$

$$= 54{,}749 - 47{,}880.33$$

$$= 6868.67$$

$$L_{xy} = \sum x_i y_i - \frac{(\sum x_i)(\sum y_i)}{n}$$

$$= 262.93 - \frac{(1137)(6.05)}{27}$$

$$= 262.93 - 254.77$$

$$= 8.16$$

$$b = \frac{L_{xy}}{L_{xx}}$$

$$= \frac{8.16}{6868.67}$$

$$= 0.0012$$

$$a = \frac{\sum y_i - b \sum x_i}{n}$$

$$= \frac{6.05 - 0.0012(1137)}{27}$$

$$= \frac{6.05 - 1.364}{27}$$

$$= \frac{4.686}{27}$$

$$= 0.174$$

Thus, the regression line is given by $y = 0.174 + 0.0012x$.

**11.2** The expected LVEF $= 0.174 + 0.0012(45) = 0.174 + 0.054 = 0.228$.

**11.3** We must first compute $L_{yy}$. We have

$$L_{yy} = \sum y_i^2 - \frac{(\sum y_i)^2}{n}$$

$$= 1.522 - \frac{(6.05)^2}{27}$$

$$= 1.522 - 1.356$$

$$= 0.166$$

We now compute the regression and residual sum of squares and mean square:

$$\text{Reg SS} = \frac{L_{xy}^2}{L_{xx}} = \frac{(8.16)^2}{6868.67} = 0.0097 = \text{Reg MS}$$

$$\text{Res SS} = 0.166 - 0.0097 = 0.156$$

$$\text{Res MS} = \frac{0.156}{25} = 0.0062$$

Finally, the $F$ statistic is given by $\lambda = \text{Reg MS}/\text{Res MS} = 0.0097/0.0062 = 1.56 \sim F_{1,25}$ under $H_0$. Since $F_{1,25,.95} > F_{1,30,.95} = 4.17 > 1.56$, it follows that $p > 0.05$. Therefore, we accept $H_0$ and conclude that there is no significant relationship between LVEF and age.

**11.4** $R^2 = \text{Reg SS}/\text{Total SS} = 0.0097/0.166 = 0.058$.

**11.5** It means that only 5.8% of the variance in LVEF is explained by age.

**11.6** We need to compute the standard error of the estimated slope as follows:

$$se(b) = \sqrt{\frac{\text{Res MS}}{L_{xx}}}$$

$$= \sqrt{\frac{0.0062}{6868.67}}$$

$$= 0.0010$$

Thus, the t statistic is given by

$$\gamma = \frac{b}{se(b)}$$

$$= \frac{0.0012}{0.0010}$$

$$= 1.20 \sim t_{25} \text{ under } H_0$$

Since $t_{25,.975} = 2.060 > \gamma$, it follows that $p > 0.05$, and we accept $H_0$ at the 5% level.

**11.7** $se(b) = 0.0010$ as given in Problem 11.6. The standard error of the intercept is given by

$$se(a) = \sqrt{\text{Res MS}\left(\frac{1}{n} + \frac{\bar{x}^2}{L_{xx}}\right)}$$

$$= \sqrt{0.0062\left[\frac{1}{27} + \frac{(1137/27)^2}{6868.67}\right]}$$

$$= \sqrt{0.0062(0.0370 + 0.2582)}$$

$$= \sqrt{(0.0062)(0.2952)}$$

$$= 0.043$$

**11.8** A 95% confidence interval for the slope is given by

$$b \pm t_{25,.975}\text{se}(b) = 0.0012 \pm 2.060(0.0010)$$

$$= 0.0012 \pm 0.0021$$

$$= (-0.0009, 0.0033)$$

A 95% confidence interval for the intercept is given by

$$a \pm t_{25,.975}\text{se}(a) = 0.174 \pm 2.060(0.043)$$

$$= 0.174 \pm 0.089$$

$$= (0.085, 0.263)$$

**11.20** We refer to Table 11 under $r = 0.34$ to obtain $z = 0.354$.

**11.26** We have the test statistic

$$T_s = \frac{r_s\sqrt{n-2}}{\sqrt{1-r_s^2}}$$

$$= \frac{0.4\sqrt{28}}{\sqrt{1-0.4^2}}$$

$$= \frac{0.4(5.292)}{\sqrt{0.84}}$$

$$= \frac{2.117}{0.917}$$

$$= 2.309 \sim t_{28} \text{ under } H_0$$

We are performing a one-tailed test. Thus, the critical value $= t_{28,.95} = 1.701 < T_s$. Therefore, we reject $H_0$ at the 5% level and conclude that the rank correlation is significantly greater than 0.

**11.27** Since $t_{28,.975} = 2.048$, $t_{28,.99} = 2.467$, and $2.048 < 2.309 < 2.467$, the one-tailed $p$-value is given by $1 - 0.99 < p < 1 - 0.975$, or $0.01 < p < 0.025$.

**11.28** Since $n < 10$, we must use the exact tables for the Spearman rank correlation coefficient. We refer to Table 12 under $n = 8$ and note that the two-tailed critical value for $\alpha = 0.10$ and 0.05 are 0.643 and 0.738, respectively. Since $0.643 < 0.7 < 0.738$, it follows that the two-tailed $p$-value is given by $0.05 \leqslant p < 0.10$. Therefore, the one-tailed $p$-value is given by $0.025 \leqslant p < 0.05$.

**11.33** Let $y =$ duration of hospitalization and $x =$ age. We must compute

$$L_{xx} = \sum_{i=1}^{n}(x_i - \bar{x})^2 = \sum_{i=1}^{n}x_i^2 - \frac{\left(\sum_{i=1}^{n}x_i\right)^2}{n}$$

$$= 52{,}217 - \frac{(1031)^2}{25} = 9698.56$$

$$L_{xy} = \sum_{i=1}^{n}(x_i - \bar{x})(y_i - \bar{y}) = \sum_{i=1}^{n}x_iy_i - \frac{\left(\sum_{i=1}^{n}x_i\right)\left(\sum_{i=1}^{n}y_i\right)}{n}$$

$$= 9869 - \frac{(1031)(215)}{25} = 1002.40$$

The least squares coefficients are then given by

$$b = L_{xy}/L_{xx} = 1002.40/9698.56 = 0.103$$

$$a = \frac{\sum_{i=1}^{n}y_i - b\sum_{i=1}^{n}x_i}{n} = \frac{215 - 0.103(1031)}{25} = 4.35$$

Thus, the regression line is $y = 4.35 + 0.103x$.

**11.34** To test for the significance of this relationship, we must assume an underlying model of the form

$$y_i = \alpha + \beta x_i + e_i \quad \text{where } e_i \sim N(0, \sigma^2)$$

Furthermore, under $H_0: \beta = 0$, whereas under $H_1: \beta \neq 0$. We set up the ANOVA table as follows:

$$\text{Regression SS} = L_{xy}^2/L_{xx} = (1002.40)^2/9698.56 = 103.60$$

$$\text{Total SS} = L_{yy} = \sum_{i=1}^{n}(y_i - \bar{y})^2 = \sum_{i=1}^{n}y_i^2 - \frac{\left(\sum_{i=1}^{n}y_i\right)^2}{n}$$

$$= 2633 - (215)^2/25 = 784$$

$$\text{Residual SS} = \text{Total SS} - \text{Regression SS}$$

$$= 784 - 103.6 = 680.4$$

*ANOVA Table*

|  | SS | df | MS | F statistic |
|---|---|---|---|---|
| Regression | 103.60 | 1 | 103.60 | 3.50 |
| Residual | 680.40 | 23 | 29.58 | |
|  | 784.00 | 24 | | |

We test for significance by noting that

$$\lambda = \text{Regression MS/Residual MS} = 3.50 \sim F_{1,23} \text{ under } H_0.$$

Since

$$F_{1,23,.95} > F_{1,30,.95} = 4.17 > \lambda$$

it follows that $p > 0.05$. Also, since

$$F_{1,23,.90} < F_{1,20,.90} = 2.97 < \lambda$$

it follows that $p < 0.10$. Thus, the $p$-value is given by $0.05 < p < 0.10$, and there is only a trend toward significance in this case.

**11.35** $R^2$ is defined as Regression SS/Total SS = $103.6/784 = 0.132$.

**11.40** We compute the correlation coefficient between THW and BW in each of the two groups. We first have the following summary statistics ($x = $ THW, $y = $ BW):

| Left heart disease | Normal |
|---|---|
| $\sum_{i=1}^{11} x_i = 4950$ | $\sum_{i=1}^{10} x_i = 3170$ |
| $\sum_{i=1}^{11} x_i^2 = 2{,}421{,}650$ | $\sum_{i=1}^{10} x_i^2 = 1{,}024{,}850$ |
| $\sum_{i=1}^{11} y_i = 611.70$ | $\sum_{i=1}^{10} y_i = 562.3$ |
| $\sum_{i=1}^{11} y_i^2 = 35{,}350.49$ | $\sum_{i=1}^{10} y_i^2 = 32{,}816.33$ |
| $\sum_{i=1}^{11} x_i y_i = 280{,}031.50$ | $\sum_{i=1}^{10} x_i y_i = 181{,}462$ |
| $L_{xx} = 194{,}150$ | $L_{xx} = 19{,}960$ |
| $L_{yy} = 1334.41$ | $L_{yy} = 1198.20$ |
| $L_{xy} = 4766.50$ | $L_{xy} = 3212.9$ |
| $r = L_{xy}/(L_{xx}L_{yy})^{1/2}$ | $r = L_{xy}/(L_{xx}L_{yy})^{1/2}$ |
| $= 0.296$ | $= 0.657$ |
| $\lambda = r\sqrt{n-2}/\sqrt{1-r^2}$ | $\lambda = r\sqrt{n-2}/\sqrt{1-r^2}$ |
| $= 0.296(3)/\sqrt{1-0.296^2}$ | $= 0.657\sqrt{8}/\sqrt{1-0.657^2}$ |
| $= 0.93 \sim t_9, \text{ NS}$ | $= 2.465 \sim t_8, 0.02$ |
| | $< p < 0.05$ |

Thus, there is a significant association between total heart weight and body weight in the normal group but not in the left heart disease group. This confirms what we saw graphically in Problem 2.7.

**11.79** We test the hypotheses $H_0: \rho = 0$ vs. $H_1: \rho \neq 0$. We use the test statistic

$$\lambda = \frac{r\sqrt{n-2}}{\sqrt{1-r^2}} \sim t_{n-2} \text{ under } H_0$$

In this case

$$r = \frac{L_{xy}}{\sqrt{L_{xx}L_{yy}}}$$

We have

$$L_{xx} = 451{,}350 - \frac{(2980)^2}{20} = 7330$$

$$L_{yy} = 351{,}350 - \frac{(2620)^2}{20} = 8130$$

$$L_{xy} = 390{,}825 - \frac{(2980)(2620)}{20} = 445$$

Thus,

$$r = \frac{445}{\sqrt{7330 \times 8130}} = \frac{445}{7719.64} = 0.058$$

The test statistic

$$\lambda = \frac{0.058\sqrt{18}}{\sqrt{1-(0.058)^2}} = \frac{0.246}{0.998} = 0.246 \sim t_{18}$$

Since $t_{18,.975} = 2.101$, this is clearly not statistically significant, and there is no significant correlation between the mother and father's bp, which is what we would expect on purely genetic grounds.

**11.80** We wish to compute

$$r_{yt} = \frac{L_{yt}}{\sqrt{L_{yy} \times L_{tt}}}$$

We have

$$L_{tt} = 210{,}850 - \frac{(2030)^2}{20} = 4805$$

$$L_{yt} = 269{,}550 - \frac{(2620)(2030)}{20} = 3620$$

and

$$r = \frac{3620}{\sqrt{8130 \times 4805}} = \frac{3620}{6250.17} = 0.579$$

We want to test the null hypothesis $H_0 : \rho = 0.5$ vs. the alternative $H_1 : \rho \neq 0.5$. We use the Fisher $z$ test, giving us

$$z = \tfrac{1}{2}[\ln(1 + r) - \ln(1 - r)] = \tfrac{1}{2}[\ln(1.579) - \ln(0.421)]$$

$$= \tfrac{1}{2}(0.4568 + 0.8651) = 0.661$$

Also, from Table 11 we have $z_0 = 0.549$. We use the test statistic

$$\lambda = (z - z_0)\sqrt{n - 3} \sim N(0, 1) \text{ under } H_0$$

Thus,

$$\lambda = \sqrt{17}(0.661 - 0.549) = 0.462 \sim N(0, 1)$$

The $p$-value $= 2 \times [1 - \Phi(0.462)] = 0.64$. We thus accept $H_0$ that $\rho = 0.5$.

**11.81** The mother and first-born child were both living in the same environment, which might explain all or part of the observed correlation of blood pressure.

**11.82** We use the model $t = \alpha + \beta y + e$. We wish to test the null hypothesis that $\beta = 0$ vs. the alternative hypothesis that $\beta \neq 0$. We have

$$b = \frac{L_{ty}}{L_{yy}}$$

where

$$L_{ty} = 3620$$

$$L_{yy} = 8130 \qquad \text{from Problems 11.79 and 11.80}$$

Thus,

$$b = \frac{3620}{8130} = 0.445$$

Furthermore,

$$a = \frac{\sum_{i=1}^{20} t_i - b \sum_{i=1}^{20} y_i}{20} = \frac{2030 - 0.445(2620)}{20} = 43.2$$

We thus have the linear relation $t = 43.2 + 0.445y$.

**11.83** We wish to test the hypothesis $H_0 : \beta = 0$ vs.

$H_1 : \beta \neq 0$. We use the test statistic

$$\lambda = \frac{\text{Reg MS}}{\text{Res MS}} \sim F_{1, n-2} \text{ under } H_0$$

We have

$$\text{Reg MS} = \frac{(L_{ty})^2}{L_{yy}} = \frac{(3620)^2}{8130} = 1611.86 = \text{Reg SS}$$

$$\text{Res MS} = \frac{L_{tt} - \text{Reg SS}}{18} = \frac{L_{tt} - 1611.86}{18}$$

Thus,

$$\text{Res MS} = \frac{4805 - 1611.86}{18} = 177.40 = s_{t \cdot y}^2$$

and

$$\lambda = \frac{1611.86}{177.40} = 9.09 \sim F_{1, 18} \text{ under } H_0$$

Since $F_{1, 18, .99} = 8.29$, $F_{1, 18, .995} = 10.22$, we have $0.005 < p < 0.01$, and there is a significant relationship between the mother and child's bp.

**11.84** We can predict the child's bp from the mother's bp from the relationship in Problem 11.82. We have $E(t) = 43.2 + 0.445 \times 130 = 101.1$ mm.

**11.85** In this case $E(t) = 43.2 + 0.445 \times 150 = 110.0$ mm.

**11.86** In this case $E(t) = 43.2 + 0.445 \times 170 = 118.9$ mm.

**11.87** The standard errors are given by the formula

$$se = \sqrt{s_{t \cdot y}^2 \left[ \frac{1}{n} + \frac{(y - \bar{y})^2}{L_{yy}} \right]} = \sqrt{177.40 \left[ \frac{1}{20} + \frac{(y - \bar{y})^2}{8130} \right]}$$

We have

$$\bar{y} = \frac{2620}{20} = 131$$

Thus, for $y = 130, 150,$ and $170$ mm, we have, respectively,

$$se(130) = \sqrt{177.40 \left[ \frac{1}{20} + \frac{(130 - 131)^2}{8130} \right]} = 2.98$$

$$se(150) = \sqrt{177.40 \left[ \frac{1}{20} + \frac{(150 - 131)^2}{8130} \right]} = 4.09$$

$$se(170) = \sqrt{177.40 \left[ \frac{1}{20} + \frac{(170 - 131)^2}{8130} \right]} = 6.49$$

**11.88** The three standard errors are not the same because the standard error increases the further the value of the mother's bp is from the mean bp for all mothers (131). Thus, the *se* corresponding to 130 is smallest, whereas the *se* corresponding to 170 is largest.

**11.89** To test for the independent effect of the father's bp on the child's bp after controlling for the effect of the mother's bp, we should test the hypothesis $H_0: \beta_1 = 0$, $\beta_2 \neq 0$ vs. $H_1: \beta_1 \neq 0, \beta_2 \neq 0$. Similarly, to test for the independent effect of the mother's bp on the child's bp after controlling for the effect of the father's bp, we should test the hypothesis $H_0: \beta_2 = 0, \beta_1 \neq 0$ vs. $H_1: \beta_2 \neq 0, \beta_1 \neq 0$.

**11.90** We compute the following test statistics:

$$\text{Father:}\quad \gamma_1 = b_1/se(b_1) = 0.4150/0.1248$$

$$= 3.33 \sim t_{17}, 0.001 < p < 0.01$$

$$\text{Mother:}\quad \gamma_2 = b_2/se(b_2) = 0.4226/0.1185$$

$$= 3.57 \sim t_{17}, 0.001 < p < 0.01$$

Thus, each parent's bp is significantly associated with the child's bp after controlling for the other spouse's bp.

**11.91** We have from Problems 11.79 and 11.80 that

$$s_t^2 = \frac{L_{tt}}{n-1} = \frac{4805}{19} = 252.89$$

$$s_x^2 = \frac{L_{xx}}{n-1} = \frac{7330}{19} = 385.79$$

$$s_y^2 = \frac{L_{yy}}{n-1} = \frac{8130}{19} = 427.89$$

The standardized regression coefficients are given by

Father: $b_s = b \times s_x/s_t$

$$= 0.4150 \times \sqrt{\frac{385.79}{252.89}} = 0.513$$

Mother: $b_s = b \times s_y/s_t$

$$= 0.4226 \times \sqrt{\frac{427.89}{252.89}} = 0.550$$

The standardized coefficients represent the increase in the number of standard deviations in the child's bp we would expect per standard deviation increase in the parent's bp after controlling for the other spouse's bp.

**11.92** The correlation is given by

$$r = \frac{L_{xy}}{\sqrt{L_{xx} \times L_{yy}}}$$

We have

$$L_{xy} = -4.12 - \frac{(2.38)(-15.55)}{8} = 0.506$$

$$L_{xx} = 1.31 - \frac{(2.38)^2}{8} = 0.602$$

$$L_{yy} = 30.71 - \frac{(-15.55)^2}{8} = 0.485$$

Thus,

$$r = \frac{0.506}{\sqrt{(0.602)(0.485)}} = 0.936$$

**11.93** We use the test statistic

$$\lambda = \frac{r\sqrt{n-2}}{\sqrt{1-r^2}} \sim t_{n-2} \text{ under } H_0$$

In this case

$$\lambda = \frac{0.936\sqrt{6}}{\sqrt{1-0.936^2}} = \frac{2.293}{0.352} = 6.51 \sim t_6 \text{ under } H_0$$

We refer to the *t* table and find that $t_{6,.9995} = 5.959 < \lambda$, which implies that $p < 0.001$. Thus, there is a highly significant association between the lung cancer mortality rate and average cigarette consumption over a 40-year period.

**11.94** It is also of interest to fit a regression line to these data of the form $y = a + bx$, where

$$b = \frac{L_{xy}}{L_{xx}} = \frac{0.506}{0.602} = 0.841$$

$$a = \frac{\sum_{i=1}^{8} y_i - b \sum_{i=1}^{8} x_i}{8} = \frac{-15.55 - 0.841(2.38)}{8} = -2.19$$

Thus, the regression line is $y = -2.19 + 0.841x$.

**11.95** No. It is unnecessary, since the *t* test in Problem 11.93 based on the correlation coefficient and the *F* test based on the regression coefficient are equivalent.

**11.96** The expected $\log_{10}$(mortality rate) $= -2.19 + 0.841 \times \log_{10}(1) = -2.19$. Thus, the expected mortality rate $= 10^{-2.19} = 0.00646$, or 646 deaths per 100,000.

**11.97** The variables are expressed in the log scale because the relationship between mortality rate and cigarette consumption is most likely to be linear when each is expressed in this scale rather than in the raw scale.

# *C*hapter 12

**12.1** Bartlett's test for homogeneity of variance.

**12.2** The test statistic is given by

$$\lambda^* = \sum_{i=1}^{3} [(n_i - 1) \ln(s^2/s_i^2)]/C \sim \chi_2^2 \text{ under } H_0$$

where $s^2$ is the pooled variance estimate. We have

$$s^2 = \frac{9(16)^2 + 9(16)^2 + 9(9)^2}{27}$$

$$= \frac{5337}{27}$$

$$= 198$$

$$C = 1 + \frac{1}{3(2)}\left(\frac{1}{9} + \frac{1}{9} + \frac{1}{9} - \frac{1}{27}\right)$$

$$= 1 + \frac{1}{6}\left(\frac{8}{27}\right) = 1.049$$

$$\lambda^* = \frac{9\ln\left(\frac{198}{256}\right) + 9\ln\left(\frac{198}{256}\right) + 9\ln\left(\frac{198}{81}\right)}{1.049}$$

$$= \frac{9(-0.257 - 0.257 + 0.894)}{1.049}$$

$$= \frac{9(0.380)}{1.049}$$

$$= \frac{3.420}{1.049}$$

$$= 3.26 \sim \chi_2^2 \text{ under } H_0$$

Since $\chi_{2,.95}^2 = 5.99 > \lambda^*$, it follows that we accept $H_0$ at the 5% level. Since $\chi_{2,.75}^2 = 2.77$, $\chi_{2,.90}^2 = 4.61$, and $2.77 < 3.26 < 4.61$, it follows that $1 - 0.90 < p < 1 - 0.75$, or $0.10 < p < 0.25$.

**12.3** Since the variances are not significantly different, we can use a one-way ANOVA.

**12.4** The test statistic is given by $\lambda =$ Between MS/Within MS $\sim F_{k-1, n-k}$ under $H_0$. We have

$$\text{Between SS} = 10(74)^2 + 10(56)^2 + 10(55)^2$$

$$- \frac{[10(74) + 10(56) + 10(55)]^2}{30}$$

$$= 54,760 + 31,360 + 30,250 - 114,083.33$$

$$= 116,370 - 114,083.33$$

$$= 2286.7$$

$$\text{Between MS} = \frac{2286.7}{2} = 1143$$

Within MS $= s^2 = 198$ (from Problem 12.2)

Therefore,

$$\lambda = \frac{1143}{198} = 5.77 \sim F_{2,27} \text{ under } H_0$$

Since $F_{2,27,.95} < F_{2,20,.95} = 3.49 < \lambda$, it follows that $p < 0.05$, and we reject $H_0$ at the 5% level.

**12.5** We use the test statistic $\delta = (\bar{y}_1 - \bar{y}_2)/\sqrt{s^2(1/n_1 + 1/n_2)} \sim t_{n-k}$ under $H_0$. The results are given as follows for each pair of groups.

| Groups compared | Test statistic | | p-value |
|---|---|---|---|
| STD, LAC | $\delta = \dfrac{74 - 56}{\sqrt{198(1/10 + 1/10)}}$ | $= \dfrac{18}{6.293} = 2.86 \sim t_{27}$ | $0.001 < p < 0.01$ |
| STD, VEG | $\delta = \dfrac{74 - 55}{6.293}$ | $= \dfrac{19}{6.293} = 3.02 \sim t_{27}$ | $0.001 < p < 0.01$ |
| LAC, VEG | $\delta = \dfrac{56 - 55}{6.293}$ | $= \dfrac{1}{6.293} = 0.16 \sim t_{27}$ | NS |

**12.6** This contrast is a comparison of the general vegetarian population with the general nonvegetarian population. We compute the test statistic

$$\lambda = \frac{L}{se(L)} \sim t_{n-k} \text{ under } H_0$$

$$= \frac{0.7(56) + 0.3(55) - 74}{\sqrt{198[(0.7)^2/10 + (0.3)^2/10 + (-1)^2/10]}}$$

$$= \frac{-18.3}{\sqrt{31.284}}$$

$$= \frac{-18.3}{5.593} = -3.27 \sim t_{27} \text{ under } H_0$$

Since $t_{27,.995} = 2.771$, and $t_{27,.9995} = 3.690$, it follows that $0.001 < p < 0.01$, and we reject $H_0$ and conclude that among premenopausal women, the general vegetarian population has a significantly lower protein intake than the general nonvegetarian population.

**12.13** We refer to Table 13 under $\alpha = 0.01$, $c = 5$, $d = 30$ to obtain $q_{5,30,.99} = 5.05$.

**12.16** We first compare groups 1–3, where 1 = STD, 2 = LAC, 3 = VEG. We have the studentized range statistic

$$q = \frac{74 - 55}{\sqrt{\frac{198}{2} \times \left(\frac{1}{10} + \frac{1}{10}\right)}}$$

$$= \frac{19}{4.450} = 4.27 > q_{3,24,.95} = 3.53 > q_{3,27,.95}$$

Therefore, $p < 0.05$, and we conclude that some of the means are significantly different. We now compare

groups 1–2 and 2–3. We have the following computations:

$$\text{Groups 1–2: } q = \frac{74 - 56}{4.450} = \frac{18}{4.450} = 4.04 > q_{2,24,.95}$$

$$= 2.92 > q_{2,27,.95}$$

$$\text{Groups 2–3: } q = \frac{56 - 55}{4.450} = \frac{1}{4.450} = 0.22 < q_{2,30,.95}$$

$$= 2.89 < q_{2,27,.95}$$

Therefore, we conclude that groups 1 and 2 are significantly different, whereas groups 2 and 3 are not. In summary, we conclude that the protein intake of the standard American diet group is significantly higher than the lactovegetarian and vegetarian groups, whereas there is no significant difference between the latter two groups.

**12.20** The two-way analysis of variance.

**12.21** We use the method of unweighted means since max $n_{ij}$/min $n_{ij} = 10/6 = 1.7 \leqslant 2$. The two-way table of means by dietary group and menopausal status is presented as follows:

| | | | Menopausal status | | |
| | | | Pre-menopausal | Post-menopausal | $y_{i.}^{*}$ |
|---|---|---|---|---|---|
| Dietary group | STD | Mean | 74 | 75 | 149 |
| | | sd | 16 | 9 | |
| | | n | 10 | 10 | |
| | LAC | Mean | 56 | 57 | 113 |
| | | sd | 16 | 13 | |
| | | n | 10 | 10 | |
| | VEG | Mean | 55 | 47 | 102 |
| | | sd | 9 | 17 | |
| | | n | 10 | 6 | |
| | | $y_{.j}^{*}$ | 185 | 179 | 364 |

The row and column sums of squares and mean squares are given by

$$\text{Row SS} = \frac{149^2 + 113^2 + 102^2}{2} - \frac{(149 + 113 + 102)^2}{3 \times 2}$$

$$= 22{,}687 - 22{,}082.67 = 604.33$$

$$\text{Row MS} = \frac{604.33}{2} = 302.17$$

Col SS $= \dfrac{185^2 + 179^2}{3} - \dfrac{(185 + 179)^2}{3 \times 2}$

$\quad = 22{,}088.67 - 22{,}082.67 = 6.00 =$ Col MS

To compute the Error MS, we need to compute $n_h$, where

$1/n_h = \dfrac{(1/10 + 1/10 + \cdots + 1/6)}{6} = 0.1111$

$n_h = 9.0$

Thus,

Error MS $= \dfrac{9(16)^2 + 9(9)^2 + \cdots + 5(17)^2}{50(9)}$

$\quad = \dfrac{9032}{450} = 20.071$

We compute the test statistics to identify significant row and column effects. We have

$\lambda_{\text{ROW}} = \dfrac{302.17}{20.071} = 15.06 \sim F_{2,50}$ under $H_0$

$\lambda_{\text{COL}} = \dfrac{6.00}{20.071} = 0.30 \sim F_{1,50}$ under $H_0$

Since $\lambda_{\text{ROW}} = 15.06 > F_{2,40,.95} = 3.23 > F_{2,50,.95}$, it follows that $p < 0.05$ and there are significant row effects. Since $\lambda_{\text{COL}} = 0.30 < F_{1,60,.95} = 4.00 < F_{1,50,.95}$, it follows that $p > 0.05$ and there are no significant column effects. In summary, there are significant differences in protein intake between different dietary groups but not between different menopausal groups.

**12.22** We have that

Int SS $= 74^2 + 75^2 + \cdots + 47^2$

$\qquad - \dfrac{(74 + 75 + \cdots + 47)^2}{6} - 604.33 - 6.00$

$\quad = 22{,}720 - \dfrac{364^2}{6} - 610.33$

$\quad = 22{,}720 - 22{,}082.67 - 610.33 = 27.00$

Int MS $= \dfrac{27.00}{2} = 13.50$

Furthermore,

$\lambda_{\text{INT}} = \dfrac{13.50}{20.071} = 0.67 \sim F_{2,50}$ under $H_0$

Since $\lambda_{\text{INT}} = 0.67 < F_{2,60,.95} = 3.15 < F_{2,50,.95}$, it follows that $p > 0.05$ and there are no significant interaction effects.

**12.23** In this instance the interaction effect, if it were present, would indicate that the differences in protein intake among diet groups are not the same for premenopausal and postmenopausal women. Since the interaction effect was not significant, it indicates that the diet group differences are similar for premenopausal and postmenopausal women.

**12.24** A one-way ANOVA is appropriate here because the three groups are classified according to only one variable—alcohol consumption.

**12.25** We first perform Bartlett's test for homogeneity of variance to ensure that we can validly use the overall $F$ test for a one-way ANOVA. We have the test statistic

$$\lambda^* = \dfrac{\lambda}{c} \sim \chi^2_{k-1} \text{ under } H_0$$

where

$$\lambda = \sum_{i=1}^{k} (n_i - 1) \ln \left( \dfrac{s^2}{s_i^2} \right)$$

$$c = 1 + \dfrac{1}{3(k-1)} \left[ \left( \sum_{i=1}^{k} \dfrac{1}{n_i - 1} \right) - \dfrac{1}{n - k} \right]$$

We have

$s^2 =$ Within MS $= \dfrac{22(25.3)^2 + 14(21.9)^2 + 11(30.3)^2}{47}$

$\quad = \dfrac{30{,}895.51}{47}$

$\quad = 657.35$

Thus,

$\lambda = 22 \ln \left[ \dfrac{657.35}{(25.3)^2} \right] + 14 \ln \left[ \dfrac{657.35}{(21.9)^2} \right] + 11 \ln \left[ \dfrac{657.35}{(30.3)^2} \right]$

$\quad = 0.585 + 4.413 - 3.675$

$\quad = 1.323$

$$c = 1 + \frac{1}{3(2)}\left(\frac{1}{22} + \frac{1}{14} + \frac{1}{11} - \frac{1}{47}\right) = 1.031$$

$$\lambda^* = \frac{1.323}{1.031} = 1.28 \sim \chi_2^2 \text{ under } H_0$$

Since $\chi_{2,.95}^2 = 5.99 > \lambda^*$, it follows that $p > 0.05$. Thus, the variances are not significantly different, and we can validly use the $F$ test to test for overall differences between means. We use the test statistic

$$\lambda = \frac{\text{Between MS}}{\text{Within MS}} \sim F_{k-1,n-k} \text{ under } H_0$$

We have

$$\text{Between MS} = \frac{(205.6)^2 23 + (182.7)^2 15 + (199.8)^2 12}{2}$$

$$- \frac{[(205.6)(23) + (182.7)15 + (199.8)12]^2}{50(2)}$$

$$= \frac{1,951,971.11 - 1,947,114.31}{2}$$

$$= \frac{4856.80}{2} = 2428.40$$

Within MS $= s^2 = 657.35$

Thus,

$$\lambda = \frac{\text{Between MS}}{\text{Within MS}} = \frac{2428.40}{657.35} = 3.69 \sim F_{2,47} \text{ under } H_0$$

Since $F_{2,47,.95} < F_{2,40,.95} = 3.23 < \lambda$, it follows that $p < 0.05$, and there is an overall significant difference between groups.

*12.26* We first order the three groups from highest to lowest cholesterol level as given in Table A.24.

**Table A.24** *Association between cholesterol level and alcohol consumption*

| Group number | Group name | Mean | n |
|---|---|---|---|
| 1 | Nondrinkers | 205.6 | 23 |
| 2 | Heavy drinkers | 199.8 | 12 |
| 3 | Light drinkers | 182.7 | 15 |

We then compare groups 1–3 using the $q$ statistic in **(12.15)** as follows:

$$q = \frac{205.6 - 182.7}{\sqrt{\frac{657.35}{2}\left(\frac{1}{23} + \frac{1}{15}\right)}} = \frac{22.9}{6.02} = 3.80$$

**Table A.25** *Comparison of specific groups using the method of multiple comparisons*

| Groups compared | Test statistic | | Reference value | Statistically significant (yes/no) |
|---|---|---|---|---|
| 1–2 | $q = \dfrac{205.6 - 199.8}{\sqrt{\dfrac{657.35}{2}\left(\dfrac{1}{23} + \dfrac{1}{12}\right)}}$ | $= \dfrac{5.8}{6.46} = 0.90$ | $q_{2,47,.95} = 2.85^*$ | No |
| 2–3 | $q = \dfrac{199.8 - 182.7}{\sqrt{\dfrac{657.35}{2}\left(\dfrac{1}{12} + \dfrac{1}{15}\right)}}$ | $= \dfrac{17.1}{7.02} = 2.44$ | 2.85 | No |

$^*q_{2,47,.95}$ is approximated by $\dfrac{(\frac{1}{47} - \frac{1}{60})q_{2,40,.95} + (\frac{1}{40} - \frac{1}{47})q_{2,60,.95}}{\frac{1}{40} - \frac{1}{60}}$

$$= \frac{(0.0046)(2.86) + (0.0037)(2.83)}{(0.0083)} = 2.85$$

We compare this value to $q_{3,47,.95}$, since we are comparing three groups and $s^2$ is estimated with 47 $df$. We have that $q_{3,47,.95} < q_{3,40,.95} = 3.44 < 3.80$. Thus, groups 1 and 3 are significantly different. We now compare each pair of groups, as given in Table A.25.

Thus, neither of these comparisons are significant, and we can only say that nondrinkers (group 1) have significantly higher cholesterol levels than light drinkers (group 3).

**12.39** A one-way ANOVA should be used on these data because there is only one effect that distinguishes the groups, namely, the mother's smoking status during pregnancy.

**12.40** Table A.26 shows the basic statistics for the four groups.

We test for the homogeneity of the variances using Bartlett's test. We have the test statistic

$$\lambda^* = \sum_{i=1}^{k} (n_i - 1) \ln(s^2/s_i^2)/c \sim \chi_{k-1}^2 \text{ under } H_0$$

$$s^2 = \frac{6(0.925) + 4(0.833) + 6(1.299) + 7(0.518)}{23} = 0.883$$

$$\lambda^* = \left[ 6 \ln\left(\frac{0.883}{0.925}\right) + 4 \ln\left(\frac{0.883}{0.833}\right) + 6 \ln\left(\frac{0.883}{1.299}\right) \right.$$

$$\left. + 7 \ln\left(\frac{0.883}{0.518}\right) \right] \bigg/ c = 1.372/c$$

$$c = 1 + \frac{1}{3(3)} \left[ \frac{1}{6} + \frac{1}{4} + \frac{1}{6} + \frac{1}{7} - \frac{1}{23} \right] = 1 + \frac{1}{9}(0.683)$$

$$= 1.076$$

$$\lambda^* = \frac{1.372}{1.076} = 1.275 \sim \chi_3^2 \text{ under } H_0$$

Since $\chi_{3,.95}^2 = 7.81 > \lambda^*$, it follows that $p > 0.05$. Thus, we accept the null hypothesis that the four within-sample population variances are the same.

**12.41** We perform a one-way ANOVA. We have

$$\text{Between SS} = \frac{\sum_{i=1}^{4} y_{i.}^2}{n_i} - \frac{y_{..}^2}{n}$$

$$= \frac{53.1^2}{7} + \frac{36.2^2}{5} + \frac{44.3^2}{7} + \frac{48.1^2}{8} - \frac{181.7^2}{27}$$

$$= 1234.446 - 1222.774$$

$$= 11.672$$

$$\text{Total SS} = \sum_{i=1}^{4} \sum_{j=1}^{n_i} y_{ij}^2 - \frac{y_{..}^2}{n}$$

$$= 7.5^2 + \cdots + 5.4^2 - \frac{181.7^2}{27}$$

$$= 1254.750 - 1222.774$$

$$= 31.976$$

$$\text{Within SS} = \text{Total SS} - \text{Between SS}$$

$$= 31.976 - 11.672$$

$$= 20.304$$

Thus, the ANOVA table is as follows:

|  | SS | df | MS | F stat | p-value |
|---|---|---|---|---|---|
| Between | 11.672 | 3 | 3.891 | 4.41 | $0.01 < p < 0.025$ |
| Within | 20.304 | 23 | 0.883 |  |  |
|  | 31.976 | 26 |  |  |  |

***Table A.26*** *Relationship between smoking habit during pregnancy and birthweight*

| Group | Mean | sd | Variance | n |
|---|---|---|---|---|
| Nonsmoker (NON) | 7.59 | 0.962 | 0.925 | 7 |
| Ex-smoker (EX) | 7.24 | 0.913 | 0.833 | 5 |
| Light current (CUR $< 1$) | 6.33 | 1.140 | 1.299 | 7 |
| Heavy current (CUR $\geqslant 1$) | 6.01 | 0.720 | 0.518 | 8 |
| Overall | 6.73 |  |  | 27 |

Since

$$F_{3,23,.975} < F_{3,20,.975} = 3.86 < 4.41$$

it follows that $p < 0.025$. Also, since

$$F_{3,23,.99} > F_{3,30,.99} = 4.51 > 4.41$$

it follows that $p > 0.01$. Therefore, we have $0.01 < p < 0.025$, and we accept the alternative hypothesis that the four population means are different.

**12.42** We can test for each difference between two groups by computing the appropriate $t$ statistic as follows:

$$\lambda = \frac{\bar{x}_i - \bar{x}_j}{\sqrt{s^2\left(\dfrac{1}{n_i} + \dfrac{1}{n_j}\right)}}$$

These are given in Table A.27.

Thus, there are significant differences between the nonsmokers and each group of current smokers but not between nonsmokers and ex-smokers. There are also significant differences between ex-smokers and heavy

current smokers but not between ex-smokers and light current smokers. Finally, there are no significant differences between the two groups of current smokers.

**12.43** We first use the procedure in **(12.15)** to look at the group of four means using the test statistic

$$q = \frac{7.59 - 6.01}{\sqrt{\dfrac{0.883}{2}\left(\dfrac{1}{7} + \dfrac{1}{8}\right)}} = \frac{1.58}{0.344} = 4.593$$

We compare $q$ with $q_{4,23,.95} < q_{4,20,.95} = 3.96 < q$. Thus, some of the means are significantly different. We now look at subgroups of three means. In particular, we look at the subgroup (CUR $\geq 1$, CUR $< 1$, EX) using the test statistic

$$q = \frac{7.24 - 6.01}{\sqrt{\dfrac{0.883}{2}\left(\dfrac{1}{5} + \dfrac{1}{8}\right)}} = \frac{1.23}{0.379} = 3.245$$

Since $q_{3,23,.95} > q_{3,24,.95} = 3.53 > q$, we declare these three means as not significantly different. We next look at the subgroup of means (CUR $< 1$, EX, NON) using

**Table A.27**  *Comparison of specific groups relating smoking habit and birthweight (t tests)*

| Groups compared | Test statistic | | p-value |
|---|---|---|---|
| NON EX | $\lambda = \dfrac{7.59 - 7.24}{\sqrt{0.883(\frac{1}{7} + \frac{1}{5})}}$ | $= \dfrac{0.35}{0.550} = 0.64 \sim t_{23}$ | NS |
| NON CUR $< 1$ | $\lambda = \dfrac{7.59 - 6.33}{\sqrt{0.883(\frac{1}{7} + \frac{1}{7})}}$ | $= \dfrac{1.26}{0.502} = 2.51 \sim t_{23}$ | $0.01 < p < 0.02$ |
| NON CUR $\geq 1$ | $\lambda = \dfrac{7.59 - 6.01}{\sqrt{0.883(\frac{1}{7} + \frac{1}{8})}}$ | $= \dfrac{1.58}{0.486} = 3.25 \sim t_{23}$ | $0.001 < p < 0.01$ |
| EX CUR $< 1$ | $\lambda = \dfrac{7.24 - 6.33}{\sqrt{0.883(\frac{1}{5} + \frac{1}{7})}}$ | $= \dfrac{0.91}{0.550} = 1.65 \sim t_{23}$ | NS |
| EX CUR $\geq 1$ | $\lambda = \dfrac{7.24 - 6.01}{\sqrt{0.883(\frac{1}{5} + \frac{1}{8})}}$ | $= \dfrac{1.23}{0.536} = 2.29 \sim t_{23}$ | $0.02 < p < 0.05$ |
| CUR $< 1$ CUR $\geq 1$ | $\lambda = \dfrac{6.33 - 6.01}{\sqrt{0.883(\frac{1}{7} + \frac{1}{8})}}$ | $= \dfrac{0.32}{0.486} = 0.66 \sim t_{23}$ | NS |

the test statistic

$$q = \frac{7.59 - 6.33}{\sqrt{\dfrac{0.883}{2}\left(\dfrac{1}{7} + \dfrac{1}{7}\right)}} = \frac{1.26}{0.355} = 3.549$$

We note that

$$q_{3,23,.95} \approx \frac{(\frac{1}{23} - \frac{1}{24})q_{3,20,.95} + (\frac{1}{20} - \frac{1}{23})q_{3,24,.95}}{(\frac{1}{20} - \frac{1}{24})}$$

$$= \frac{(0.0018)(3.58) + 0.0065(3.53)}{0.0083} = 3.541$$

Thus, since $q > q_{3,23,.95}$, it follows that the group of three means is significantly different.

However, we already know that (CUR < 1 and EX) are not significantly different, because they are part of the subgroup (CUR ≥ 1, CUR < 1, EX), which was tested previously. The only remaining exercise is to test if EX and NON are significantly different, using the following test statistic

$$q = \frac{7.59 - 7.24}{\sqrt{\dfrac{0.883}{2}\left(\dfrac{1}{7} + \dfrac{1}{5}\right)}} = \frac{0.35}{0.389} = 0.900$$

Since $q_{2,23,.95} > q_{2,24,.95} = 2.92 > q$, these two means are not significantly different. The results can be summarized in Figure A.7.

| CUR ≥ 1 | CUR < 1 | EX | NON |
|---------|---------|-----|------|

**Figure A.7**

Thus, the only significant differences are between nonsmokers and each of the groups of current smokers.

**12.44** The only difference between the results using the multiple comparison procedures in **(12.16)** and the pairwise $t$ tests in **(12.13)** is that the ex-smokers and heavy current smokers are significantly different ($0.02 < p < 0.05$) with the $t$ tests but not with the multiple comparisons.

**12.45** We wish to look at the contrast

$$L = 0\bar{y}_2 + 0.5\bar{y}_3 + 1.3\bar{y}_4$$

However, the sum of the coefficients here adds up to 1.8 rather than 0. If we subtract $1.8/3 = 0.6$ from each coefficient, then we will have an appropriate contrast of the form

$$L = -0.6\bar{y}_2 + (0.5 - 0.6)\bar{y}_3 + (1.3 - 0.6)\bar{y}_4$$

$$= 0.6\bar{y}_2 - 0.1\bar{y}_3 + 0.7\bar{y}_4$$

$$= -0.6(7.24) - 0.1(6.33) + 0.7(6.01) = -0.77$$

We wish to test the hypothesis $H_0: E(L) = 0$ vs. $H_1: E(L) \neq 0$, where under $H_0: E(L) = 0$ and

$$Var(L) = s^2 \left[\frac{(0.6)^2}{n_2} + \frac{(0.1)^2}{n_3} + \frac{(0.7)^2}{n_4}\right]$$

$$= 0.883\left(\frac{0.36}{5} + \frac{0.01}{7} + \frac{0.49}{8}\right) = 0.119$$

$$se(L) = 0.345$$

Thus, we have the test statistic

$$\lambda = \frac{L}{se(L)} = \frac{-0.77}{0.345} = -2.232 \sim t_{23} \text{ under } H_0$$

Since $t_{23,.975} = 2.069$, $t_{23,.99} = 2.500$, it follows that $0.02 < p < 0.05$. Thus, there is a significant trend among ever smokers, with a lower mean birthweight as the current number of cigarettes smoked per day increases.

**12.60** A two-way ANOVA is appropriate here because the 80 patients can be classified by two parameters: (1) instruction for weight reduction (yes/no) and (2) instruction for meditation (yes/no).

**12.61** We use the method of unweighted means. First, we rearrange the data in the format of a $2 \times 2$ table (Table A.28) giving the sum of the means in each row ($y_{i.}^*$) and each column ($y_{.j}^*$) in the margins.

We now compute the Row, Column, and Interaction SS and MS as follows:

$$\text{Row SS} = \frac{13.9^2 + 6.0^2}{2} - \frac{(13.9 + 6.0)^2}{2 \times 2}$$

$$= 114.605 - 99.003$$

$$= 15.60 = \text{Row MS}$$

$$\text{Column SS} = \frac{13.5^2 + 6.4^2}{2} - \frac{(13.5 + 6.4)^2}{2 \times 2}$$

$$= 111.605 - 99.003$$

$$= 12.60 = \text{Column MS}$$

**Table A.28** *Effect of counseling for weight reduction and/or meditation on the change in diastolic bp*

| | | | Instruction in meditation | | |
| --- | --- | --- | --- | --- | --- |
| | | | Yes | No | $Y_i^*$ |
| | | Mean | 8.6 | 5.3 | 13.9 |
| | Yes | sd | 6.2 | 5.4 | |
| | | n | 20 | 20 | |
| Instruction in weight reduction | | | | | |
| | | Mean | 4.9 | 1.1 | 6.0 |
| | No | sd | 7.0 | 6.5 | |
| | | n | 20 | 20 | |
| | | $y_i^*$ | 13.5 | 6.4 | 19.9 |

Interaction SS $= (8.6)^2 + \cdots + (1.1)^2$

$$-\frac{(8.6 + \cdots + 1.1)^2}{4} - 15.60 - 12.60$$

$$= 127.27 - \frac{(19.9)^2}{4} - 28.20$$

$$= 127.27 - 99.00 - 28.20$$

$$= 0.07 = \text{Interaction MS}$$

Finally, we compute the Error MS to perform our significance tests. Since the sample size of each group is the same, we have $n_h = 20$. Thus,

$$\text{Error MS} = \frac{19[(6.2)^2 + (5.4)^2 + (7.0)^2 + (6.5)^2]}{76(20)}$$

$$= \frac{(6.2)^2 + (5.4)^2 + (7.0)^2 + (6.5)^2}{4(20)}$$

$$= 1.986$$

We test for row (weight reduction instruction) effects using the following test statistic:

$$\lambda_{\text{ROW}} = \frac{\text{Row MS}}{\text{Error MS}} = \frac{15.60}{1.986} = 7.85 \sim F_{1,76} \text{ under } H_0$$

Since

$$F_{1,76,.99} < F_{1,60,.99} = 7.08 < 7.85$$

it follows that $p < 0.01$. Similarly, since

$$F_{1,76,.995} > F_{1,120,.995} = 8.18 > 7.85$$

it follows that $p > 0.005$. Thus, $0.005 < p < 0.01$, and there is a significant effect of weight reduction instruction on reduction of blood pressure after controlling for the effect of meditation.

**12.62** We test for column (meditation instruction) effects using the following test statistic:

$$\lambda_{\text{COLUMN}} = \frac{\text{Column MS}}{\text{Error MS}} = \frac{12.60}{1.986}$$

$$= 6.34 \sim F_{1,76} \text{ under } H_0$$

Since

$$F_{1,76,.975} < F_{1,60,.975} = 5.29 < 6.34$$

it follows that $p < 0.025$. Similarly, since

$$F_{1,76,.99} > F_{1,120,.99} = 6.85 > 6.34$$

it follows that $p > 0.01$. Thus, $0.01 < p < 0.025$, and there is a significant effect of meditation instruction on reduction of blood pressure after controlling for the effect of weight reduction.

**12.63** We test for an interaction effect between weight reduction instruction and meditation instruction. We use the test statistic

$$\lambda_{\text{INT}} = \frac{\text{Interaction MS}}{\text{Error MS}} = \frac{0.07}{1.986} = 0.04 \sim F_{1,76} \text{ under } H_0$$

Since $F_{1,76,.95} > F_{1,120,.95} = 3.92 > 0.04$, it follows that $p > 0.05$, and there is no interaction effect between the two types of instruction. Thus, the effect of weight reduction is similar in patients who do and do not receive meditation instruction.

*Flowchart for appropriate methods of statistical inference*

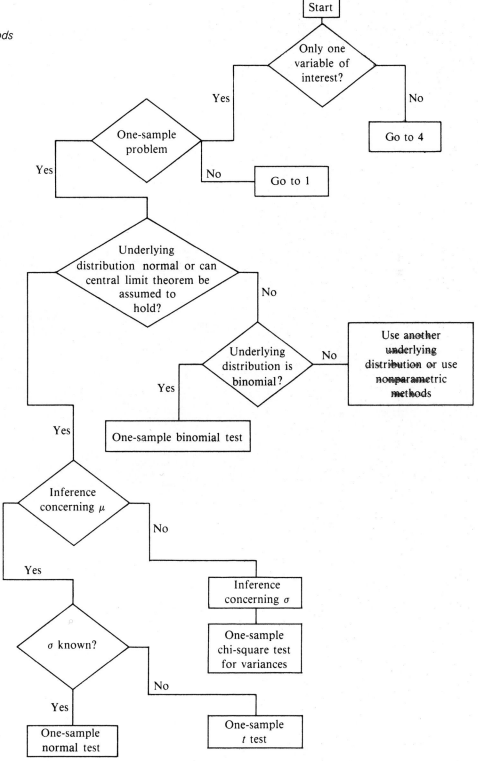

*Flowchart for appropriate methods of statistical inference (continued)*

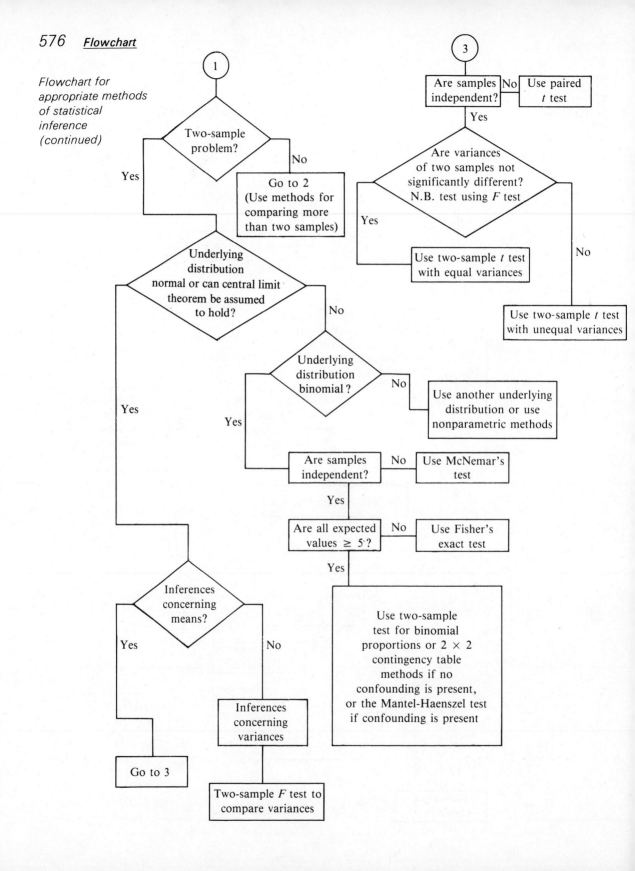

*Flowchart for appropriate methods of statistical inference (continued)*

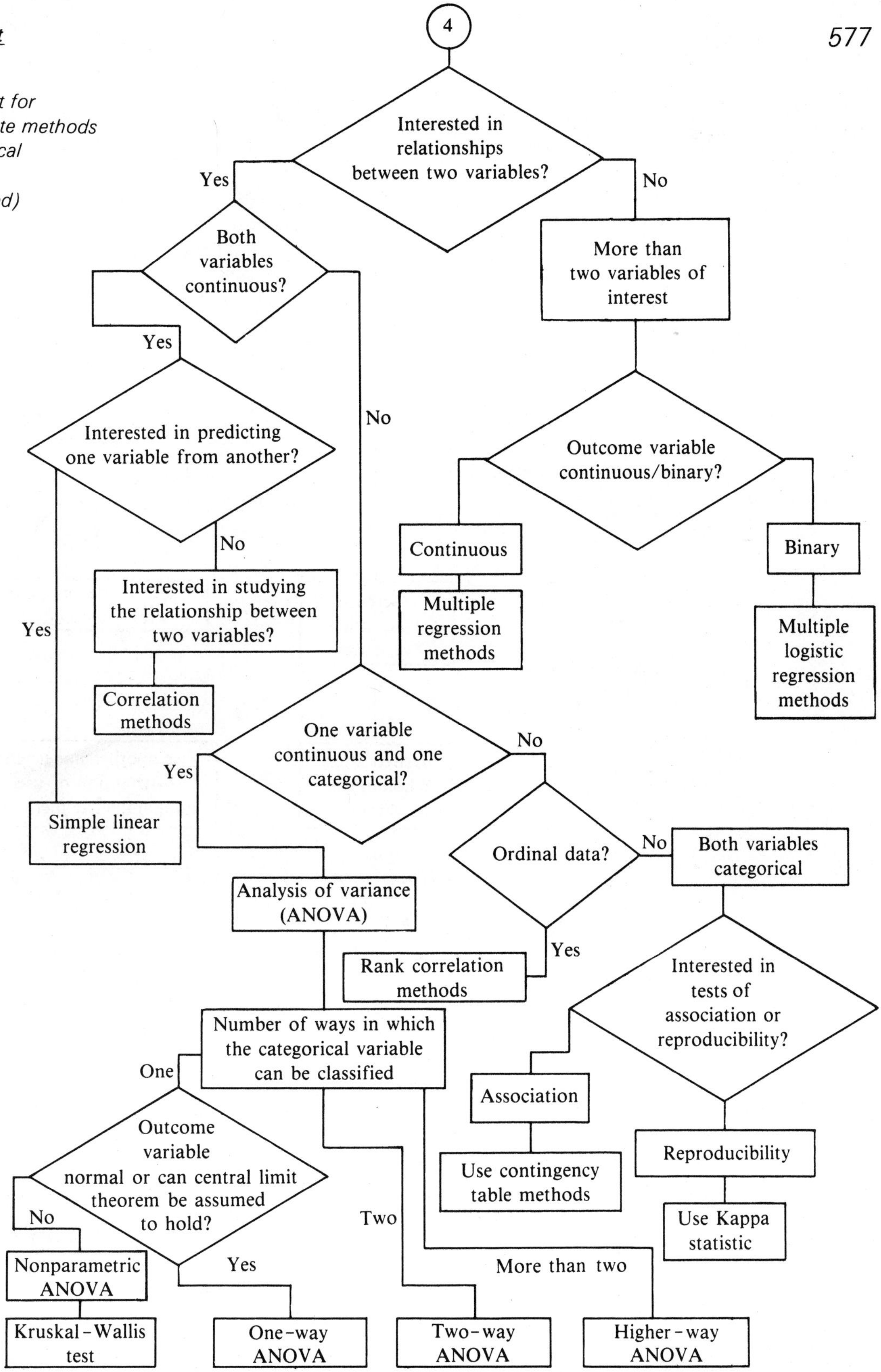

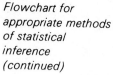

*Flowchart for appropriate methods of statistical inference (continued)*

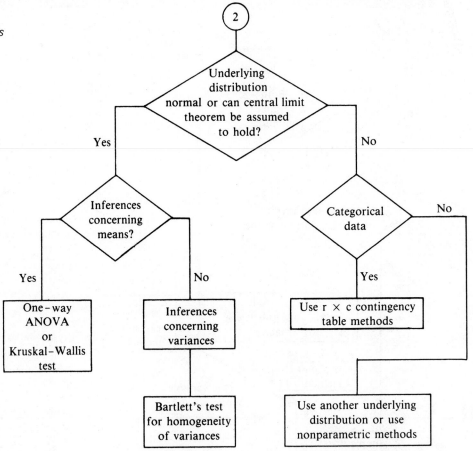

# Index

# Index of Applications